PULMONARY AND CARDIAC IMAGING

LUNG BIOLOGY IN HEALTH AND DISEASE

Executive Editor

Claude Lenfant
*Director, National Heart, Lung and Blood Institute
National Institutes of Health
Bethesda, Maryland*

1. Immunologic and Infectious Reactions in the Lung, *edited by Charles H. Kirkpatrick and Herbert Y. Reynolds*
2. The Biochemical Basis of Pulmonary Function, *edited by Ronald G. Crystal*
3. Bioengineering Aspects of the Lung, *edited by John B. West*
4. Metabolic Functions of the Lung, *edited by Y. S. Bakhle and John R. Vane*
5. Respiratory Defense Mechanisms (in two parts), *edited by Joseph D. Brain, Donald F. Proctor, and Lynne M. Reid*
6. Development of the Lung, *edited by W. Alan Hodson*
7. Lung Water and Solute Exchange, *edited by Norman C. Staub*
8. Extrapulmonary Manifestations of Respiratory Disease, *edited by Eugene Debs Robin*
9. Chronic Obstructive Pulmonary Disease, *edited by Thomas L. Petty*
10. Pathogenesis and Therapy of Lung Cancer, *edited by Curtis C. Harris*
11. Genetic Determinants of Pulmonary Disease, *edited by Stephen D. Litwin*
12. The Lung in the Transition Between Health and Disease, *edited by Peter T. Macklem and Solbert Permutt*
13. Evolution of Respiratory Processes: A Comparative Approach, *edited by Stephen C. Wood and Claude Lenfant*
14. Pulmonary Vascular Diseases, *edited by Kenneth M. Moser*
15. Physiology and Pharmacology of the Airways, *edited by Jay A. Nadel*
16. Diagnostic Techniques in Pulmonary Disease (in two parts), *edited by Marvin A. Sackner*
17. Regulation of Breathing (in two parts), *edited by Thomas F. Hornbein*
18. Occupational Lung Diseases: Research Approaches and Methods, *edited by Hans Weill and Margaret Turner-Warwick*
19. Immunopharmacology of the Lung, *edited by Harold H. Newball*
20. Sarcoidosis and Other Granulomatous Diseases of the Lung, *edited by Barry L. Fanburg*
21. Sleep and Breathing, *edited by Nicholas A. Saunders and Colin E. Sullivan*

22. *Pneumocystis carinii* Pneumonia: Pathogenesis, Diagnosis, and Treatment, *edited by Lowell S. Young*
23. Pulmonary Nuclear Medicine: Techniques in Diagnosis of Lung Disease, *edited by Harold L. Atkins*
24. Acute Respiratory Failure, *edited by Warren M. Zapol and Konrad J. Falke*
25. Gas Mixing and Distribution in the Lung, *edited by Ludwig A. Engel and Manuel Paiva*
26. High-Frequency Ventilation in Intensive Care and During Surgery, *edited by Graziano Carlon and William S. Howland*
27. Pulmonary Development: Transition from Intrauterine to Extrauterine Life, *edited by George H. Nelson*
28. Chronic Obstructive Pulmonary Disease: Second Edition, Revised and Expanded, *edited by Thomas L. Petty*
29. The Thorax (in two parts), *edited by Charis Roussos and Peter T. Macklem*
30. The Pleura in Health and Disease, *edited by Jacques Chrétien, Jean Bignon, and Albert Hirsch*
31. Drug Therapy for Asthma: Research and Clinical Practice, *edited by John W. Jenne and Shirley Murphy*
32. Pulmonary Endothelium in Health and Disease, *edited by Una S. Ryan*
33. The Airways: Neural Control in Health and Disease, *edited by Michael A. Kaliner and Peter J. Barnes*
34. Pathophysiology and Treatment of Inhalation Injuries, *edited by Jacob Loke*
35. Respiratory Function of the Upper Airway, *edited by Oommen P. Mathew and Giuseppe Sant'Ambrogio*
36. Chronic Obstructive Pulmonary Disease: A Behavioral Perspective, *edited by A. John McSweeny and Igor Grant*
37. Biology of Lung Cancer: Diagnosis and Treatment, *edited by Steven T. Rosen, James L. Mulshine, Frank Cuttitta, and Paul G. Abrams*
38. Pulmonary Vascular Physiology and Pathophysiology, *edited by E. Kenneth Weir and John T. Reeves*
39. Comparative Pulmonary Physiology: Current Concepts, *edited by Stephen C. Wood*
40. Respiratory Physiology: An Analytical Approach, *edited by H. K. Chang and Manuel Paiva*
41. Lung Cell Biology, *edited by Donald Massaro*
42. Heart–Lung Interactions in Health and Disease, *edited by Steven M. Scharf and Sharon S. Cassidy*
43. Clinical Epidemiology of Chronic Obstructive Pulmonary Disease, *edited by Michael J. Hensley and Nicholas A. Saunders*
44. Surgical Pathology of Lung Neoplasms, *edited by Alberto M. Marchevsky*
45. The Lung in Rheumatic Diseases, *edited by Grant W. Cannon and Guy A. Zimmerman*
46. Diagnostic Imaging of the Lung, *edited by Charles E. Putman*

47. Models of Lung Disease: Microscopy and Structural Methods, *edited by Joan Gil*
48. Electron Microscopy of the Lung, *edited by Dean E. Schraufnagel*
49. Asthma: Its Pathology and Treatment, *edited by Michael A. Kaliner, Peter J. Barnes, and Carl G. A. Persson*
50. Acute Respiratory Failure: Second Edition, *edited by Warren M. Zapol and Francois Lemaire*
51. Lung Disease in the Tropics, *edited by Om P. Sharma*
52. Exercise: Pulmonary Physiology and Pathophysiology, *edited by Brian J. Whipp and Karlman Wasserman*
53. Developmental Neurobiology of Breathing, *edited by Gabriel G. Haddad and Jay P. Farber*
54. Mediators of Pulmonary Inflammation, *edited by Michael A. Bray and Wayne H. Anderson*
55. The Airway Epithelium, *edited by Stephen G. Farmer and Douglas Hay*
56. Physiological Adaptations in Vertebrates: Respiration, Circulation, and Metabolism, *edited by Stephen C. Wood, Roy E. Weber, Alan R. Hargens, and Ronald W. Millard*
57. The Bronchial Circulation, *edited by John Butler*
58. Lung Cancer Differentiation: Implications for Diagnosis and Treatment, *edited by Samuel D. Bernal and Paul J. Hesketh*
59. Pulmonary Complications of Systemic Disease, *edited by John F. Murray*
60. Lung Vascular Injury: Molecular and Cellular Response, *edited by Arnold Johnson and Thomas J. Ferro*
61. Cytokines of the Lung, *edited by Jason Kelley*
62. The Mast Cell in Health and Disease, *edited by Michael A. Kaliner and Dean D. Metcalfe*
63. Pulmonary Disease in the Elderly Patient, *edited by Donald A. Mahler*
64. Cystic Fibrosis, *edited by Pamela B. Davis*
65. Signal Transduction in Lung Cells, *edited by Jerome S. Brody, David M. Center, and Vsevolod A. Tkachuk*
66. Tuberculosis: A Comprehensive International Approach, *edited by Lee B. Reichman and Earl S. Hershfield*
67. Pharmacology of the Respiratory Tract: Experimental and Clinical Research, *edited by K. Fan Chung and Peter J. Barnes*
68. Prevention of Respiratory Diseases, *edited by Albert Hirsch, Marcel Goldberg, Jean-Pierre Martin, and Roland Masse*
69. *Pneumocystis carinii* Pneumonia: Second Edition, Revised and Expanded, *edited by Peter D. Walzer*
70. Fluid and Solute Transport in the Airspaces of the Lungs, *edited by Richard M. Effros and H. K. Chang*
71. Sleep and Breathing: Second Edition, Revised and Expanded, *edited by Nicholas A. Saunders and Colin E. Sullivan*
72. Airway Secretion: Physiological Bases for the Control of Mucous Hypersecretion, *edited by Tamotsu Takishima and Sanae Shimura*
73. Sarcoidosis and Other Granulomatous Disorders, *edited by D. Geraint James*

74. Epidemiology of Lung Cancer, *edited by Jonathan M. Samet*
75. Pulmonary Embolism, *edited by Mario Morpurgo*
76. Sports and Exercise Medicine, *edited by Stephen C. Wood and Robert C. Roach*
77. Endotoxin and the Lungs, *edited by Kenneth L. Brigham*
78. The Mesothelial Cell and Mesothelioma, *edited by Marie-Claude Jaurand and Jean Bignon*
79. Regulation of Breathing: Second Edition, Revised and Expanded, *edited by Jerome A. Dempsey and Allan I. Pack*
80. Pulmonary Fibrosis, *edited by Sem Hin Phan and Roger S. Thrall*
81. Long-Term Oxygen Therapy: Scientific Basis and Clinical Application, *edited by Walter J. O'Donohue, Jr.*
82. Ventral Brainstem Mechanisms and Control of Respiration and Blood Pressure, *edited by C. Ovid Trouth, Richard M. Millis, Heidrun F. Kiwull-Schöne, and Marianne E. Schläfke*
83. A History of Breathing Physiology, *edited by Donald F. Proctor*
84. Surfactant Therapy for Lung Disease, *edited by Bengt Robertson and H. William Taeusch*
85. The Thorax: Second Edition, Revised and Expanded (in three parts), *edited by Charis Roussos*
86. Severe Asthma: Pathogenesis and Clinical Management, *edited by Stanley J. Szefler and Donald Y. M. Leung*
87. *Mycobacterium avium*–Complex Infection: Progress in Research and Treatment, *edited by Joyce A. Korvick and Constance A. Benson*
88. Alpha 1–Antitrypsin Deficiency: Biology • Pathogenesis • Clinical Manifestations • Therapy, *edited by Ronald G. Crystal*
89. Adhesion Molecules and the Lung, *edited by Peter A. Ward and Joseph C. Fantone*
90. Respiratory Sensation, *edited by Lewis Adams and Abraham Guz*
91. Pulmonary Rehabilitation, *edited by Alfred P. Fishman*
92. Acute Respiratory Failure in Chronic Obstructive Pulmonary Disease, *edited by Jean-Philippe Derenne, William A. Whitelaw, and Thomas Similowski*
93. Environmental Impact on the Airways: From Injury to Repair, *edited by Jacques Chrétien and Daniel Dusser*
94. Inhalation Aerosols: Physical and Biological Basis for Therapy, *edited by Anthony J. Hickey*
95. Tissue Oxygen Deprivation: From Molecular to Integrated Function, *edited by Gabriel G. Haddad and George Lister*
96. The Genetics of Asthma, *edited by Stephen B. Liggett and Deborah A. Meyers*
97. Inhaled Glucocorticoids in Asthma: Mechanisms and Clinical Actions, *edited by Robert P. Schleimer, William W. Busse, and Paul M. O'Byrne*
98. Nitric Oxide and the Lung, *edited by Warren M. Zapol and Kenneth D. Bloch*
99. Primary Pulmonary Hypertension, *edited by Lewis J. Rubin and Stuart Rich*
100. Lung Growth and Development, *edited by John A. McDonald*

101. Parasitic Lung Diseases, *edited by Adel A. F. Mahmoud*
102. Lung Macrophages and Dendritic Cells in Health and Disease, *edited by Mary F. Lipscomb and Stephen W. Russell*
103. Pulmonary and Cardiac Imaging, *edited by Caroline Chiles and Charles E. Putman*
104. Gene Therapy for Diseases of the Lung, *edited by Kenneth L. Brigham*

ADDITIONAL VOLUMES IN PREPARATION

Inhalation Delivery of Therapeutic Peptides and Proteins, *edited by Lex A. Adjei and Pramod K. Gupta*

Treatment of the Hospitalized Cystic Fibrosis Patient, *edited by David M. Orenstein and Robert C. Stern*

Dyspnea, *edited by Donald A. Mahler*

$Beta_2$-Agonists in Asthma Treatment, *edited by Romain Pauwels and Paul M. O'Byrne*

Oxygen, Gene Expression, and Cellular Function, *edited by Donald J. Massaro and Linda Clerch*

Asthma and Immunological Diseases in Pregnancy and Early Infancy, *edited by Michael Schatz, Robert S. Zeiger, and Henry Claman*

Self-Management of Asthma, *edited by Harry Kotses and Andrew Harver*

Asthma in the Elderly, *edited by Robert A. Barbee and John W. Bloom*

The opinions expressed in these volumes do not necessarily represent the views of the National Institutes of Health.

PULMONARY AND CARDIAC IMAGING

Edited by

Caroline Chiles

*Bowman Gray School of Medicine–
Wake Forest University
Winston-Salem, North Carolina*

Charles E. Putman

*Duke University Medical Center
Durham, North Carolina*

MARCEL DEKKER, INC.   NEW YORK • BASEL • HONG KONG

Library of Congress Cataloging-in-Publication Data

Pulmonary and cardiac imaging / edited by Caroline Chiles, Charles E. Putman.
    p. cm. — (Lung biology in health and disease ; v. 103)
    Includes bibliographical references and indexes.
    ISBN 0-8247-9743-4 (hardcover : alk. paper)
    1. Cardiopulmonary system—Imaging. 2. Cardiopulmonary system—Diseases—Diagnosis. I. Chiles, Caroline. II. Putman, Charles E. (Charles Edgar). III. Series.
    [DNLM: 1. Lung Diseases—diagnosis. 2. Cardiovascular Diseases—diagnosis. 3. Diagnostic Imaging—methods. 4. Thoracic Diseases—diagnosis. 5. Thoracic Injuries—diagnosis. W1 LU62 v.103 1997 / WF 600 P9803 1997]
RC702.P85 1997
616.2'40754—dc21
DNLM/DLC
for Library of Congress   97-722
                                                                                                            CIP

The publisher offers discounts on this book when ordered in bulk quantities. For more information, write to Special Sales/Professional Marketing at the address below.

This book is printed on acid-free paper.

Copyright © 1997 by Marcel Dekker, Inc. All Rights Reserved.

Neither this book nor any part may be reproduced or transmitted in any form or by any means, electronic or mechanical, including photocopying, microfilming, and recording, or by any information storage and retrieval system, without permission in writing from the publisher.

Marcel Dekker, Inc.
270 Madison Avenue, New York, New York 10016

Current printing (last digit):
10 9 8 7 6 5 4 3 2 1

PRINTED IN THE UNITED STATES OF AMERICA

INTRODUCTION

Medical historians correctly assert that the art of medicine became more of a science with the advent of instruments that extended the range of the human senses. However, over the years, this development has fueled some debates because of the new relationship between the observer and the object under observation.

The question of how we perceive what is real has puzzled observers since at least the time of ancient Greece. Plato, in his famous "Allegory of the Cave" (Book VII of the Republic, circa 360 B.C.), compared the perceptions of persons who were permitted to see only the shadows of objects reflected on the walls of a dimly lit cave to those of persons who were allowed to see the actual objects, but still within the limited light available in the cave, and finally to those of persons who were permitted to exit the cave and see those same objects in the full light of day. At each transition, the old view of reality was discarded in favor of a new one based on an improved ability to perceive.

This allegory is, in a way, the history of the art and science of medical diagnosis. In the world of imaging, physicians have long left behind the shadows of Roentgen's days and have now emerged from the cave to see with the full illumination of the sun. Here, the sun is computed tomography, positron emission tomography, and magnetic resonance imaging.

Francis Henry Williams of Boston is credited with establishing the first x-ray picture detecting the enlargement of the heart and with first describing the use of fluoroscopy to study heart and lung disease, in 1896, only one year after Roentgen's monumental discovery. Although the observations of Williams can hardly be compared to those of a caveman, there is no question that today's sun is bright and may be bewildering. Plato knew this, as shown by the following dialogue from the "Allegory of the Cave":

> FIRST SPEAKER: Anyone who has common sense will remember that the bewilderments of the eyes are of two kinds, and arise from the caves, either from coming out of the light or from going into the light, which is true of the mind's eye, quite as much as of the bodily eye; and he who remembers this when he sees anyone whose vision is perplexed and weak, will not be too ready to laugh; he will first ask whether that soul of man has come out of the brighter light, and is unable to see because unaccustomed to the dark, or having turned from darkness to the day is dazzled by excess of light.
> SECOND SPEAKER: That ... is a very just distinction.
> FIRST SPEAKER: But then, if I am right, certain professors of education must be wrong when they say that they cannot put a knowledge into the soul which was not there before, like sight into blind eyes.

Only seven years ago, the series of monographs Lung Biology in Health and Disease presented *Diagnostic Imaging of the Lung* (1990). Since then, major steps, if not leaps, have occurred in the power of imaging to enhance medicine. The editors of this volume, Caroline Chiles and Charles E. Putman, set out to "provide [their] clinical and research colleagues with an update of current imaging modalities and their applications to pulmonary and cardiac medicine, from the perspectives of both patient care and research." They, and the authors of the chapters, have fully met their goals in the most scholarly fashion. This volume is a landmark in the series of monographs, one from which the patients will be the great beneficiaries.

Claude Lenfant, M.D.
Bethesda, Maryland

PREFACE

> Knowledge advances by steps, and not by leaps.
> —Lord Macauley (1800–1859)

Radiology, like knowledge in general, seems to advance by steps, and not by leaps. Since the discovery of the x-ray 100 years ago, radiographic imaging has provided physicians with the ability to make diagnoses noninvasively and to monitor the course of disease. The last century has seen step-by-step advances as new technologies join the ranks of the x-ray. Radionuclide imaging, ultrasonography, computed tomography, magnetic resonance imaging, and positron emission tomography are now widely accepted imaging modalities. It is a daily challenge to the physician to remain versed in each of these technologies and to know how best to apply these imaging tools to answer the diagnostic question at hand. A major role of the radiologist is to act as a consultant to clinicians in the most effective and least costly implementation of imaging studies. Communication between physicians is of great importance for the provision of optimal patient care at the least cost to society. Communication within the research arena is also of great importance, to help imaging research develop diagnostic tools that ultimately result in improvements in patient care. Technology assessment and outcomes research require a team of researchers who can objectively evaluate the costs and benefits of imaging. In this text, it has been our goal to provide our clinical and research colleagues with an update of current imaging modalities and their applications to pulmonary and cardiac medicine, from the perspectives of both patient care and research.

We have divided the text into two sections. The first section, Pulmonary Imaging, is organized primarily according to disease. Ten chapters include reviews of infection in immunocompromised patients (AIDS and non-AIDS), trauma, bronchogenic carcinoma, metastatic disease, lung transplantation, emphysema, chronic infiltrative lung disease, pulmonary hemorrhage, and complications of thoracic surgery. Two chapters are devoted to techniques, one on digital imaging, and another on interventional procedures within the thorax. Two anatomical areas, the pleural space and the airways, are discussed separately.

The second section, Cardiac Imaging, is organized primarily on an anatomical basis. An overview of cardiac imaging and chapters devoted to the coronary circulation, the pulmonary circulation, the aorta, and the pericardium are included. The remaining chapters deal with congenital heart diseases in the adult patient and cardiovascular interventional procedures.

We are indebted to the contributors; all are widely respected specialists in pulmonary and cardiac imaging who have shared with us their vast clinical experiences. These chapters are concisely written and amply illustrated with cases from the authors' personal teaching files. It is our hope that the reader will be able to apply this knowledge to clinical practice and to research and teaching programs.

We thank Dr. Claude Lenfant, the Executive Editor of the Lung Biology in Health and Disease series, for the opportunity to contribute the radiologist's perspective.

Caroline Chiles
Charles E. Putman

CONTRIBUTORS

Denise R. Aberle, M.D. Associate Professor and Section Chief, Thoracic Imaging, Department of Radiological Sciences, UCLA School of Medicine, Los Angeles, California

Poonam Batra, M.D., F.A.C.R., F.C.C.P. Professor of Clinical Radiology, Department of Radiological Sciences, UCLA School of Medicine, Los Angeles, California

Lawrence M. Boxt, M.D., F.A.C.C. Professor and Section Chief, Cardiac Radiology, Department of Radiology, Columbia University College of Physicians and Surgeons, and Columbia–Presbyterian Medical Center, New York, New York

Lynn S. Broderick, M.D. Assistant Professor, Department of Surgery, Indiana University School of Medicine, University Hospital, Indianapolis, Indiana

Paul Burrowes, M.D., F.R.C.P.C. Clinical Assistant Professor, University of Calgary, and Department of Diagnostic Imaging, Foothills Hospital, Calgary, Alberta, Canada

J. Jeffrey Carr, M.D. Assistant Professor of Radiology, Division of Radiologic Sciences, Bowman Gray School of Medicine–Wake Forest University, Winston-Salem, North Carolina

Caroline Chiles, M.D. Associate Professor of Radiology and Section Chief, Thoracic Imaging, Department of Radiology, Bowman Gray School of Medicine–Wake Forest University, Winston-Salem, North Carolina

Robert H. Choplin, M.D. Professor of Radiology, Department of Radiology, Bowman Gray School of Medicine–Wake Forest University, Winston-Salem, North Carolina

Craig L. Coblentz, M.D., F.R.C.P.C. Associate Professor of Radiology, Department of Diagnostic Radiology, McMaster University Medical Centre, Hamilton, Ontario, Canada

Dewey J. Conces, Jr., M.D. Professor of Radiology, Department of Radiology, Indiana University School of Medicine, University Hospital, Indianapolis, Indiana

Lynn Coppage, M.D. Assistant Professor, Department of Radiology, Medical University of South Carolina, Charleston, South Carolina

Joseph E. Cox, M.D. Fellow in Thoracic Imaging, Department of Radiology, Bowman Gray School of Medicine–Wake Forest University, Winston-Salem, North Carolina

Carole J. Dennie, M.D. Department of Diagnostic Radiology, Ottawa Civic Hospital, Ottawa, Ontario, Canada

Jeremy J. Erasmus, M.D., M.B.B.Ch. Assistant Professor, Department of Radiology, Duke University Medical Center, Durham, North Carolina

S. Melanie Greaves, M.R.C.P., F.R.C.R. Visiting Assistant Professor, Department of Radiological Sciences, UCLA School of Medicine, Los Angeles, California

Thomas E. Hartman, M.D. Assistant Professor of Radiology, Department of Diagnostic Radiology, Mayo Clinic and Mayo Foundation, Rochester, Minnesota

George G. Hartnell, F.R.C.R. Director of Cardiovascular and Interventional Radiology, Department of Radiological Sciences, Deaconess Hospital, and Associate Professor of Radiology, Harvard Medical School, Boston, Massachusetts

Stephen J. Herman, M.D., F.R.C.P. Associate Professor, Department of Medical Imaging, University of Toronto, and Staff Radiologist, Department of Radiology, The Toronto Hospital, Toronto, Ontario, Canada

Bob Hu, M.D. Stanford University School of Medicine, Stanford, California

Erik J. Kilgore, M.D. Resident Physician, Department of Radiology, Bowman Gray School of Medicine–Wake Forest University, Winston-Salem, North Carolina

Contributors

Jeffrey S. Klein, M.D. Chief of Thoracic Imaging, Department of Radiology, University of Vermont School of Medicine, Burlington, Vermont

Ann N. Leung, M.D. Assistant Professor and Section Chief, Thoracic Imaging, Department of Radiology, Stanford University Medical Center, Stanford, California.

Kerry M. Link, M.D. Associate Professor, Department of Radiology, Bowman Gray School of Medicine–Wake Forest University, Winston-Salem, North Carolina

John H. M. MacGregor, M.D., F.R.C.P.C. Clinical Associate Professor, Department of Diagnostic Radiology, University of Calgary, Foothills Hospital, Calgary, Alberta, Canada

John R. Mayo, M.D. Assistant Professor, Department of Radiology, University of British Columbia and Vancouver Hospital and Health Sciences Centre, Vancouver, British Columbia, Canada

Naeem Merchant, M.D. Stanford University School of Medicine, Stanford, California

Paul L. Molina, M.D. Assistant Professor, Department of Radiology, University of North Carolina School of Medicine, Chapel Hill, North Carolina

Nestor L. Müller, M.D., Ph.D. Professor, Department of Radiology, University of British Columbia and Vancouver Hospital and Health Sciences Centre, Vancouver, British Columbia, Canada

Glenn E. Newman, M.D. Associate Professor of Radiology, Assistant Professor of Surgery, Department of Radiology, Duke University Medical Center, Durham, North Carolina

Robert J. Optican, M.D. Director of Cardiopulmonary Imaging, Department of Radiology, Baptist Memorial Hospital, Memphis, Tennessee

Edward F. Patz, Jr., M.D. Associate Professor of Radiology, Department of Radiology, Duke University Medical Center, Durham, North Carolina

Steven L. Primack, M.D. Assistant Professor, Department of Radiology, Oregon Health Sciences University, Portland, Oregon

Charles E. Putman, M.D. Senior Vice President for Research Administration and Policy and James B. Duke Professor of Radiology, Department of Medicine, Duke University Medical Center, Durham, North Carolina

Tony P. Smith, M.D. Professor of Radiology, Department of Radiology, Duke University Medical Center, Durham, North Carolina

H. William Strauss, M.D. Stanford University School of Medicine, Stanford, California

Robert D. Tarver, M.D., F.A.R.C. Professor of Radiology, Department of Radiology, Indiana University School of Medicine, Wishard Memorial Hospital, Indianapolis, Indiana

James G. Warner, Jr., M.D. Assistant Professor, Department of Cardiology, Bowman Gray School of Medicine–Wake Forest University, Winston-Salem, North Carolina

Lewis Wexler, M.D. Professor of Radiology and Medicine, Department of Radiology, Stanford University School of Medicine, Stanford, California

CONTENTS

Introduction Claude Lenfant   *iii*
Preface   *v*
Contributors   *vii*

Part I: Pulmonary Imaging

1. Thoracic Imaging: 1896–Present   3

Caroline Chiles and Charles E. Putman

I.	The Discovery of the X-Ray	3
II.	The Emergence of Chest Radiography	5
III.	Tomography of the Chest	7
IV.	Advances in Film Technology	8
V.	Digital Imaging and Teleradiology	8
VI.	Cross-Sectional Imaging of the Chest	10
VII.	Health Care Costs and Chest Imaging	11
VIII.	Clinical Efficacy of Diagnostic Imaging	13
IX.	Research and Training in Chest Imaging	15

X.	Conclusion	16
	References	16

2. Pulmonary Disease in the Immunocompromised Host (Non-AIDS) — 19

Ann N. Leung and Nestor L. Müller

I.	Introduction	19
II.	Role of Imaging	20
III.	Infection	20
IV.	Drug-Induced Lung Disease	30
V.	Pulmonary Edema	32
VI.	Diffuse Alveolar Hemorrhage	32
VII.	Recurrence or Extension of Underlying Neoplasm	32
VIII.	Posttransplantation Lymphoproliferative Disorder	35
	References	36

3. Pulmonary Disease in the Immunocompromised Host (AIDS) — 41

S. Melanie Greaves and Poonam Batra

I.	Introduction	41
II.	Infectious Complications	42
III.	Neoplastic Complications	56
IV.	Nonneoplastic, Noninfectious Complications	64
V.	Interventional Radiology in AIDS Patients	65
	References	65

4. Diagnostic Imaging of Bronchogenic Carcinoma — 69

Jeremy J. Erasmus and Edward F. Patz, Jr.

I.	Introduction	69
II.	Screening	70
III.	Pathological Classification	70
IV.	Radiologic Features	71
V.	Diagnosis	81
VI.	Staging	84
VII.	Summary	96
	References	96

5. Metastatic Disease to the Chest from Extrathoracic Primary Malignancy   105

Lynn Coppage

I.	Introduction	105
II.	Frequency	105
III.	Mechanisms of Spread	107
IV.	Radiographic Appearance	107
V.	Detection	116
VI.	Summary	121
	References	121

6. Radiology of Chest Trauma   127

Joseph E. Cox and Paul L. Molina

I.	Introduction	127
II.	Chest Wall Trauma	128
III.	Pleural Space Injuries	132
IV.	Mechanisms of Chest Injury	137
V.	Parenchymal Lung Injuries	139
VI.	Tracheobronchial Rupture	145
VII.	Esophageal Injury	147
VIII.	Diaphragmatic Injury	148
	References	152

7. Radiology of Thoracic Surgical Complications   159

Robert D. Tarver, Lynn S. Broderick, and Dewey J. Conces, Jr.

I.	Introduction	159
II.	General Problems	160
III.	Aortic Surgery	167
IV.	Coronary Artery Bypass Surgery	167
V.	Pulmonary Resection Complications	172
VI.	Esophageal Surgery	185
VII.	Complications of Mediastinal Tumor Surgery	187
VIII.	Thoracic Transplant Surgery	189
	References	194

8. High-Resolution Computed Tomography of Chronic Infiltrative Lung Disease   199

Thomas E. Hartman

I.	Introduction	199
II.	Usual Interstitial Pneumonia	200
III.	Asbestosis	202
IV.	Sarcoidosis	203
V.	Silicosis and Coal Workers Pneumoconiosis	203
VI.	Pulmonary Langerhans Cell Histiocytosis	205
VII.	Lymphangiomyomatosis	207
VIII.	Extrinsic Allergic Alveolitis	209
IX.	Alveolar Proteinosis	210
X.	Lymphangitic Carcinomatosis	212
XI.	Chronic Eosinophilic Pneumonia	212
XII.	Conclusion	213
	References	215

9. Pulmonary Hemorrhage   219

Steven L. Primack

I.	Introduction	219
II.	Imaging Techniques	219
III.	Focal Pulmonary Hemorrhage	221
IV.	Diffuse Pulmonary Hemorrhage	227
	References	240

10. Diseases of the Airways   245

S. Melanie Greaves and Denise R. Aberle

I.	Introduction	245
II.	Focal or Central Lesions	246
III.	Bronchiectasis	249
IV.	Small Airways	259
V.	Functional Imaging	265
	References	271

11. Emphysema   275

Carole J. Dennie and Craig L. Coblentz

I.	Introduction	275
II.	Pathology and Pathogenesis	276

III.	Pathological-Radiologic Correlation	280
IV.	Radiology	280
V.	Conclusion	293
	References	293

12. Radiologic Assessment After Lung Transplantation   297

Stephen J. Herman

I.	Introduction	297
II.	Reimplantation Response	298
III.	Acute Rejection	299
IV.	Bronchiolitis Obliterans	305
V.	Airway Complications	307
VI.	Infections	309
VII.	Lymphoproliferative Disorders	310
VIII.	Pulmonary and Cardiac Changes	311
IX.	Omentum	313
X.	Postransbronchial Biopsy Changes	314
XI.	Summary	315
	References	315

13. Imaging of the Pleura   321

Paul Burrowes and John H. M. MacGregor

I.	Introduction	321
II.	Imaging of Pleural Fluid	323
III.	Empyema	327
IV.	Focal Pleural Diseases	330
V.	Diffuse Pleural Diseases	333
VI.	Role of Imaging in Diffuse Pleural Thickening	338
	References	338

14. Thoracic Interventional Procedures   343

Jeffrey S. Klein

I.	Transthoracic Needle Biopsy	343
II.	Thoracic Drainage Procedures	355
	References	362

15. Digital Imaging of the Chest   369

Erik J. Kilgore and Robert H. Choplin

I.	Introduction	369
II.	Advantages and Limitations	370
III.	Image Quality	370
IV.	Characteristics of a Digital Image	371
V.	Image Acquisition	373
VI.	Image Processing	384
VII.	Display	385
VIII.	Transmission and Storage	386
	References	387

16. Imaging of the Pulmonary Circulation   389

Tony P. Smith and Glenn E. Newman

I.	Introduction	389
II.	Chest Radiograph	390
III.	Nuclear Scintigraphy	392
IV.	Computed Tomography	400
V.	Magnetic Resonance Imaging	404
VI.	Sonography	412
VII.	Pulmonary Angiography	413
VIII.	Summary	415
	References	415

Part II: Cardiac Imaging

17. Imaging the Coronary Circulation   423

Lawrence M. Boxt

I.	Introduction	423
II.	Magnetic Resonance Coronary Arteriography	426
III.	Echocardiography	432
IV.	Coronary Artery Calcification and Very Rapid Computed Tomography	436
V.	Intravascular Ultrasound	439
	References	441

18. Imaging of the Pericardium — 445

J. Jeffrey Carr, James G. Warner, Jr., and Kerry M. Link

I.	General Background	445
II.	Imaging Anatomy of the Pericardium	447
III.	Pericardial Abnormalities and Their Imaging	452
IV.	Summary	471
	References	472

19. Adult Congenital Heart Disease — 475

Robert J. Optican

I.	Introduction	475
II.	Techniques	476
III.	Specific Lesions	488
IV.	Postoperative Imaging of Congenital Heart Disease	502
V.	Summary	505
	References	505

20. The Thoracic Aorta — 507

John R. Mayo

I.	Introduction	507
II.	Imaging Techniques	508
III.	Aortic Diseases and Imaging Algorithms	516
IV.	Summary	530
	References	530

21. Interventional Techniques in Cardiac Diagnosis and Treatment — 535

George G. Hartnell

I.	Introduction	535
II.	Interventional Diagnostic Techniques	536
III.	Interventional Therapeutic Techniques	541
IV.	Mechanical Coronary Recanalization	548
V.	Balloon Valvuloplasty	555
	References	562

22. Advances in Cardiac Imaging   **571**

Lewis Wexler, H. William Strauss, Naeem Merchant, and Bob Hu

I.	Introduction	571
II.	Brief History of Cardiac-Imaging Modalities and Current Indications	572
III.	Recent Advances and Potential Applications of Newer-Imaging Modalities	587
IV.	Conclusion	595
	References	596

Author Index   *603*
Subject Index   *643*

PULMONARY AND CARDIAC IMAGING

Part One

PULMONARY IMAGING

1

Thoracic Imaging: 1896–Present

CAROLINE CHILES
Bowman Gray School of Medicine–Wake Forest University
Winston-Salem, North Carolina

CHARLES E. PUTMAN
Duke University Medical Center
Durham, North Carolina

I. The Discovery of the X-Ray

On Friday, November 8, 1895, Wilhelm Conrad Roentgen (1845–1923), a 50-year-old professor of physics at the University of Wurzburg in Germany, worked in his laboratory, repeating experiments with a cathode ray tube previously described by a young German physicist, Philip Lenard (1862–1947) (1–3). The tube was a glass bulb from which most of the air had been evacuated. Two electrodes, a cathode and an anode, were positioned inside the tube. The electrodes were connected to an external high-voltage supply. As the electric current was turned on, the glass walls of the cathode ray tube glowed brightly. Just as Lenard had done, Roentgen wrapped the tube with thick black paper to shield his eyes from the light and to prevent ultraviolet rays from interfering with his experiments.

Roentgen, similar to Lenard and other physicists of his time, used a variety of phosphors in the form of crystals to study ultraviolet and cathode rays. They held glass vials of crystals close to a window in the cathode ray tube to observe their fluorescence. Lenard recorded the ultraviolet and cathode ray fluorescence of many crystals and, in a laboratory notebook in May 3, 1893, described barium platinocyanide as showing as brilliant greenish fluorescence (3).

As Roentgen duplicated the experiments previously described by Lenard, a sheet of cardboard covered with barium platinocyanide crystals lay on Roentgen's workbench, a meter away from the cathode ray tube. After shielding the cathode ray tube, Roentgen noticed a persistent glow from the barium platinocyanide screen. When Roentgen turned off the cathode ray tube, the screen stopped glowing. When the cathode ray tube was turned back on, the screen began to glow again. The scientific thinking of Roentgen's time was that cathode rays traveled only a few centimeters and were unable to pass through the glass walls of the tube. Since the screen lay a meter away, Roentgen deduced that a different type of ray was responsible.

Roentgen placed his hand between the cathode ray tube and the screen and saw the outline of the bones of his hand as they blocked the rays from hitting the crystals. As he reported to the Society of the Physico-Medical Society of Wurzburg on December 28, 1895,

> If one holds a hand between the discharge apparatus and the screen, one can see the dark shadows of the bones surrounded by the faint shadow image of the hand.

This observation represents the birth of radiology. On December 22, 1895, Roentgen placed his wife's hand on a photographic plate and, with a 15-min exposure, produced the first radiograph, an image that clearly showed the bones and soft tissues of her hand and the ring on her finger. Because Roentgen did not know the exact source of these rays, he referred to them as "x-rays" (*x strahlen*) to distinguish them from other types of rays (4).

News of Roentgen's discovery reached America by transatlantic cable. His description of x-rays was reported in the *New York Sun* on January 6, 1896, only 3 days after it appeared in the Vienna press. Scientific magazines quickly reported the discovery, which appeared in *Scientific American* on January 25, 1896, and in *Science* on January 31, 1896; a full translation of Roentgen's text was printed in the February 14, 1896, issue. Accompanying the translation in February were letters and comments from three American researchers who, within a matter of weeks, had begun to experiment with this new "ray." Edwin B. Frost of Dartmouth College in Hanover, New Hampshire, described making a radiograph of a patient with a fracture of the ulna—the first documented medical use of x-rays in the United States (5).

Early investigators initially used x-rays for fluoroscopy (a term coined by inventor Thomas Edison). Images on expensive photographic film were made only to document what was seen fluoroscopically. Because of the low output of the early x-ray tubes and the relative insensitivity of photographic film, long exposure times were required to produce an image.

In 1901, Roentgen received the first Nobel Prize in physics for his work. The next 20 years saw immediate acceptance of x-rays by the medical community, among whom x-rays were primarily used for evaluating skeletal fractures and for observing foreign bodies. Unfortunately, the hazards of x-rays were not appreciated, and side effects of exposure to x-rays ranged from edema and dermatitis, to necrosis and eventual amputation of fingers and hands. Many early workers also died of cancer and leukemia, likely the result of radiation exposure (6).

II. The Emergence of Chest Radiography

In 1882, Robert Koch published a manuscript on the etiology of tuberculosis, proving that it was a contagious disease. At the turn of the century, tuberculosis was widespread and devastating; it accounted for at least 15% of all reported deaths (7). Advanced tuberculosis was untreatable, however, and the ability to detect early disease was limited. Recognition of patients with tuberculosis was considered important so that they could be given appropriate sanitarium care, or could at least be taught to avoid spreading the infection. The primary screening tools at that time were medical history and physical examination (8). "Moist rales" heard in the apices of the lungs were considered evidence of tuberculous infection.

Francis H. Williams (1852–1936) practiced medicine in Boston, Massachusetts, at the turn of the century and was among those who believed that improved survival of patients with tuberculosis depended on early recognition and treatment (7). When news of the discovery of the x-ray reached him in early 1896, his interest in chest medicine prompted him to consider applying the x-ray to examination of the chest. He was an 1874 graduate of the Massachusetts Institute of Technology (MIT), and his engineering background placed him in a unique position to combine fluoroscopy and x-rays with chest medicine. He began a series of clinical studies, transporting patients from Boston City Hospital to the MIT physics laboratory for fluoroscopy of the chest, as early as April 1896. During that year, he described successful fluoroscopic localization of tuberculosis in the *Medical and Surgical Reports of the Boston City Hospital*. By 1896, he had collected more than 100 volumes containing notes and drawings concerning fluoroscopic examination of patients with tuberculosis. By 1897, he reported that tuberculosis could be detected earlier with fluoroscopy than by auscultation and percussion and that fluoroscopy also allowed greater estimation of the extent of lung involvement (9,10).

Williams understood the benefit of pathological correlation. He made radiographic images of the lungs of autopsy specimens, comparing the radiographic findings with observations made at autopsy. He also emphasized the importance of comparing normal and abnormal:

> When both sides are diseased the opportunity for direct comparison with the normal is lost, and one is obliged to depend upon a recollection of the normal in an individual of the same build (6).

In his 1897 paper in the *Medical and Surgical Reports of the Boston City Hospital,* Williams summarized his 12 months of initial experience with fluoroscopy and radiography of the chest:

> [B]y x-ray examinations of the chest we gain assistance in recognizing a density greater than normal in tuberculosis, pneumonia, infarction, edema, congestion of the lungs, in aneurysm, and in new growths.... The distribution, location, and amount of this increase in density which the fluoroscope shows assist us in some cases to differentiate these diseases and conditions. Diminution of the normal density, which is the result of emphysema and pneumothorax, is indicated by the position and movement of the diaphragm; a certain curve of the diaphragm is characteristic of this latter condition (6).

Owing to the expense of producing a photographic image, most physicians employed fluoroscopy to detect disease. In 1910, the American Roentgen Ray Society recommended charges of 25–100 dollars for an examination of the chest, a price not far from current fee structures (11).

Cigarette production and smoking rapidly became popular in the first half of the 20th century, and lung cancer and emphysema became a focus of chest fluoroscopy as well. Williams's description of a patient with emphysema in 1896 paints a picture that is very familiar today:

> The pulmonary area is more extensive and brighter than in health, and reaches not only lower down, but higher up in the chest. The diaphragm is lower down in the thorax, and its excursion is restricted in the upper part of its usual movement.... The lower position of the diaphragm gives the axis of the heart ... this vertical direction, and is one of the reasons why this organ when looked at from side to side, is at greater distance from the sternum in emphysema than in health (7,12).

By 1905, Dr. Chevalier Jackson, at Jefferson Hospital in Philadelphia, had developed a method of examining the tracheobronchial tree. He blew dry bismuth powder through a tube into the tracheobronchial tree, creating the first bronchograms (6). This procedure was not widely accepted because of reports of bismuth poisoning, and it was replaced in 1922, when Drs. Jean-Athannase Sicard and Jacques Forestier in Paris announced visualization of the tracheobronchial tree with the use of an iodine-containing oil called Lipiodol. Bronchography, in 1925, was described as beneficial in several diseases, including bronchiectasis, bronchial stenosis, bronchopleural fistula, and bronchogenic carcinoma. Dr. Louis Clerf of Jefferson Hospital reported that

> The extent of involvement of a primary malignant growth of the bronchus can often be accurately determined for the information of the surgeon ... (6).

As is still true a century later, many physicians worried about the effect of this technology on the clinical skills of chest percussion and auscultation. Although many physicians in the early part of the 20th century doubted the usefulness of chest radiography in the diagnosis of cardiac and pulmonary disease, the chest radiograph represented a technological advance at a time when people looked to technology to greatly improve their lives and eliminate human suffering (11). The public was perhaps more accepting of this technological development than were some members of the medical community; however, the costs of radiological procedures limited their use.

During World War II, mass screening with chest radiography became possible, as the costs of the procedure were borne by the United States government. By 1942, all recruits were radiographed as part of the induction physical (13). Approximately 1% of the population had sufficient radiographic evidence of tuberculosis to warrant rejection from the armed services (13). Since the number of calcified lymph nodes and pulmonary parenchymal nodules determined rejection from the military, patients with histoplasmosis undoubtedly were rejected as well. Screening radiographs were made with either a 35-mm unit or a 4 × 5-in photofluorographic unit. Military radiologists used magnifying lenses to interpret the images.

Screening for tuberculosis was soon extended to civilian groups, particularly those working in war-related industries. The United States Public Health Service sponsored mobile vans that brought free chest radiography to the general population. As the incidence of tuberculosis declined after the discovery of streptomycin, mass screening was discouraged and was finally discontinued in the early 1970s (8). Meanwhile, public acceptance of the chest radiograph as a screening tool for disease had been firmly established.

III. Tomography of the Chest

The early radiologist recognized that many areas of the body were obscured by overlying bones. Separation of bones from soft tissues on radiographs required the development of tomography, also known as laminography or planigraphy. Many American and European inventors worked simultaneously on developing the device. The first workable American tomographic machine was developed in 1936 by Dr. J. Robert Andrews at Cleveland University Hospital, in association with Robert J. Stava of the Picker X-Ray Corporation (6). The principle behind tomography lies in the reciprocal motion between the x-ray beam and the film relative to the patient. As the x-ray beam is moved from right to left, for example, the film is moved from left to right. The x-ray beam blurs the detail of the parts of the body closest to it; the moving film blurs the detail of the parts of the body closest to it. A single plane of the body remains in focus, allowing visualization of areas normally obscured by overlying bones. The thickness of the tomographic "slice" is controlled by the operator and varies from a few millimeters to a centimeter or more.

Tomography was primarily used for chest imaging for quite some time, since it provided superior evaluation of the mediastinum and hila, as well as areas of lung obscured by overlying ribs. Before the development of computed tomography (CT), conventional tomography was used to detect hilar and mediastinal lymphadenopathy in patients with lymphoma or carcinoma. Tomography was also very useful in the detection of pulmonary nodules. The slices of the chest as seen by conventional tomography could be acquired in almost any imaging plane. Lung tomograms were typically coronal; the pulmonary hila were evaluated with oblique tomograms.

IV. Advances in Film Technology

Although the physical principles of chest radiography are much the same as they were 100 years ago, there has been tremendous improvement in the quality of the chest film. The radiographic film and intensifying screens of several decades ago were not as sensitive to x-rays as is the film of today. The chest radiograph taken 50 years ago was a very high-contrast examination obtained at 70–80 kilovoltage peaks (kVp); the lungs appear very black, and the mediastinum and bones are very white. As a result, many radiologists in the past used fluoroscopy much more frequently than it is used today. The human eye was able to make observations under fluoroscopy that could not, at that time, be successfully recorded on radiographic film. Much of the information was lost. The radiographic film of today, on the other hand, is a much more sensitive film used in conjunction with higher kilovoltage peaks and with intensifying screens that are matched to the film and to the kilovoltage used. Film is dedicated for use in the chest, for example, or for use in the abdomen or the extremities.

The major hurdle to overcome in producing a high-quality radiographic image of the chest is the different attenuation of the x-ray beam by the heart and mediastinum relative to the attenuation by the lungs. More energy is required to penetrate the heart and mediastinum than to penetrate the lungs. One approach to this problem has been the development of a radiographic film that has two emulsions, one optimized for the mediastinum, and one optimized for the lungs (InSight Thoracic Imaging System by Kodak). The mediastinum emulsion is paired with an intensifying screen matched to its characteristics; the lung emulsion, on the other side of the film, is paired with its own intensifying screen (14,15). This design provides more clinically useful detail of the mediastinum, as well as of the pulmonary parenchyma superimposed on the diaphragm and heart (15,16). In addition, the radiation dose is lower than the radiation dose associated with conventional radiographic film.

V. Digital Imaging and Teleradiology

Storage phosphor digital imaging replaces the traditional film-intensifying screen combination with a reusable imaging plate coated with a photosensitive phosphor material. The x-rays that reach the plate create a latent image, which is converted to a digital image by a scanning laser beam. A 2000 × 2000 × 10-bit pixel array creates an image that can be manipulated to provide optimal contrast in both the lungs and the mediastinum (17–19). Storage phosphor imaging, or computed radiography, is used with increasing frequency for portable films, since this technology provides consistently high film quality with conventional mobile generators. The digital nature of this examination permits its ready transmission over telephone lines from one computer monitor to another, including monitors placed within the intensive care units. Digital imaging has the advantages of not only providing high film quality, but also of transferring information more rapidly from the radiology department to the clinical area.

Teleradiology is the transmission of radiologic images from one location to another. Teleradiology was originally used for interpretation of images obtained in remote sites where no radiologist was available. As teleradiology has become more widely accepted, it has been used for off-hours consultation, for transmission and display of images in intensive care units, and to provide subspecialist interpretation of radiologic studies performed at remote sites. Teleradiology may ultimately help in improving the efficiency of radiologists by rapid transmission and display of images from hospitals and clinics to a subspecialist radiologist at a single site. The ability to transmit digital images is a major factor in the drive to develop an "all-digital" radiology department. The results for the clinician will be the increasing availability of subspecialist interpretation of images and the potential for improved communication in radiology reporting. As the costs of these systems decrease and the data transmission rates increase, radiologic images linked with the verbal radiology report will ultimately be rapidly available to the referring physician.

Many imaging modalities, including computed radiography, CT, magnetic resonance (MR) imaging, and ultrasonography, are already in a digital format, and the data can be directly captured for transmission. Conventional radiographs, in an analog format, can be converted to a digital output by means of a laser digitizer. The laser digitizers currently in use scan a conventional chest radiograph in 6–10 seconds, converting it into a digital format with a spatial resolution of 1684 × 2048 × 12 bits. The digital data are then transmitted over a communication link to a workstation. The communication links currently available include standard telephone lines, dedicated T-1 lines, digital microwave service, and fiber-optic cables. Telephone line transmission is slow, but inexpensive and widely available. A T-1 line is a dedicated line placed between two points; it offers transmission rates of 1.522 Mbits/sec, and the cost is established on the basis of the distance between the two points (20) Dedicated T-1 lines are practical for two hospitals transmitting many images when the distance between the two hospitals is not great. Microwave links and fiber optics will provide even faster transmission rates as they become more widely used.

The digital data are transmitted to an image server at the receiving hospital that is linked with a diagnostic workstation. The diagnostic workstation consists of a computer and a monitor, on which the images are displayed. Observer performance on tests of teleradiology transmission and interpretation is in part linked to the characteristics of the monitor. Spatial resolutions of monitors used for primary interpretation should be at least 1024 × 1536 pixels; superior resolution is available in 2560 × 2048 pixels and 4096 × 4096 pixels. The luminance of the cathode ray tube (CRT) also affect observer performance in comparison studies with film interpretation on viewboxes (21). The CRT displays generate a luminescence of 50–60 ft-L, compared with 200–400 ft-L for view boxes (22).

The archiving of images is of critical importance. Digital data can be compressed, either reversibly or irreversibly, to decrease storage requirements. Long-term storage is currently achieved with optical jukeboxes, which have data capacities on the order of 140 Gbytes.

Teleradiology systems currently in use include the least-expensive, lowest-resolution systems transmitting images over standard telephone lines for off-hours image review by an on-call radiologist. The primary interpretation of the images is often done at a later time with review of the hard-copy images. Teleradiology systems for primary interpretation are more likely to implement dial-up digital service, T-1 lines, or fiber optics for rapid transmission to a workstation with high-resolution display, and optical-archiving capabilities.

The radiology reading room will one day consist of computers and banks of monitors, rather than view boxes and alternators.

VI. Cross-Sectional Imaging of the Chest

The first extensive research on CT was performed by Sir Godfrey Newbold Hounsfield in England in the late 1960s. Hounsfield was a senior research scientist at EMI Central Research Laboratories in Middlesex, England. His early laboratory machine required 9 days to acquire the data and another 2½ hr to reconstruct the data into an image (23). The first clinical scanner was constructed by EMI in 1970–1971. In 1972, CT was introduced for clinical imaging, and the first clinical trials were performed by neuroradiologist James Ambrose at the Atkinson Morley's Hospital in south London (24). Each slice acquisition required 8 min. The prolonged scan time and the water bath configuration of the gantry limited scanning to the brain (23). The images were crude by today's standards, with an 80 × 80 matrix, but showed abnormalities within the brain more clearly than they had ever been shown with a noninvasive technique.

The first CT scanner in North America was installed at the Mayo Clinic in June 1973 (24). As the second-generation scanner was somewhat faster, scanning was extended to cover the body as well. During the 1970s and 1980s, subsequent generations of CT scanners not only became capable of acquiring data more rapidly, but also provided superior spatial resolution. Shorter scan times allowed imaging of the lungs with breath-holding. Pulmonary imaging has been taken to a higher level with the introduction of high-resolution CT, providing great anatomical detail on 1.0-mm–thick slices.

Hounsfield has been immortalized by the use of the term Hounsfield units (HU) to describe attenuation values of tissues within the image; he also received the 1979 Nobel Prize in physiology or medicine (25). He shared the prize with Allan MacLeod Cormack, who had derived a mathematical theory for image reconstruction in the late 1950s (26).

Helical, or spiral, CT is a further improvement in CT imaging. Helical CT of the thorax provides a contiguous data set of multiple slices, typically obtained in one breath-hold. This technique ensures that no information is lost as a result of changes in breathing patterns. With conventional CT scanners, there is always the possibility that one image slice will be obtained in a shallow inspiration, and the next slice in a deeper inspiration, and that the small pulmonary nodule or mediastinal lymph node will not be recorded. The problem of respiratory-associated misregistration is solved by helical CT, which allows continuous data acquisition over multiple rotations while the patient is simultaneously transported continuously through the scanner (27). The spacing between slices can be varied during image reconstruction to optimize data interpretation. This has improved detection of pulmonary nodules and enhanced confidence in the diagnosis of pulmonary nodules on CT (28). The fast-imaging rate not only allows a single breath-hold acquisition of data, but also allows optimization of vascular enhancement with intravenous contrast material administration. As a result, pulmonary vascular and thoracic aorta abnormalities (including pulmonary emboli and thoracic aorta dissections) are seen to better advantage with helical scanners than with conventional CT scanners.

VII. Health Care Costs and Chest Imaging

In 1992, 14% of our gross national product went for health care (29). The amount of money that the public is willing to spend on national health care has been reached, or perhaps surpassed. The current move to managed care has many implications for clinicians and radiologists alike. For the individual interested in chest imaging, the move toward managed care has both advantages and disadvantages. The chest radiograph remains a relatively inexpensive means of evaluating the chest. As a screening tool and in the monitoring of disease, the chest radiograph provides a tremendous amount of information about both cardiac and pulmonary disease. Research directed toward determining the efficacy of screening chest radiographs (e.g., annual physical examinations and preoperative chest radiographs) will benefit patients as well as health care providers. More expensive-imaging modalities, including CT, angiography, MR imaging, and positron emission tomography (PET), on the other hand, face a more difficult challenge. More expensive technologies will be required to provide accurate information that cannot be obtained by any less expensive method.

As radiology has become more complex, there has been a shift toward organ–system subspecialization, and toward subspecialist radiologists communicating primarily with clinicians in similar areas. The chest radiologist works as part of a team with pulmonologists, cardiothoracic surgeons, and cardiologists; the neuroradiologist communicates primarily with neurosurgeons and neurologists. In a managed care system, a primary care physician functions as a gatekeeper and assumes a continuing role in the care of the patient. As a result, radiologists will work with primary care physicians with increasing frequency and will be more involved in the imaging decisions during the workup of patients (30).

In 1990, an estimated 260–300 million radiologic procedures, the equivalent of 1.0–1.3 procedures for each man, woman, and child, were performed in the United States, including both diagnostic and therapeutic procedures (31). Payments for these procedures represented 3.5% of national spending on personal health care in the United States. Although expensive high-tech equipment within the radiology department has been cited as one of the factors in rising health care costs, the number of procedures and the percentage of health care spending that it represents suggest that many other factors must be involved. Ensuring that the radiologic studies performed for each patient represent the best diagnostic strategy for that patient is common sense; it seems unlikely that limiting access to radiologic services would have a significant effect on current health care costs.

Radiologists have, in the past, performed radiologic procedures on the request of the referring clinician, with variable levels of input into the diagnostic workup. Under managed care, greater emphasis is placed on ensuring that the diagnostic workup of a patient is performed in the most cost-effective manner. To aid in this goal, the American College of Radiology (ACR) put together a task force to develop patient care guidelines. Ten expert panels of radiologists were formed and were organized according to body systems. Fourteen representatives from national specialty organizations acted as consultants to these panels. Their goal was to identify appropriate and economical diagnostic-imaging strategies that should be used for a patient, given the patient's presenting condition, and to develop appropriateness criteria that would be nationally accepted and scientifically based. The American College of Radiology Appropriateness Criteria for Imaging and Treatment Decisions were published in 1995 (32). Each diagnostic-imaging study that might come under consideration for a given clinical condition is ranked on a scale from 1 to 9, in which 9 represents a "most appropriate" examination. For example, in the staging of bronchogenic carcinoma, the posteroanterior (PA) and lateral chest radiographs are considered most appropriate (9), a CT scan of the thorax including the adrenal glands receives a score of 8, and an appropriateness level of 6 is assigned to the radionuclide bone scan. As radiology is an ever-changing specialty, these criteria are scheduled to undergo periodic review and revision. The categories are now very broad. These appropriateness criteria will be even more valuable, as the patient with lung cancer, for example, can be categorized on the basis of cell type, clinical evidence of systemic disease, and so on.

VIII. Clinical Efficacy of Diagnostic Imaging

Radiology is a very visual science, which is reflected in the scientific radiology literature over the last 100 years. Since Roentgen described the appearance of the bones and soft tissues of his hand in 1895, radiologists have published reports of radiologic observations as they pertain to both normal anatomy and disease. With the introduction of each new imaging modality, research in radiology was dominated by case studies linking new observations to pathological and physiological events. The health care reform currently under way has promoted greater interest in other types of research: technology assessment and outcomes research (33). The goal of radiologists will always be to provide high-quality images and accurate diagnoses, but radiologists are now viewing this goal within a more global framework. The expanded goal goes beyond technical quality of a radiograph, or diagnostic accuracy of the interpretation, to clinical efficacy. How does diagnostic imaging affect patient care? What is the ultimate benefit to patients and to society of diagnostic imaging?

A six-tiered model of efficacy has been adapted by Fryback and Thornbury to help evaluate the clinical efficacy of diagnostic imaging (34,35). These six levels describe the areas in which diagnostic imaging must be analyzed to determine its ultimate value. Level 1, technical efficacy, describes the physical properties of a diagnostic image, including spatial resolution, signal/noise ratio, and image contrast. These sorts of studies are performed with phantoms and allow comparison of one system with another. Level 2 describes diagnostic accuracy efficacy: within a case series, what percentage of diagnoses are correct? Studies of this type compare sensitivity and specificity, or the area under the receiver–operating–characteristic (ROC) curve to compare one imaging modality with another. An overwhelming majority of radiology research studies during the last 20 years have been of technical efficacy and diagnostic accuracy.

The four remaining levels of efficacy include the effect of diagnostic imaging on patient care and on society. Level 3 is diagnostic-thinking efficacy. Studies in this group analyze the change in the physician's diagnostic certainty or differential diagnosis as a result of the image information. To show efficacy at this level, the diagnostic examination must influence the physician toward an alternative course of action from what would have been done without the imaging information. Level 4, therapeutic efficacy, includes the number of times that the planned therapy was altered by the diagnostic imaging information, or the percentage of times a medical procedure was avoided because of imaging findings. Level 5, patient–outcome efficacy, examines the change in quality-adjusted life expectancy, the morbidity or medical procedures avoided, or the cost per quality-adjusted life years saved with the diagnostic imaging information. Level 6 studies determine, from the societal viewpoint, the cost-effectiveness of diagnostic imaging. These studies determine whether the cost of a given imaging technology to society, as a whole, is acceptable.

The time between the introduction of a new technology, CT, for example, and the determination of its value to society is quite long. There is increasing financial pressure for earlier evaluation of diagnostic-thinking efficacy and therapeutic efficacy. To achieve this within the shortest possible time period requires collaboration among investigators and a multiple center prospective study with attention to the ultimate outcome of the patient.

A good example of how radiology research proceeds is the use of chest CT in the investigation of traumatic aortic rupture . Conventional CT was introduced into clinical practice in 1973, and multiple generations of improved scanners appeared during the next 20 years. Spiral CT was introduced into clinical practice in 1989, and studies were performed with phantoms over the next several years to determine spatial resolution, noise characteristics, and artifacts as a function of kilovoltage peaks, milliamperes, section-thickness, and table-feed speed (27,36). These are level 1 studies of technical efficacy. Beginning in 1990, many radiologists began to screen trauma patients with chest CT to detect mediastinal hematoma. Prospective studies using both CT and aortography produced both proponents and opponents of screening CT (37–40). These studies determined the percentage of correct diagnoses in a case series and, therefore, are level 2, diagnostic accuracy–efficacy, studies.

A metanalysis, compiling ten published reports of CT for detection of aortic rupture after blunt chest trauma, appeared in 1995 (41). Six diagnostic strategies combining chest radiography, CT, and aortography were established. By using existing data, the effectiveness, expressed as survival to hospital discharge, and the costs incurred to society were calculated for each diagnostic strategy. This study determined that, in the cohort undergoing CT for the evaluation of other injuries, triage to aortography based on CT findings of mediastinal hematoma, disruption of the aortic contour, or an intimal flap, yielded equivalent survival at a lower cost than triage based on the chest radiograph. For the cohort not undergoing CT, immediate aortography yielded the highest survival, but at a high cost (2.2 million dollars per life saved) compared with that of CT screening before aortography (242,000 dollars per life saved). This study is a level 6 study, as it includes a benefit–cost analysis from a societal viewpoint.

These types of studies are necessary for a wide variety of clinical conditions and imaging modalities. Within the ever-changing field of radiology, one must constantly reevaluate these studies, because new technology brings with it changes in both costs and effectiveness.

IX. Research and Training in Chest Imaging

Holding down health care costs has become primary focus for legislators, health care workers, hospital administrators, and patients alike. Hospitals affiliated with medical schools, resident-training programs, and research laboratories have higher overhead costs as a result of these programs. In the past, the higher costs of health care at academic institutions has been justified by the level of care they provided. Now, in an attempt to compete with community hospitals for patients in this era of managed care contracts, academic hospitals will need to reexamine costs incurred by physician-training programs, as well as research programs.

An example of technology development and research that will come under critical review during this period of cost containment is the PET scanner. In addition to applications in the brain, PET scanners have tremendous potential in chest imaging for the diagnosis, staging, and management of both primary and metastatic malignancies. Positron emission tomography uses derivatives of biologically active compounds labeled with positron emitters. The most commonly used compound for PET imaging at present is [^{18}F] fluorodeoxyglucose (FDG), which is used as a marker of glucose metabolism. Because of the high metabolic rate of malignant tumors, increased uptake of FDG allows recognition of both the primary malignancy and the sites of spread. This physiological method of imaging is different from conventional radiography and CT, which show anatomical detail and structural changes with a high degree of resolution. The use of PET does not replace CT, but instead, provides tissue-specific information that helps distinguish malignant from benign lesions.

Several factors may account for the fact that PET has not yet been incorporated into mainstream medicine (42). The positron-emitting isotopes used most frequently in PET imaging have extremely short half-lives, on the order of minutes to hours; centers with PET scanners must maintain cyclotrons or have access to regional cyclotrons for the production of isotopes. [The half-life of fluorine 18 is 110 min.] Because of the complexity of PET, operating a PET scanner and cyclotron also requires a staff of physicians, physicists, and technicians trained in this field. Capital expenses for the installation of a PET facility are estimated to be 5–7 million dollars; annual operating expenses average another 2 million dollars per year. Since each scan requires 1–2 hr to complete, only a limited number of scans can be performed each day. The average charge for each procedure, therefore, is approximately 2 thousand dollars.

Positron emission tomography suffers the misfortune of being developed at a time when any new procedure is expected to provide a high level of accuracy, with more cost-effectiveness than currently available technologies (43). New technologies are held to a higher standard than were previously developed technologies, including CT, ultrasonography, and MR imaging. For PET to develop to its full potential, it will have to survive the lean years, during which it is not widely accepted clinically and is seen largely as a research tool. To continue PET research, academic centers must be able to afford the installation and maintenance of PET facilities. Two sources of revenue are required: (1) compensation for cases for which PET has proved clinical efficacy and (2) funding for basic research and clinical trials so that other areas of clinical efficacy can be discovered.

Positron emission tomography is just one example of emerging technology in radiology. Other emergent technologies include MR spectroscopy, magnetic source imaging, electrical impedance tomography (EIT), and noninvasive infrared scanning. In view of the contributions of CT, ultrasonography, and MR imaging to patient care and the rapidity with which these imaging modalities have become incorporated into the standard of care, it is clear that resources must be provided to allow development of technologies that will take diagnostic imaging into the 21st century.

X. Conclusion

The 20th century has witnessed rapid advances in the field of diagnostic imaging. The last 25 years alone have seen the development of CT, MR imaging, and PET. Computer technology has made many of these advances possible. It is impossible to predict where we will be in another 25 years. Film is likely to be obsolete, and digital imaging will provide the media for diagnosis, whether the images are generated by x-rays, sound waves, protons, or positrons. A new imaging method will have likely joined the ranks of chest radiography, CT, MR, ultrasonography, and PET to give us perhaps a more tissue-specific or more physiological approach to diagnosis. Although the effect of these advances in diagnostic imaging may not equal that of a therapeutic cure, the ability to recognize disease at an earlier stage and to help direct appropriate therapy will always have a positive influence on patient care.

Radiology research must now focus on clinical efficacy, including technology assessment and outcomes research. It is our hope that these studies will allow the ongoing development of imaging technology and, ultimately, improve the level of care we can provide to our patients.

References

1. Patton DD. Roentgen and the "new light." I. Roentgen and Lenard. Invest Radiol 1992; 27:408–414.
2. Patton DD. Roentgen and the "new light"—Roentgen's moment of discovery. Part 2: The first glimmer of the "new light." Invest Radiol 1993; 28:51–58.

3. Patton DD. Roentgen and the "new light"—Roentgen's moment of discovery. Part 3: The genealogy of Roentgen's barium platinocyanide screen. Invest Radiol 1993; 28:954–961.
4. Kotzur IM. W C. Roentgen: a new type of ray. Radiology 1994; 193:329–332.
5. Linton OW. News of x-ray reaches America days after announcement of Roentgen's discovery. AJR 1995; 165:571–472.
6. Brecher R, Brecher E. The Rays: A History of Radiology in the United States and Canada. Baltimore: Williams & Wilkins, 1969.
7. Greene R. Imaging the respiratory system in the first few years after discovery of the x-ray: contributions of Francis H. Williams, M.D. AJR 1992; 159:1–7.
8. Haygood TM. Chest screening and tuberculosis in the United States. Radiographics 1994; 14:1151–1166.
9. Williams FH. The roentgen rays in thoracic diseases. Am J Med Sci 1897; 114:665–687
10. Singh SP, Nath H. Early radiology of pulmonary tuberculosis. AJR 1994; 162:846.
11. Gurney JW. Why chest radiography became routine. Radiology 1995; 195:245–246
12. Williams FH. The Roentgen Rays in Medicine and Surgery. New York: Macmillan, 1901.
13. Haygood TM. Briggs JE. World War II military led the way in screening chest radiography. Milit Med 1992; 157:113–116.
14. Glazer HS, Muka E, Sagel SS, Jost RG. New techniques in chest radiography. Radiol Clin North Am 1994; 32:711–729.
15. Swenson SJ, Gray JE, Brown LR, Aughenbaugh GL, Harms GF, Stears J. A new asymmetric screen–film combination for conventional chest radiography: evaluation in 50 patients. AJR 1992; 160:483–486.
16. Gray JE, Stears JG, Swenson SJ, Bunch PC. Evaluation of resolution and sensitometric characteristics of an asymmetric screen–film imaging system. Radiology 1993; 188:537–539.
17. Schaefer CM, Greene R, Oestmann JW, et al. Digital storage phosphor imaging versus conventional film radiography in CT-documented chest disease. Radiology 1990; 174:207–210.
18. Chotas HG, Floyd CE Jr, Dobbins JT III, Ravin CE. Digital chest radiography with photostimulable storage phosphors: signal-to-noise ratio as a function of kilovoltage with matched exposure risk. Radiology 1993; 186:395–398.
19. Niklason LT, Chan H-P, Cascade PN, Chang CL, Chee PW, Mathews JF. Portable chest imaging: comparison of storage phosphor digital, asymmetric screen–film, and conventional screen–film systems. Radiology 1993; 186:387–393.
20. Dwyer SJ, Stewart BK, Sayre JW, Honeyman JC. Wide area network strategies for teleradiology systems. Radiographics 1992; 12:567–576.
21. Goldberg MA, Rosenthal DI, Chew FS, Blickman JG, Miller SW, Mueller PR. New high-resolution teleradiology system: prospective study of diagnostic accuracy in 685 transmitted clinical cases. Radiology 1993; 186:429–434.
22. Dwyer SJ, Stewart BK, Sayre JW, et al. Performance characteristics and image fidelity of grey-scale monitors. Radiographics 1992; 12:765–772.
23. Hounsfield GN. Computerized transverse axial scanning (tomography): Part I. Description of system. Br J Radiol 1973; 46:1016–1022.
24. Baker HL Jr. Historical vignette: introduction of computed tomography in North America. AJNR 1993; 14:283–287.

25. Hounsfield GN. Computed medical imaging. Nobel lecture, December 9, 1979. J Comput Assist Tomogr 1980; 4:665–674.
26. DeChiro G, Brooks RA. The 1979 Nobel Prize in physiology or medicine. J Comput Assist Tomogr 1980; 4:241–245.
27. Kalender WA, Seissler W, Klotz E, Vock P. Spiral volumetric CT with single-breath-hold technique, continuous transport, and continuous scanner rotation. Radiology 1990; 176:181–183.
28. Buckley JA, Scott WW Jr, Siegelman SS, et al. Pulmonary nodules: effect of increased data sampling on detection with spiral CT and confidence in diagnosis. Radiology 1995; 196:395–400.
29. Sunshine JH, Evens RG. The challenge of managed care and managed competition. AJR 1994; 162:767–771.
30. Thrall JH. The radiologist in the 1990s: new practice expectations and management responsibilities. AJR 1994; 163:11–15.
31. Sunshine JH, Mabry MR, Bansal S. The volume and cost of radiologic services in the United States in 1990. AJR 1991; 157:609–613.
32. American College of Radiology Appropriateness Criteria for Imaging and Treatment Decisions. Reston VA: American College of Radiology, 1995.
33. Hillman BJ. Outcomes research and cost-effectiveness analysis for diagnostic imaging. Radiology 1994; 193:307–310.
34. Fryback DG, Thornbury JR. The efficacy of diagnostic imaging. Med Decis Making 1991; 11:88–94.
35. Thornbury JR. Clinical efficacy of diagnostic imaging: love it or leave it. AJR 1994; 162:1–8.
36. Polacin A, Kalender WA, Marchal G. Evaluation of section sensitivity profiles and image noise in spiral CT. Radiology 1992; 185:29–35.
37. Richardson P, Mirvis SE, Scorpio R, Dunham CM. Value of CT in determining the need for angiography when findings of mediastinal hemorrhage are equivocal. AJR 1991; 156:272–279.
38. Raptopoulos V, Sherman RG, Phillips DA, Davidoff A, Silva WE. Traumatic aortic tear: screening with chest CT. Radiology 1992; 182:667–673.
39. Morgan PW, Goodman LR, Aprahamian C, Foley WD, Lipchik EO. Evaluation of traumatic aortic injury: does dynamic contrast-enhanced CT play a role? Radiology 1992; 182:661–666.
40. Risher RG, Chasen MH, Lamik N. Diagnosis of injuries of the aorta and brachiocephalic arteries caused by blunt chest trauma: CT vs aortography. AJR 1994; 162:1047–1052.
41. Hunink MGM, Bos JJ. Triage of patients to angiography for detection of aortic rupture after blunt chest trauma: cost-effectiveness analysis of using CT. AJR 1995; 165:27–36.
42. Conti PS, Keppler JS, Halls JM. Positron emission tomography: a financial and operational analysis. AJR 1994; 162:1279–1286.
43. Young IR. Review of modalities with a potential future in radiology. Radiology 1994; 192:307–317.

2

Pulmonary Disease in the Immunocompromised Host (Non-AIDS)

ANN N. LEUNG

Stanford University Medical Center
Stanford, California

NESTOR L. MÜLLER

University of British Columbia
and Vancouver Hospital and Health
 Sciences Centre
Vancouver, British Columbia, Canada

I. Introduction

The *immunocompromised state* may be defined as any condition in which the response of a host to a foreign antigen is subnormal (1). Although congenital and acquired immunodeficiency syndromes and hematological malignancies may directly cause an impairment in one or more mechanisms of host defense, in most immunocompromised patients, subnormal resistance is iatrogenic. Immunosuppression is a direct result of medical treatment in patients receiving chemotherapy for malignancies, cyclosporine for organ transplantation, and steroids and cytotoxic drugs for nonmalignant disorders.

Pulmonary complications are a common cause of morbidity and mortality in the immunocompromised host. Infections account for 75% of cases; in the remaining one-quarter cases, causes are noninfectious and include drug-induced lung disease, recurrence of underlying disease, posttransplantation lymphoproliferative disorder, and unrelated processes, such as pulmonary edema (2,3). Expeditious evaluation of pulmonary symptoms in the immunocompromised host is critical, because respiratory disease in this susceptible population may progress rapidly to respiratory failure. Prompt diagnoses, leading to institution of specific therapy, are important factors in patient survival (4).

II. Role of Imaging

In the assessment of pulmonary complications in the immunocompromised host, imaging studies are performed to (1) detect an abnormality, (2) aid in the differential diagnosis, (3) guide to the appropriate diagnostic procedure, and (4) evaluate the response to therapy (5). Because of its low cost and availability, chest radiography remains the most widely used imaging technique. However, several limitations in the efficacy of radiographs have been recognized: in up to 10% of symptomatic patients, results of radiographs may be normal; even when abnormalities are detected, confident specific diagnoses are seldom possible.

The use of computed tomography (CT) and, more specifically, high-resolution CT (HRCT) can significantly influence the diagnostic workup and management of pulmonary complications in the immunocompromised host. *High-resolution CT*, defined as 1- to 2-mm–collimation CT reconstructed using a high-spatial–resolution algorithm, provides superior demonstration of the presence, extent, and distribution of parenchymal abnormalities in comparison with either chest radiography or conventional CT. The HRCT scan allows more sensitive detection of abnormalities in patients with normal or questionable radiographic findings (6–8), may provide a confident diagnosis (9–12), and can guide to the optimal type and site of biopsy (12,13).

III. Infection

Infections account for 75% of pulmonary complications in the immunocompromised host; this percentage increases to greater than 90% if the patient has either severe neutropenia (a neutrophil count of $< 500/mm^3$) or if the lung process is focal (2). Important clinical factors to be considered in formulation of the differential diagnosis are (1) the primary disease and associated immune defect, (2) the use of empiric antimicrobial therapy, and (3) the typical temporal pattern of infection in specific disease states.

Immunodeficiency can result from alterations in the absolute number or function of granulocytes, or from impairment in the cell-mediated (T-lymphocyte) or humoral (B-lymphocyte) immune defense mechanisms. Recognition of the general category of immune dysfunction can help predict the most likely causative organisms. Empiric, broad-spectrum antibiotics have become the standard of care for febrile, neutropenic patients (14); nonresponse to empiric therapy usually indicates the presence of resistant bacteria, atypical pneumonias, such as those caused by *Legionella* or *Nocardia*, fungi, or viruses (1). For several groups of immunodeficient patients, the cause of immunosuppression can be reliably predicted to allow recognition of the most likely infectious pathogens (1,15,16). For example, in the bone marrow transplant population, time lines have been established that focus the differential diagnosis on pathogens that are likely to occur at sequential points in the transplantation process. During the first month posttransplantation, neutropenia predisposes to bacterial and fungal infections; with recovery of neutrophil count in the second month, viruses, particularly cytomegalovirus, play an increasingly important role in causing pulmonary complications (16).

A. Bacterial Infections

Immunocompromised patients are susceptible to community-acquired and nosocomial bacterial pneumonias, as well as to infection by more opportunistic bacteria, such as *Nocardia asteroides* and *Listeria monocytogenes*, that less often cause disease in normal hosts. *Streptococcus pneumoniae* and *Haemophilus influenzae* are common pathogens in patients with humoral defects or asplenia, whereas gram-negative bacteria (*Pseudomonas, Klebsiella, Escherichia coli, Enterobacter* species) and *Staphylococcus aureus* frequently cause infection in neutropenic patients.

Radiographically, the appearance of bacterial pneumonia is similar in both the immunocompromised and normal hosts. Focal areas of consolidation in a segmental or lobar distribution are typically seen; multilobar and bilateral involvement may also occur (17). Cavitation indicating the presence of a necrotizing pneumonia is characteristic of gram-negative organisms (Fig. 1). Diagnosis of bacterial infections is usually made on the basis of sputum cultures or response to empiric treatment.

Nocardia asteroides

Nocardia asteroides is a gram-positive bacterium that causes infection in patients with defective cell-mediated immunity. The most common predisposing conditions are organ transplantation, hematological malignancy, and use of corticosteroids (18). The radiographic manifestations usually consist of focal abnormalities, ranging from single or multiple pulmonary nodules to areas of consolidation with cavitation. Nocardial infection may extend into the pleural space and cause empyema and chest wall involvement. On CT, peripheral pulmonary nodules or focal airspace consolidation with internal low attenuation or cavitation may be present (Fig. 2; 19). Invasive procedures, such as percutaneous biopsy and bronchoscopy, are often required to establish the diagnosis of nocardiosis, as the yield of sputum examination and culture is low (20).

Legionella pneumophila

Legionella pneumonia also occurs in the setting of decreased cell-mediated immunity. Infection with *Legionella* commonly cause extrapulmonary symptoms involving the gastrointestinal, renal, and central nervous systems. Patients may have abdominal pain, diarrhea, hematuria, proteinuria, confusion, and neurological

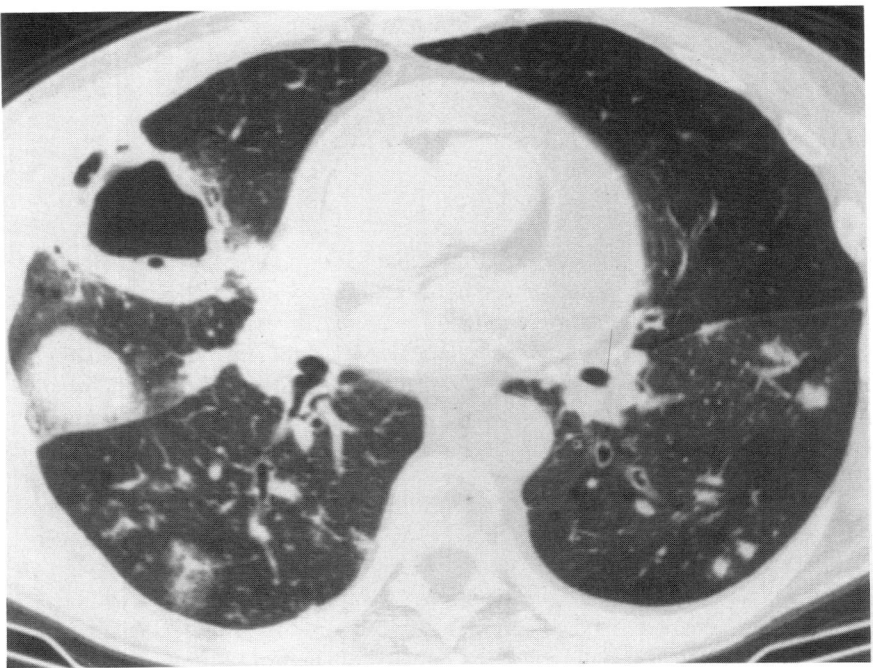

Figure 1 Pseudomonal infection in a 52-year-old woman with rheumatoid arthritis: The HRCT scan demonstrates focal areas of consolidation, with cavitation in the right middle lobe associated with multiple smaller nodules in the lower lobes bilaterally. Pyogenic pericardial involvement was proved by pericardiocentesis.

deficits. Peripheral patchy or segmental consolidation is the usual presenting radiographic pattern (21,22). Rapid progression to lobar involvement and spread to noncontiguous ipsilateral and contralateral sites are common (21,23). There is a propensity for lower lobe involvement, and pleural effusions occur in approximately 50% of patients (21,23). Cavitary lesions, although infrequent in the normal host, occur in the setting of immunosuppression (21,23). The indirect (IFA) immunofluorescent test is the most commonly used test to detect legionella infection. Appropriate treatment by erythromycin decreases the case fatality rate from 80% in nontreated immunosuppressed patients to 25% (21).

Septic Embolism

Immunocompromised patients, particularly those with long-term indwelling catheters, are predisposed to developing septic emboli. The most common organisms cultured are *S. aureus* and streptococci (24). The characteristic radiographic

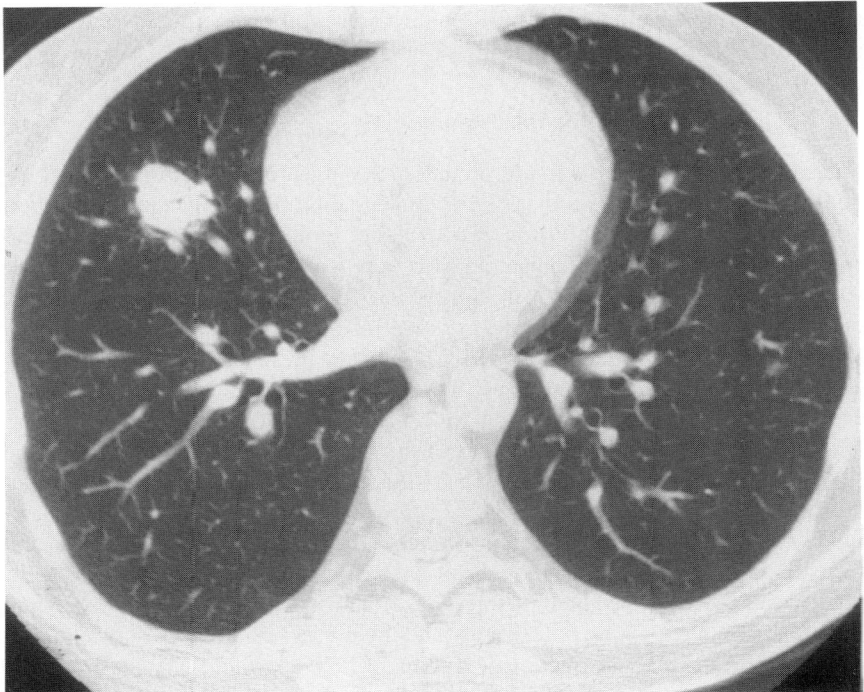

Figure 2 Pulmonary nocardiosis in a 42-year-old bone marrow transplant recipient: The HRCT scan demonstrates a well-circumscribed nodule with central cavitation in the right middle lobe.

findings, consisting of multiple, round or wedge-shaped opacities in the periphery of the lung, are identified in the minority of cases (11). A CT scan is more specific than radiography in the diagnosis of septic emboli (11,25). On a CT scan, septic emboli appear as heterogeneous, subpleural, wedge-shaped opacities, or as multiple pulmonary nodules, with or without cavitation, often associated with a feeding vessel (11,25).

Mycobacterium tuberculosis

Tuberculosis occurs with increased frequency in immunosuppressed patients with deficient T-cell lymphocyte function. The prevalence of mycobacterial disease is highest in patients with hematological malignancies, cancers of the lung and head and neck, and organ transplant recipients (15,26). As most infections are due to reactivation, the features of postprimary disease are common: focal upper lobe abnormalities, with or without cavitation. Atypical multilobar or miliary patterns occurring in patients in whom infection develops after chemotherapy are associated with a poor prognosis (26).

B. *Pneumocystis carinii* Pneumonia

Pneumocystis carinii is the major protozoal pathogen in immunosuppressed patients. In the 1970s, *Pneumocystis carinii* pneumonia (PCP) was the most important cause of pulmonary infection in patients receiving immunosuppressive therapy for transplantation or malignancy, particularly lymphoma and acute lymphocytic leukemia. With the institution of routine prophylaxis for patients at risk, the prevalence of PCP declined until the advent of the acquired immunodeficiency syndrome (AIDS) era. In contrast with the subacute presentation typical of AIDS-related infection, PCP in the non-AIDS, immunocompromised host is usually acute, with high-grade fever, dyspnea, and hypoxemia (27).

The radiographic manifestations of disease are dependent on the stage and severity of infection. In early stages, a diffuse, perihilar reticular or reticulonodular pattern is present, with associated ground-glass opacification (28). In later stages or in more severe disease, homogeneous, bilateral consolidation may occur. Unusual manifestations that have been described include asymmetric or focal involvement, nodules, and cavitation (29). Pleural effusions and lymphadenopathy are uncommon. Chest radiographs may be normal in up to 10% of patients.

On CT, the most characteristic finding of PCP is *ground-glass attenuation*, defined as areas of increased parenchymal attenuation, without obscuration of the underlying vascular structures (Fig. 3). The distribution of ground-glass attenuation may be diffuse and homogeneous, or geographic, with relatively normal secondary pulmonary lobules adjacent to diseased ones (7,8). A superimposed reticular pattern with interlobular septal thickening is present in 18–50% of patients (7,8). Cystic lesions, which are predominantly subcortical and upper lobe in distribution, likely represent pneumatoceles and predispose to pneumothorax (30).

Diagnosis of PCP is made on the basis of morphological identification of the organism in either induced sputum or bronchoalveolar lavage fluid. Treated infection has a survival rate of 65–75% (14,27).

C. Fungal Infections

With the development of effective chemoprophylaxis and empiric therapy for bacterial infections and PCP, invasive fungi have emerged as a major cause of infectious morbidity and mortality in immunocompromised patients. Fungal infections occur in the setting of neutropenia and impaired cellular immunity; predisposing conditions include hematological malignancies, particularly leukemia, bone marrow transplantation, and steroid administration.

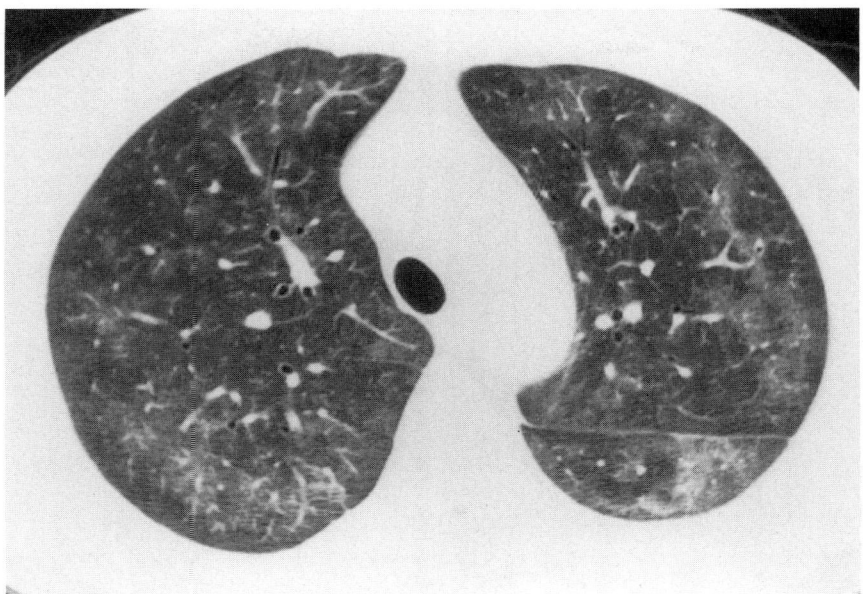

Figure 3 *Pneumocystis carinii* pneumonia in a 56-year-old renal transplant recipient: The HRCT scan at the level of the aortic arch demonstrates bilateral areas of ground-glass attenuation.

Invasive Aspergillosis

Aspergillus is the most common fungal opportunistic invader of the lung. Inhalation of the ubiquitous spores is believed to be the portal of entry in susceptible hosts (31). The radiologic patterns of disease closely reflect the pathogenesis of infection. In the early stages of the angioinvasive form of disease, a relatively well-circumscribed area of consolidation appears as the fungal infection spreads from small membranous and respiratory bronchiole lumens to the adjacent parenchyma; more extensive parenchymal opacification, sometimes in a characteristic wedge-shaped pattern, develops as the fungi invade adjacent vessels, leading to thrombosis and hemorrhagic infarction (31). On CT, the angioinvasive stage manifests as a nodule surrounded by ground-glass attenuation (CT halo sign) representing the nidus of fungal infection and adjacent area of hemorrhagic infarction, respectively (Fig. 4; 32,33). In the recovery phase of infection, cavitation of the nodule will occur (air-crescent sign) usually coincident with clinical improvement and resolution of neutropenia.

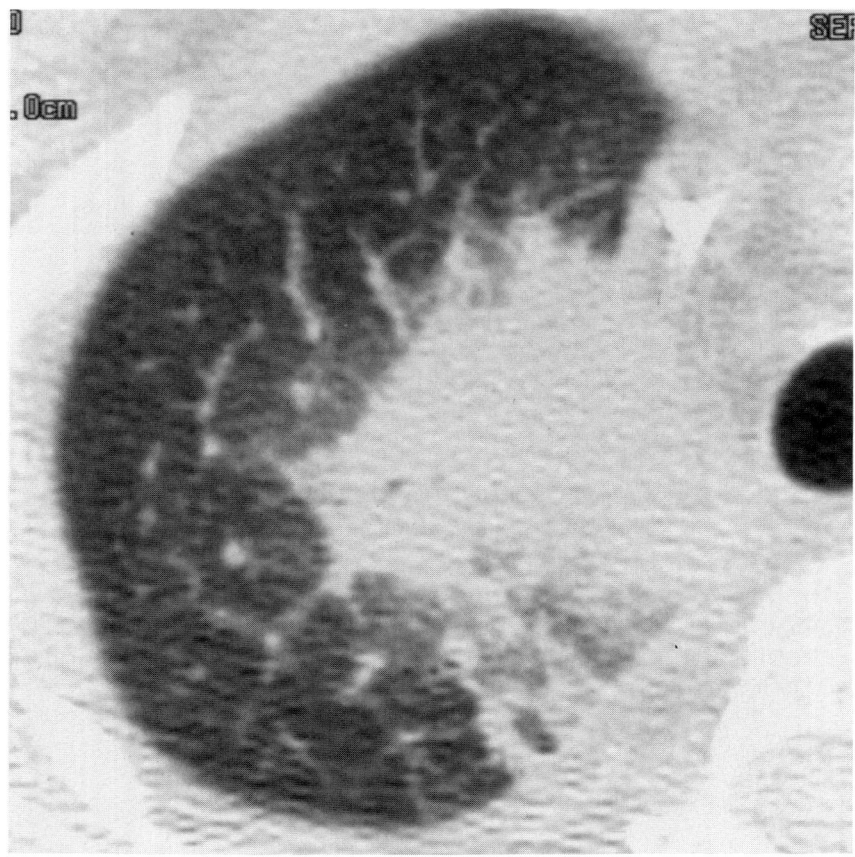

Figure 4 Angioinvasive aspergillosis in 25-year-old woman with acute myeloblastic leukemia: A HRCT scan of the right upper lobe demonstrates a peripheral mass with surrounding halo of ground-glass attenuation.

Diagnosis of angioinvasive aspergillosis is often problematic. Early recognition and treatment of infection is critical to survival and may be facilitated by the presence of a CT halo sign. However, this finding is nonspecific and may be present in other opportunistic infections (34). Sputum cultures yield aspergilli in only 8–34% of patients (35), and diagnosis usually necessitates an invasive procedure, such as bronchoscopy or percutaneous biopsy.

Invasive aspergillosis of the airways occurs less commonly than the angioinvasive form of disease. Diagnosis is based on pathological demonstration of organisms deep to the basement membrane. Radiographic findings are nonspecific; mostly commonly, ill-defined 3- to 5-mm nodules or areas of consolidation are found (36). The main findings on CT consist of consolidation in a peribronchial or lobar distribution, often associated with centrilobular nodules (Fig. 5; 36).

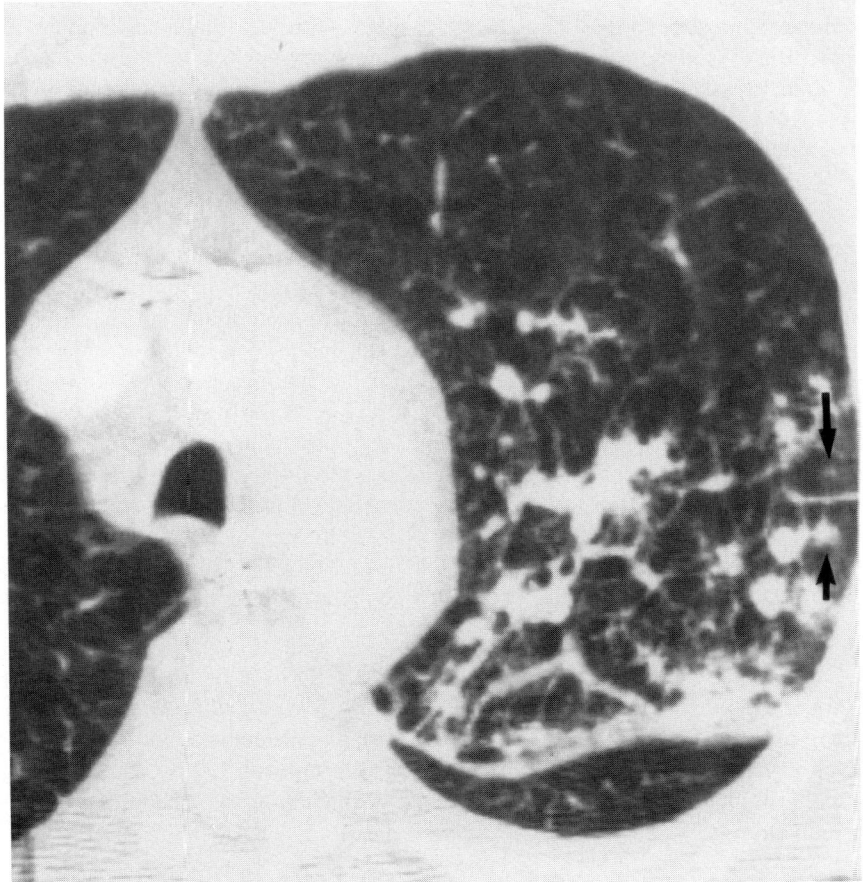

Figure 5 Airway invasive aspergillosis in a 59-year-old man, immunosuppressed due to long-term corticosteroid therapy for chronic obstructive pulmonary disease: A HRCT scan of the left upper lobe shows patchy, peribronchial consolidation associated with centrilobular nodules (arrows).

Mucormycosis

Mucorales are ubiquitous saphrophytic fungi that are an uncommon, but important cause of infection in immunosuppressed patients. The most common predisposing conditions are hematological malignancy, diabetes, and steroid administration. The presentation is of an acute, fulminant illness, with symptoms of cough, fever, and variable sputum production; pleuritic chest pain is often present (37). Because of a shared propensity for vascular invasion and subsequent parenchymal infarction, mucormycosis and aspergillosis have similar radiographic manifestations: nodular, lobular, or wedge-shaped abnormalities, with or without development of cavitation (37). Antemortem diagnosis is infrequently made, but is best achieved through invasive procedures, as sputum cultures are usually noncontributory. Management consists of correction of the cause of immunosuppression, conservative surgery, and antifungal therapy.

Candidiasis

Candida species are common human saprophytes, being found normally in the gastrointestinal tract and mucocutaneous regions. Increased colonization predisposing to infection occurs with prolonged administration of antibiotics. Pulmonary candidiasis may develop by oropharyngeal aspiration or, more commonly, by hematogenous dissemination. Chest radiographic findings may vary from unilateral, segmental, or lobar consolidation, to bilateral, diffuse, homogeneous or patchy, ill-defined opacities (38). On CT, the most characteristic finding is a nodular pattern of disease (10,39). Nodules may be single or multiple and nodule size varies from 5 to 20 mm (39). An associated halo of ground-glass attenuation is seen in 60% of cases (10).

Transbronchial, percutaneous, or open-lung biopsy, with histopathological confirmation of lung invasion, is the only reliable method of diagnosis (40).

D. Viral Infections

Herpes group viruses are the most important cause of viral pulmonary infection in the immunocompromised host. With depression of cell-mediated immunity, reactivation from the latent state can occur, causing clinical disease. Predisposing conditions include organ and bone marrow transplantation and use of immunosuppressive drugs.

Cytomegalovirus

Cytomegalovirus (CMV) pneumonia occurs almost exclusively in immunosuppressed patients. Radiographically, findings are variable and range from a reticulonodular pattern to airspace consolidation, the distribution of which may be extensive and bilateral or lobar (41,42). Pleural effusions may be associated. The most common pattern on CT consists of multiple nodules of 1–5 mm associated with areas of ground-glass attenuation (Fig. 6; 10,39). This small-nodular pattern correlates well with pathological findings seen in early CMV pneumonia, which consist of multiple, small hemorrhagic nodules scattered randomly in lung parenchyma and accompanied by varying degrees of diffuse alveolar damage.

Definitive diagnosis of CMV pneumonia necessitates studies of tissue or fluid obtained from the lung by bronchoscopy or open-lung biopsy. Fluorescent antibody staining of cultures (shell vial method) allows presumptive diagnosis within 24 h and has 80–100% sensitivity of that of culture (35).

Herpes Simplex Virus

Both Herpes simplex virus types I (HSV-I) and II (HSV-II) can cause pneumonitis. The HSV-I type is transmitted by close personal contact through saliva or droplet inhalation and is commonly associated with oral disease; HSV-II is congenitally or sexually transmitted and is associated with severe disseminated disease in the neonate and genital herpes in the adult. The radiographic manifestations of herpes simplex pneumonitis are dependent on the mode of spread: endobronchial or hematogenous. Focal or multifocal parenchymal abnormalities are the most com-

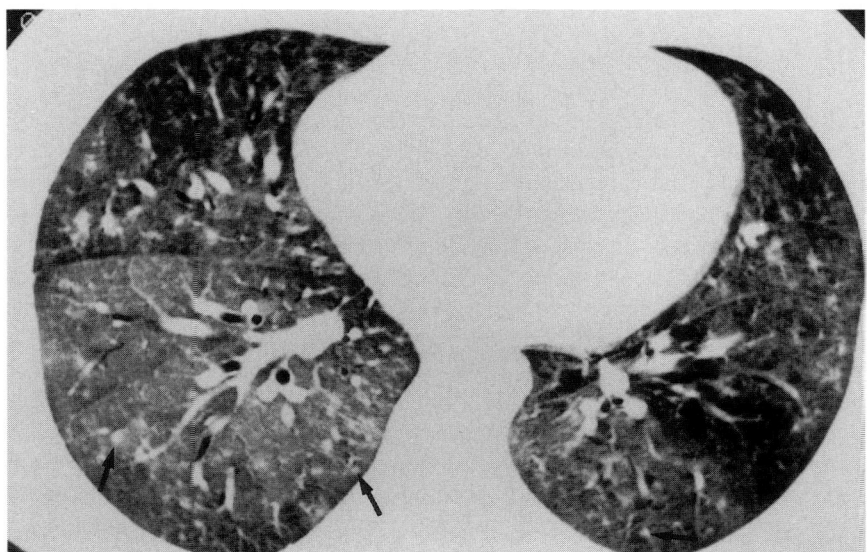

Figure 6 Cytomegalovirus pneumonitis in a 20-year-old bone marrow transplant recipient: The HRCT scan demonstrates diffuse areas of ground-glass attenuation with scattered small pulmonary nodules (arrows).

mon finding in patients in whom contiguous spread of infection occurs from ulcerative lesions in the upper airway into the lung parenchyma (43). Hematogenous dissemination, which occurs specifically in immunocompromised hosts, causes a diffuse interstitial pattern. On CT, multiple pulmonary nodules of 3–20 mm are seen in a diffuse distribution associated with sparse patchy areas of ground-glass attenuation and consolidation (39). Pathologically, this pattern has been correlated with hemorrhagic nodules, with surrounding areas of diffuse alveolar damage (39).

Diagnosis of herpes simplex virus pneumonia is dependent on viral isolation from the lung. The diagnosis may be suggested by the presence of associated facial, oral, or esophageal lesions.

Varicella–Zoster Virus

In immunocompromised patients, chickenpox (varicella) and shingles (herpes zoster) may be associated with a life-threatening respiratory infection. Presumptive diagnosis of varicella–zoster pneumonia can be made in the presence of characteristic skin lesions. Radiographically, patchy, diffuse, airspace consolidation occurs, which may be peribronchial in distribution. *Acinar densities*, defined as 5- to 10-mm, ill-defined opacities, are the most characteristic finding (44,45). Lymphadenopathy and pleural effusions are uncommon.

IV. Drug-Induced Lung Disease

Cytotoxic drug administration will cause pulmonary complications in up to 20% of patients (46). Three distinct clinical syndromes with radiologic correlates have been described. Chronic pneumonitis or fibrosis is the most common and has been associated with virtually all categories of cytotoxic drugs capable of causing lung injury (47). Patients present with a subacute illness, characterized by dyspnea, fever, and nonproductive cough. Radiographic findings generally are consistent with a progressive pulmonary fibrosis and consist of a reticular or reticulonodular pattern predominantly affecting the subpleural and basilar regions (48). On HRCT, irregular linear opacities, with architectural distortion and/or consolidation, are present (49).

Hypersensitivity lung disease has been associated with bleomycin, methotrexate, and procarbazine (47). Presentation is acute, with nonspecific respiratory signs and symptoms developing several hours to days after drug administration. Peripheral eosinophilia may be associated (47). A spectrum of radiographic abnormalities may occur, ranging from a fine reticulonodular pattern, to acinar consolidation. On a HRCT scan, patchy bilateral areas of ground-glass attenuation are the predominant finding (Fig. 7; 49).

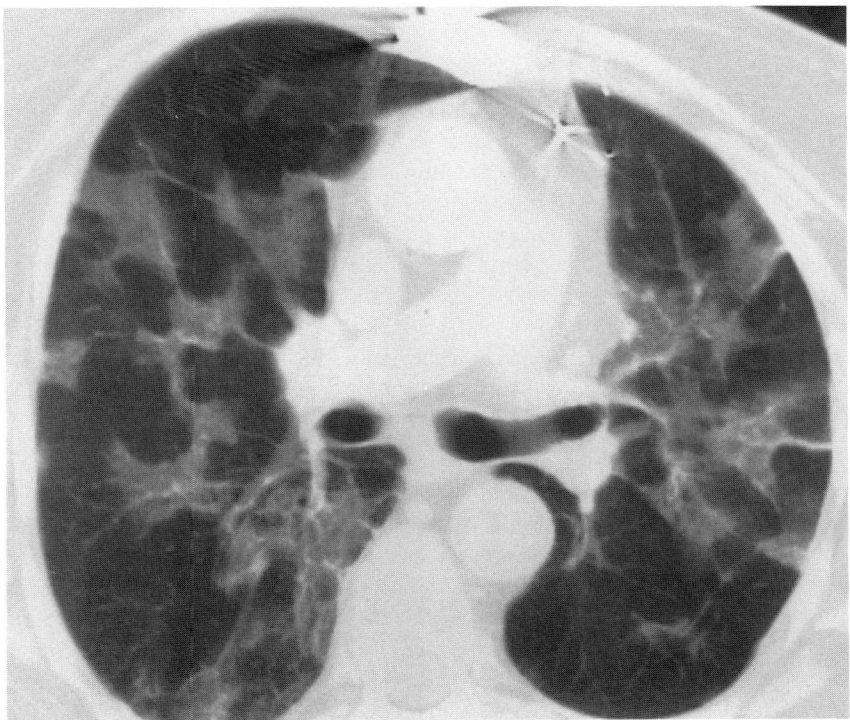

Figure 7 Hypersensitivity reaction in a 79-year-old woman with rheumatoid arthritis receiving methotrexate: This HRCT scan shows a geographic distribution of ground-glass attenuation with a patchwork pattern of normal and diseased secondary pulmonary lobules.

Noncardiogenic pulmonary edema is the least common of the three clinical syndromes and may occur with administration of cytosine arabinoside, methotrexate, and cyclophosphamide (47). Presentation is acute with symptoms and radiographic findings identical with other causes of pulmonary edema (46,47). On HRCT, widespread airspace consolidation is present that may have a dependent distribution (49).

Diagnosis of a drug-induced lung disease is usually made on the basis of empiric correlation: drug administration resulting in a characteristic reaction after an appropriate latent period (50). Putative diagnosis should be accepted only after exclusion of other causes.

V. Pulmonary Edema

Pulmonary edema may be classified etiologically as either *cardiogenic* (elevated microvascular pressure) or *noncardiogenic* (increased vascular permeability). Aside from primary cardiac diseases, other causes for pulmonary edema in the immunocompromised patient include drug-induced cardiac dysfunction and fluid overload. Although the radiographic manifestations of pulmonary edema are well recognized, they are also nonspecific and, in select clinical settings, may be indistinguishable from other pulmonary complications. The CT findings that are characteristic of edema include enlarged pulmonary vessels, dependent areas of parenchymal opacification (51), and interlobular septal thickening (52). Early edema, manifest as bilateral areas of ground-glass attenuation, may be indistinguishable from an opportunistic infection or drug-induced lung disease.

VI. Diffuse Alveolar Hemorrhage

Diffuse alveolar hemorrhage (DAH) affects specific immunosuppressed patient groups. In leukemic patients, alveolar hemorrhage is the most common noninfectious cause of radiographic abnormalities (53). It affects 20% of bone marrow transplant patients, usually presents within the first 2 weeks posttransplantation, and its occurrence is associated with onset of marrow recovery (54). The clinical presentation is acute, with nonspecific symptoms such as dyspnea and fever; platelet cell counts are usually below $50,000/\mu L$, and hemoptysis is rare (54,55). The radiographic findings of DAH may be reticular or alveolar in pattern (56). Diffuse involvement usually occurs with middle and lower lung zonal predominance (56). On CT, the predominant finding is ground-glass attenuation, sometimes seen in association with fine nodules (Fig. 8).

The diagnosis of DAH is based on characteristic bronchoalveolar lavage findings consisting of progressively bloodier aliquots of lavage fluid aspirated from sequential saline instillations. Diagnosis requires exclusion of infectious causes of pulmonary hemorrhage, such as invasive aspergillosis or candidiasis. High-dose corticosteroid therapy is associated with improved survival (57).

VII. Recurrence or Extension of Underlying Neoplasm

Metastatic involvement of the lung occurs in one-third of patients who die of cancer (2). The most common radiographic findings consist of multiple pulmonary nodules of varying size that show a basilar predominance. Lymphangitic carcinomatosis (LC) is characterized by metastatic tumor growth in the pulmonary lymphatics; adenocarcinomas are the usual histological type, with the most common primary sites being lung, breast, and gastrointestinal tract. The radio-

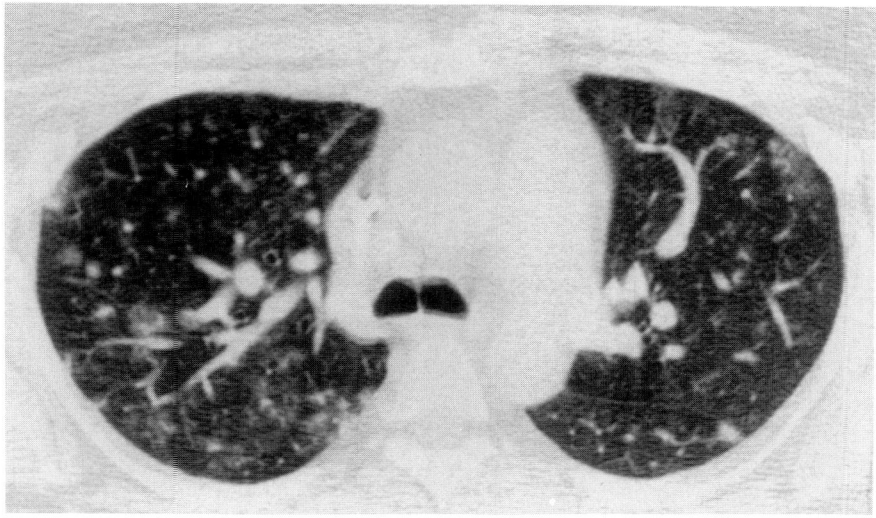

Figure 8 Diffuse alveolar hemorrhage in a 35-year-old bone marrow transplant recipient: The HRCT scan of the upper lobes demonstrates patchy areas of ground-glass attenuation associated with scattered nodules.

graphic findings of LC are nonspecific and consist of a reticulonodular or reticular pattern, with thickened interlobular septa (Kerley lines) (58). Lymphadenopathy and effusion may be associated. On HRCT, a characteristic pattern of nodular thickening of the bronchovascular bundles and interlobular septa occurs (Fig. 9; 59,60). In patients with focal involvement, CT may be helpful as a guide to the most favorable biopsy site.

At time of initial presentation, pulmonary involvement occurs in 4 and 12% of patients with non-Hodgkin's and Hodgkin's lymphoma, respectively (61). Eventually, 20–60% of patients will develop parenchymal involvement (62,63). The radiographic manifestations of parenchymal lymphoma may consist of multiple pulmonary nodules or masses, areas of airspace consolidation, or a reticulonodular pattern (Fig. 10; 64). Relapses involving the parenchyma are infrequently associated with development of intrathoracic lymphadenopathy in patients who have previously received mediastinal and hilar radiation therapy (65).

Leukemic infiltration of lung, causing symptomatic, radiographically apparent disease is unusual. When present, it is usually seen in the setting of uncontrolled leukemia, with a peripheral blast count exceeding 40% of circulating leukocytes (66). Radiographically, diffuse, bilateral reticular or reticulonodular

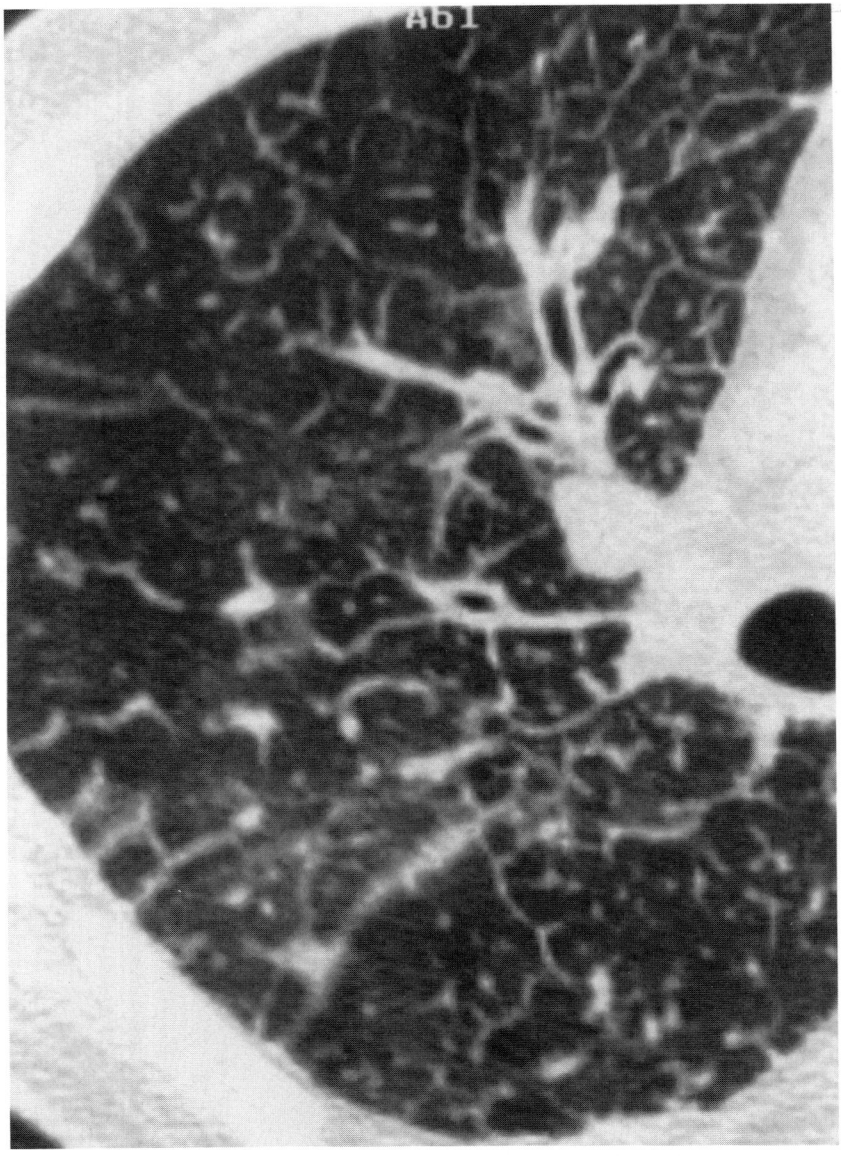

Figure 9 Lymphangitic carcinomatosis in a 62-year-old man with history of colonic adenocarcinoma: This HRCT scan at the level of the bronchus intermedius demonstrates nodular thickening of the bronchovascular bundles and interlobular septa.

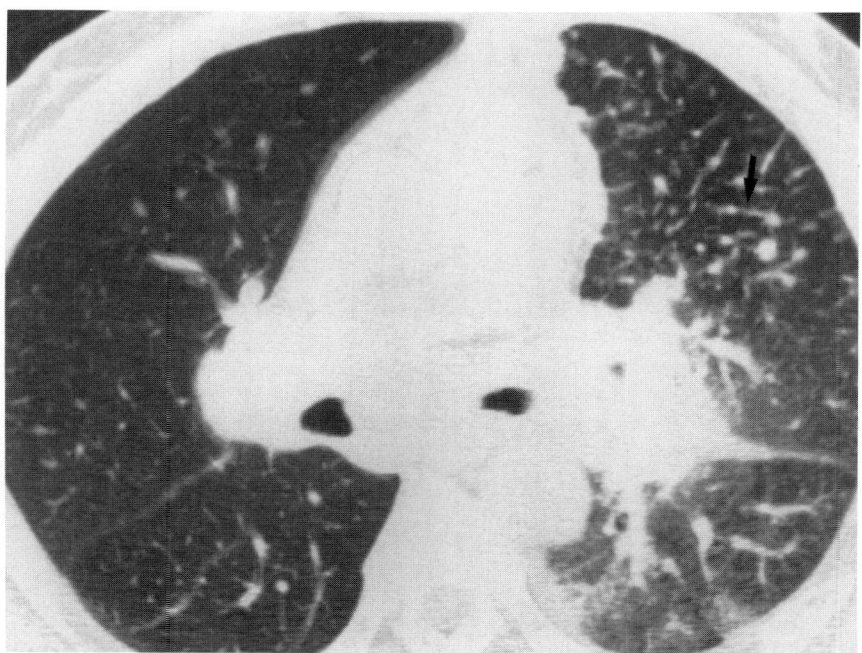

Figure 10 Recurrence of large cell lymphoma in a 63-year-old man, who had previously received only chemotherapy: A HRCT scan at the level of the bronchus intermedius demonstrates left hilar and subcarinal lymphadenopathy; nodular thickening of interlobular septa (arrow) in the left upper lobe indicates the presence of parenchymal involvement.

patterns are seen; localized abnormalities simulating bacterial pneumonia may also occur (66).

VIII. Posttransplantation Lymphoproliferative Disorder

Posttransplantation lymphoproliferative disorder (PTLD) affects approximately 2% of all organ allograft recipients, frequencies varying dependent on the type of organ transplanted and the nature and severity of accompanying immunosuppressive regimen (67). Heart and heart–lung transplant recipients have the highest overall incidence (68). PTLD arises as a direct sequela of immunosuppression and is believed to be induced by Epstein-Barr virus infection in almost all patients (67). There is a spectrum of disease, ranging from mild, polyclonal lymphoid

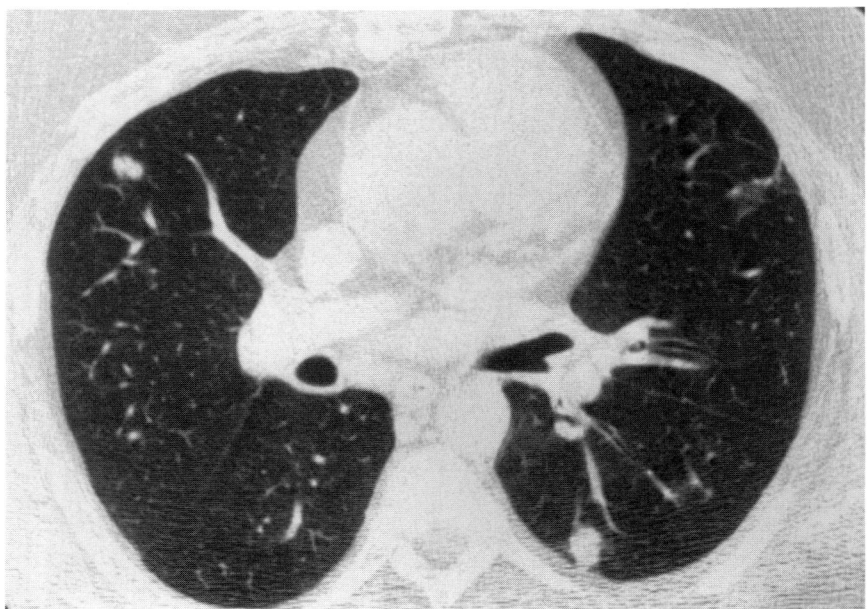

Figure 11 Posttransplantation lymphoproliferative disorder in a 32-year-old heart transplant recipient: This HRCT scan at the level of the bronchus intermedius shows two well-circumscribed pulmonary nodules in the right upper and left lower lobes respectively; no associated lymphadenopathy was present.

hyperplasia, to monoclonal disease and frank lymphoma. The time between transplantation and onset of disease may vary from 1 month to several years.

Nodules are the most common pulmonary manifestation of PTLD; nodules may be single or multiple, are usually well circumscribed, and are of variable size (Fig. 11; 69,70). Less commonly, areas of airspace consolidation are present. Lymphadenopathy occurs in 48% of patients and selectively involves the paratracheal, anterior mediastinal, and aortic–pulmonary nodes (70). Other potential sites of intrathoracic involvement include the thymus and pericardium.

Reduction in immunosuppression may result in complete resolution of disease. Localized disease detected in the early posttransplantation period appears to have the best prognosis (67,71).

References

1. Shelhamer JH, Toews GB, Masur H, et al. Respiratory disease in the immunosuppressed patient. Ann Intern Med 1992; 117:415–431.

2. Rosenow EC III, Wilson WR, Cockerill FR III. Pulmonary disease in the immunocompromised host, part I. Mayo Clin Proc 1985; 60:473–487.
3. Rosenow EC III, Wilson WR, Cockerill FR III. Pulmonary disease in the immunocompromised host, part 2. Mayo Clin Proc 1985; 60:611–631.
4. Ognibene FP, Pass HI, Roth JA, Shelhamer JH, Milne ENC. Role of imaging and interventional techniques in the diagnosis of respiratory disease in the immunocompromised host. J Thorac Imaging 1988; 3:1–20.
5. McLoud TC, Naidich DP. Thoracic disease in the immunocompromised patient. Radiol Clin North Am 1992; 30:525–554.
6. Bellamy EA, Husband JE, Blaquiere RM, Law MR. Bleomycin-related lung damage: CT evidence. Radiology 1985; 156:155–158.
7. Bergin CJ, Wirth RL, Berry GJ, Castellino RA. *Pneumocystis carinii* pneumonia: CT and HRCT observations. J Comput Assist Tomogr 1990; 14:756–759.
8. Kuhlman JE, Kavuru M, Fishman EK, Siegelman SS. *Pneumocystis carinii* pneumonia: spectrum of parenchymal CT findings. Radiology 1990; 175:711–714.
9. Barloon TJ, Galvin JR, Mori M, Stanford W, Gingrich RD. High-resolution ultrafast CT in the clinical management of febrile bone marrow transplant patients with normal or nonspecific chest roentgenograms. Chest 1991; 99:928–933.
10. Janzen DL, Padley SPG, Adler BD, Müller NL. Acute pulmonary complications in immunocompromised non-AIDS patients: comparison of diagnostic accuracy of CT and chest radiology. Clin Radiol 1993; 47:159–165.
11. Huang R, Naidich DP, Lubat E, Shinella R, Garay SM, McCauley DI. Septic pulmonary emboli: CT-radiographic correlation. AJR 1989; 153:41–45.
12. Mori M, Galvin JR, Barloon TJ, Gingrich RD, Stanford W. Fungal pulmonary infections after bone marrow transplantation: evaluation with radiography and CT. Radiology 1991; 178:721–726.
13. Janzen DL, Adler BD, Padley SPG, Müller NL. Diagnostic success of bronchoscopic biopsy in immunocompromised patients with acute pulmonary disease: predictive value of disease distribution as shown in CT. AJR 1993; 160:21–24.
14. Freifeld AG. The antimicrobial armamentarium. Hematol Oncol Clin North Am 1993; 7:813–839.
15. Rubin RH, Ferraro MJ. Understanding and diagnosing infectious complications in the immunocompromised host: current issues and trends. Hematol Oncol Clin North Am 1993; 7:795–812.
16. Dichter JR, Levine SJ, Shelhamer JH. Approach to the immunocompromised host with pulmonary symptoms. Hematol Oncol Clin North Am 1993; 7:887–912.
17. Valdivieso M, Gil-Extremera B, Zornoza J, Rodriguez V, Bodey GP. Gram-negative bacillary pneumonia in the compromised host. Medicine 1977; 56:241–254.
18. Beaman BL, Beaman L. *Nocardia* species: host–parasite relationships. Clin Microbiol Rev 1994; 7:213–264.
19. Yoon HK, Im J-G, Ahn JM, Han MC. Pulmonary nocardiosis: CT findings. J Comput Assist Tomogr 1995; 19:52–55.
20. Simpson GL, Stinson EB, Egger MJ, Remington JS. Nocardial infections in the immunocompromised host: a detailed study in a defined population. Rev Infect Dis 1981; 3:492–507.
21. Ching WTW, Meyer RD, Legionella infections. Infect Dis Clin North Am 1987; 1:595–614.

22. Kroboth FJ, Yu VL, Reddy SC, Yu AC. Clinicoradiographic correlation with the extent of Legionnaire disease. AJR 1983; 141:263–268.
23. Saravolatz LD, Burch KH, Fisher E, et al. The compromised host and Legionnaire's disease. Ann Intern Med 1979; 90:533–537.
24. Jaffe RB, Koschmann EB. Septic pulmonary emboli. Radiology 1970; 96:527–532.
25. Kuhlman JE, Fishman EK, Teigen C. Pulmonary septic emboli: diagnosis with CT. Radiology 1990; 174:211–213.
26. Kaplan MH, Armstrong D, Rosen P. Tuberculosis complicating neoplastic disease: a review of 201 cases. Cancer 1974; 33:850–858.
27. Godeau B, Coutant-Perronne V, Huong DLT, et al. *Pneumocystis carinii* pneumonia in the course of connective tissue disease: report of 34 cases. J Rheumatol 1994; 21:246–251.
28. Feinberg SB, Lester RG, Burke B. The roentgen findings in *Pneumocystis carinii* pneumonia. Radiology 1961; 76:594–599.
29. Doppman JL, Geelhoed GW, Vita VTD. Atypical radiographic features in *Pneumocystis carinii* pneumonia. Radiology 1975; 114:39–44.
30. Feuerstein IM, Archer A, Pluda JM, et al. Thin-walled cavities, cysts, and pneumothorax in *Pneumocystis carinii* pneumonia: further observations with histopathologic correlation. Radiology 1990; 174:697–702.
31. Fraser RS. Pulmonary aspergillosis: pathologic and pathogenetic features. Pathol Annu 1993; 28:231–277.
32. Kuhlman JE, Fishman EK, Siegelman SS. Invasive pulmonary aspergillosis in acute leukemia: characteristic findings on CT, the CT halo sign, and the role of CT in early diagnosis. Radiology 1985; 157:611–614.
33. Hruban RH, Meziane MA, Zerhouni EA, Wheeler PS, Dumler JS, Hutchins GM. Radiologic–pathologic correlation of the CT halo sign in invasive pulmonary aspergillosis. J Comput Assist Tomogr 1987; 11:534–536.
34. Primack SL, Hartman TE, Lee KS, Müller NL. Pulmonary nodules and the CT halo sign. Radiology 1994; 190:513–515.
35. McCabe RE. Diagnosis of pulmonary infections in immunocompromised patients. Med Clin North Am 1988; 72:1067–1089.
36. Logan PM, Primack SL, Miller RR, Müller NL. Invasive aspergillosis of the airways: radiographic, CT, and pathologic findings. Radiology 1994; 193:383–388.
37. Bigby TD, Serota ML, Tierney LM Jr, Matthay MA. Clinical spectrum of pulmonary mucormycosis. Chest 1986; 89:435–439.
38. Buff SJ, McLelland R, Gallis HA, Matthay R, Putman CE. *Candida albicans* pneumonia: radiographic appearance. AJR 1982; 138:645–648.
39. Brown MJ, Miller RR, Müller NL. Acute lung disease in the immunocompromised host: CT and pathologic examination findings. Radiology 1994; 190:247–254.
40. Walsh TJ. Management of immunocompromised patients with evidence of an invasive mycosis. Hematol Oncol Clin North Am 1993; 7:1003–1026.
41. Abdallah PS, Mark JBD, Merigan TC. Diagnosis of cytomegalovirus pneumonia in compromised hosts. Am J Med 1976; 61:326–332.
42. Schulman LL. Cytomegalovirus pneumonitis and lobar consolidation. Chest 1987; 91:558–561.
43. Ramsey PG, Fife KH, Hackman RC, Meyers JD, Corey L. Herpes simplex virus

pneumonia: clinical, virologic, and pathologic features in 20 patients. Ann Intern Med 1982; 97:813–820.
44. Endress ZF, Schnell FR. Varicella pneumonitis. Radiology 1956; 66:723–725.
45. Triebwasser JH, Harris RE, Bryant RE, Rhoades ER. Varicella pneumonia in adults. Medicine 1967; 46:409–423.
46. Snyder LS, Hertz MI. Cytotoxic drug-induced lung injury. Semin Respir Infect 1988; 3:217–228.
47. Cooper JAD Jr, White DA, Matthay RA. Drug-induced pulmonary disease, part I: Cytotoxic drugs. Am Rev Respir Dis 1986; 133:321–340.
48. Aronchick JM, Gefter WB. Drug-induced pulmonary disorders. Semin Roentgenol 1995; 30:18–34.
49. Padley SPG, Adler B, Hansell DM, Müller NL. High-resolution computed tomography of drug-induced lung disease. Clin Radiol 1992; 46:232–236.
50. Irey NS. Tissue reactions to drugs. Am J Pathol 1976; 82:617–647.
51. Hedlund LW, Vock P, Effmann EL, Lischko MM, Putman CE. Hydrostatic pulmonary edema: an analysis of lung density changes by computed tomography. Invest Radiol 1984; 19:254–262.
52. Swensen S, Aughenbaugh GL, Brown LR. High-resolution computed tomography of the lung. Mayo Clin Proc 1989; 64:1284–1294.
53. Tenholder MF, Hooper RG. Pulmonary infiltrates in leukemia. Chest 1980; 78:468–473.
54. Robbins RA, Linder J, Stahl MG, et al. Diffuse alveolar hemorrhage in autologous bone marrow transplant recipients. Am J Med 1989; 87:511–518.
55. Bodey GP, Powell RD Jr, Hersh EM, Yeterian A, Freireich EJ. Pulmonary complications of acute leukemia. Cancer 1966; 19:781–793.
56. Witte RJ, Gurney JW, Linder J, et al. Diffuse pulmonary alveolar hemorrhage after bone marrow transplantation: radiographic findings in 39 patients. AJR 1991; 157:461–464.
57. Metcalf JP, Rennard SI, Reed EC, et al. Corticosteroids as adjunctive therapy for diffuse alveolar hemorrhage associated with bone marrow transplantation. Am J Med 1994; 96:327–334.
58. Janower ML, Blennerhaset JB. Lymphangitic spread of metastatic cancer to the lung. Radiology 1971; 101:267–273.
59. Stein MG, Mayo J, Müller N, Aberle DR, Webb MR, Gamsu G. Pulmonary lymphangitic spread of carcinoma: appearance on CT scans. Radiology 1987; 162:371–375.
60. Munk PL, Müller NL, Miller RR, Ostrow DN. Pulmonary lymphangitic carcinomatosis: CT and pathologic findings. Radiology 1988; 166:705–709.
61. Filly R, Blank N, Castellino RA. Radiographic distribution of intrathoracic disease in previously untreated patients with Hodgkin's disease and non-Hodgkin's lymphoma. Radiology 1976; 120:277–281.
62. Rosenberg SA, Diamond HD, Jaslowitz B, Craver LF. Lymphosarcoma: a review of 1269 cases. Medicine 1961; 40:31–84.
63. McDonald JB. Lung involvement in Hodgkin's disease. Thorax 1977; 32:664–667.
64. Blank N, Castellino RA. The intrathoracic manifestations of the malignant lymphomas and the leukemias. Semin Roentgenol 1980; 15:227–245.

65. Costello P, Mauch P. Radiographic features of recurrent intrathoracic Hodgkin's disease following radiation therapy. AJR 1979; 133:201–206.
66. Kovalski R, Hansen-Flaschen J, Lodato RF, Pietra GG. Localized leukemic pulmonary infiltrates: diagnosis by bronchoscopy and resolution with therapy. Chest 1990; 97:674–678.
67. Craig FE, Gulley ML, Banks PM. Posttransplantation lymphoproliferative disorders. Am J Clin Pathol 1993; 99:265–276.
68. Penn I. Incidence and treatment of neoplasia after transplantation. J Heart Lung Transplant 1993; 12:S328–S336.
69. Harris KM, Schwartz ML, Slasky BS, Nalesnik M, Makowka L. Posttransplantation cyclosporine-induced lymphoproliferative disorders: clinical and radiologic manifestations. Radiology 1987; 162:697–700.
70. Dodd GD III, Ledesma-Medina J, Baron RL, Fuhrman CR. Posttransplant lymphoproliferative disorder: intrathoracic manifestations. Radiology 1992; 184:65–69.
71. Bragg DG, Chor PJ, Murray KA, Kjeldsberg CR. Lymphoproliferative disorders of the lung: histopathology, clinical manifestations, and imaging features. AJR 1994; 163:273–281.

3

Pulmonary Disease in the Immunocompromised Host (AIDS)

S. MELANIE GREAVES and POONAM BATRA

UCLA School of Medicine
Los Angeles, California

I. Introduction

The acquired immunodeficiency syndrome (AIDS) results from infection with the human immunodeficiency virus (HIV). This infection progressively impairs cell-mediated and humoral immunity primarily by the destruction of helper (CD4) T lymphocytes. The resulting immune suppression leads to opportunistic infections, neoplasms, and premature death (1). An estimated 17 million people have been infected with HIV worldwide since the recognition of the disease in 1981, and, approximately 6000 new individuals become infected every day (2). In 1993, AIDS became the leading cause of death among adults aged 25–44 yr in the United States (3). The HIV disease affects homosexual and bisexual men (43%), intravenous drug abusers (32%), heterosexual contacts (10%), transfusion recipients (1%), hemophiliacs (0.6%), and infants through perinatal transmission (1%). Approximately 12% of infected individuals have no identifiable risk factors (4). Throughout the course of HIV disease, the lung is a major target organ for multiple infections and malignancies, and pulmonary complications occur in up to 80% of these patients (Table 1).

Table 1 Common Radiographic Patterns in AIDS: Differential Diagnosis

Pattern	Disease[a]
Interstitial lung disease	PCP
	PCP + other infections
	KS
	LIP, NIP
Focal consolidation	Pyogenic bacteria
	TB
	Fungi
Nodules or masses	KS
	Septic emboli
	TB
	Fungi
	Lymphoma
	Cancer
Cavitary lesions or cysts	Septic emboli
	Bacterial infection
	TB (early in course of HIV infection)
	Fungi
	PCP
Intrathoracic adenopathy	TB/NTMB
	KS
	Lymphoma
	Fungi
	Cancer
Pleural effusions	KS
	Lymphoma
	Pyogenic bacteria
	TB
Normal chest radiograph	PCP
	Disseminated TB/NTMB

[a]PCP, *Pneumocystis carinii* pneumonia; KS, Kaposi's sarcoma; LIP, lymphocytic interstitial pneumonia; NIP, nonspecific interstitial pneumonia; TB, tuberculosis; HIV, Human immunodeficiency virus; NTMB, nontuberculous mycobacteria.

II. Infectious Complications

Patients with AIDS are susceptible to a variety of mycobacterial, bacterial, fungal, and parasitic pulmonary infections. Simultaneous infection with multiple organisms is common and may make precise radiologic diagnosis difficult.

A. Pneumocystis carinii Pneumonia

Pneumocystis carinii pneumonia (PCP) is the most common pulmonary infection in patients with AIDS, and approximately 60–80% of HIV-seropositive individuals will acquire this infection in the course of their disease. The risk of developing PCP increases as the CD4 count falls (patients typically have CD4 cell counts of fewer than $200/mm^3$). Pneumocystis pneumonia may present with either acute or relatively indolent symptoms, consisting of shortness of breath, cough and fever.

Chest radiographs in patients with PCP typically demonstrate diffuse, bilateral, fine reticular and granular opacification (Fig. 1; 5). Dense consolidation may eventually supervene and be indistinguishable from the adult respiratory distress syndrome. Lymphadenopathy and pleural effusions are uncommon and their presence should prompt the search for additional complications such as tuberculosis, lymphoma, or Kaposi's sarcoma (KS). Unfortunately, the appearance of PCP is frequently nonspecific, and a wide variety of atypical appearances have been described, including an upper lobe distribution, focal alveolar consolidation, miliary nodules, and a solitary nodule (5–7). Several of these atypical manifestations, particularly disseminated disease and upper lobe involvement, have been associated with prophylactic pentamidine therapy (8,9). The radiologic diagnosis may be further complicated by multiorganism infection or concurrent neoplastic disease, and it should also be appreciated that up to 10% of patients with documented PCP will have a normal chest radiograph (5).

Computed tomography (CT) has been more sensitive than chest radiography in the diagnosis of PCP. Therefore, it may be useful in those patients strongly suspected of having PCP in the setting of a normal or equivocal chest radiograph. Both CT and high-resolution CT (HRCT) commonly demonstrate bilateral ground-glass airspace disease that does not obscure underlying vessels (Fig. 2). Thickened septal lines within the areas of ground-glass opacification may also be present. Abnormalities are frequently patchy in distribution, and this multifocality is more easily appreciated on HRCT than on chest radiography. Pleural effusions and significant lymphadenopathy are uncommon (10).

Cystic lung lesions are now a well-recognized complication of AIDS. The radiologic terminology in the literature is confusing, as these lesions are variably described as thin-walled cystic lesions, pneumatoceles, and premature bullous damage (11). Most cystic lesions have been described in association with PCP, and the presence of organisms and inflammatory exudate within cyst walls appears to implicate *P. carinii* directly in their pathogenesis (12). In one study, pulmonary cysts were detected in 34% of patients with proved PCP. Most cysts were multiple and were most commonly found in the upper lungs (13). Cystic lesions have also been described in intravenous drug abusers and in HIV-infected patients without documented PCP infection; smoking and other unidentified insults may be ac-

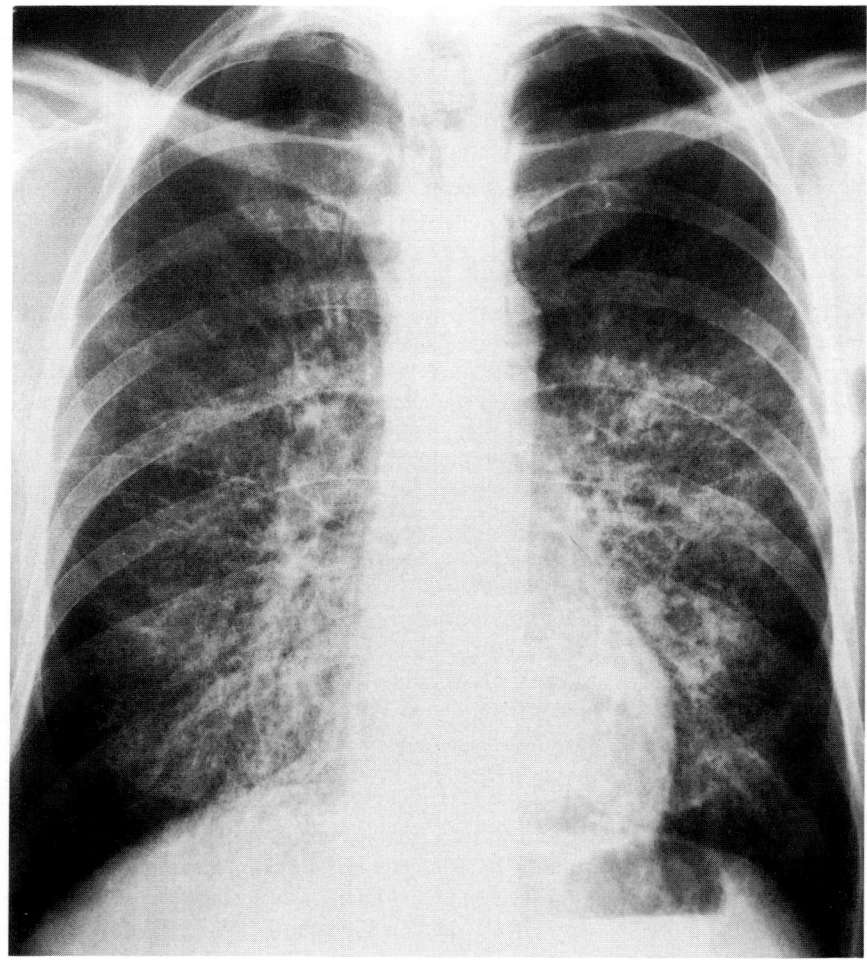

Figure 1 A 44-year-old man infected with PCP: The chest radiograph shows bilateral perihilar fine reticular and granular opacification typical of this infection. Note the absence of lymphadenopathy and pleural effusions.

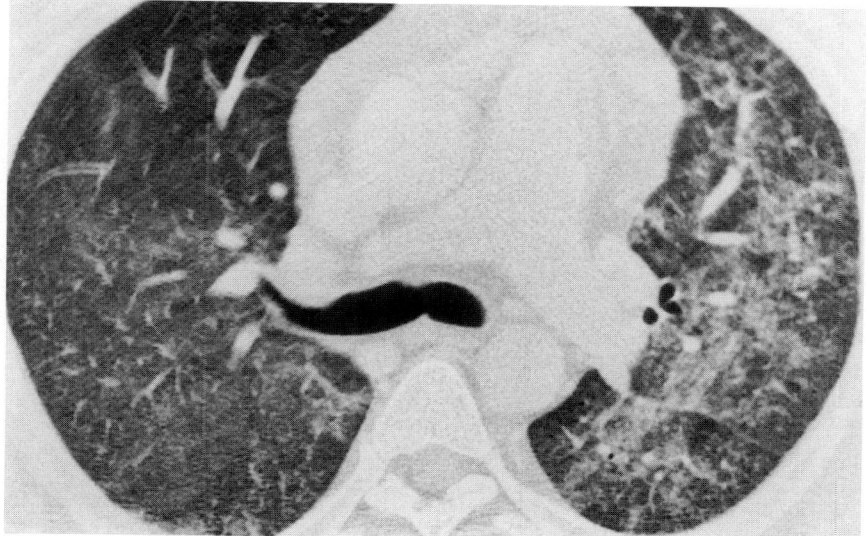

Figure 2 A 30-year-old man with PCP: This HRCT scan reveals bilateral ground-glass opacification and consolidation that is most severe in the left lung.

countable for these cases (14). Patients with cysts have a higher incidence of complicating pneumothorax than those without (Fig. 3). A pneumothorax complicating PCP is characteristically difficult to treat and worsens the patient's prognosis (12,13). The natural history of cystic lesions appears variable, some may persist for many months, although, most eventually resolve (13).

B. Bacterial Pneumonia

Although HIV infection primarily affects cell-mediated immunity, the humoral immune system is also involved, and it is now well established that patients with AIDS are more susceptible to acute and recurrent bacterial pneumonias than is the general population. Pulmonary bacterial infections are estimated to account for up to 10% of cases of AIDS-related pneumonias (15). Early in the course of HIV the most common organisms causing infection are *Streptococcus pneumoniae* and *Haemophilus influenzae*. As immunosuppression increases, severe infections with *Staphylococcus aureus* and gram-negative bacteria may occur (Fig. 4; 16).

The presentation of community-acquired bacterial pneumonias in HIV patients is very similar to that in the general population, although diagnosis may be difficult owing to the presence of additional infections or neoplasms. The onset of disease is characteristically acute, and most patients present with fever and

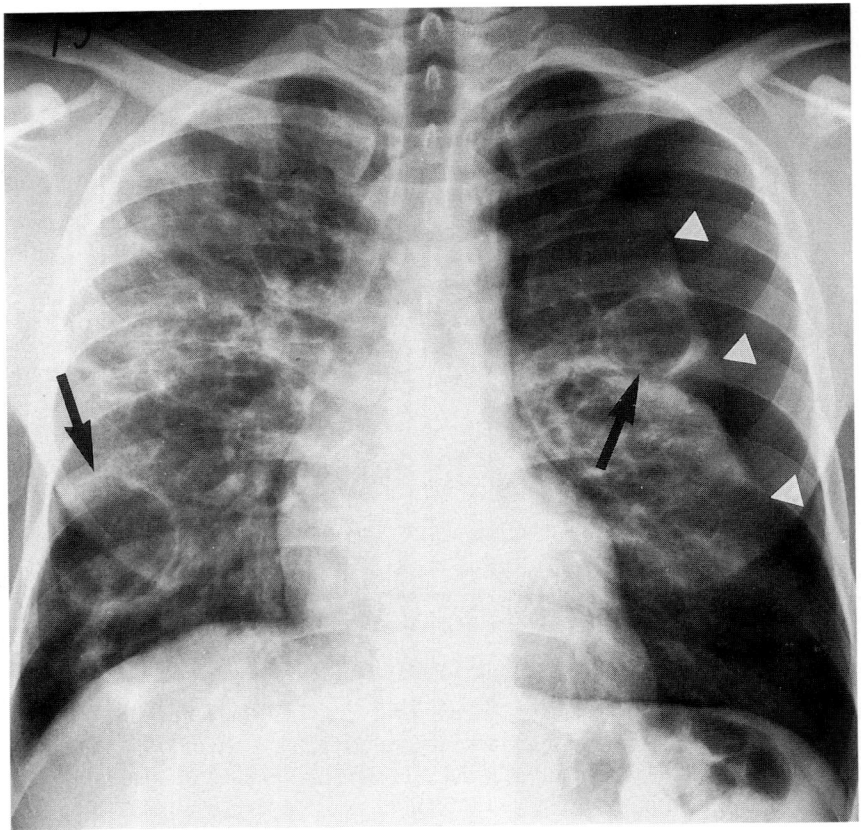

Figure 3 A 27-year-old man with PCP: This PA chest radiograph demonstrates bilateral reticular opacities, numerous pneumatoceles (arrows), and a large left pneumothorax (arrowheads).

productive cough (15). Bacteremia, particularly secondary to *S. pneumoniae*, is common. Chest radiographs are invariably abnormal, demonstrating segmental, lobar, or multifocal consolidation. Pulmonary cavitation, intrathoracic lymphadenopathy, and pleural effusions are uncommon. As response to appropriate treatment is generally rapid, slow resolution should prompt consideration of other pathogens, such as PCP.

Those AIDS patients who have a history of intravenous drug abuse may present with septic emboli, recurrent staphylococcal infections, lung abscesses, and empyemas. Radiologic appearances are similar to those in immunocompetent individuals.

While uncommon, pneumonias caused by *Nocardia* species have also been described in the HIV-infected population. Chest radiographs in these patients generally reveal lobar or multilobar consolidation, although, a solitary mass, multiple nodules, or pleural effusions have also been reported (16).

C. Pulmonary Tuberculosis

The incidence of pulmonary tuberculosis (TB) had been declining in the United States until 1984, when the disease showed a resurgence that has been partly attributed to the HIV epidemic (17). The HIV-infected individuals have an increased incidence of TB, estimated at 8% per year. Tuberculosis may be the first indication of HIV seropositivity, as it occurs earlier in the course of the disease than other opportunistic infections and malignancies. In most patients the infection is fully responsive to treatment, and the prognosis is good. Nonetheless, the high prevalence of TB-infected AIDS patients and the emergence of multiple drug-resistant strains has serious public health implications because, unlike other opportunistic infections, TB can be transmitted to an otherwise healthy individual (18). Its early diagnosis, therefore, is of paramount importance.

The radiographic manifestations of TB are dependent on the degree of immunosuppression. Early in the course of HIV infection, when the CD4 cell count is higher than $200/mm^3$, the patient is able to mount an effective cell-mediated response to the disease. The chest radiographic findings of upper lobe cavitary consolidation are indistinguishable from those of pulmonary TB in immunocompetent individuals. As the CD4 count decreases, chest radiographic abnormalities are increasingly reminiscent of primary TB. Characteristic findings include, intrathoracic lymphadenopathy, middle or lower lobe parenchymal consolidation, pulmonary nodules, and pleural effusions (Fig. 5; 19,20). Patients with low CD4 counts are also more likely to have normal or equivocal chest radiographs (19) and negative skin tests. In advanced HIV disease, TB is usually widely disseminated, with involvement of multiple organs (21). The finding of low attenuation lymph nodes with peripheral rim enhancement on contrast enhanced thoracic CT has been associated with mycobacterial infection. Although low-attenuation nodes may be found in other infections, particularly those caused by fungi and atypical mycobacteria, their presence may warrant empirical antituberculous therapy pending culture results (22).

D. Nontuberculous Mycobacterial Infections

Infection with nontuberculous mycobacteria (NTMB), particularly *Mycobacterium avium-intracellulare* (MAI) and *M. kansasii*, is common in patients with AIDS. These organisms are ubiquitous in the environment, and entry is believed to

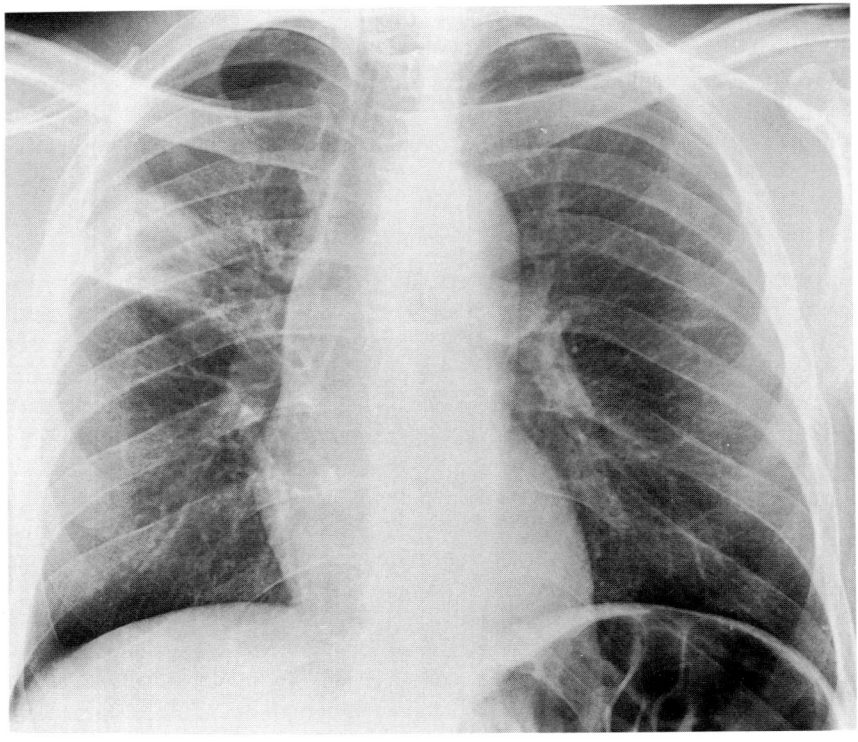

(a)

Figure 4 A 32-year-old man with pseudomonal pneumonia: (a) Digital chest radiograph and (b) CT scan reveal cavitary right upper lobe consolidation consistent with a necrotizing pneumonia.

be through the gastrointestinal tract. They are low in virulence and, therefore, are usually found in advanced cases of AIDS when the CD4 cell count is fewer than 50/mm^3 (23).

In patients with AIDS, MAI infection is almost always a disseminated disease with organisms present in blood, sputum, and bone marrow cultures. It presents with nonspecific symptoms, such as persistent fever, weight loss, chronic diarrhea, and abdominal pain. Respiratory symptoms usually are not prominent, and the chest radiographs are typically normal, even when sputum is positive. Pulmonary involvement, if present, may result in mediastinal or hilar lymphadenopathy and possibly pleural effusions. It is unclear whether MAI produces

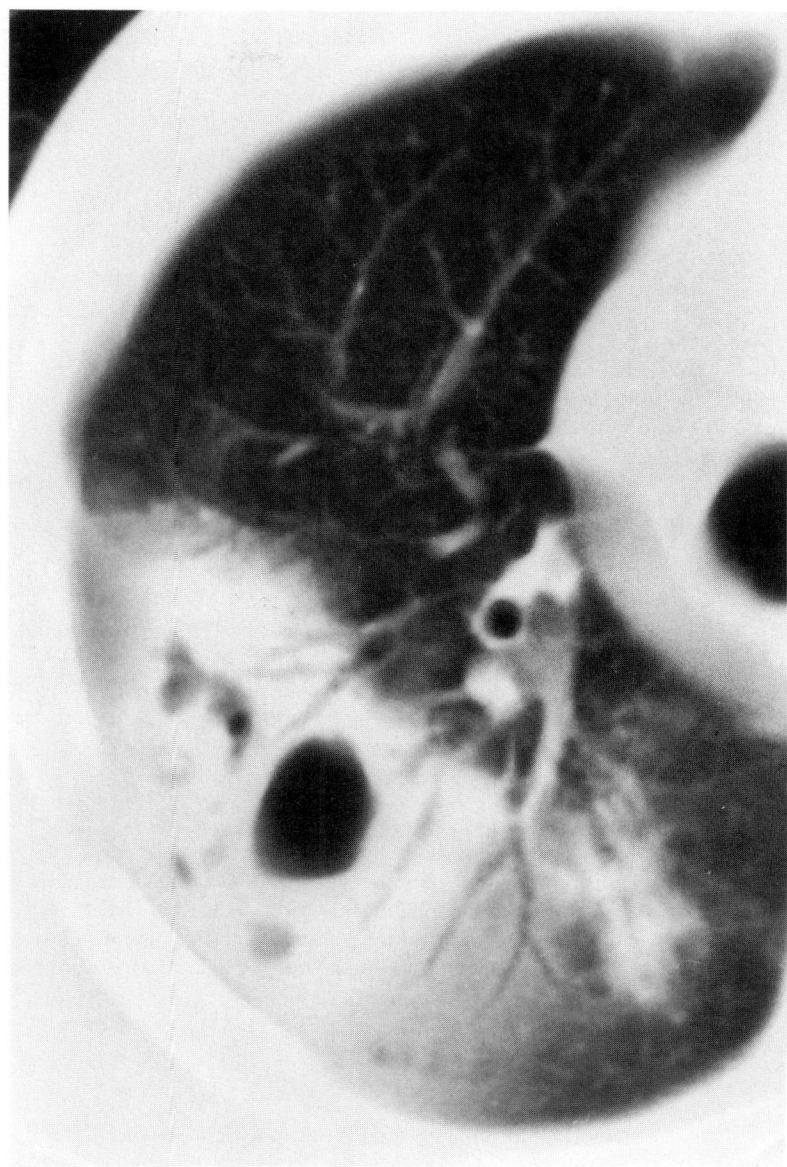

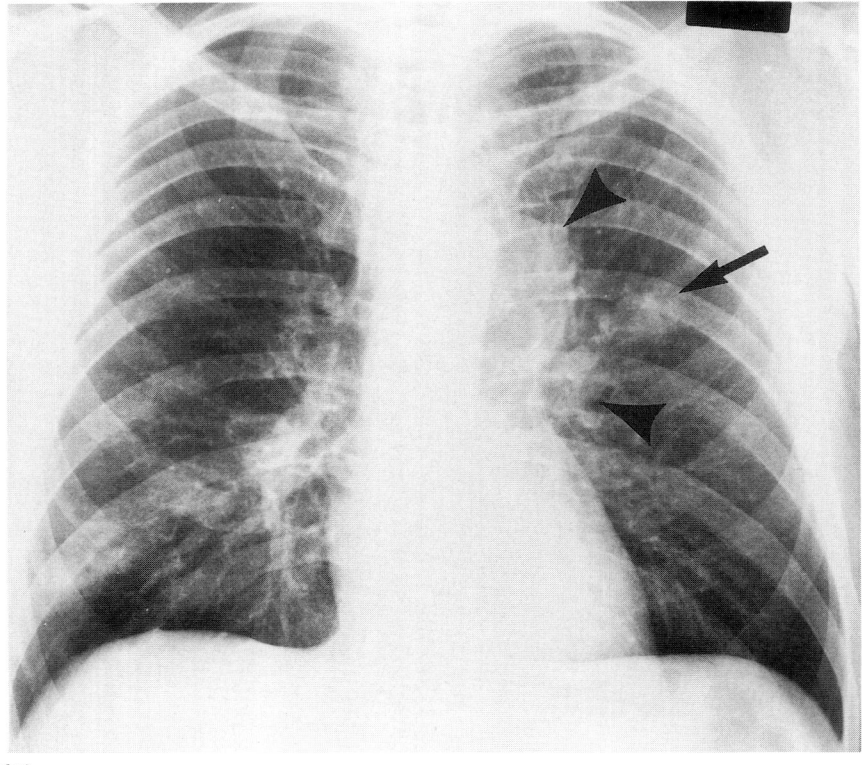

(a)

Figure 5 A 48-year-old man with tuberculosis: (a) The PA chest radiograph shows left hilar and mediastinal lymphadenopathy (arrowheads), with an ill-defined nodular opacity in the left perihilar region (arrow). (b) Contrast-enhanced thoracic CT scan demonstrates mediastinal lymphadenopathy in the aortopulmonary window (arrow). The affected nodes have central low attenuation and peripheral rim enhancement. (c) Lung windows reveal miliary nodules that are not appreciated on the chest radiograph (arrows). (Courtesy of Dr. Eric Hart, Los Angeles.)

radiologically characterizable parenchymal abnormalities, as patients with pulmonary MAI frequently have coexisting pulmonary disease (24,25).

In contrast with MAI, *M. kansasii* is an important cause of treatable pulmonary disease in AIDS patients. Most patients have disease confined to the lungs, although disseminated infection does occur. Chest radiographs may demonstrate either diffuse, reticulonodular interstitial disease, or upper lobe nodular opacifica-

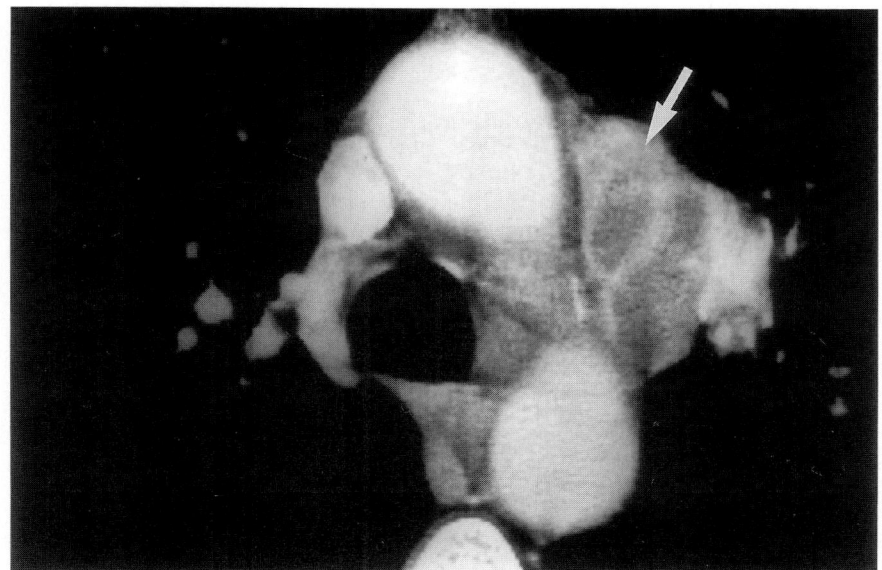

(b)

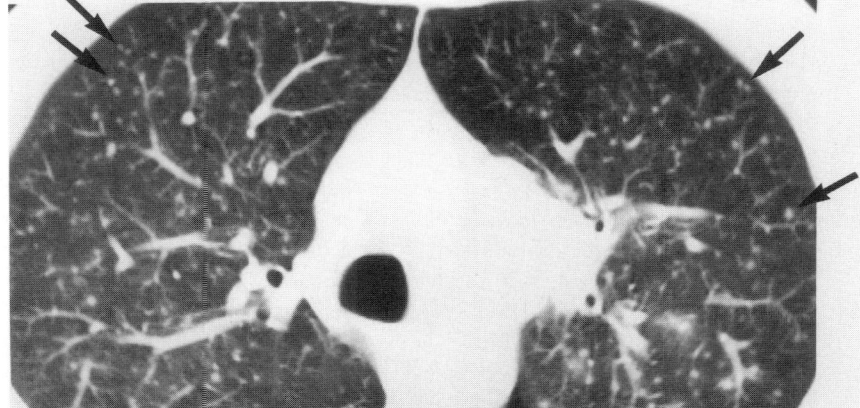

(c)

tion. Cavitary lesions appear common and the disease may mimic reactivated TB (Fig. 6; 26).

E. Fungal Pneumonias

Fungal pneumonias are less common than PCP and bacterial infections, but represent a significant cause of morbidity and mortality in the AIDS population. Cryptococcosis is the most common fungal infection to involve the lung; histoplasmosis, coccidioidomycosis, aspergillosis, and blastomycosis are less frequently seen.

Cryptococcosis most commonly presents as a meningitis, the pulmonary infection being relatively silent. Cryptococcal pneumonia in AIDS patients has an incidence of up to 15%. Abnormalities on chest radiographs in these patients include single or multiple nodules that may cavitate, parenchymal consolidation, and interstitial disease. Lymphadenopathy and effusions may be present, but do not appear to be prominent features (27,28). A CT scan may help in further evaluation of these patients (29), although its contribution to a specific diagnosis is doubtful.

Histoplasmosis has a worldwide distribution, but is endemic to North America. In contrast with infected immunocompetent patients, AIDS patients develop disseminated disease. The most common chest radiographic abnormality in these patients is diffuse, miliary nodularity (Fig. 7), although, less commonly, a linear interstitial pattern is present. Focal airspace disease has been described, but is less common than in immunocompetent patients with acute pulmonary histoplasmosis. Lymphadenopathy and pleural effusions are uncommon (30).

Coccidioidomycosis is endemic to the southwestern United States. The HIV-infected patients are at high risk in these areas for severe progressive infection with the fungus. It usually presents as a wasting illness, with respiratory symptoms reported in up to 75% of cases. Chest radiographs in most AIDS patients demonstrate a reticulonodular pattern of disease (31).

Pulmonary aspergillosis is a relatively rare cause of symptomatic pulmonary disease in patients with AIDS, as defense against this infection does not depend primarily on T cells. Those with aspergillosis are often taking corticosteroids or have therapy-induced neutropenia. Radiologically the disease may manifest as chronic cavitary upper lobe disease, resembling noninvasive aspergillosis in patients without AIDS. This form of infection has a significant risk of fatal hemoptysis. Invasive aspergillosis is seen either as focal alveolar opacities (Fig. 8) or bilateral interstitial, or alveolar disease. An obstructive form of aspergillosis has also been described, in which fungal casts or bronchial pseudomembranes obstruct the airways (32).

Blastomycosis is an uncommon opportunistic infection in patients with AIDS. The disease may be limited to the lungs and pleura, or may be disseminated; those patients with disseminated disease have a high mortality, despite

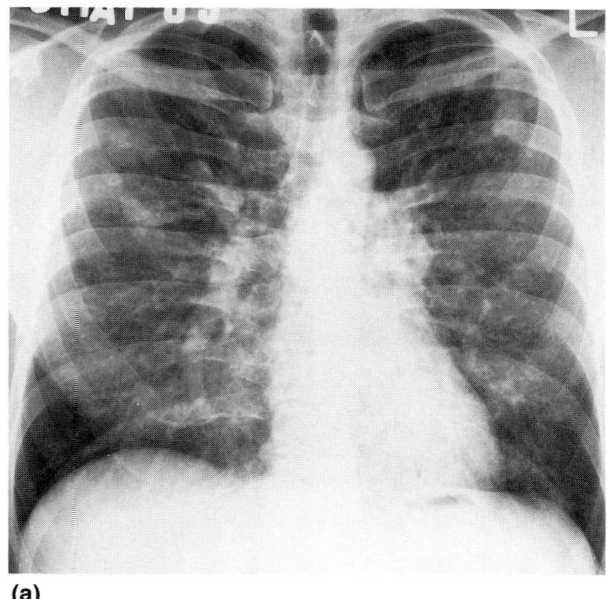

(a)

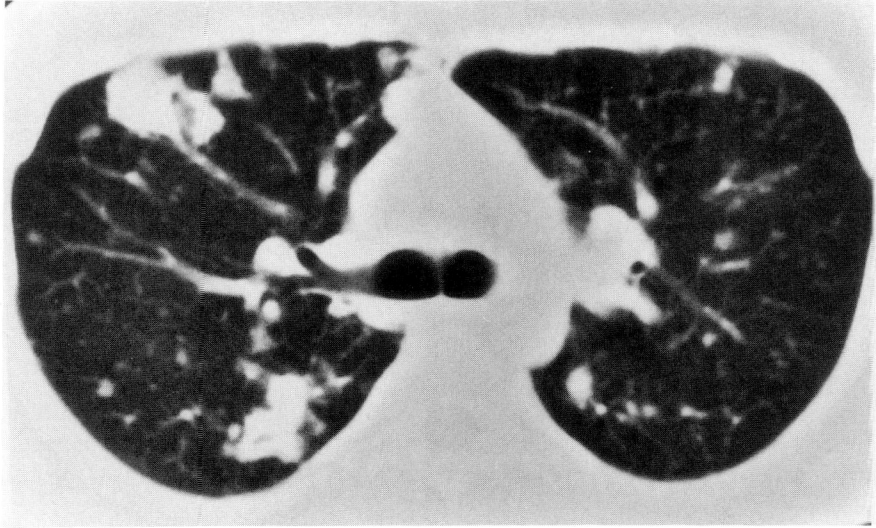

(b)

Figure 6 A 34-year-old man with *M. kansasii*: (a) The PA chest radiograph and (b) CT scan demonstrate bilateral pulmonary nodules and left hilar lymphadenopathy.

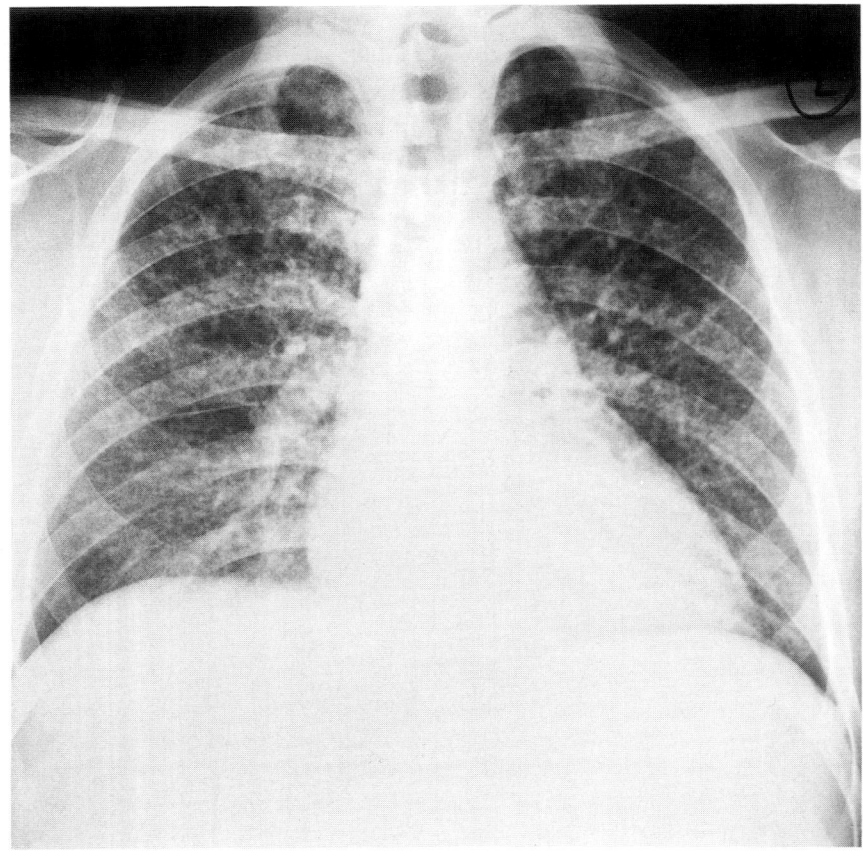

Figure 7 A 31-year-old man with disseminated histoplasmosis: The chest radiograph demonstrates bilateral miliary pulmonary nodules. (Courtesy of Dr. Kathleen Brown, Los Angeles.)

antifungal therapy. Radiologic features are varied, but include miliary or diffuse interstitial disease, focal lobar consolidation, which may be cavitary, and pulmonary nodules (33).

F. Viral Pneumonias

The clinical significance of viruses in HIV-related pulmonary disease is frequently unclear, although they may cause fatal pneumonias. Herpes viruses are the most commonly recognized, particularly cytomegalovirus (CMV).

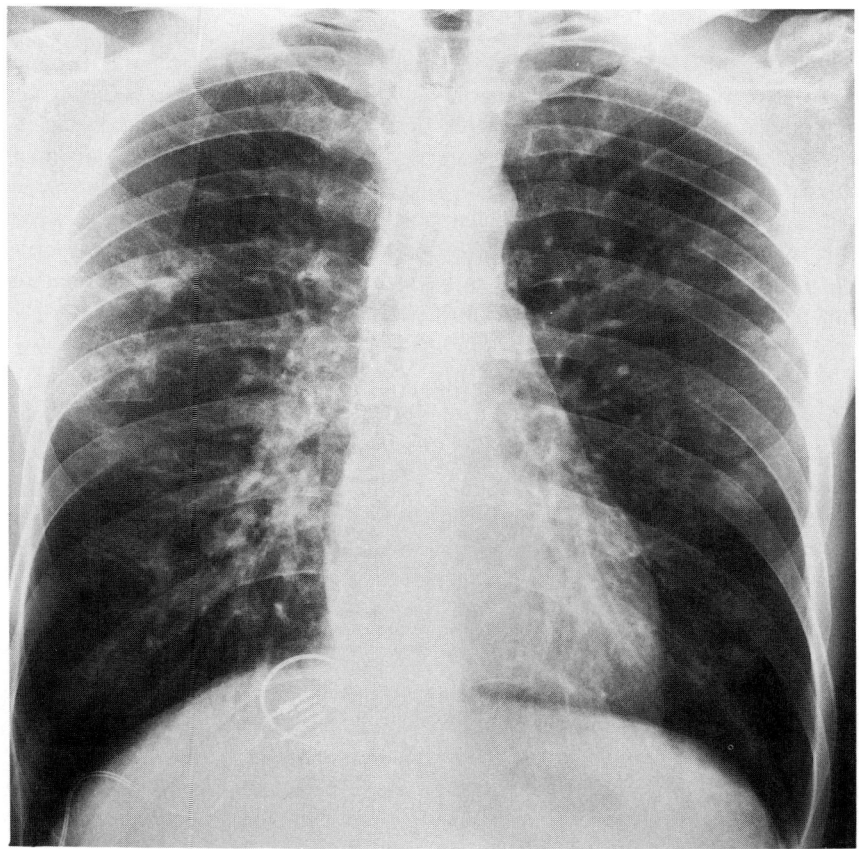

Figure 8 A 32-year-old man with invasive aspergillosis: The chest radiograph shows scattered bilateral pulmonary nodules predominantly within the upper lungs.

Although CMV can frequently be isolated from the lungs of AIDS patients, the significance of this finding, relative to clinically important pulmonary disease, is still controversial. Documented CMV pneumonitis frequently coexists with other diseases, particularly PCP and pulmonary KS, and its pathogenic role may be difficult to determine (34). The spectrum of CMV-related pulmonary parenchymal abnormalities on CT is broad and nonspecific. Findings include ground-glass opacification, consolidation, interstitial disease, nodules or masses, and bronchiectasis (35).

G. Parasitic Infections

Toxoplasma gondi is usually associated with central nervous system involvement in AIDS patients; however, pulmonary disease has also been reported. Chest radiographs are nonspecific, but may demonstrate coarse bilateral nodular opacities. Less commonly, a reticulonodular pattern may be observed that is indistinguishable from PCP (36).

A hyperinfection syndrome has been described in HIV-positive patients infected with *Strongyloides stercoralis*. The migration of large numbers of larvae through the lungs produces dyspnea, wheezing, and cough, and reticulonodular opacities may be seen on chest radiographs (37).

III. Neoplastic Complications

A defective immune system predisposes AIDS patients to neoplastic disease. Kaposi's sarcoma is the most frequent neoplasm found in AIDS patients, with lymphoma a close second. Radiologic diagnosis is often difficult as concurrent infection may distort or mask the typical imaging features of these malignancies.

A. Kaposi's Sarcoma

Kaposi's sarcoma is a multicentric neoplasm that arises from endothelial cells and currently affects approximately 20% of AIDS patients (38). It has a marked tendency to appear in homosexual and bisexual men with AIDS, and up to 51% of these individuals have KS, although its incidence is declining (39). Recent studies have implicated one of the herpes viruses as a cofactor for disease development. Cutaneous or visceral involvement nearly always precedes respiratory involvement, although pulmonary KS can develop in up to 13% of patients with no cutaneous lesions (40).

Pulmonary KS is a late feature of AIDS and is usually diagnosed when the CD4 cell count is fewer than $100/mm^3$ (40). Patients generally present with dyspnea, nonproductive cough, and fever. Pulmonary KS affects the parenchyma, tracheobronchial tree, pleura, and lymph nodes, either individually or in combination. The tumor typically extends peripherally along the bronchovascular interstitium and, in its earliest stage, produces peribronchial thickening in a perihilar distribution. With disease progression small nodules are produced by extension of the tumor into adjacent parenchyma, and coalescent consolidation may supervene (Fig. 9; 41,42). Pleural effusions and septal lines are also features of this disease. Most effusions are small; however, large effusions have been described, and occasionally, massive chylothorax does occur.

Radiologically, gross mediastinal and hilar lymphadenopathy is uncommon, although nodal involvement has been found in up to 50% of patients at autopsy (Fig. 10). A staging system, based on chest radiographs, has recently been devised by Gruden et al. (40). Stage 0 represents normal parenchyma, stage 1— isolated bronchial wall thickening; stage 2—small nodules, with or without findings of stage 1 disease; and stage 3—large nodules or frank consolidation. Kerley B lines and pleural effusions are not included in the staging. The disease appears to advance along these stages, in that peribronchial thickening progresses to perihilar consolidation, and nodules enlarge and become ill-defined. The timing of progression varies extensively from patient to patient. The staging system correlates with bronchoscopic grading, in that a visible estimate of tracheobronchial lesions on bronchoscopy will usually indicate the extent of underlying parenchymal disease. However, significant parenchymal disease may occur in the absence of visible tracheobronchial disease.

Chest radiography, therefore, is important in the initial investigation and follow-up of these patients. It should be realized that all these findings are relatively nonspecific and are sometimes difficult to differentiate from abnormalities caused by infection and lymphoma. Findings on CT are very similar to those on chest radiographs, although CT enables more accurate assessment of disease extent (43,44).

Combined thallium and gallium scintigraphy may be useful in the diagnosis of pulmonary KS in patients with AIDS and in its differentiation from infection and lymphoma. The KS lesions appear to take up thallium, but not gallium. Infections tend to be gallium-avid, but thallium-negative, and lymphomas are both thallium- and gallium-avid (45).

B. Lymphoma

The incidence of AIDS-related lymphoma (ARL) is increasing and it is currently detected in 2–5% of AIDS patients. The characteristics of ARL are very similar to transplant-related lymphomas, in that most are aggressive B-cell non-Hodgkin's lymphomas (46). The most common histological types are large-cell immunoblastic and small-cell noncleaved; the immunoblastic form tends to occur late in the disease when the CD4 cell count is fewer than $100/mm^3$.

At the time of diagnosis, the disease is usually widely disseminated and approximately 30% of patients will present with extranodal disease alone (46). This lymphoma usually affects the central nervous system, gastrointestinal tract, liver, spleen, and bone marrow. The incidence of thoracic involvement varies in the literature, ranging from 6 to 31% of patients (46,47). Radiologically, pleural effusions and pulmonary involvement may be seen in combination or alone. Effusions may be bilateral or unilateral and are frequently recurrent. There is no predominant pattern of parenchymal involvement, with disease manifesting as multiple nodules, interstitial disease, or consolidation (Fig. 11). Lymphadenopathy may be present, but is rarely as prominent as that seen in immunocompetent

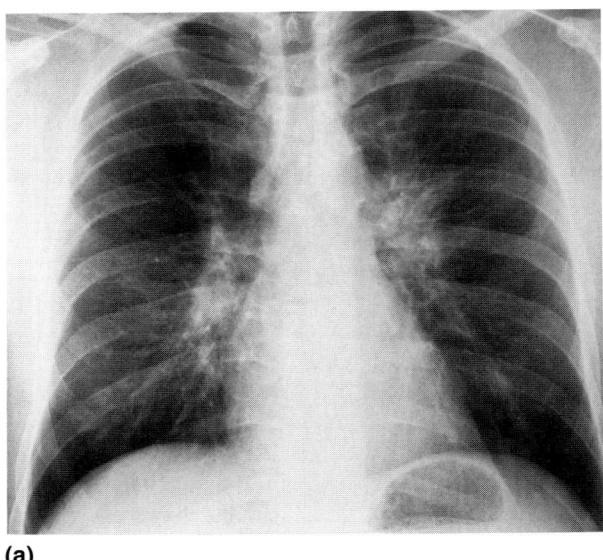
(a)

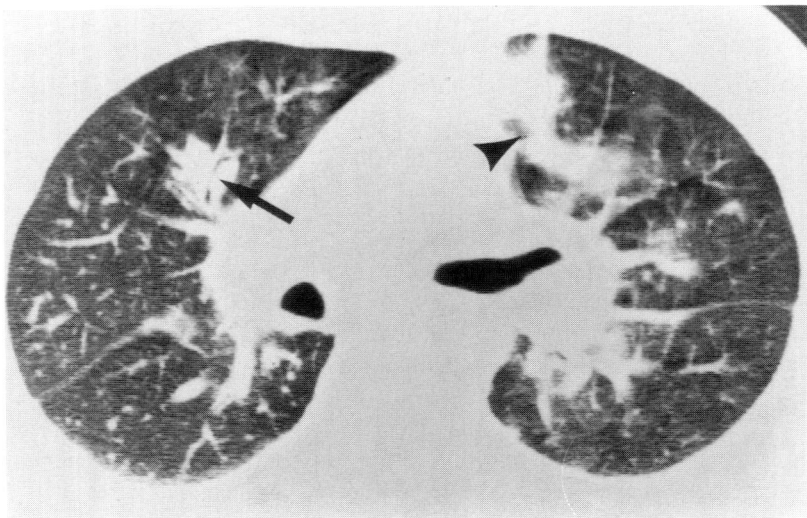
(b)

Figure 9 A 31-year-old man with pulmonary Kaposi's sarcoma: (a) PA chest radiograph demonstrates coarse bilateral linear opacities radiating from the hila. Also note the bilateral hilar and aortopulmonary window lymphadenopathy. (b) A CT scan confirms the peribronchial distribution of this disease (arrow). More confluent perihilar consolidation is seen in the left upper lobe (arrowhead).

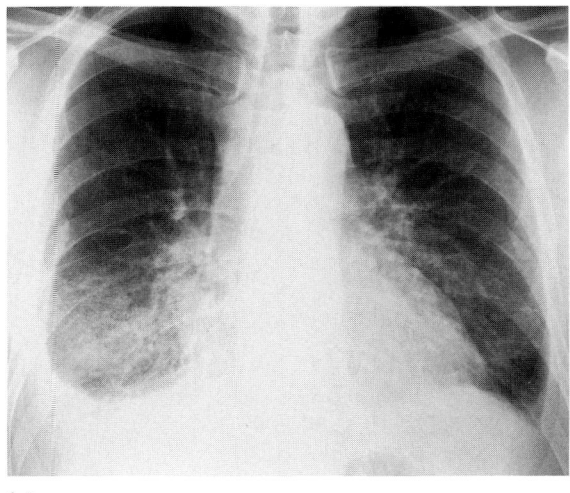

Figure 10 A 51-year-old man with pulmonary Kaposi's sarcoma: (a) PA chest radiograph shows subtle hilar and mediastinal lymphadenopathy, predominantly right basal interstitial disease, and bilateral small pleural effusions. (b) The soft-tissue CT image confirms the presence of the right hilar and mediastinal lymphadenopathy (arrows) and the pleural effusions.

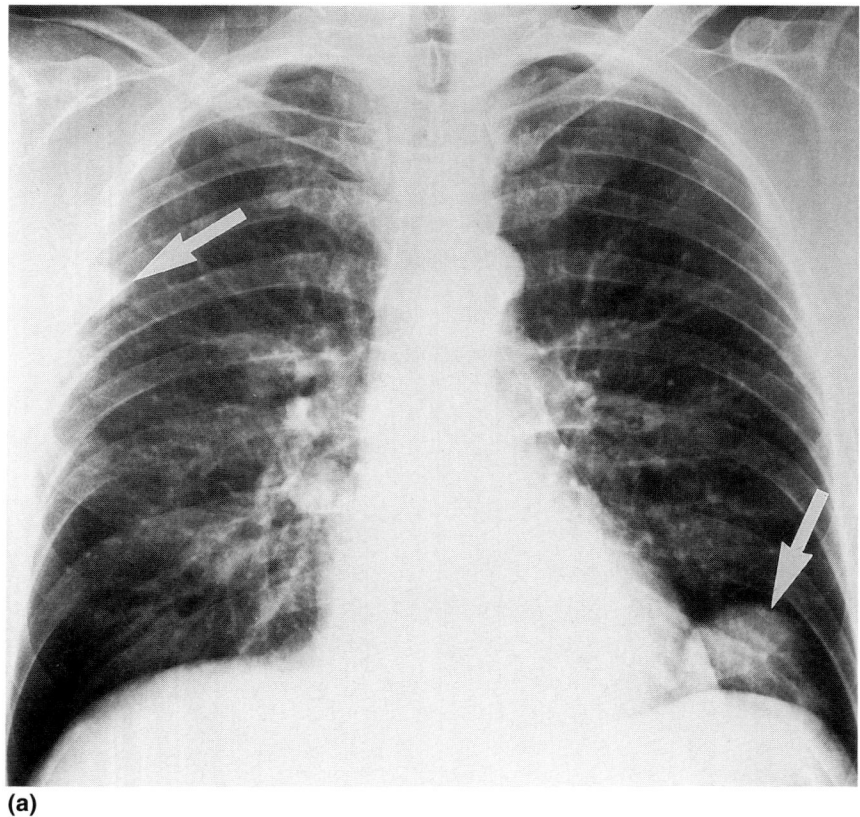

(a)

Figure 11 A 49-year-old man with AIDS-related non-Hodgkin's lymphoma: (a) The PA chest radiograph and (b) CT scan show multiple bilateral well-defined pulmonary nodules (arrows).

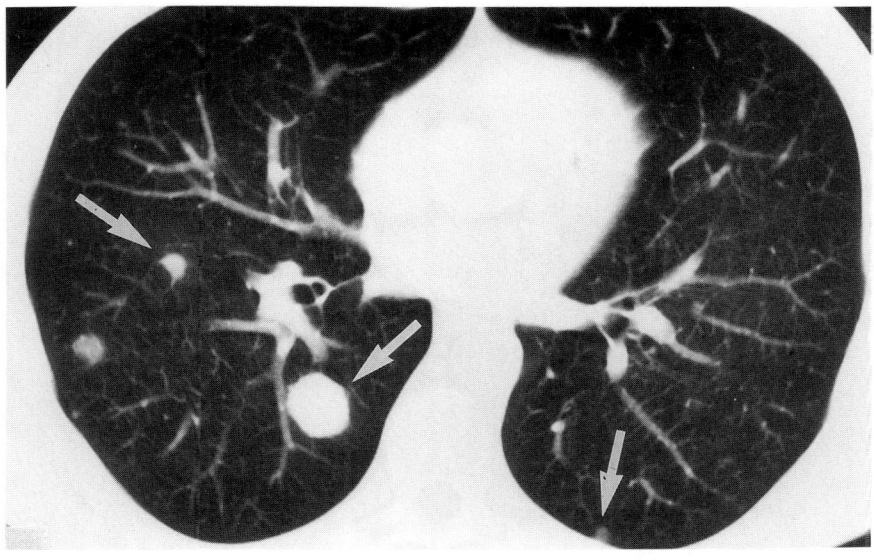

(b)

patients with lymphoma. Differentiation from infection and KS is, therefore, difficult, and tissue diagnosis is often necessary (47,48).

C. Bronchogenic Carcinoma

The possibility that primary lung carcinoma may occur with increased frequency in HIV-infected individuals is still under debate. Reported cases do, however, suggest that they appear to develop bronchogenic carcinoma at a younger age, and that their prognosis is more dismal than that of uninfected patients with lung carcinoma. Most patients have a smoking history, and a variety of cell types have been described, although adenocarcinoma appears to occur with greater frequency than in the general population (49).

Radiographic findings are generally indistinguishable from those of lung carcinoma in non-AIDS patients, and chest radiographs typically demonstrate a central or peripheral mass, often seen in an upper lobe (Fig. 12). Extensive pleural disease in the absence of a definable primary lung lesion may also occur. Prompt diagnosis in HIV-seropositive patients is problematic, as a primary lung cancer may simulate, or be misinterpreted as AIDS-related infectious or neoplastic disease (50). A CT scan may be more sensitive than chest radiography in the diagnosis of bronchogenic carcinoma, particularly if extensive pleural disease is present (49). It may also provide additional information enabling accurate tumor staging.

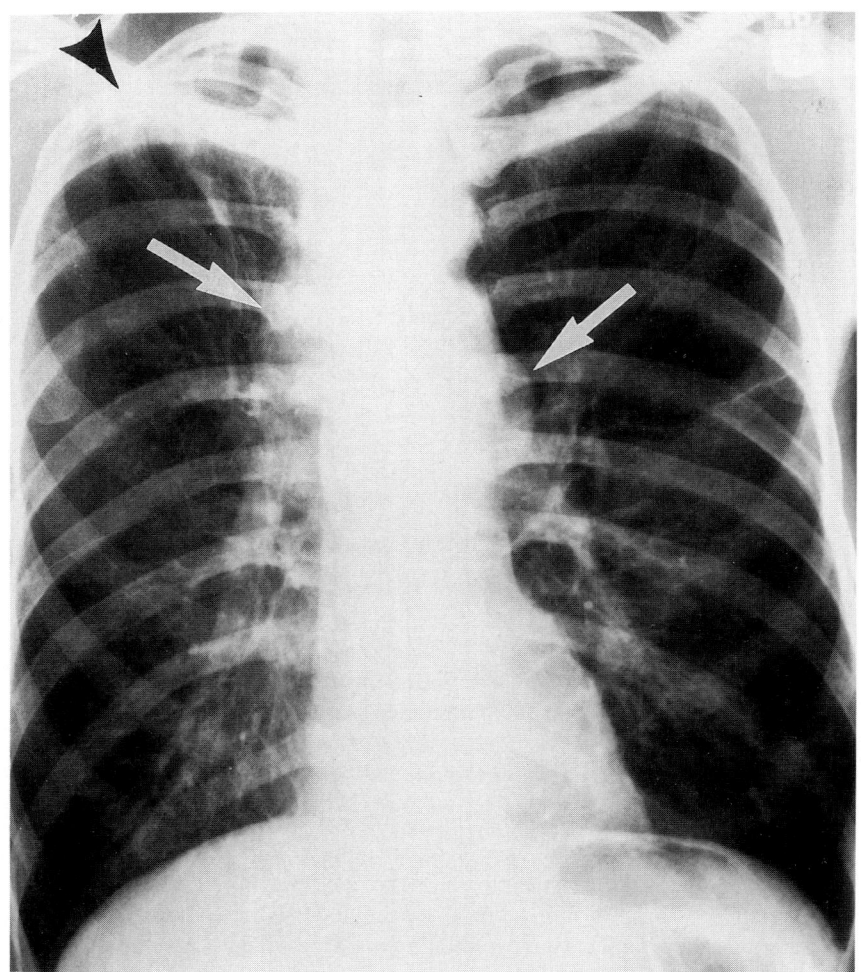

Figure 12 A 46-year-old male smoker with pulmonary adenocarcinoma and AIDS: The PA chest radiograph demonstrates an irregular opacity at the right apex that is partially obscured by the clavicle (arrowhead). There is extensive bilateral paratracheal and aortopulmonary window lymphadenopathy (arrows). Hyperinflation and vascular attenuation is consistent with pulmonary emphysema.

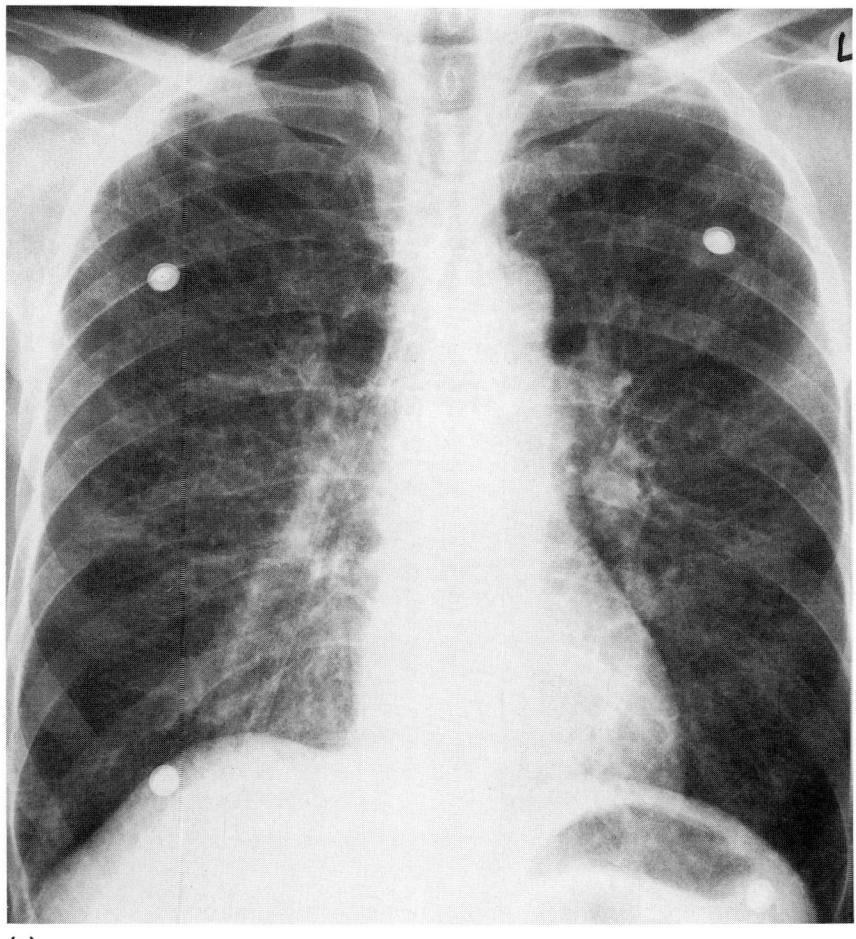

(a)

Figure 13 A 52-year-old male smoker with nonspecific interstitial pneumonitis, who presented with a dry cough and dyspnea. Bronchoscopy and biopsy failed to demonstrate an identifiable pathogen. (a) The chest radiograph shows bilateral fine interstitial disease, radiologically indistinguishable from PCP. Note the bullous apical changes, possibly caused by a combination of smoking and previous PCP infection. (b) The CT scan demonstrates bilateral interstitial opacities, with patchy ground-glass opacification that is most marked in the posterior lungs.

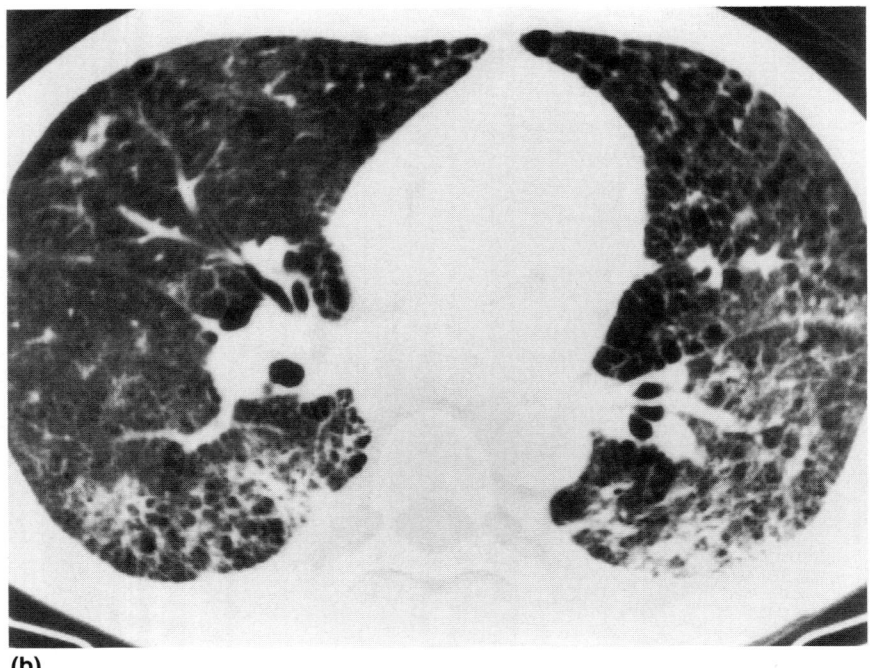

(b)

Figure 13 (Continued)

IV. Nonneoplastic, Noninfectious Complications

A. Lymphocytic Interstitial Pneumonia

Lymphocytic interstitial pneumonia (LIP) refers to infiltration of the interstitium by small benign-appearing lymphocytes and plasma cells. The LIP complicating HIV infection is seen most commonly in children and is an AIDS-defining illness in those younger than 13 years. An uncommon disease in adult AIDS patients, it typically presents with a nonproductive cough and progressive dyspnea (51). Chest radiographs classically demonstrate fine or coarse reticular interstitial disease, with or without foci of patchy consolidation. It is usually indolent, remaining stable in appearance throughout the course of HIV infection. Because the radiologic and presenting clinical features are similar to PCP, biopsy is required to confirm the diagnosis and to exclude infection (52).

B. Nonspecific Interstitial Pneumonia

A substantial number of lung biopsies in AIDS patients reveal diffuse alveolar damage and infiltration of the interstitium by a mixed mononuclear cell infiltrate in the absence of a recognizable pathogen. The clinical presentation is frequently very similar to that of PCP, with cough, dyspnea, and fever. Chest radiographs may demonstrate a pattern of diffuse interstitial disease also indistinguishable from PCP (Fig. 13). Pleural effusions do occur, but are uncommon. Approximately 50% of patients have a normal chest radiograph. Nonspecific interstitial pneumonia is usually self-limiting or stabilizes without specific therapy (53).

V. Interventional Radiology in AIDS Patients

Fluoroscopically guided transthoracic needle aspiration (TNA) is useful for diagnosing diffuse parenchymal lung disease in AIDS patients, with a reported diagnostic yield of 87.5%. The incidence of complicating pneumothorax appears higher in this group of patients compared with the usual biopsy population (54). Use of TNA has also proved effective (diagnostic yield of 84%) and safe for diagnosing focal lung and mediastinal lesions in AIDS patients, using fluoroscopic or CT guidance (55). When performed with CT guidance, bullae and lung cysts can be avoided, and pneumothorax rates are similar to that of TNA in non-AIDS patients. Mediastinoscopy and open-lung biopsy, therefore, should be reserved for those patients in whom the results of TNA are negative (55).

References

1. Batra P. AIDS: immunological abnormalities following human immunodeficiency virus infection. J Thorac Imaging 1991; 6:1–5.
2. Global Program on AIDS, World Health Organization. World AIDS Day Newsletter. Geneva: World Health Organization, Global Program on AIDS. 1994;(2):1.
3. Centers for Disease Control (CDC) update: NCHS. Annual summary of births, marriages, Divorces and deaths: United States 1993. Hyattsville Maryland: US Department of Health and Human Services, Public Health Service. Monthly vital statistics report, 1994; 42:18–20.
4. Centers for Disease Control (CDC) update: Update. Acquired immunodeficiency syndrome—United States 1994. MMWR 1995; 44:64–67.
5. DeLorenzo LJ, Huang CT, Stone DJ. Roentgenographic patterns of *Pneumocystis carinii* pneumonia in 104 patients with AIDS. Chest 1987; 91:323–327.
6. Wasser LS, Brown E, Talavera W. Miliary PCP in AIDS. Chest 1989; 96:693–695.
7. Barrio JL, Suarez M, Rodriguez JL, Saldana MJ, Pitchenik AE. *Pneumocystis carinii* pneumonia presenting as cavitating and noncavitating solitary pulmonary nodules in patients with the acquired immunodeficiency syndrome. Am Rev Respir Dis 1985; 134:1094–1096.

8. Abd AG, Nierman DM, Ilowite JS, Pierson RN, Bell ALL. Bilateral upper lobe *Pneumocystis carinii* pneumonia in a patient receiving inhaled pentamidine prophylaxis. Chest 1988; 94:329–31.
9. Pilon VA, Echols RM, Celo JS, Elmendorf SL. Disseminated *Pneumocystis carinii* infection in AIDS. N Engl J Med 1987; 316:1410–1411.
10. Bergin CJ, Wirth RL, Berry GJ, Castellino RA. *Pneumocystis carinii* pneumonia: CT and HRCT observations. J Comput Assist Tomogr 1990; 14:756–759.
11. Kuhlman JE, Knowles MC, Fishman EK, Siegelman SS. Premature bullous damage in AIDS: CT diagnosis. Radiology 1989; 173:23–26.
12. Feuerstein IM, Archer A, Pluda JM, et al. Thin-walled cavities, cysts, and pneumothorax in *Pneumocystis carinii* pneumonia: further observations with histopathologic correlation. Radiology 1990; 174:697–702.
13. Chow C, Templeton PA, White CS. Lung cysts associated with *Pneumocystis carinii* pneumonia: radiographic characteristics, natural history and complications. AJR 1993; 161:527–531.
14. Gurney J, Bates FT. Pulmonary cystic disease: comparison of *Pneumocystis carinii* pneumatoceles and bullous emphysema due to intravenous drug abuse. Radiology 1989; 173:27–31.
15. Meduri GU, Stein DS. Pulmonary manifestations of acquired immunodeficiency syndrome. Clin Infect Dis 1992; 14:98–113.
16. Daley CL. Bacterial pneumonia in HIV-infected patients. Semin Respir Infect 1993; 8:104–115.
17. Bloch AB, Rieder HL, Kelly GD, Cauthen GM, Hayden CH, Snider DE. The epidemiology of tuberculosis in the United States. Semin Respir Infect 1989; 4:157–170.
18. Barnes PF, Bloch AB, Davidson PT, Snider DE. Tuberculosis in patients with human immunodeficiency virus infection. N Engl J Med 1991; 324:1644–1650.
19. Greenberg SD, Frager D, Suster B, Walker S, Stavropoulos C, Rothpearl A. Active pulmonary tuberculosis in patients with AIDS: spectrum of radiographic findings (including a normal appearance). Radiology 1994; 193:115–119.
20. Keiper MD, Beumont M, Elshami A, Langlotz CP, Miller W. CD4 lymphocyte count and the radiographic presentation of pulmonary tuberculosis. A study of the relationship between these factors in patients with the human immunodeficiency virus infection. Chest 1995; 107:74–80.
21. Fischl MA, Daikos GL, Uttamchandani RB, et al. Clinical presentation and outcome of patients with HIV infection and tuberculosis caused by multiple drug resistant bacilli. Ann Intern Med 1992; 117:184–190.
22. Pastores SM, Naidich DP, Aranda CP, McGuinnes G, Rom WN. Intrathoracic adenopathy associated with pulmonary tuberculosis in patients with human immunodeficiency virus infection. Chest 1993; 103:1433–37.
23. Wallace JM, Hannah J. *Mycobacterium avium-intracellulare* infection found at autopsy in patients with the acquired immunodeficiency syndrome (AIDS). Am Rev Respir Dis 1989; 131:A224.
24. Aronchick JM, Miller WT. Disseminated nontuberculous mycobacterial infections in immunosuppressed patients. Semin Roentgenol 1993; 28:150–157.

25. Marinelli DL, Albelda SM, Willianms TM, Kern JA, Iozzo RV, Miller WT. Nontuberculous mycobacterial infection in AIDS: clinical, pathologic and radiographic features. Radiology 1986; 160:77–82
26. Levine B, Chaisson RE. *Mycobacterium kansasii*: a cause of treatable pulmonary disease associated with advanced human immunodeficiency virus (HIV) infection. Ann Intern Med 1991; 114:861–868.
27. Khoury MB, Godwin JD, Ravin CE, Gallis HA, Halvorsen RA, Putman CE. Thoracic cryptococcosis: immunologic competence and radiologic appearance. AJR 1984; 141:893–896.
28. Miller WT, Edelman JM, Miller WT. Cryptococcal pulmonary infection in patients with AIDS: radiographic appearance. Radiology 1990; 175:725–728.
29. Sider L, Westcott MA. Pulmonary manifestations of cryptococcosis in patients with AIDS: CT features. J Thorac Imaging 1994; 9:78–84.
30. Conces DJ, Stockberger SM, Tarver RD, Wheat LJ. Disseminated histoplasmosis in AIDS: findings on chest radiographs. AJR 1993; 160:15–19.
31. Galgiani JN, Ampel NM. *Coccidioides immitis* in patients with human immunodeficiency virus infections. Semin Respir Infect 1990; 5:151–154.
32. Miller WT Jr, Sais GJ, Frank I, Gefter WB, Aronchick JM, Miller WT. Pulmonary aspergillosis in patients with AIDS. Clinical and radiographic correlations. Chest 1994; 105:37–44.
33. Pappas PG, Pottage JC, Powderly WG, et al. Blastomycosis in patients with the acquired immunodeficiency syndrome. Ann Intern Med 1992; 116:847–853.
34. Wallace JM, Hannah J. Cytomegalovirus pneumonitis in patients with AIDS. Chest 1987; 92:198–203.
35. McGuinness G, Scholes JV, Garay SM, Leitman BS, McCauley DI, Naidich DP. Cytomegalovirus pneumonitis: spectrum of parenchymal CT findings with pathologic correlation in 21 AIDS patients. Radiology 1994; 192:451–459.
36. Goodman PC, Schnapp LM. Pulmonary toxoplasmosis in AIDS. Radiology 1992; 184:791–793.
37. Makris AN, Sher S, Bertoli C, Latour MG. Pulmonary strongyloidiasis: an unusual opportunistic pneumonia in a patient with AIDS. AJR 1993; 161:545–547.
38. Rothenberg R, Woelfel M, Stoneburner R, et al. Survival with acquired immunodeficiency syndrome. N Engl J Med 1987; 317:1297–1302.
39. Katz MH, Hessol NA, Buchbinder SP, Hirozawa A, O'Malley P, Holmberg SD. Temporal trends of opportunistic infections and malignancies in homosexual men with AIDS. J Infect Dis 1994; 170:198–202.
40. Gruden JF, Huang L, Webb WR, Gamsu G, Hopewell PC, Sides DM. AIDS-related Kaposi sarcoma of the lung: radiographic findings and staging system with bronchoscopic correlation. Radiology 1995; 195:545–552.
41. Sivit CJ, Schwartz AM, Rockoff SD. Kaposi's sarcoma of the lung in AIDS: radiologic–pathologic analysis. AJR 1987; 148:25–28.
42. Davis SD, Henschke CI, Chamides BK, Westcott JL. Intrathoracic Kaposi sarcoma in AIDS patients: radiographic–pathologic correlation. Radiology 1987; 163:495–500.
43. Naidich DP, Tarras M, Garay SM, Birnbaum B, Rybak BJ, Schinella R. Kaposi's sarcoma: CT–radiographic correlation. Chest 1989; 96:723–728.

44. Wolff SD, Kuhlman JE, Fishman EK. Thoracic Kaposi sarcoma in AIDS: CT findings. J Comput Assist Tomogr 1993; 17:60–62.
45. Lee VW, Fuller JD, O'Brian MJ, Parker DR, Cooley TP, Liebman HA. Pulmonary Kaposi sarcoma in patients with AIDS: scintigraphic diagnosis with sequential thallium and gallium scanning. Radiology 1991; 180:409–412.
46. Kaplan LD, Abrams DI, Feigal E, et al. AIDS-associated non-Hodgkin's lymphoma in San Francisco. JAMA 1989; 261:719–724.
47. Sider L, Weiss AJ, Smith MD, VonRoenn JH, Glassroth J. Varied appearance of AIDS-related lymphoma in the chest. Radiology 1989; 171:629–632.
48. Heitzman ER. Pulmonary neoplastic and lymphoproliferative disease in AIDS: a review. Radiology 1990; 177:347–351.
49. White CS, Haramati LB, Elder KH, Karp J, Belani CP. Carcinoma of the lung in HIV-positive patients: findings on chest radiographs and CT scans. AJR 1995; 164:593–597.
50. Fishman JE, Schwartz DS, Sais GJ, Flores MR, Sridhar KS. Bronchogenic carcinoma in HIV-positive patients: findings on chest radiographs and CT scans. AJR 1995; 164:57–61.
51. Morris JC, Rosen MJ, Marchevsky A, Teirstein AS. Lymphocytic interstitial pneumonia in patients at risk for the acquired immune deficiency syndrome. Chest 1987; 91:63–67.
52. Oldham SAA, Castillo M, Jacobson FL, Mones JM, Saldana MJ. HIV-associated lymphocytic interstitial pneumonia: radiologic manifestations and pathologic correlation. Radiology 1989; 170:83–87.
53. Simmons JT, Suffredini AF, Lack EE, et al. Nonspecific interstitial pneumonitis in patients with AIDS: radiologic features. AJR 1987; 149:265–268.
54. Wallace JM, Batra P, Gong H, Ovenfors CO. Percutaneous needle lung aspiration for diagnosing pneumonitis in the patients with acquired immunodeficiency syndrome (AIDS). Am Rev Respir Dis 1985; 131:389–392.
55. Gruden JF, Klein JS, Webb WR. Percutaneous transthoracic needle biopsy in AIDS: analysis in 32 patients. Radiology 1993; 189:567–571.

4

Diagnostic Imaging of Bronchogenic Carcinoma

JEREMY J. ERASMUS and EDWARD F. PATZ, JR.
Duke University Medical Center
Durham, North Carolina

I. Introduction

Bronchogenic carcinoma has become a significant health problem of the 20th century. Whereas only several hundred cases were reported in the literature before 1900, an estimated 172,000 new cases will be diagnosed this year in the United States alone (1,2). It is the most common malignancy in the Western World, and the leading cause of cancer-related death, accounting for 34% of all cancer deaths in men and 22% in women (2).

Seventy-five percent of cases will occur in patients in their fifth and sixth decades of life, with a male/female ratio of 2:1 in 1984, decreased from 7:1 in 1964 (3,4). In the United States, 80–90% of lung cancers are attributable to cigarette smoking, and smokers have at least a 25-fold or greater chance of developing lung cancer than nonsmokers (1,3,5). Involuntary smoke exposure (passive smoking) also appears responsible for an increased risk of lung cancer, accounting for 2000–4000 cases annually (4,6).

It is estimated that 14,000 lung cancer deaths are caused annually in the United States by radon, making it the second most important cause of lung cancer (4). Individuals exposed to asbestos have an approximately 10 times increased risk for developing lung cancer, and those with asbestos exposure and a smoking history have up to a 90 times increased risk (3,7). Additional risk factors include exposure to chromium, arsenic, nickel, chlorethyl methyl ether, and radiation (1,3,4,8,9). Tuberculosis, peripheral pulmonary scars, lipoid pneumonia, and interstitial fibrosis have been suggested to increase the risk of lung cancer; however, the data are inconclusive and are frequently derived from case series, rather than epidemiological investigations (4).

The vast majority of lung cancers are detected initially on chest radiographs. They have many different radiologic manifestations that often depend on the cell type and stage at presentation. This review will focus on imaging bronchogenic carcinoma, including screening, diagnosis, and staging evaluation.

II. Screening

Lung cancer continues to have a dismal overall 5-year survival rate of 14%, despite recent advances in treatment options (10). This poor prognosis reflects the advanced stage of disease at presentation in the vast majority of patients with non–small-cell carcinoma (10). Thus, in an effort to detect lesions at an early stage and improve survival, several large prospective lung cancer screening studies using chest radiographs and sputum cytological studies have been performed (11–13). Although screening initially appeared to result in earlier detection and improved survival, further analysis demonstrated lead time bias, and length bias, changed the eventual outcome with no overall reduction in mortality associated with screening (11,14). It is now generally accepted that chest film screening for the early detection of lung cancer is not effective. The American Cancer Society policy advocates primary prevention, but not routine radiographic surveys (15,16). More recently, however, the data from these studies have been reanalyzed and may provide some justification for chest radiography as a screening modality in high-risk groups (16–18). A new trial supported by the National Cancer Institute (NCI) proposes randomizing approximately 150,000 patients again to reexamine the usefulness of screening chest radiographs for early lung cancer detection.

III. Pathological Classification

Bronchogenic carcinomas constitute more than 95% of all tumors in the thorax (19,20). These neoplasms are divided into two fundamental categories, non–small-cell lung carcinoma (NSCLC), and small-cell lung carcinoma (SCLC). The rationale for this general distinction is that it provides both therapeutic and prognostic information. Further classification by histological appearance has been suggested by the World Health Organization (WHO), although up to 45% of all lung cancers demonstrate more than one cell type (Table 1; 20–23).

Table 1 WHO Pathological Classification of Lung Tumors

Non–small-cell lung carcinoma (NSCLC)
1. Squamous cell carcinoma
    a. Variant: spindle cell carcinoma
2. Adenocarcinoma
    a. Acinar adenocarcinoma
    b. Papillary adenocarcinoma
    c. Bronchioloalveolar carcinoma
    d. Solid carcinoma with formation of mucus
3. Large-cell undifferentiated carcinoma
    a. Variant: giant cell carcinoma
    b. Variant: clear cell carcinoma
4. Adenosquamous carcinoma

Small-cell carcinoma (SCLC)
   a. Oat cell carcinoma
   b. Intermediate cell type
   c. Combined oat cell carcinoma

Carcinoid tumor

Bronchial gland carcinomas
   a. Adenoid cystic carcinoma
   b. Mucoepidermoid carcinoma

IV. Radiologic Features

Lung cancer is often considered in the differential diagnosis of a variety of thoracic abnormalities. Although the typical, classic radiographic appearance is that of a spiculated, irregular lung mass, many tumors will have a spectrum of radiologic findings. Specific cell types often share common radiographic features, but most patients still require a tissue diagnosis, particularly to differentiate non–small-cell carcinoma from small-cell carcinoma.

A. Non–Small-Cell Carcinoma

Squamous Cell Carcinoma

The relative incidence of squamous cell carcinoma has been decreasing, and now constitutes 25% of lung cancer (24). There is marked variation in differentiation, probably contributing to the range in biological behavior (25). Most squamous cell carcinomas are slow-growing with late metastasis, predominately to the liver, adrenal glands, kidneys, and bones (19,26).

Most squamous cell carcinomas occur in central bronchi, although one-third of tumors occur beyond the segmental bronchi (19,27,28). Endobronchial masses

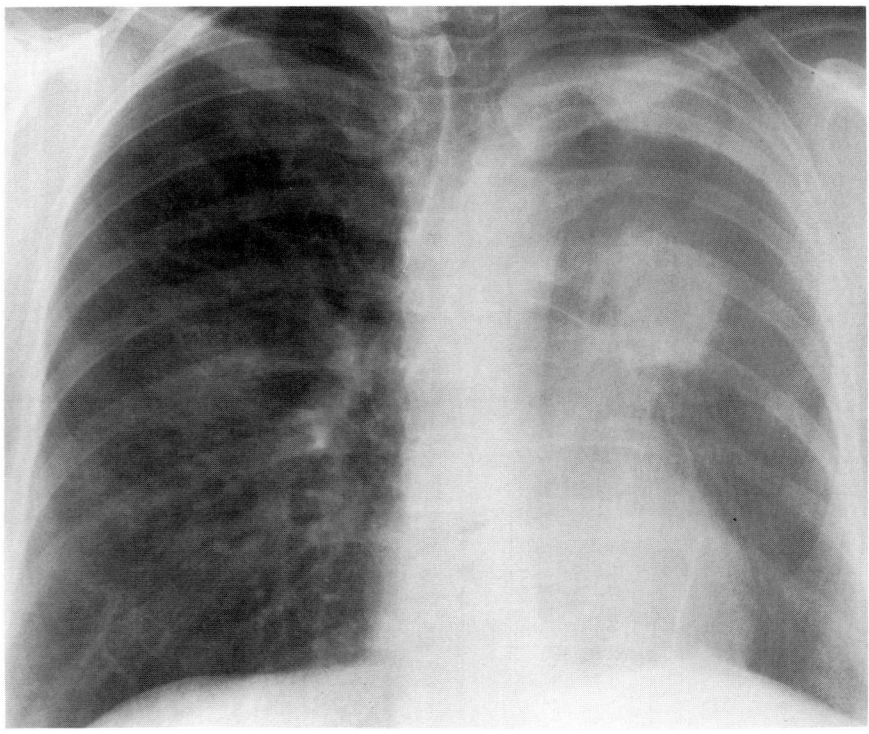

(a)

Figure 1 Squamous cell carcinoma: (a) A posteroanterior (PA) chest radiograph demonstrates a left hilar mass with left upper lobe collapse. (b) CT shows the obstructing mass within the left upper lobe bronchus with associated collapse.

may result in distal postobstructive pneumonia or atelectasis in up to 50% of cases (19,28,29; Fig. 1). Atelectasis is most often segmental or lobar, and it may obscure the underlying mass (19,29). Mucoid impaction, bronchiectasis, and hyperinflation are additional findings of a central obstructing neoplasm (Fig. 2; 19,27,30,31). These tumors may also have local extension into the chest wall or mediastinum, causing bone destruction, superior vena cava (SVC) syndrome, and phrenic or recurrent laryngeal nerve paralysis (19,20,32).

Tumors usually range in size from 1 to 10 cm, although peripheral lesions are usually larger (28). It is the most common lung tumor to cavitate, and this occurs in 10–20% of cases (19,28). The frequency of cavitation increases with histological grade of malignancy and is more common in large peripheral squamous cell carcinomas (30%) (27,33). Cavitation is characteristically eccentric,

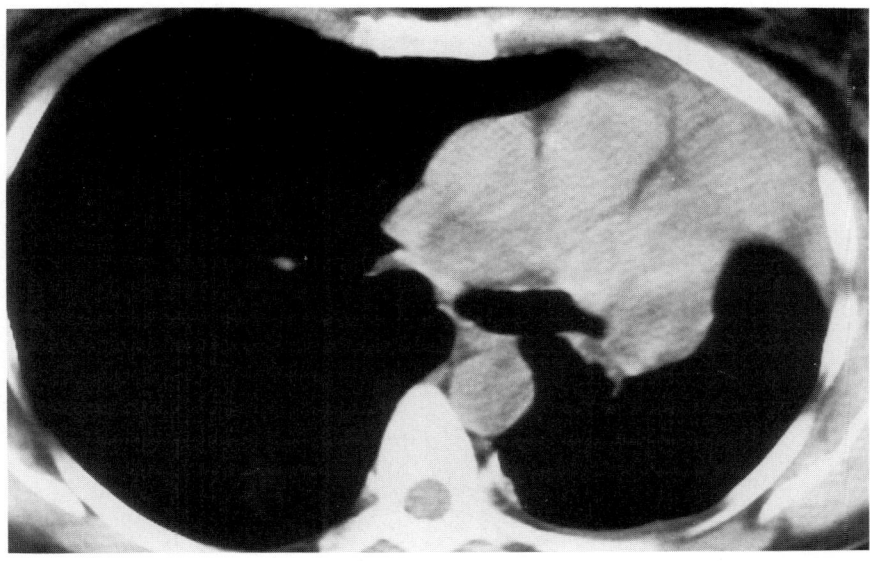

(b)

and the walls are usually thick and irregular, ranging in size from 0.5 to 3 cm. Rarely, extensive necrosis may result in very thin walls (Fig. 3; 19). Squamous cell carcinoma has been the most common histological type for a Pancoast or superior sulcus tumor (19). Asymmetry of more than 8 mm of apical pleural thickening may be an important finding, especially when associated with chest wall pain, brachial or laryngeal nerve paralysis, or bony destruction (Fig. 4; 19).

Adenocarcinoma

The incidence of adenocarcinoma is increasing and is now the most common lung cancer cell type, constituting 25–30% of all cases (24). It is subdivided into four subtypes: acinar, papillary, solid, and bronchioloalveolar, although stage at presentation is the most important factor in determining treatment and prognosis.

Adenocarcinoma typically presents as a peripheral, solitary pulmonary nodule, usually smaller than 4 cm, with hilar (18%) and, less commonly, mediastinal metastases (2%) (28,34). More recently, a higher incidence of more centrally located adenocarcinomas (28–40%) has been reported, with increased hilar and mediastinal lymph node metastases (40 and 27%, respectively; 27,34).

Adenocarcinomas often have uniform growth rates; thus, lesions are usually round or oval (19). They tend to have well-defined margins, although this cannot be used to predict lack of aggressiveness (27). Infiltrating edges, with distortion of

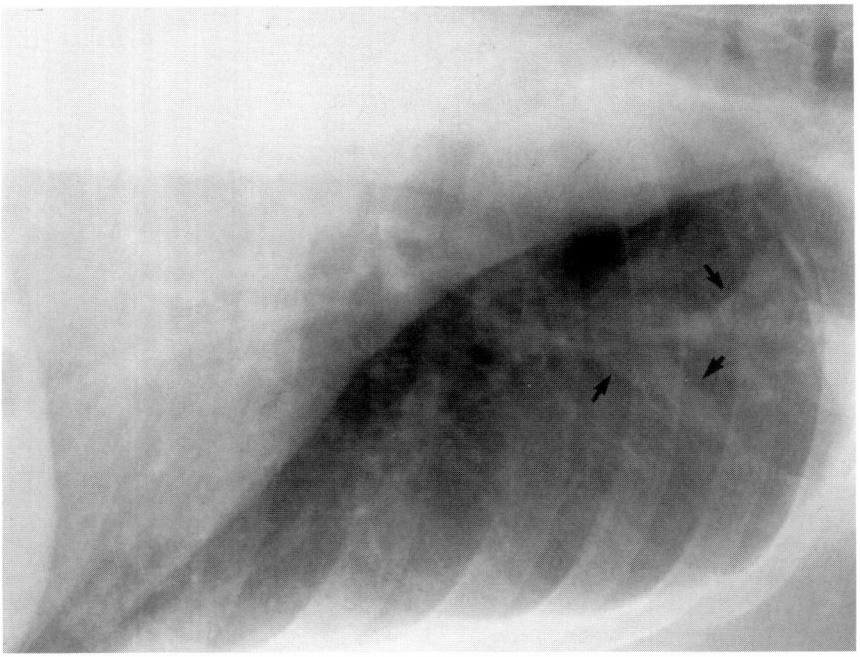

(a)

Figure 2 Squamous cell carcinoma: (a) PA chest radiograph demonstrates a branching, tubular opacity in the left upper lobe (arrows). (b,c) Sequential CT images demonstrate a small central mass and dilated, more distal mucoid impacted bronchi.

adjacent vessels, has been described as sunburst or corona radiata appearance and is due to fibrosis and parenchymal invasion at the margins (19,27). This finding occurs rarely with benign lesions and is suggestive of malignancy. Retraction of the adjacent pleura can occur with peripheral carcinomas (35). This pleural tag or pleuroparenchymal tail can occur with both benign and other malignant abnormalities (35).

Eccentric, amorphous calcification within the lesion is extremely rare on chest radiographs, although it has been observed in up to 6% of all cancers on computed tomography (CT) scans (36; Fig. 5). Calcification is probably due to engulfment of a preexisting granuloma or associated with scar carcinomas (5,34,37). Approximately 5% of peripheral tumors, the majority of which are adenocarcinomas, are thought to arise in preexisting scars (27,34,38,39).

Bronchioloalveolar cell carcinoma (BAC) is a subset of adenocarcinomas that have been described as both solitary or multifocal in origin (32). They

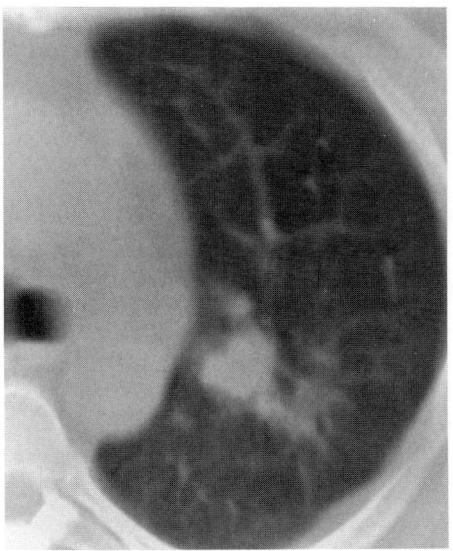

(b)

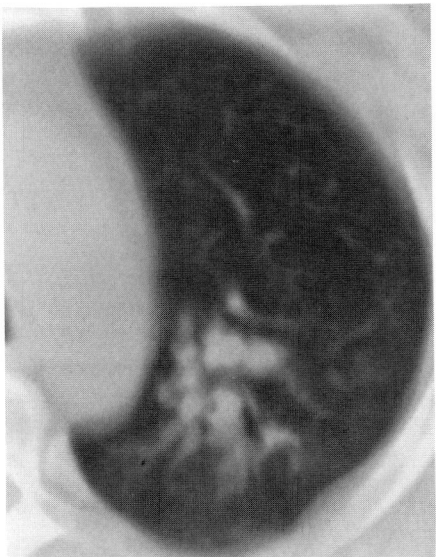

(c)

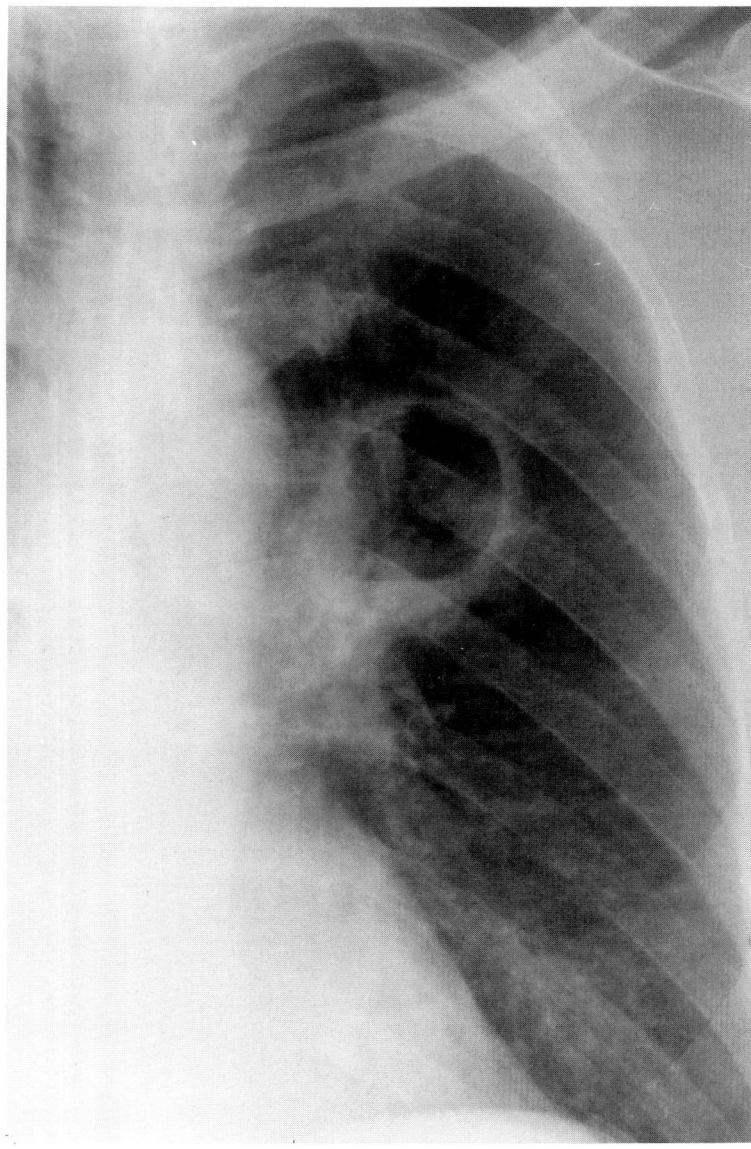

(a)

Figure 3 Squamous cell carcinoma: (a,b) PA and lateral chest radiographs demonstrate a thin-walled cavitary left upper lobe mass.

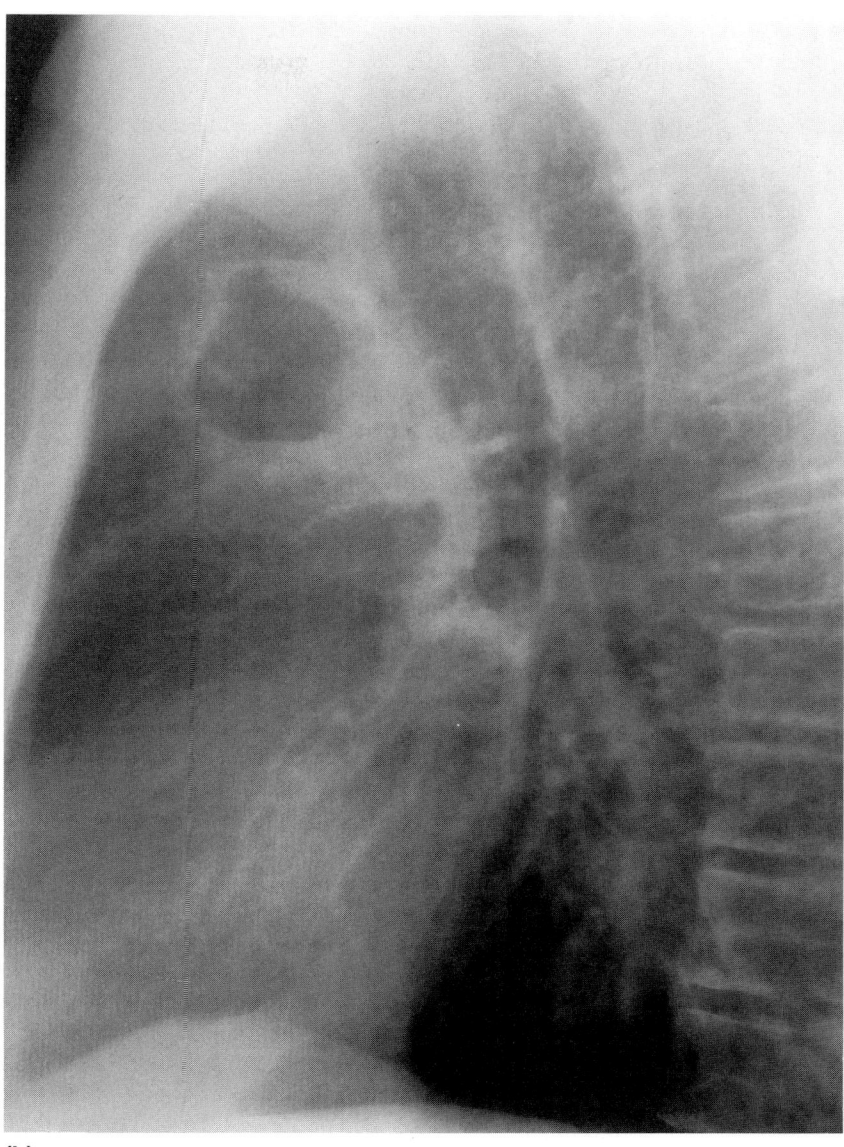
(b)

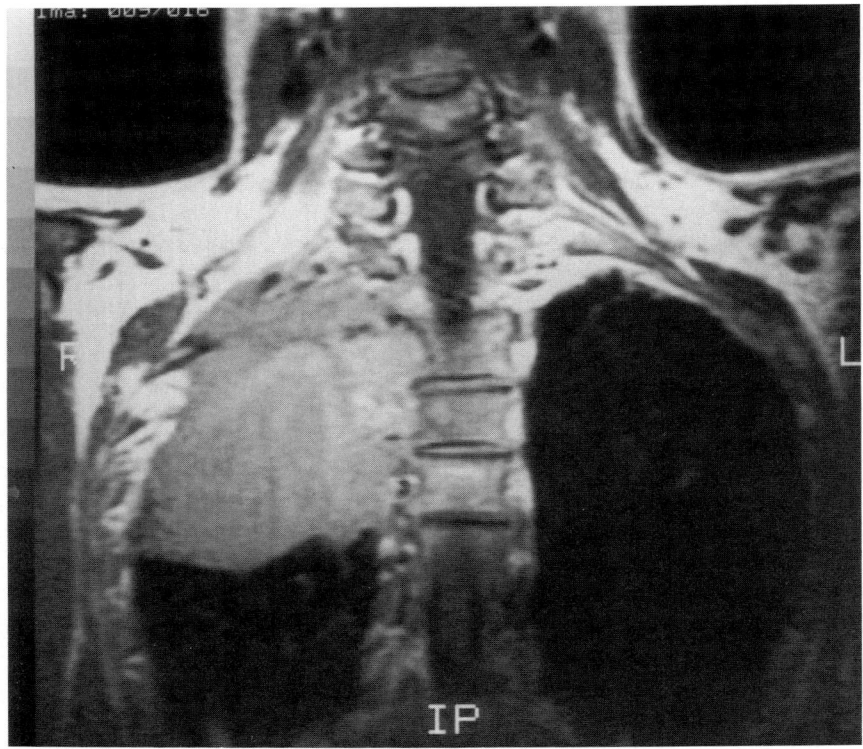

Figure 4 Squamous cell carcinoma: Coronal T1-weighted MR demonstrates a right apical mass with chest wall infiltration consistent with a Pancoast tumor.

constitute 1.5–10% of all lung cancers and have a variety of biological, clinical, and radiographic features. Clinical features that may distinguish BAC from other lung cancers are (9,20,40–43)

1. Younger age at presentation
2. Equal distribution between men and women
3. Copious watery sputum (bronchorrhea; 43,44)
4. Association with parenchymal scarring or fibrosis (19,41) (higher incidence in patients with progressive systemic sclerosis; 45)
5. Higher incidence in nonsmokers (46)

The most common radiographic finding is a well-circumscribed, solitary nodule (60%), the size of which may remain unchanged over several years (27,43,43,47). Bronchioloalveolar carcinomas, similarly to most adenocarcinomas,

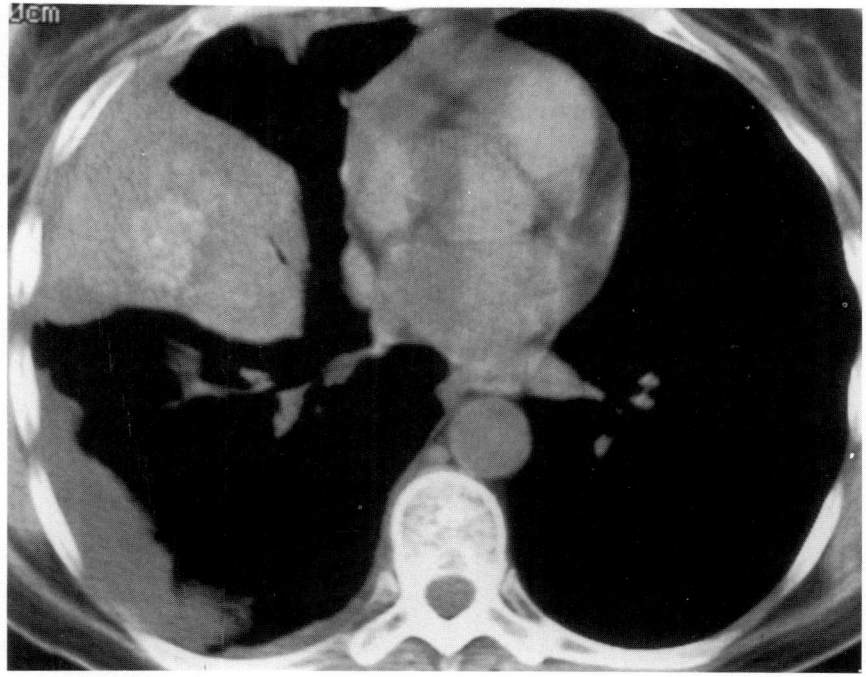

Figure 5 Adenocarcinoma: CT image demonstrates a large peripheral mass with extensive amorphous calcification.

are usually peripheral (40,48). Pseudocavitation, the presence of small, focal low-attenuation regions within or surrounding the periphery of the nodule and air bronchograms are more commonly associated with these tumors than with other cell types.

The diffuse form may present as multiple nodular opacities, varying in size, and involving one or both lungs (15%) (Fig. 6; 19,20,27,41,43,44,47,48). Focal, poorly defined opacities, or multiple scattered opacities, resembling pneumonia (10%) (27), may coalesce into lobar, and rarely complete, lung opacification (19; Fig. 7). Some patients will have reticulonodular opacities resembling interstitial lung disease. Other radiographic findings associated with parenchymal disease are hilar and mediastinal metastases (18%), pleural effusions (1–10%), atelectasis (3%), and rarely, pneumothorax (19,48).

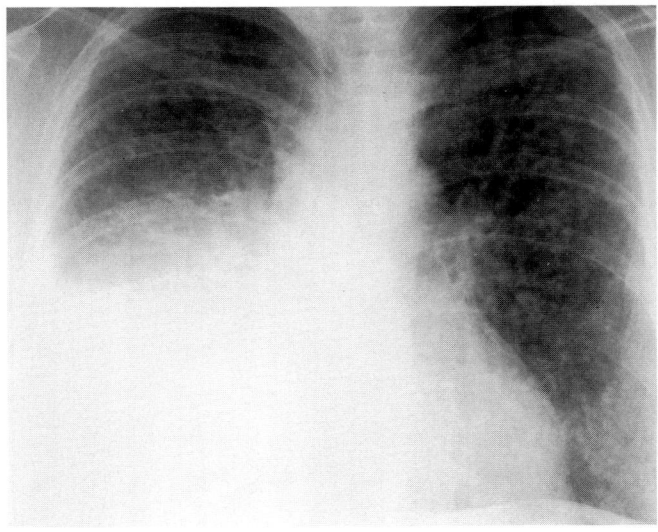

(a)

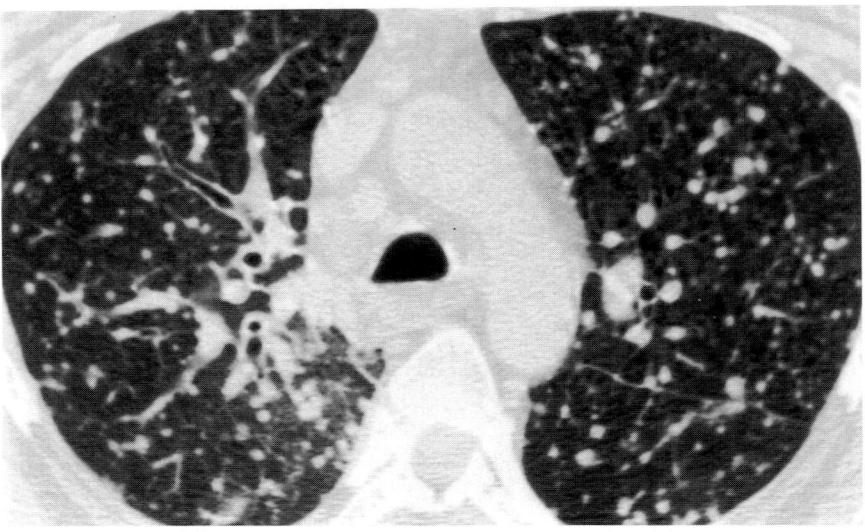

(b)

Figure 6 Adenocarcinoma: (a) PA chest radiograph demonstrates numerous, small bilateral pulmonary nodular opacities, with a large right pleural effusion. (b) CT confirms the multiple nodules of varying size.

Large-Cell Carcinoma

Approximately 10–20% of all lung cancers are large-cell carcinomas (5,19,20). Two subtypes, with varying degrees of differentiation, have been recognized: giant cell carcinoma and clear cell carcinoma. In fact, only 3% of all lung tumors can be definitively classified as giant or clear cell carcinomas (32).

Most large-cell carcinomas are large, peripheral masses, with an average size exceeding 7 cm (5,19,26–28,49,50). The margins are usually poorly defined (57–85%) (27,49). Cavitation is uncommon (6%), and rapid growth, with early lymphatic and hematogenous metastases, is common (50). Thirty-two percent will have hilar and 10% will have mediastinal adenopathy at presentation (5,19,27,28; Fig. 8).

B. Small-Cell Carcinoma

The small-cell tumors constitute approximately 20–25% of all lung cancers (5,20,51). They are thought to arise from neuroendocrine cells, contain neurosecretory granules, and may produce peptide hormones (20,32). Small-cell carcinomas consequently may be associated with paraneoplastic syndromes and hormone production, usually corticotropin (adenocorticotropic hormone; ACTH; 20). In fact, small-cell carcinomas account for 75% of clinical symptoms of ectopic hormone production (19).

Small-cell carcinomas have a high mitotic rate, demonstrate marked invasion into lung parenchyma, and rapidly spread to submucosal vessels, lymphatics, and regional lymph nodes (5). Although the tumor is often very small and may not be identified, early extensive extrathoracic metastases are common and are often present before the development of pulmonary symptoms (20,32). Liver, bone marrow, adrenal glands, and brain are frequent sites of metastatic disease (5,52). Combined radiotherapy and chemotherapy frequently result in rapid resolution of adenopathy, although recurrence is common, with a mean survival of 14 months (19,51,53).

The tumors are located centrally in 78–90% of cases (5,52). Mediastinal extension with adenopathy may be detected in up to 97% by CT when hilar adenopathy is present (54). Mediastinal adenopathy usually is extensive and may encase mediastinal structures, and 70% will have tracheobronchial compression on CT (54,55; Fig. 9). Atelectasis is usually due to massive hilar and mediastinal adenopathy, with airway compromise (5,27).

Peripheral SCLC, is often associated with hilar adenopathy (5,19,20,28). These primary neoplasms are usually small, and pleural effusion has been reported in 5–40% of cases (3,19,54,55).

V. Diagnosis

Early detection of lung cancer can be problematic, because findings may be subtle and the clinical picture nonspecific. In addition benign pulmonary abnormalities

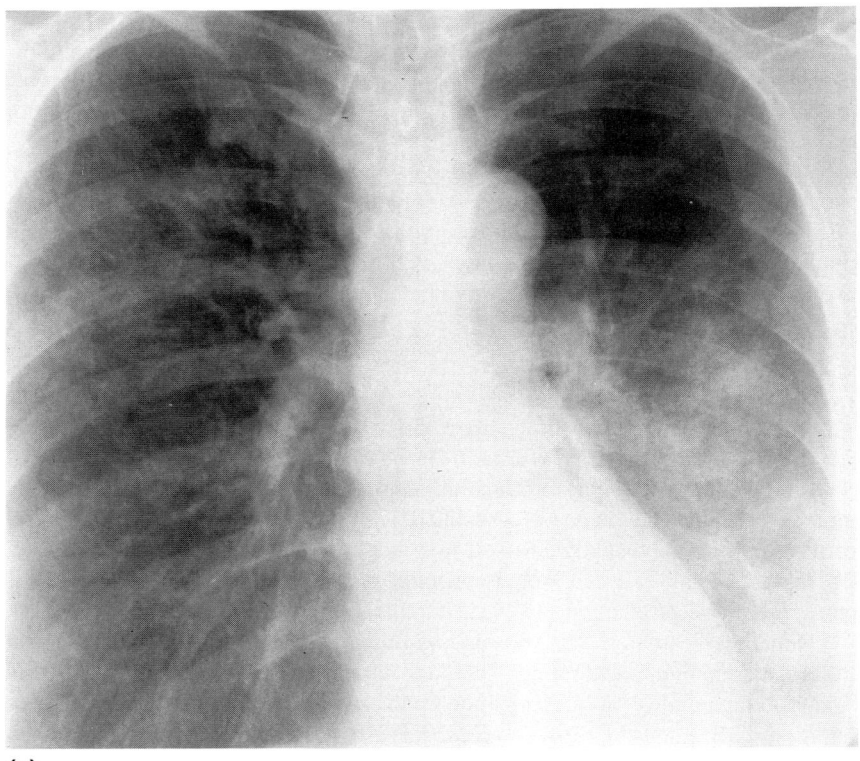

(a)

Figure 7 Bronchioloalveolar cell carcinoma: (a) A PA chest radiograph demonstrates diffuse, bilateral, poorly defined opacities, with consolidation in the left base. (b) The CT scan demonstrates bilateral nodular opacities with consolidation in the left lower lobe. The findings are consistent with transbronchial spread of disease.

may have similar anatomical or morphological features. The absence of growth over a 2-year period is reliable in determining that a nodule is benign (56). Specific patterns of calcification (central, concentric, or a stippled appearance), have traditionally been the only additional feature diagnostic of a benign lesion. Many lesions, however, are radiographically indeterminate after standard evaluation and, thus, require further workup with transthoracic needle aspirate (TTNA), bronchoscopy, or thoracotomy. Use of TTNA is optimal for peripheral nodules, although most radiographically visible lesions are amenable to biopsy if clinically indicated. This procedure can confirm a diagnosis of malignancy in 90–95% of

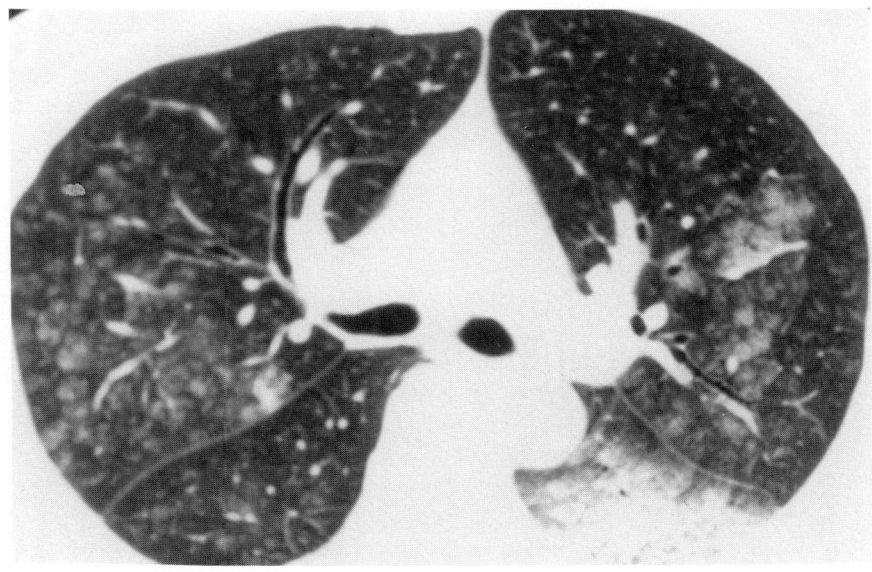

(b)

nodules larger than 2 cm and in 60% of smaller nodules (56,57). Complications, most notably pneumothorax, occur in 10–30% of patients, although only 20% of these patients eventually require a chest tube. Unfortunately, making a specific benign diagnosis is often more difficult, and a nondiagnostic biopsy is not uncommon if the lesion is benign (57). Although bronchoscopy has a low complication rate (5%), a diagnosis is obtained in only 40–80% of cases if the lesion is larger than 2 cm, and smaller nodules are less optimally evaluated (<10% diagnostic; 56,58–60).

A new alternative, positron emission tomography (PET) imaging, provides a noninvasive, physiological method to evaluate pulmonary nodules that are indeterminate with conventional imaging. Use of PET with [^{18}F]fluorodeoxyglucose (18-FDG), a d-glucose analogue, is a measure of glucose metabolism. Increased glucose utilization is a well-described property of tumor cells. The FDG-PET scan is highly accurate (sensitivity of 83–100% and specificity 80–100%) in differentiating benign from malignant focal pulmonary lesions as small as 1 cm (Fig. 10; 56,61,62). Increased uptake can be detected in some lesions smaller than 1 cm, although spatial resolution becomes a limitation. The current usefulness of PET is with lesions that are hypometabolic, virtually excluding a malignancy. There are, however, false-positive studies, (i.e., increased FDG in benign lesions, including aspergillomas, abscesses, tuberculosis, and histo-

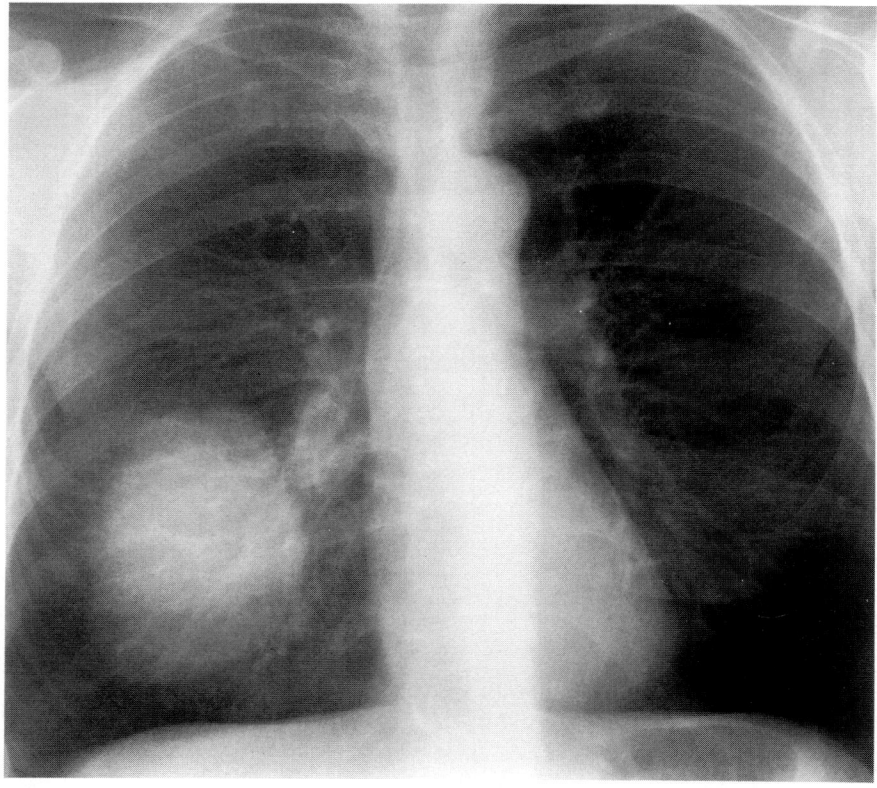

(a)

Figure 8 Large-cell carcinoma: (a) A PA chest radiograph demonstrates a large right lower lobe mass with hilar adenopathy. (b) The CT scan shows the mass with a low-attenuation, necrotic region. There are also enlarged hilar and subcarinal lymph nodes.

plasmomas; 56,61,63–66). This new technology may become the most cost-effective way to evaluate focal pulmonary lesions, although more clinical studies are needed to determine its full value.

VI. Staging

A. Non–Small-Cell Carcinoma

Once the diagnosis of bronchogenic carcinoma has been established, accurate staging becomes essential for therapeutic decisions and prognostic information.

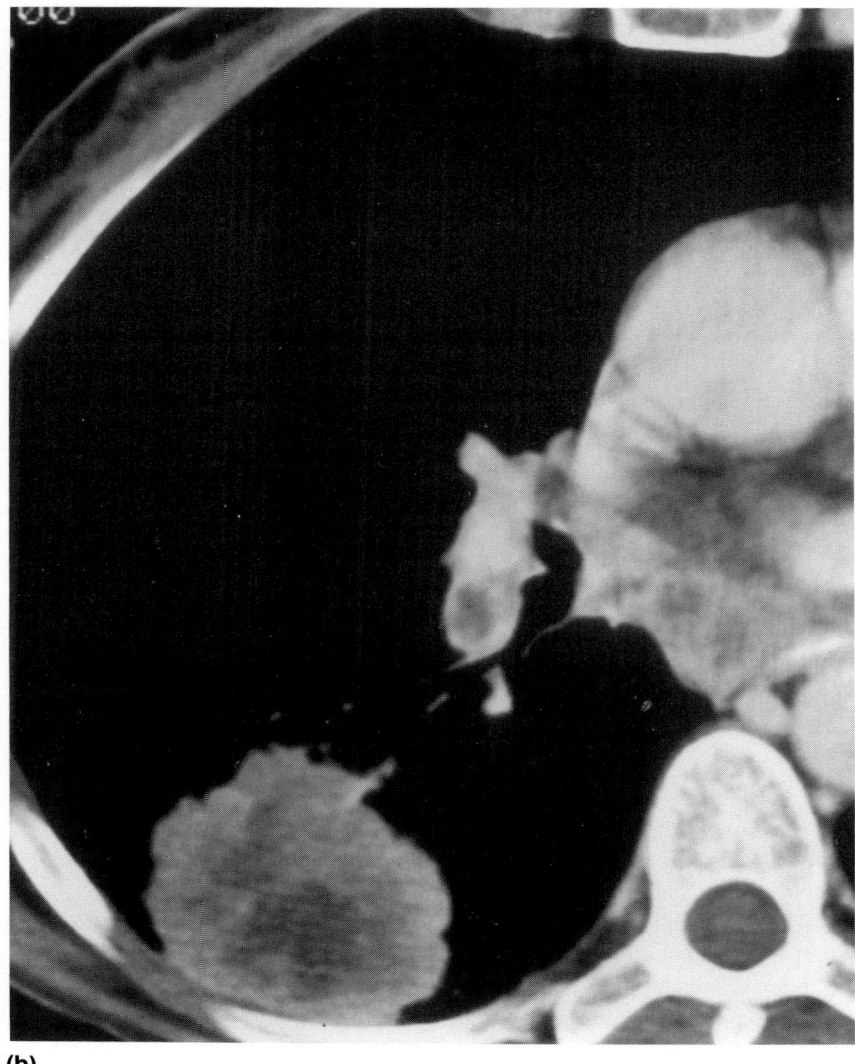

(b)

The TNM system for non–small-cell carcinoma (NSCC) enables a standardized description of the anatomical extent of disease (67–71). Radiologic studies, including chest radiographs, CT, and occasionally magnetic resonance imaging (MRI) are used together with clinical information and invasive procedures to stage patients (72). The appropriate role of imaging in NSCC management still remains

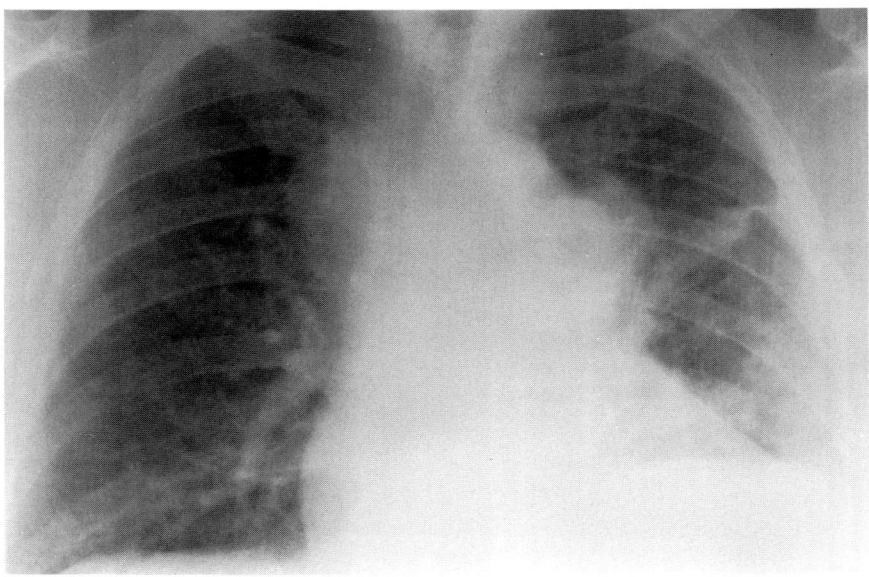

(a)

Figure 9 Small cell carcinoma: (a) Chest PA radiograph with lobular enlargement of the left hilum and mediastinum caused by extensive adenopathy. There is a small left upper lobe mass and a left effusion. (b,c) The CT scan shows low-attenuation mediastinal adenopathy with encasement of the left pulmonary artery and diffuse narrowing of the left main bronchus.

somewhat controversial, although the purpose of imaging is to accurately differentiate stage I–IIIa (potentially resectable) from stage IIIb–IV (nonresectable) cancer and limit unnecessary interventional procedures (72–74).

The American Joint Committee on Cancer (AJCC) International Staging System 8 for Lung Cancer (67,68) reflects revision and unification of earlier staging recommendations of the AJCC and the Internationale Union Contere Le Cancer (UICC) (67,68,71). The system has two main components: (1) cell typing and (2) description of the anatomical extent of malignancy.

Radiologic stage is described by using descriptors for the primary tumor and its local extent (i.e., size, location, and absence or presence of pleural, chest wall, or mediastinal invasion [T], presence or absence of hilar/mediastinal lymph node involvement [N], and extrathoracic metastatic disease [M]; 67,68).

Local Disease (T Status)

Radiologic assessment of the anatomical extent of lung cancer is essential in determining the appropriate use of bronchoscopy, mediastinoscopy, or percutane-

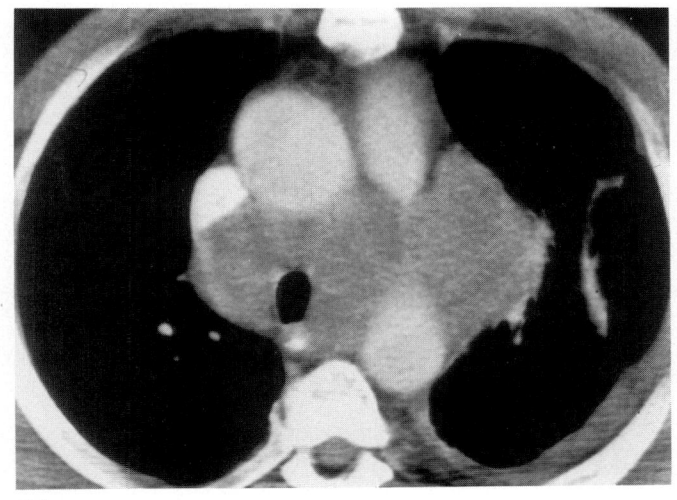

(b)

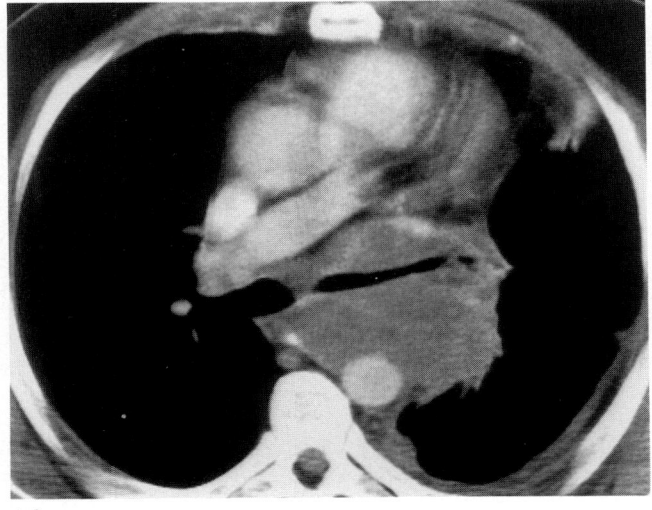

(c)

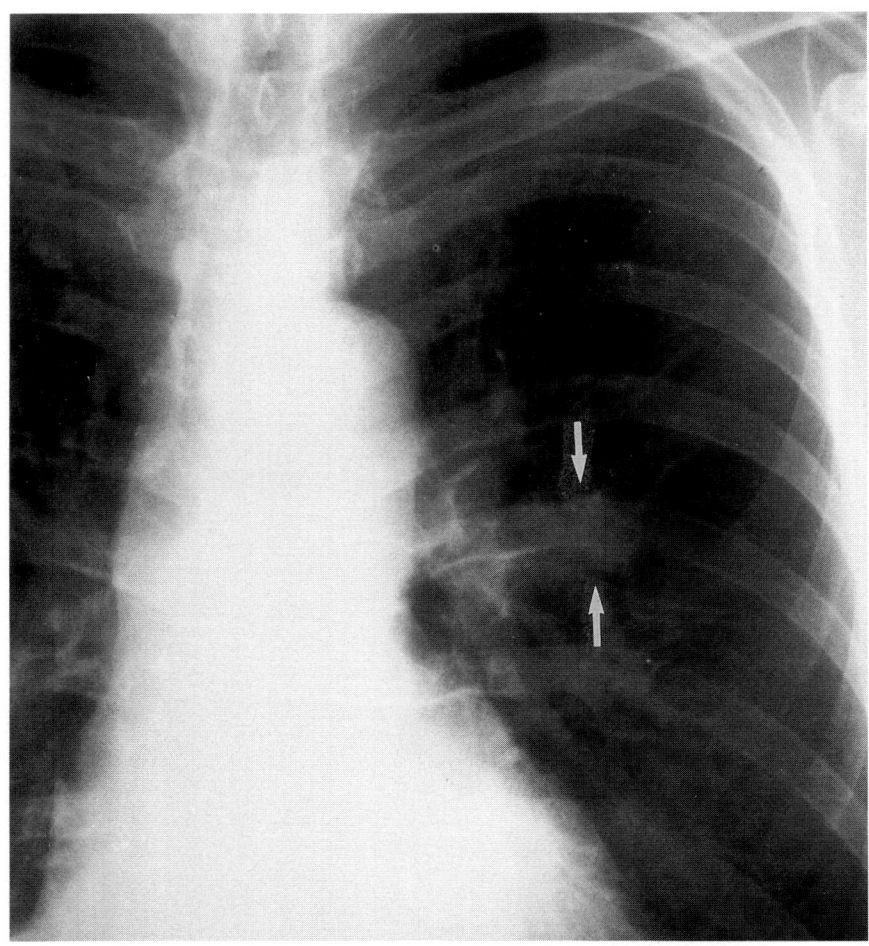

(a)

Figure 10 Adenocarcinoma: (a) A PA chest radiograph demonstrates a 1.5-cm left midlung nodule (arrows). (b) The CT image confirms the lingular nodule with somewhat irregular margins. (c) Axial FDG–PET image at the same level demonstrates increased activity within the nodule consistent with a malignancy.

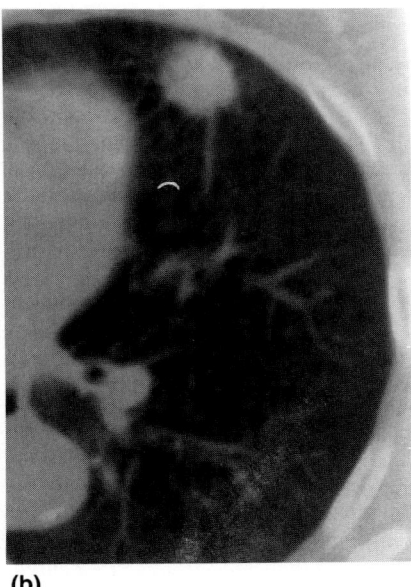

(b)

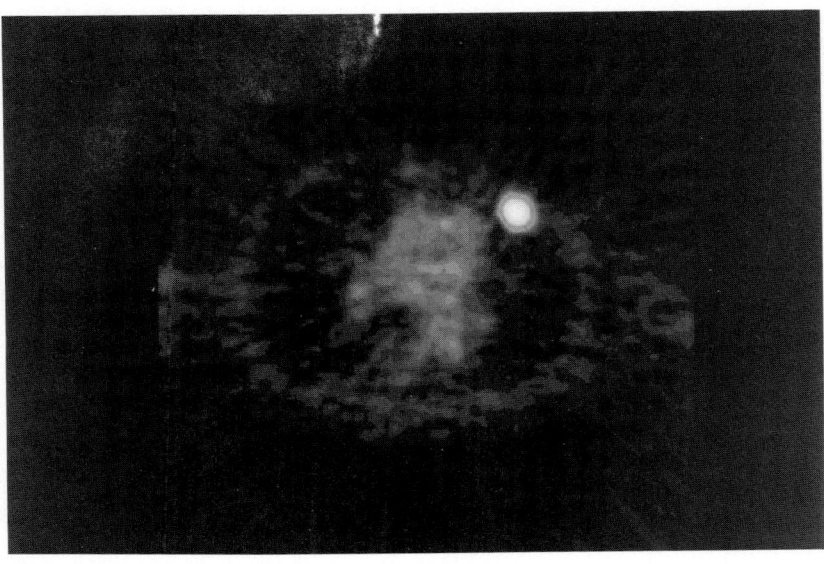

(c)

ous biopsy. Local invasion occurs in 8% of cases when the primary tumor is peripheral and contiguous with the chest wall (75). Limited local invasion is resectable, and defining peripheral tumor spread will influence the decision to perform an extrapleural dissection (tumor confined to parietal pleura) or an en bloc resection of lung and chest wall (75–79). Plain radiographs, CT, and MRI findings are often suggestive, but may not be definitive in confirming chest wall or local mediastinal invasion, unless a chest wall mass, rib destruction, or gross encasement of mediastinal structures is present (75,80,81). Additional useful MRI and CT findings that may indicate chest wall invasion include (76,77,82)

1. Tumor–pleura contact extending over more than 3 cm
2. An obtuse angle at the tumor–pleura interface
3. Thickening of the adjacent pleura
4. Increased attenuation of the extrapleural fat adjacent to the tumor

The overall accuracy of CT in confirming invasion has been reported to be 39–86% (65,75–77,82,83). Focal chest pain has a similar accuracy (85%) in determining chest wall invasion (77). Artificial pneumothorax and subsequent CT may be useful in assessing possible chest wall and mediastinal invasion. This procedure has a sensitivity of 100%, specificity of 57–80%, and accuracy of 76–100% (83,84). Limitations of the procedure include technical failure to induce pneumothoraces in the region of the hila, false-positive results associated with pleural adhesions, and poor tolerance of the procedure in patients with poor respiratory function (83,84).

An advantage of MRI in evaluating chest wall invasion is its superior soft-tissue contrast resolution and multiplanar capability (85,86). The sensitivity (63–90%) and specificity (84–86%) of MRI in diagnosing chest wall invasion is similar to CT (65,87,88). The superior contrast resolution of MRI may, however, define the extent of invasion better than CT and may be diagnostic when CT findings are equivocal (82,89). Magnetic resonance imaging is particularly useful in evaluation of superior sulcus tumors, as CT is limited by axial plane and streak artifact from the shoulders. An MRI scan can accurately assess the extent of local invasion and brachial plexus and subclavian vessel involvement (82,85,87,90–92). Vertebral body marrow invasion, a finding that would preclude resection, is also optimally assessed by MRI (91).

The CT and MRI scans have been reported to have similar accuracies in diagnosing mediastinal involvement (56–89% and 50–93%, respectively); however, MRI has recently been shown by the Radiologic Diagnostic Oncology Group (RDOG) trials to be more accurate than CT in assessing the mediastinum (82,87,93–95). T1-weighted images optimally demonstrate invasion of mediastinal fat by tumor, and mediastinal invasion adjacent to a hilar mass is easier to determine owing to the contrast between the tumor and flow void in vessels (91,96). The MRI and CT findings that are suggestive of mediastinal invasion include (80,82)

1. Obliteration of the fat plane between the descending aorta and the tumor
2. Tumor contacting more than 90° of the aortic diameter
3. Tumor–mediastinal contact extending over more than 3 cm

Most patients without these findings will have technically resectable disease (80,95).

Nodal Disease (N Status)

Both CT and MRI are often used to evaluate the hilar–mediastinal lymph nodes. Size is usually the only criterion used to distinguish normal and abnormal nodes, as morphology of lymph nodes (shape and definition) and T1/T2 signal characteristics are usually not useful (65). A short axis nodal diameter of 1 cm is often used as the upper limit of normal (97). Although CT and MRI are very accurate in demonstrating enlarged hilar nodes, this finding may be due to hyperplastic, reactive nodes, particularly if there is a postobstructive pneumonia (90,98). The accuracy of CT and MRI for detecting metastatic hilar (N1) disease is only 62–68% and 68–74%, respectively (93,99). This low accuracy of radiographic staging of N1 metastatic disease usually does not prevent surgical resection unless the person is a poor surgical candidate (65,98).

Assessment of mediastinal nodal status is also based on size, although metastatic disease can be found in normal-sized nodes, and enlarged nodes may be reactive (99,100). If mediastinal nodes are larger than 1 cm, the accuracy of CT or MRI for mediastinal nodal metastases is 56–82% and 50–82%, respectively (82,87,90,93,94,101). More accurate evaluation of metastatic lymph node disease (N2) may be possible using different a size criteria for specific American Thoracic Society (ATS) mediastinal regions (102). By using a short diameter of 13 mm as the upper limit of normal for nodes in the subcarina, precarinal, and tracheobrachial regions, and 10 mm for the remaining regions, the number of false-positive results can be markedly reduced (102). Preoperative staging of enlarged mediastinal lymph nodes may also be improved by comparing the largest nodes in the expected lymphatic drainage of the tumor with nodes in the rest of the mediastinum (103).

Current-imaging modalities are only suggestive and are not definitive for detecting the extent of disease. The limitations of chest radiographs and CT and MRI scans, which depend on morphological and anatomical findings, may be overcome by metabolic changes in tumor cells. Several studies with FDG-PET imaging have shown that it may be useful in detecting metastases (61,62). The use of PET has recently been demonstrated to be more accurate than CT in diagnosing the presence or absence of intrathoracic metastatic nodal disease (81 and 52%, respectively; Fig. 11; 61,104). Furthermore, the negative predictive value of enlarged nodes on CT that were not FDG avid was 100%, and the positive

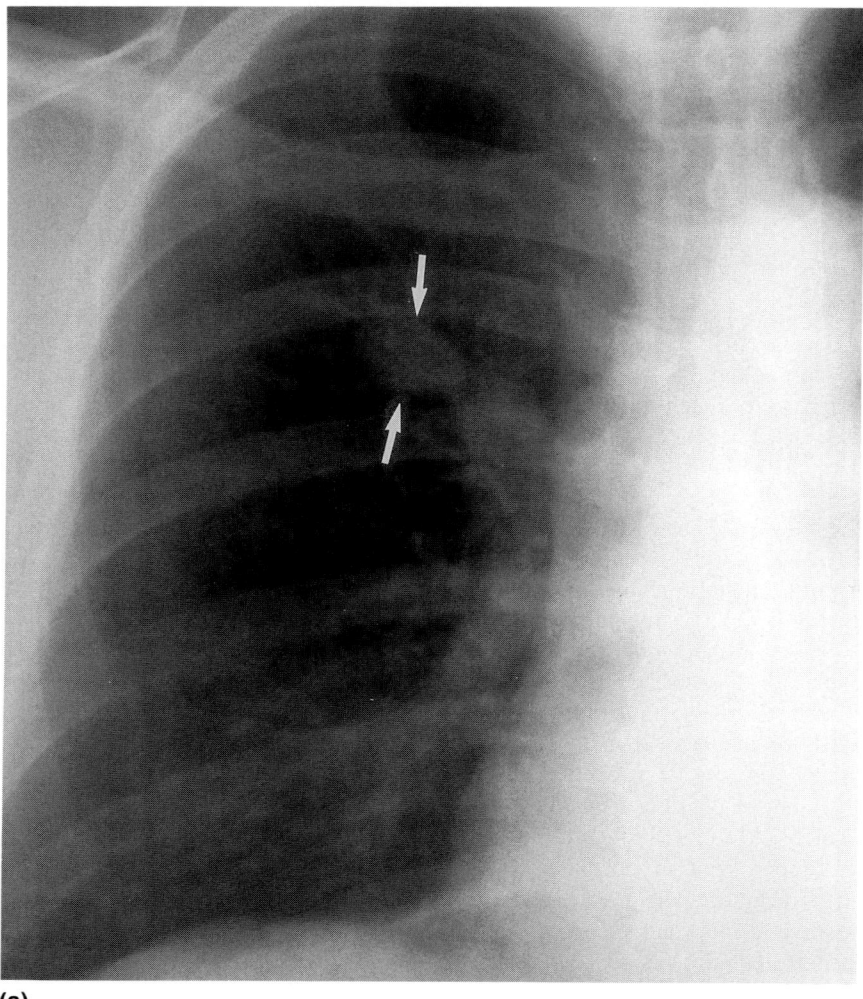

(a)

Figure 11 Squamous cell carcinoma: (a) PA chest radiograph demonstrates a 1.8-cm oval-shaped nodular opacity in the right upper lobe (arrows). There is no significant adenopathy. (b) Axial FDG–PET image demonstrates increased activity within the right upper lobe nodule. In addition, there is an area of slight increased uptake in a right paratracheal lymph node, which proved to be metastatic disease (N2) at thoracotomy.

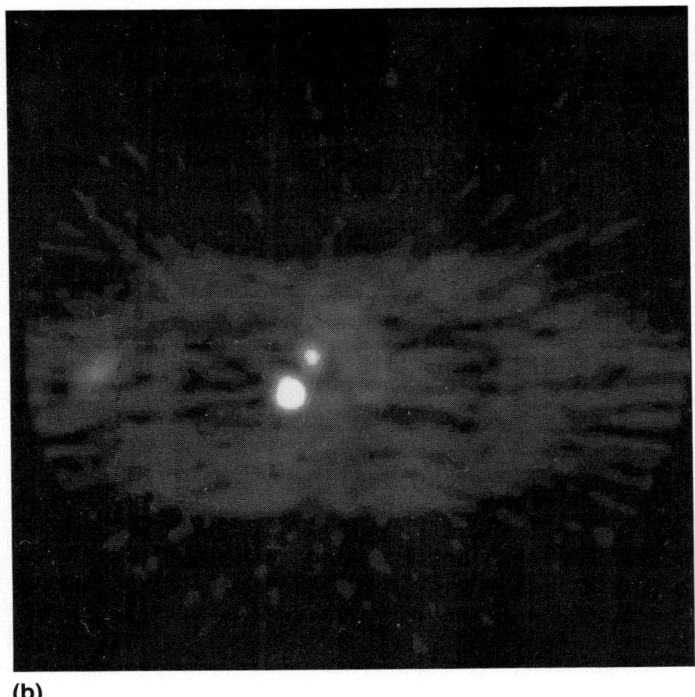

(b)

predictive values (PPV) was 100% for small nodes on CT with intense FDG uptake (105).

Metastatic Disease (M Status)

Common sites of metastases are lymph nodes, liver, adrenal glands, bones, and brain (82). Metastases to the contralateral lung also occur as a result of hematogenous dissemination and are considered M1 disease (82). Radiologic investigation of possible metastatic disease is often based on the clinical history, physical examination, and blood indices (complete blood cell counts, alkaline phosphatase, liver function tests; 73,106). Abnormal clinical and laboratory findings alone are inadequate in determining the extent of disease with an accuracy of only 49.3%, PPV of 36%, and NPV of 86.8% (107,108). If radiologic staging is performed only on the basis of symptomatology and abnormal laboratory indices, approximately 9% of patients with M1 disease will be incorrectly staged as candidates for curative resection (107). Routine radiologic evaluation for occult metastases in the absence of clinical or laboratory findings is not clearly defined (72,73,82,106).

Metastases to the central nervous system (CNS) have been reported to be a rare isolated finding in patients with NSCC and, when present, they are associated with an abnormal neurological examination (82,109). Routine CT or MRI scans of the CNS in asymptomatic patients with NSCC is controversial. Asymptomatic brain metastases occur in 2.7–9.6% of patients with NSCC and are usually associated with large-cell carcinomas and adenocarcinomas (107–110).

Patients with skeletal metastases are usually symptomatic or have laboratory abnormalities suggestive of bone metastases (107). Bone radiographs, radionuclide bone scanning with ^{99m}Tc-methylene diphosphonate (MDP) or MRI should be done to further evaluate a history of focal bone pain or elevated alkaline phosphatase (73). The detection of occult skeletal metastases by radionuclide ^{99}Tc-MDP is low (up to 4%), with a high false-positive rate (approximately 40%; 106–109). Because of these factors, routine radionuclide skeletal imaging should not be performed in NSSC.

Lung cancer has a propensity for adrenal metastases and because of the poor reliability of clinical and laboratory findings, upper abdominal imaging is often performed. The adrenal glands are easily evaluated on CT or MRI scans performed as part of the thoracic CT staging (Fig. 12). Nonfunctioning cortical adenomas occur as an incidental finding in 3–5% of the population, and approximately 10% of patients with NSCC who are being staged will have an adrenal mass (82,111,112). In the absence of extrathoracic metastases an adrenal mass is more likely to be an incidental or benign finding (82,111). Scans with CT and MRI are similar in detecting hepatic metastases, although isolated liver metastases are extremely uncommon, and routine liver imaging is not usually suggested (72,113,114).

B. Small-Cell Carcinoma

Radiologic and clinical staging of SCLC is also important to determine prognosis, and for treatment planning (115). Most oncologists use a two-stage classification proposed by the Veterans Administration Lung Cancer Study Group (VALG). This classification separates patients into limited or extensive disease and was initially proposed to determine suitability for radiotherapy (116). *Limited disease* defines tumor within a single radiotherapy port (tumor confined to the thorax). *Extensive disease* includes distant metastases and noncontiguous metastases to the contralateral lung (71,116). Long-term survival occurs primarily with limited disease and is rare with extensive disease (116). The VALG classification is not optimal, as there are subsets in the categories that have different therapeutic and prognostic implications that are not accounted for by this staging (116,117). A modified-staging system that defines clinical substages that are of prognostic importance may overcome this inadequacy (116,117).

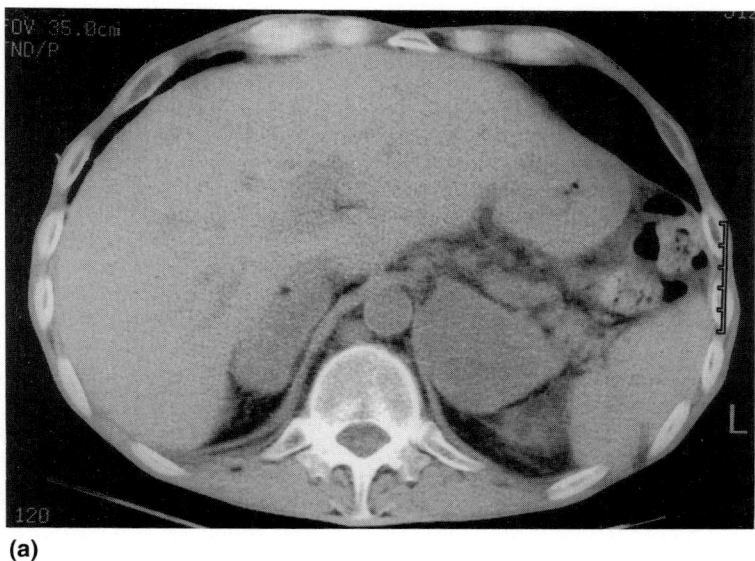

(a)

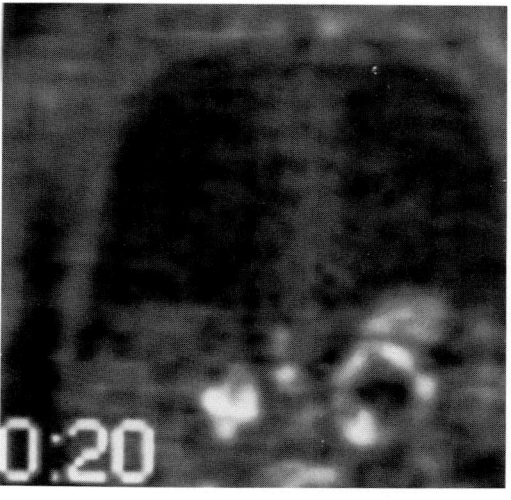

(b)

Figure 12 Metastatic adenocarcinoma: (a) Axial CT image demonstrates bilateral adrenal masses. (b) Coronal FDG–PET image demonstrates increased activity in both adrenal glands, consistent with metastatic disease.

Extensive disease is present in 60–80% of patients with SCLC at presentation (82,115,118,119). Metastatic disease commonly involves liver (22–28%), bone (30–38%), bone marrow (17–25%), brain (8–15%), and retroperitoneal lymph nodes (11%) (115,116,118–120). Conventional clinical and radiographic evaluation of extrathoracic metastatic disease usually includes bone marrow aspiration, radionuclide ^{99}Tc-MDP bone scan, and CT or MRI scans of the brain and abdomen (82,115,121). Recently, MRI has been used as a single-imaging study to assess the liver, adrenals, brain, and axial skeleton, and it staged SCLC more accurately than conventional staging (115).

Isolated bone and bone marrow metastases are uncommon and are usually associated with involvement of other organs (116,121). These patients often have no focal bone pain and alkaline phosphatase and peripheral blood findings are usually normal (116,121). Consequently, if there are extrathoracic metastases, further evaluation should include a routine radionuclide bone scan and bone marrow aspiration. An MRI scan may be more sensitive than bone scintigraphy in detecting small and rapidly growing metastases with marrow infiltration (115,122).

Liver function tests can be normal with hepatic metastases, and 25% of patients presenting with hepatic metastatic disease will not have involvement of other organs (116). Abdominal CT or ultrasound should be done routinely in the staging evaluation of SCLC (116). The MRI scan may be more sensitive than contrast-enhanced CT in detecting hepatic metastases and similar to CT in evaluation of adrenal metastases (115).

The CNS metastases are common at presentation and as a site of progressive disease (116). Routine CT or MRI evaluation of the CNS is recommended, because approximately 5% of patients with cerebral metastases are asymptomatic (123). Detection and treatment with aggressive chemotherapy and radiotherapy can decrease morbidity and improve prognosis if the brain is the only site of extrathoracic disease (116).

VII. Summary

Bronchogenic carcinoma continues to represent a major health problem in the United States. Unfortunately, survival remains dismal, despite advances in treatment options. As more is understood about basic tumor biology, molecular markers, and genetic abnormalities, newer, alternative stages in the screening, diagnosis, and treatment of lung cancer may have a significant effect on this devastating disease.

References

1. Rubin SA. Lung cancer: past, present, and future. J Thorac Imaging 1991; 7:1–8.

2. Osteen RT. Cancer Manual. 8th ed. Boston: American Cancer Society, 1990:1–576.
3. Bruderman I. Bronchogenic carcinoma. In: Baum GL, Wolinsky E, eds. Textbook of Pulmonary Diseases. 5th ed. Boston: Little, Brown & Co, 1994:1345–1391.
4. Samet JM. The epidemiology of lung cancer. Chest 1993; 103:20S–29S.
5. Filderman AE, Shaw C, Matthay RA. Lung cancer part I: etiology, pathology, natural history, manifestations, and diagnostic techniques. Invest Radiol 1986; 21:80–90.
6. Repace JL, Lowrey AH. Risk assessment methodologies for passive smoking-induced lung cancer. Risk Anal 1990; 10:27–37.
7. Saracci R. Asbestos and lung cancer: an analysis of the epidemiological evidence of the asbestos–smoking interaction. Am J Cancer 1977; 20:323–331.
8. National Research Council, Committee on the Biological Effects of Ionizing Radiation. Health risks of radon and other internally deposited alpha-emitters: BEIR IV. Washington DC: National Academy Press; 1988.
9. List AF, Doll DC, Greco FA. Lung cancer in Hodgkin's disease: association with previous radiotherapy. J Clin Oncol 1985; 3:215–221.
10. Boring CC, Squires TS, Tong T. cancer Statistics, 1993. CA 1993; 43:7–23.
11. Berlin NI, Buncher CR, Fontana RS, Frost JK, Melamed MR. Early lung detection. Am Rev Respir Dis 1984; 103:545–549.
12. Flehinger BJ, Kimmel M, Melamed MR. National history of adenocarcinoma—large cell carcinoma of the lung: conclusions from screening programs in New York and Baltimore. JNCI 1988; 80:337–344.
13. National Cancer Institute Cooperative Early Lung Cancer Group. Manual of Procedures. NIH publication 79-1972, 1979.
14. Epstein DM. The role of radiologic screening in lung cancer. Radiol Clin North Am 1990; 28:489–495.
15. Fink D. Guidelines for the cancer related checkup: recommendations and rationale. In: Textbook of Clinical Oncology. Atlanta: American Cancer Society 1991:153–176.
16. Strauss GM, Gleason RE, Sugarbaker DJ. Screening for lung cancer re-examined. A reinterpretation of the Mayo lung project randomized trial on lung cancer screening. Chest 1993; 103:337S–341S.
17. Flehinger BJ, Kimmel M, Melamed MR. The effect of surgical treatment on survival from early lung cancer. Chest 1982; 101:1013–1018.
18. Chu K, Smart C. Chest x-rays reduce lung cancer mortality [abstr]. Proc Am Soc Clin Oncol 1990; 9:59.
19. Sider L. Radiographic manifestations of primary bronchogenic carcinoma. Radiol Clin North Am 1990; 28:583–597.
20. Haque AK. Pathology of carcinoma of lung: an update on current concepts. J Thorac Imaging 1991; 7:9–20.
21. World Health Organization. The World Health Organization histological typing of lung tumours. Am J Clin Pathol 1982; 77:123–136.
22. Roggli VL, Vollmer RT, Greenberg SD, McGavran MH, Spjut HJ, Yesner R. Lung cancer heterogeneity: a blinded and randomized study of 100 consecutive cases. Hum Pathol 1985; 16:569–579.
23. Adelstein DJ, Tomashefski JF, Snow NJ, Horrigan TP, Hines JD. Mixed small cell and non–small cell lung cancer. Chest 1986; 89:699–704.

24. Vincent RG, Pickren JW, Lane WW, et al. The changing histopathology of lung cancer. Cancer 1977; 39:1647–1655.
25. Pietra GG. The pathology of carcinoma of the lung. Semin Roentgenol 1990; 25:25–33.
26. Cohen MH. Signs and symptoms of bronchogenic carcinoma. Semin Oncol 1974; 1:183–189.
27. Theros EG. Varying manifestations of peripheral pulmonary neoplasms: a radiologic–pathologic correlative study. AJR 1977; 128:893–914.
28. Byrd RB, Carr DT, Miller WE, Payne WS, Woolner LB. Radiographic abnormalities in carcinoma of the lung as related to histological cell. Thorax 1969; 24:573–575.
29. Byrd RB, Miller WE, Carr DT, Payne WS, Woolner LB. The roentgenographic appearance of squamous cell carcinoma of the bronchus. Mayo Clin Proc 1968; 43:327–332.
30. Woodring JH. Unusual radiographic manifestations of lung cancer. Radiol Clin North Am 1990; 28:599–618.
31. Felson B. Mucoid impaction (inspissated secretions) in segmental bronchial obstruction. Radiology 1979; 133:9–16.
32. Matthews MJ. Morphology of lung cancer. Semin Oncol 1974; 1:175–182.
33. Chaudhuri MR. Primary pulmonary cavitating carcinomas. Thorax 1973; 28:354–366.
34. Woodring JH, Stelling CB. Adenocarcinoma of the lung: a tumor with a changing pleomorphic character. AJR 1983; 140:657–664.
35. Hill CA. "Tail" signs associated with pulmonary lesions: critical reappraisal. AJR 1982; 139:311–316.
36. Mahoney MC, Shipley RT, Corcoran HL, Dickson BA. CT demonstration of calcification in carcinoma of the lung. AJR 1990; 154:255–258.
37. Heitzman ER. Bronchogenic carcinoma: radiologic–pathologic correlations. Semin Roentgenol 1977; 12:165–173.
38. Bakris GL, Mulopulos GP, Korchik R, Ezdinli EZ, Ro JAE, Yoon B. Pulmonary scar carcinoma. Cancer 1983; 52:493–497.
39. Limas C, Japaze H, Garcia-Bunuel R. "Scar" carcinoma of the lung. Chest 1971; 59:219–222.
40. Kuhlman JE, Fishman EK, Kuhjda FP, et al. Solitary bronchioloalveolar carcinoma: CT criteria. Radiology 1988; 167:379–382.
41. Ludington LG, Verska JJ, Howard T, Kypridakis G, Brewer LA III. Bronchiolar carcioma (alveolar cell), another great imitator; a review of 41 cases. Chest 1972; 61:622–628.
42. Metzger RA, Mulhern CB, Arger PH, Coleman BG, Epstein DM, Gefter WB. CT differentiation of solitary from diffuse bronchioloalveolar carcinoma. J Comput Assist Tomogr 1981; 5:830–833.
43. Epstein DM, Gefter WB, Miller WT. Lobar bronchioloalveolar cell carcinoma. AJR 1982; 139:463–468.
44. Miller WT, Husted J, Frieman D, Atkinson B, Pietra GG. Bronchioloalveolar carcinoma: two clinical entities with one pathologic diagnosis. AJR 1978; 130:905–912.
45. Montgomery RD, Stirling GA, Hamer NAJ. Bronchiolar carcinoma in progressive systemic sclerosis. Lancet 1964; 1:586–587.

46. Marcq M, Galy P. Bronchioloalveolar carcinoma. Am Rev Respir Dis 1973; 107:621–629.
47. Im J, Choi BI, Park JH, et al. CT findings of lobar bronchioloalveolar carcinoma. J Comput Assist Tomogr 1986; 10:320–322.
48. Hill CA. Bronchioloalveolar carcinoma: a review. Radiology 1984; 150:15–20.
49. Byrd RB, Miller WE, Carr DT, Payne WS, Woolner LB. The roentgenographic appearance of large cell carcinoma of the bronchus. Mayo Clin Proc 1968; 43:333–336.
50. Shin MS, Jackson LK, Shelton RW, Greene RE. Giant cell carcinoma of the lung. Chest 1986; 89:366–369.
51. Lewis E, Bernardino ME, Valdivieso M, Farha P, Barnes PA, Thomas JL. Computed tomography and routine chest radiography in oat cell carcinoma of the lung. J Comput Assist Tomogr 1982; 6:739–745.
52. Hansen M, Hansen HH, Dombernowsky P. Long-term survival in small cell carcinoma of the lung. JAMA 1980; 244:247–250.
53. Weiss W, Boucot KR, Cooper DA. The histopathology of bronchogenic carcinoma and its relation to growth rate, metastasis, and prognosis. Cancer 1970; 26:965–970.
54. Pearlberg JL, Sandler MA, Lewis JW Jr, Beute GH, Alpern MB. Small-cell bronchogenic carcinoma: CT evaluation. AJR 1988; 150:265–268.
55. Whitley NO, Fuks JZ, McCrea ES, et al. Computed tomography of the chest in small cell lung cancer: potential new prognostic signs. AJR 1984; 141:885–892.
56. Dewan NA, Gupta NC, Redepenning LS, Phalen JJ, Frick MP. diagnostic efficacy of PET–FDG imaging in solitary pulmonary nodules. Chest 1993; 104:997–1002.
57. Berquist TH, Bailey PB, Cortese DA, Miller WE. Transthoracic needle biopsy. Accuracy and complications in relation to location and type of lesion. Mayo Cl n Proc 1980; 55:475–481.
58. Herf SM, Suratt PM, Arora NS. Deaths and complications associated with transbronchial lung biopsy. Am Rev Respir Dis 1977; 115:708–711.
59. Fletcher EC, Levin DC. Flexible fiberoptic bronchoscopy and fluoroscopically guided transbronchial biopsy in the management of solitary pulmonary nodules. West J Med 1982; 136:477–483.
60. Wallace JM, Deutsch AL. Flexible fiberoptic bronchoscopy and percutaneous needle lung aspiration for evaluating the solitary pulmonary nodule. Chest 1982; 81:665–671.
61. Patz EF, Lowe VJ, Hoffman JM, et al. Focal pulmonary abnormalities: evaluation with F-18 fluorodeoxyglucose PET scanning. Radiology 1993; 188:487–490.
62. Gupta NC, Frank AR, Dewan NA, et al. Solitary pulmonary nodules: detection of malignancy with PET with 2-[F-18]-fluoro-2-deoxy-D-glucose. Radiology 1992; 184:441–444.
63. Strauss LG, Conti PS. The applications of PET in clinical oncology. J Nucl Med 1991; 32:623–648.
64. Kubota K, Matsuzawa T, Fujiwara T, et al. Differential diagnosis of lung tumor with positron emission tomography: a prospective study. J Nucl Med 1990; 31:1927–1933.
65. Quint LE, Francis IR, Wahl RL, Gross BH, Glazer GM. Preoperative staging of non–small-cell carcinoma of the lung: imaging methods. AJR 1995; 164:1349–1359.

66. Kubota K, Yamada S, Ishiwata K, Ito M, Ido T. Positron emission tomography for treatment evaluation and recurrence detection compared with CT in long-term follow-up cases of lung cancer. Clin Nucl Med 1992; 17:877–881.
67. Mountain CF. A new international staging system for lung cancer. Chest 1986; 89(suppl):225S–233S.
68. Mountain CF. Prognostic implications of International Staging System for Lung Cancer. Semin Oncol 1988; 15:236–245.
69. Friedman PJ. Lung cancer: update on staging classifications. AJR 1988; 150:261–264.
70. Mann H, Karwande SV. The new proposed International Staging System for Lung Cancer. Semin Ultrasound CT MR 1988; 9:34–39.
71. Stitik FP. The new staging of lung cancer. Radiol Clin North Am 1994; 32:635–647.
72. Templeton PA, Caskey CI, Zerhouni EA. Current uses of CT and MR imaging in the staging of lung cancer. Radiol Clin North Am 1990; 28:631–646.
73. Stitik FP. Staging of lung cancer. Radiol Clin North Am 1990; 28:619–630.
74. Epstein DM, Stephenson LW, Gefter WB, van der Vorde F, Aronchik JM, Miller WT. Value of CT in the preoperative assessment of lung cancer: a survey of thoracic surgeons. Radiology 1986; 161:423–427.
75. Pennes DR, Glazer GM, Wimbush KJ, Gross BH, Long RW, Orringer MB. Chest wall invasion by lung cancer: limitations of CT evaluation. AJR 1985; 144:507–511.
76. Ratto GB, Piacenza G, Frola C, et al. Chest wall involvement by lung cancer: computed tomographic detection and results of operation. Ann Thorac Surg 1991; 51:182–188.
77. Glazer HS, Duncan-Meyer J, Aronberg DJ, Moran JF, Levitt RG, Sagel SS. Pleural and chest wall invasion in bronchogenic carcinoma: CT evaluation. Radiology 1985; 157:191–194.
78. Piehler JM, Pairolero PC, Weiland LH, Offord KP, Payne WS, Bernatz PE. Bronchogenic carcinoma with chest wall invasion: factors affecting survival following en block resection. Ann Thorac Surg 1982; 34:684–691.
79. Patterson GA, Ilves R, Ginsberg RJ, Cooper JD, Tood TRJ, Pearson FG. The value of adjuvant radiotherapy in pulmonary and chest wall resection for bronchogenic carcinoma. Ann Thorac Surg 1982; 34:693–697.
80. Glazer HS, Kaiser LR, Anderson DJ, et al. Indeterminate mediastinal invasion in bronchogenic carcinoma: CT evaluation. Radiology 1989; 173:37–42.
81. Pearlberg JL, Sandler MA, Beute GH, Lewis JW Jr, Madrazo BL. Limitations of CT in evaluation of neoplasms involving chest wall. J Comput Assist Tomogr 1987; 11:290–293.
82. Klein JS, Webb WR. The radiologic staging of lung cancer. J Thorac Imaging 1991; 7:29–47.
83. Yokoi K, Mori K, Miyazawa N, Saito Y, Okuyama A, Sasagawa M. Tumor invasion of the chest wall and mediastinum in lung cancer: evaluation with pneumothorax. Radiology 1991; 181:147–152.
84. Watanabe A, Shimokata K, Saka H, Nomura F, Sakai S. Chest CT combined with artificial pneumothorax: value in determining origin and extent of tumor. AJR 1991; 156:707–710.

85. Webb WR, Sostman HD. MR imaging of thoracic disease: clinical uses. Radiology 1992; 182:621–630.
86. Rapoport S, Blair DN, McCarthy SM, Desser TS, Hammers LW, Sostman HD. Brachial plexus: correlation of MR imaging with CT and pathologic findings. Radiology 1988; 167:161–165.
87. Webb WR, Gatsonis C, Zerhouni EA, et al. CT and MR imaging in staging non-small cell bronchogenic carcinoma: report of the Radiologic Diagnostic Oncology Group. Radiology 1991; 178:705–713.
88. Padovani B, Mouroux J, Seksik L, et al. Chest wall invasion by bronchogenic carcinoma: evaluation with MR imaging. Radiology 1993; 187:33–38.
89. Haggar AM, Pearlberg JL, Froelich JW, et al. Chest-wall invasion by carcinoma of the lung: detection by MR imaging. AJR 1987; 148:1075–1078.
90. Webb WR. MR imaging in the evaluation and staging of lung cancer. Semin Ultrasound CT MR 1988; 9:53–66.
91. McLoud TC, Filion RB, Edelman RR, Shepard JO. MR imaging of superior sulcus carcinoma. J Comput Assist Tomogr 1989; 13:233–239.
92. Castagno AA, Shuman WP. MR imaging in clinically suspected brachial plexus tumor. AJR 1987; 149:1219–1222.
93. Martini N, Heelan R, Westcott J, et al. Comparative merits of conventional, computed tomographic, and magnetic resonance imaging in assessing mediastinal involvement in surgically confirmed lung carcinoma. J Thorac Cardiovasc Surg 1985; 90:639–648.
94. Musset D, Grenier P, Carette MF, et al. Primary lung cancer staging: prospective comparative study of MR imaging with CT. Radiology 1986; 160:607–611.
95. McLoud TC. CT of bronchogenic carcinoma: indeterminate mediastinal invasion. Radiology 1989; 173:15–16.
96. Webb WR, Jensen BG, Sollitto R, et al. Bronchogenic carcinoma: staging with MR compared with staging with CT and surgery. Radiology 1985; 156:117–124.
97. Glazer GM, Gross BH, Quint LE, Francis IR, Bookstein FL, Orringer MB. Normal mediastinal lymph nodes: number and size according to American Thoracic Society Mapping. AJR 1985; 144:261–265.
98. McLoud TC, Bourgouin PM, Greenberg RW, et al. Bronchogenic carcinoma: analysis of staging in the mediastinum with CT by correlative lymph node mapping and sampling. Radiology 1992; 182:319–323.
99. Glazer GM, Gross BH, Aisen AM, Quint LE, Francis IR, Orringer MB. Imaging of the pulmonary hilum: a prospective comparative study in patients with lung cancer. AJR 1985; 145:245–248.
100. Glazer GM, Orringer MB, Chenevert TL, et al. Mediastinal lymph nodes: relaxation time/pathologic correlation and implications in staging of lung cancer with MR imaging. Radiology 1988; 168:429–431.
101. Staples CA, Müller NL, Miller RR, Evans KG, Nelems B. Mediastinal nodes in bronchogenic carcinoma: comparison between CT and mediastinoscopy. Radiology 1988; 167:367–372.
102. Ikezoe J, Kadowaki K, Morimoto S, et al. Mediastinal lymph node metastases from

nonsmall cell bronchogenic carcinoma: reevaluation with CT. J Comput Assist Tomogr 1990; 14:340–344.
103. Buy J, Ghossain MA, Poirson F, et al. Computed tomography of mediastinal lymph nodes in nonsmall cell lung cancer. J Comput Assist Tomogr 1988; 12:545–552.
104. Patz EF Jr, Lowe VJ, Goodman PC, Herndon J. Thoracic nodal staging with positron emission (PET) and ^{18}F-2-fluoro-2-deoxy-D-glucose in patients with bronchogenic carcinoma. Chest 1995; 108:1617–1621.
105. Wahl RL, Quint LE, Greenough RL, Meyer CR, White RI, Orringer MB. Staging of mediastinal non–small cell lung cancer with FDG PET, CT, and fusion images: preliminary prospective evaluation. Radiology 1994; 191:371–377.
106. Little AG, Stitik FP. Clinical staging of patients with non–small cell lung cancer. Chest 1990; 97:1431–1438.
107. Salvatierra A, Baamonde C, Llamas JM, Cruz F, Lopez-Pujol J. Extrathoracic staging of bronchogenic carcinoma. Chest 1990; 97:1052–1058.
108. Quinn DL, Ostrow LB, Porter DK, Shelton DK Jr, Jackson DE Jr. Staging of non–small cell bronchogenic carcinoma. Chest 1986; 89:270–275.
109. Hooper RG, Tenholder MF, Underwood GH, Beechler CR, Spratling L. Computed tomographic scanning of the brain in initial staging of bronchogenic carcinoma. Chest 1984; 85:774–776.
110. Mintz BJ, Tuhrim S, Alexander S, Yang WC, Shanzer S. Intracranial metastases in the initial staging of bronchogenic carcinoma. Chest 1984; 86:850–853.
111. Oliver TW Jr, Bernardino ME, Miller JI, Mansour K, Greene D, Davis WA. Isolated adrenal masses in nonsmall-cell bronchogenic carcinoma. Radiology 1984; 153:217–218.
112. Sandler MA, Pearlberg JL, Madrazo BL, Gitschlag KF, Gross SC. Computed tomographic evaluation of the adrenal gland in the preoperative assessment of bronchogenic carcinoma. Radiology 1982; 145:733–736.
113. Fretz CJ, Stark DD, Metz CE, et al. Detection of hepatic metastases: comparison of contrast-enhanced CT, unenhanced MR imaging, and iron oxide-enhanced MR imaging. AJR 1990; 155:763–770.
114. Ferrucci JT. MR imaging of the liver. AJR 1988; 147:1103–1116.
115. Jelinek JS, Redmond J, Perry JJ, et al. Small cell lung cancer: staging with MR imaging. Radiology 1990; 177:837–842.
116. Abrams J, Doyle LA, Aisner J. Staging, prognostic factors, and special considerations in small cell lung cancer. Semin Oncol 1988; 15:261–277.
117. Shepherd FA, Ginsberg RJ, Haddad R, et al. Importance of clinical staging in limited small-cell lung cancer: a valuable system to separate prognostic subgroups. J Clin Oncol 1993; 11:1592–1597.
118. Mirvis SE, Whitley NO, Aisner J, Moody M, Whitacre M, Whitley JE. Abdominal CT in the staging of small-cell carcinoma of the lung: incidence of metastases and effect on prognosis. AJR 1987; 148:845–847.
119. Osterlind K, Ihde DC, Ettinger DS, et al. Staging prognostic factors in small cell carcinoma of the lung. Cancer Treat Rep 1983; 67:3–9.
120. Dunnick NR, Ihde DC, Johnston-Early A. Abdominal CT in the evaluation of small cell carcinoma of the lung. AJR 1979; 133:1085–1088.

121. Stahel RA, Ginsberg R, Havemann K, et al. Staging and prognostic factors in small cell lung cancer: a consensus report. Lung Cancer 1989; 5:119–126.
122. Mehta RC, Wilson MA, Perlman SB. False-negative bone scan in extensive metastatic disease: CT and MR findings. J Comput Assist Tomogr 1989; 13:717–719.
123. Bunn PA Jr, Rosen ST. Central nervous system manifestations of small cell lung cancer. In: Aisner J, ed. Contemporary Issues in Clinical Oncology: Lung Cancer. New York: Churchill Livingstone, 1985:287–305.

5

Metastatic Disease to the Chest from Extrathoracic Primary Malignancy

LYNN COPPAGE

Medical University of South Carolina
Charleston, South Carolina

I. Introduction

The role of chest imaging in the evaluation of extrathoracic malignancy (ETM) is complex and depends on multiple factors, including the propensity of the extrathoracic malignancy to metastasize to the thorax, time course from diagnosis, and potential for further therapy. A basic understanding of the incidence of intrathoracic involvement and mechanism of spread for specific primary tumors is necessary to plan a practical, cost-efficient, radiographic approach, both at the time of initial diagnosis and also in follow-up. Currently used imaging modalities include plain chest radiography, fluoroscopy, computed tomography (CT)—spiral volumetric, low dose, and high resolution CT (HRCT)—as well as evolving techniques, such as magnetic resonance imaging (MRI) and positron emission tomography (PET) scanning. The conventional chest radiograph and CT still remain the mainstays in the radiographic evaluation of thoracic involvement.

II. Frequency

Metastatic disease to the thorax may involve the lung parenchyma, mediastinal and hilar lymph nodes, airways, and pleura. The overall incidence of metastases to the lung parenchyma at autopsy ranges from 20 to 54% (Table 1; 1–4). The most common sources include tumors of the breast, kidney, colon, head, and neck (3,4). Other tumors (e.g., choriocarcinoma and osteosarcoma) although rare, have a higher rate of parenchymal metastases (4,5).

Metastatic involvement of hilar and mediastinal lymph nodes is less common. In a large series, intrathoracic nodal enlargement was demonstrated on conventional chest radiographs in 2.3% (6). The incidence would likely be higher if evaluated with computed tomography or at autopsy. Tumors of the genitourinary system, head and neck, and breast accounted for most cases.

Gross involvement of the major airways in patients who died of solid tumors was present in 2% of 342 patients in one study (7). Microscopic invasion of proximal and distal airways has been described in 18–50% (8,9). However, when these studies citing higher figures are reviewed to include only those patients likely to have had clinically significant airway involvement (i.e., gross central lesions), the incidence falls to less than 5%. Primary tumors, which account for most endobronchial metastases, are carcinomas of the kidney and colon–rectum (7).

Table 1 Incidence of Pulmonary Metastases

Primary	Frequency of metastases in terms of given primary (autopsy)	Frequency of metastases at presentation for a given primary	Frequency of a given primary in autopsy-identified lung metastases
Kidney	75	5	11
Osteosarcoma	75	15	1
Choriocarcinoma	75	61	
Thyroid	65	7	3.3
Melanoma	60	5	1.3
Breast	55	4	21.6
Prostate	40	5	4.1
Head and neck	30	5	10
Esophagus	20	20	1.7
Stomach	20	20	3.9
Liver	20	20	1.9
Pancreas	20	25	5.4
Colorectal	15	5	9.4
Uterus	15	5	5.8
Ovary	10	2.7	5

Source: Ref. 24.

III. Mechanisms of Spread

Mechanisms by which tumors spread to the thorax include hematogenous or lymphatic dissemination, direct extension, and rarely, endobronchial spread.

The lung has a rich vascular supply and is the first capillary bed encountered by cells of many primary cell types. The process of hematogenous dissemination, implantation, and progression to a viable parenchymal metastatic deposit is the result of complex biological and anatomical factors (10,11). Cells first detach from the tumor mass of origin and penetrate into the bloodstream, where they are transported to other capillary beds within the body. In the lungs, they become lodged in the pulmonary arterioles and capillary bed, and a small percentage become viable metastases following adhesion and penetration through the endothelium. New blood vessels, usually from the pulmonary arterial system, develop, and multiple cycles of cell division must occur before a radiographically visible nodule is detected (10).

Lymphangitic carcinomatosis (LC) is also most often the result of initial hematogenous dissemination, with subsequent invasion of the peripheral lymphatics (2,12). Hilar and mediastinal lymph nodes may become secondarily infiltrated, or nodal involvement may be the result of direct spread through lymphatic channels (13,14).

Knowledge of "typical" modes of spread of different histological types of tumors is helpful in formulating a diagnostic and follow-up imaging plan. The ETMs can be divided into three main categories: (1) those that tend to metastasize first to the lungs, (2) those that typically seed other organs first, and (3) those that independently spread to the lungs and other organs (15,16). Therefore, in the search for metastatic spread, intrathoracic involvement with tumors in category 1 (e.g., osteosarcoma) can be expected as an early manifestation, and routine screening for pulmonary metastases will have a higher yield than with category 2 malignancies (e.g., prostate carcinoma), for which pulmonary disease typically follows other organ (bone) involvement (17). Simultaneous metastatic disease (category 3) is seen in multiple malignancies, including cancer of the breast, kidney, rectum, and bladder.

IV. Radiographic Appearance

A. Parenchyma

The most common radiographic appearance of parenchymal metastatic disease is one of multiple spherical nodules of varying size, located in the periphery or subpleural region of the lungs (3,19). Metastatic foci range in size from miliary to greater than 5 cm, with most smaller than 5 mm (3). The lung bases are involved to a greater degree in most instances; however, alterations in blood flow in a given patient may change this typical distribution (20). On thin-section CT image, a vascular connection to a metastatic lesion may be seen when the feeding vessel runs parallel to the imaging plane. This appearance on CT correlated closely with experimental studies that demonstrated a pulmonary circulation as principal blood supply to metastatic lesions (versus a primary bronchial circulation in bronchogenic carcinomas; 21).

Typically, the margins appear well defined on plain chest radiographs and conventional CT, a feature helpful in distinguishing metastatic foci from primary lung carcinoma, in which the margins tend to be spiculated. "Shaggy" or ill-defined metastatic deposits, presumably owing to hemorrhage, have been described in patients with choriocarcinoma (22)—although this is a relatively unusual appearance—in metastatic Kaposi's sarcoma, and in a variety of other malignancies following chemotherapy (20). A recent study, correlating the appearance of pulmonary metastases on HRCT with histopathological sections in patients who had received chemotherapy and subsequently died, demonstrates a spectrum in margin characteristics for a variety of cell types (23).

Even though metastatic nodules typically vary in size, a uniform miliary pattern (suggestive of disseminated tuberculosis or other granulomatous disease) can be seen with medullary carcinoma of the thyroid and, on occasion, with other ETMs, such as breast, melanoma, and serous carcinoma of the ovary (24). Large, "cannonball" metastases bring to mind colorectal carcinoma, renal cell carcinoma, sarcomas, and melanoma, among others (Fig. 1).

Spontaneous cavitation of parenchymal metastases occurs in less than 4%, most frequently in squamous cell types, although sarcomas and adenocarcinomas may cavitate as well (25). Cavitation is more common following chemotherapy. Wall thickness and contour are not always reliable indicators of benignity or malignancy. Most cavities of neoplastic origin have thick and irregular walls; however, thin to nearly imperceptible walls (which can be seen only on CT), have been described in cases of metastatic testicular teratoma and transitional cell carcinoma of the bladder following chemotherapy (26,27). Spontaneous pneumothorax is unusual, but does occur, primarily with sarcomatous tumors, and is presumably the result of necrosis of a pleural-based metastasis and extension through the visceral pleura (Fig. 2; 28).

Radiographically visible calcification or ossification of metastases is rare, but has been described with osteosarcoma, chondrosarcoma, and a variety of other malignancies (29). In osteosarcoma, the mechanism relates to bone formation in the osteoid matrix produced by the tumor cells. Dystrophic calcification is a second mechanism that occurs in metastatic foci following chemotherapy (Fig. 3) and in the production of psammoma bodies in tumors, such as papillary carcinoma of the thyroid. A third mechanism, mucoid calcification, has been described in mucinous adenocarcinomas of the gastrointestinal tract and breast (29). The demonstration of calcified nodules in a patient with a known ETM can be prop-

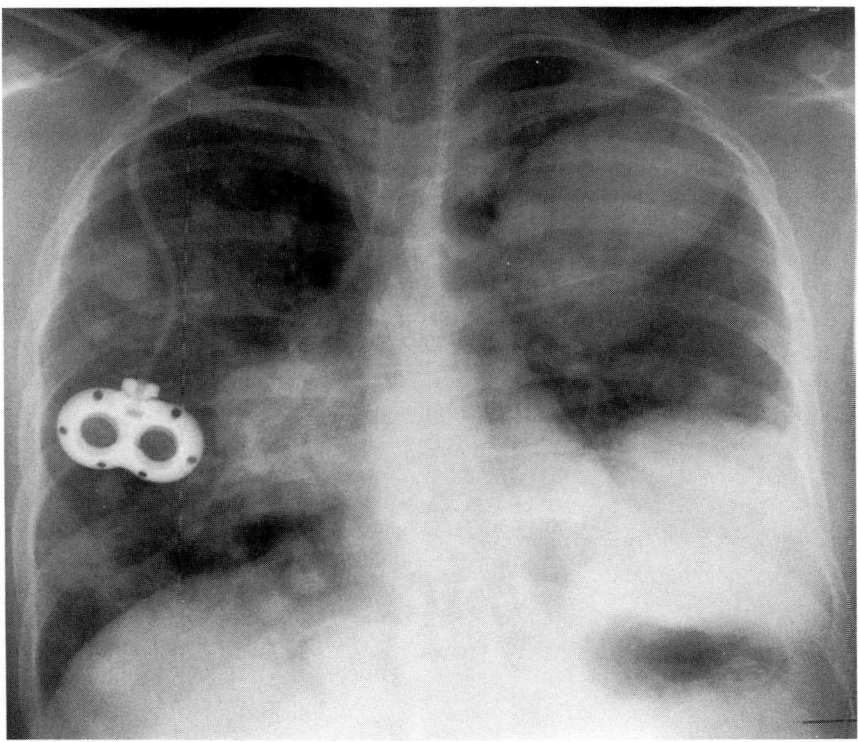

Figure 1 "Cannonball" metastases, synovial cell sarcoma: Posteroanterior chest radiograph in a 29-year-old woman with metastatic synovial cell sarcoma demonstrates multiple parenchymal nodules, including cannonball size (larger than 3 cm) masses.

lematic. If prior radiographs are available and reveal stability, a benign etiology, such as granulomatous disease, can be assumed. However, this is often not the case, and analysis of the pattern of calcification may be helpful. Central, laminated, popcorn, or eggshell calcifications are considered benign. This is best characterized on a thin-section CT image. However, there is overlap between these classic "benign" patterns and the appearance of some calcified or ossified metastatic lesions. Therefore, in a patient with a known ETM, the presence of new or enlarging calcified nodules may necessitate biopsy if confirmation of metastatic disease will alter therapy.

Metastatic parenchymal nodules and mediastinal lymph nodes demonstrating low attenuation on CT (-8 to 8 Hounsefield units; HU) have been observed in patients with testicular carcinoma (30) or sarcoma (Fig. 4), either before or after

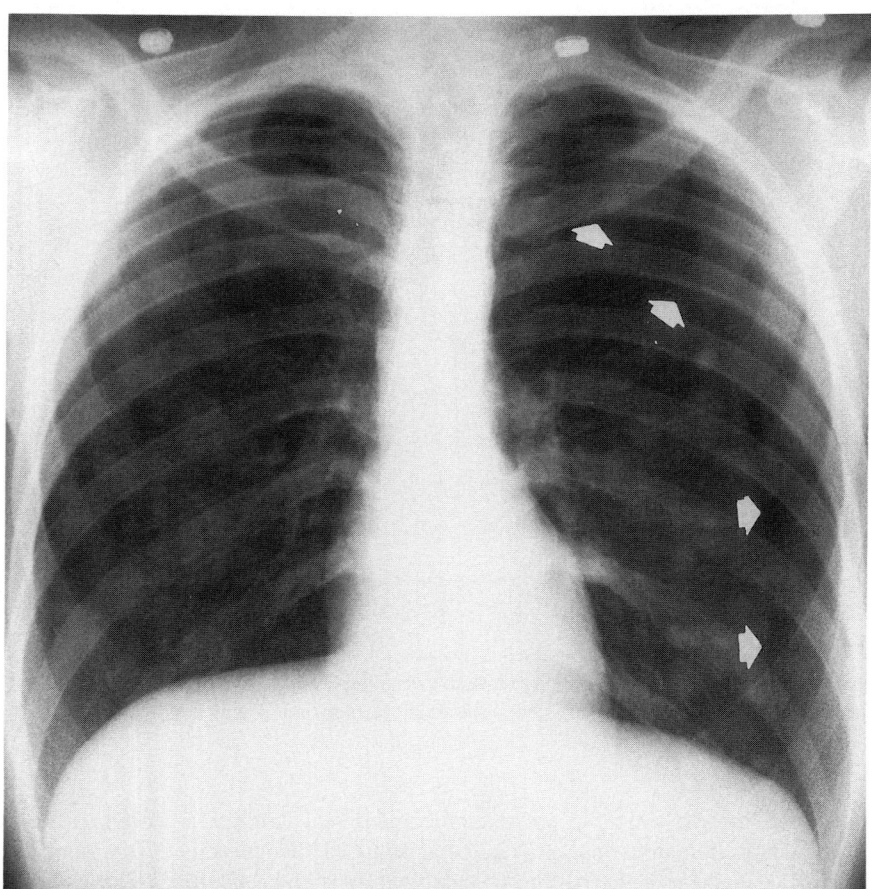

Figure 2 Spontaneous pneumothorax in a patient with metastatic leiomyosarcoma: Frontal view coned to the left hemithorax in a 56-year-old woman presenting with chest pain and a history of leiomyosarcoma demonstrates multiple cavitary metastases and a spontaneous pneumothorax (arrows). On the right, metastatic lesions and a smaller pneumothorax were also present.

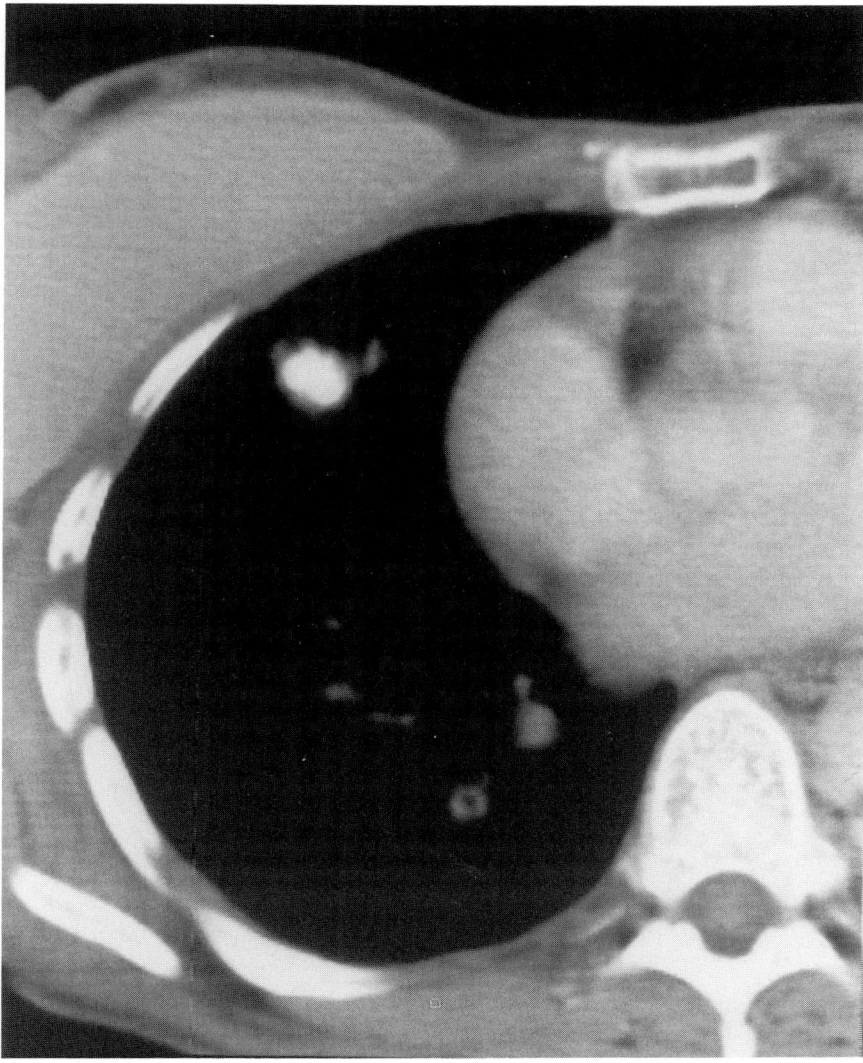

Figure 3 Dystrophic calcification, treated adenocarcinoma: Serial CT scans in a patient receiving chemotherapy for metastatic adenocarcinoma of the breast revealed progressive calcification in multiple parenchymal metastatic foci, such as the densely calcified nodule in the middle lobe. Failure to review the previous examinations could lead to an erroneous interpretation of multiple, benign, calcified granulomata.

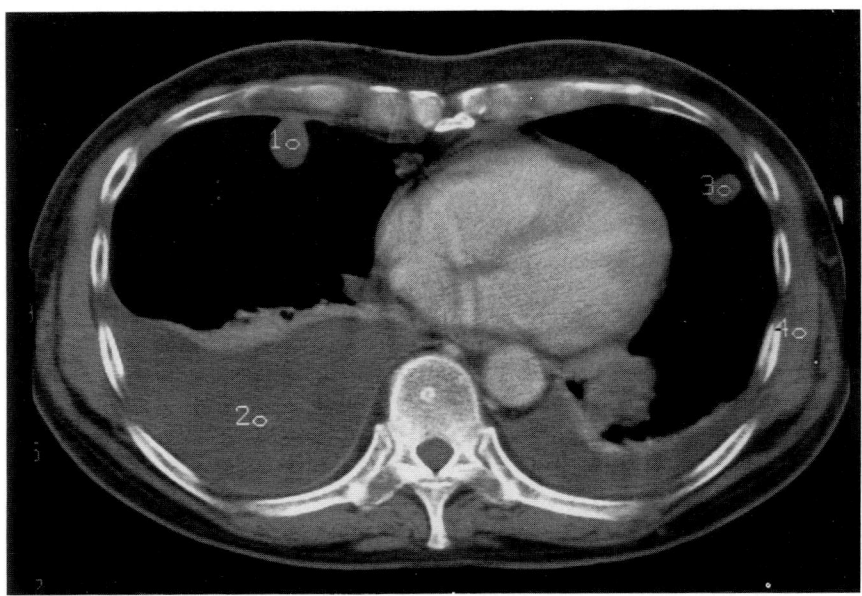

Figure 4 Low-attenuation metastases, soft-tissue sarcoma: Axial CT image through the lower thorax in this 66-year-old man with metastatic sarcoma reveals bilateral pleural effusions and low-density parenchymal nodules measuring 6–23 Hounsefield units (HU) (pleural fluid 6 HU and muscle 39 HU).

treatment. This has been ascribed to necrosis or cystic degeneration of the metastatic foci, or to lipid-laden macrophages within necrotic tumor (30).

B. Differential Diagnosis

Although the presence of multiple spherical nodules in a patient with a known ETM is highly suggestive of metastatic disease, other possible etiologies should be considered and correlated with relevant history and examination. Many patients are immunocompromised following chemotherapy; therefore, opportunistic infections are common in this setting. Metastatic lesions may mimic pulmonary infarction and organizing pneumonia when irregular in configuration and located in a subpleural area (3,19). Albeit unusual, certain chemotherapeutic agents, notably bleomycin and methotrexate, have been associated nodular parenchymal opacities (20,24,31).

On occasion, metastatic nodules will initially decrease in size in response to therapy, but then remain stable. These may contain residual tumor cells, indicating a partial response, or they may be "sterilized," with fibrous tissue seen only on histopathological examination (32,33). The two may coexist in the same patient (34). In patients with testicular carcinoma, maturation to cystic teratomas has occurred following chemotherapy (35).

In the patient with a known ETM, the development of new solitary, pulmonary nodule presents a diagnostic challenge. Depending on the histological type of the primary tumor, the patient's age and smoking history, the incidence of a primary lung cancer may exceed that of a solitary metastasis. In a study of 800 patients with a known ETM and a new pulmonary nodule, 63% of the lesions represented a primary lung neoplasm, 25% had a solitary metastasis, and 1.4% had a benign etiology (36). In most patients, the diagnosis can be made with percutaneous biopsy under fluoroscopic or CT guidance.

C. Intrathoracic Lymph Nodes

Hilar or mediastinal adenopathy, resulting from metastatic disease, is indistinguishable from adenopathy from a variety of causes, including metastatic bronchogenic carcinoma, lymphoma, sarcoidosis, and other granulomatous diseases. The pattern of intrathoracic adenopathy varies with the tumor type and respective lymphatic drainage. In a study (6) of 25 patients with nodal involvement from a variety of ETMs, hilar and right paratracheal lymph nodes were involved with the greatest frequency, whereas enlarged subcarinal and posterior mediastinal lymph nodes were infrequently observed on conventional chest radiographs. Unilateral hilar adenopathy was present in 8 of 25 (32%) patients, with or without mediastinal adenopathy, and bilateral hilar adenopathy was present in 7 of 25 (28%). Enlarged right paratracheal lymph nodes were noted in 60% (Fig. 5). Posterior mediastinal or subcarinal involvement was noted in only 2 patients (6). In a more recent study (37), in which 200 patients with testicular seminoma were evaluated with chest radiographs and CT, the subcarinal and posterior mediastinal nodal stations were most frequently involved, followed by the right paratracheal chain. In a retrospective review (38) of 50 patients with infradiaphragmatic malignancies and presumed thoracic nodal disease, on the basis of enlarged lymph nodes or malignant pattern of calcification on CT, the right paratracheal chain was involved in 82%, followed by the subcarinal group in 62%, the posterior mediastinal chain in 52%, and the aorticopulmonary window in 50%. Although these studies cite relatively infrequent involvement of anterior intrathoracic nodes, reports of patients with breast cancer reveal a high incidence of internal mammary adenopathy, a finding that influences surgical approach in operable patients and has a negative influence on 10-year survival statistics (39). The second anterior

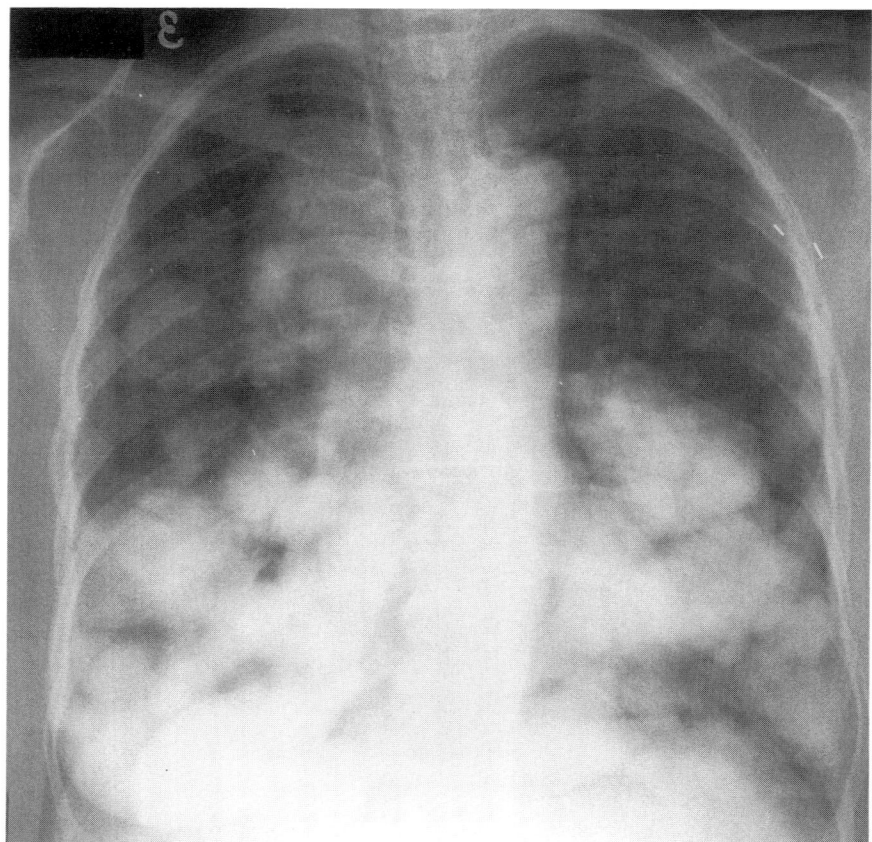

Figure 5 Mediastinal and parenchymal metastatic disease, breast carcinoma: Posteroanterior chest radiograph in a patient with a history of breast carcinoma (note left mastectomy defect and axillary surgical clips) and papillary carcinoma of the thyroid demonstrates bulky right paratracheal lymphadenopathy and widespread parenchymal nodules of varying size. Percutaneous biopsy of a peripheral lung nodule was consistent with metastases from the breast primary.

intercostal space is most commonly affected, although contiguous involvement of multiple levels is observed in a significant percentage of patients (40).

In the foregoing studies, the incidence of concomitant parenchymal nodules again varied among tumor types, from 17% in the patients with testicular seminoma, to 58% in those with infradiaphragmatic malignancies (37,38).

D. Pleural and Pericardial Metastases

Carcinomas of the lung account for 36% of malignant pleural effusions, breast for 25%, lymphoma for 10%, and ovarian and gastric for 5% each. Up to 7% of patients with malignant effusions have an unknown primary site at the time of diagnosis (41). Approximately 50% of all patients with breast carcinoma will develop a malignant pleural effusion during the course of their disease, and the pleura will be the only site of recurrence in some of these (42,43). Metastatic involvement of the pleura most commonly manifests as an effusion, although nodular pleural studding may be observed. Subtle pleural implants are best demonstrated on contrast-enhanced CT scans on which they appear as small, enhancing soft-tissue masses that typically make obtuse angles with the chest wall (44). Diffuse unilateral pleural involvement can mimic mesothelioma (Fig. 6).

Metastatic disease to the pericardium is often not detected clinically, but is discovered only at autopsy. It generally presents as a pericardial effusion, with distinct soft tissue pericardial nodules, rarely detected on echocardiographic or on CT scans. Neoplasms known to affect the pericardium include breast and lung carcinoma, melanoma, lymphoma, and leukemia (45).

E. Endobronchial Metastases

Metastatic involvement of the proximal airways may result from direct endobronchial implantation by hematogenous spread, or secondary invasion from adjacent metastatic foci in the lung parenchyma or lymph nodes. Although far less common than primary squamous cell carcinoma or adenoid cystic carcinoma, metastatic tracheal tumor deposits have been associated with a wide variety of tumors, including those of the colon or rectum, kidney, breast, prostate, and melanoma (46). The radiographic presentation of major airway involvement is indistinguishable from that of a central bronchogenic carcinoma, in which atelectasis (of a lung, lobe, or segment) or postobstructive pneumonia are frequent findings. A rounded endobronchial lesion is seen less often (Fig. 7). Contrast-enhanced CT scanning accurately distinguishes benign from malignant causes of atelectasis (47,48). It is a reliable-imaging modality for evaluating the proximal airways and is considered superior to MRI because of higher spatial resolution (49). Studies that compare the efficacy of CT with fibroscopic bronchoscopy in the evaluation of bronchial neoplasms show that CT findings correlated with bronchoscopic findings in 81–90% of patients with documented malignancy (50,51).

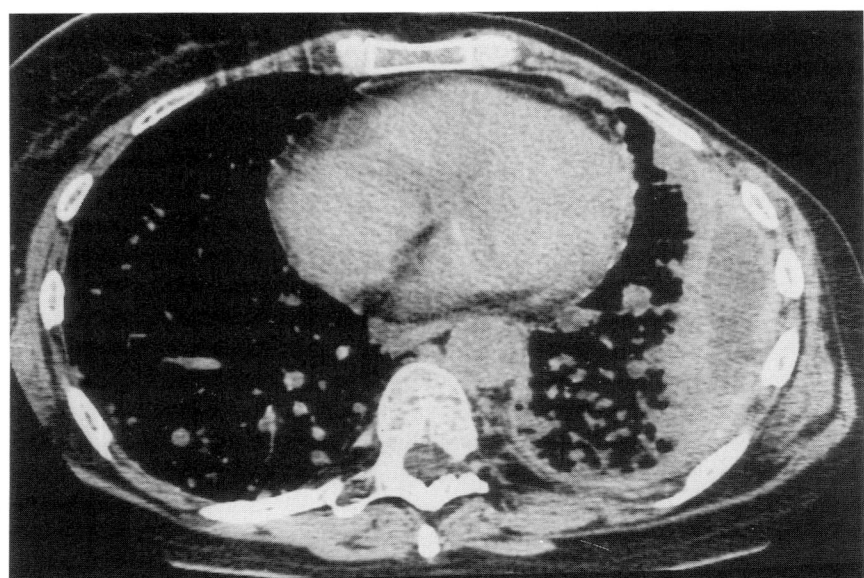

Figure 6 Metastatic pleural disease mimicking mesothelioma: Thin-section axial CT image through the lower hemithorax in a patient with metastatic breast carcinoma reveals a left mastectomy defect. Extensive unilateral nodular pleural thickening and effusion, with associated reduction in volume of the left hemithorax, mimics the appearance of mesothelioma. Bilateral parenchymal metastatic deposits were also present.

For optimal evaluation of the airways, routine 8- or 10-mm consecutive images should be followed by thin sections through the specific region of abnormality. A satisfactory alternative is 5-mm consecutive scans through the hilar regions (46). In addition to intraluminal abnormalities, CT will demonstrate the extent of spread into the mediastinum or hila, which may alter the therapeutic approach. Palliative treatment consists of surgery, external beam radiotherapy, or laser therapy, alone or in combination.

V. Detection

Initial-screening examination is the standard posteroanterior (PA) and lateral chest radiograph and comparison with prior examinations, if available. If new or enlarging nodules are detected and compatible in appearance with parenchymal metastases, no further imaging may be necessary. However, if the abnormality on the chest radiograph is questionable and the documentation of metastatic disease will

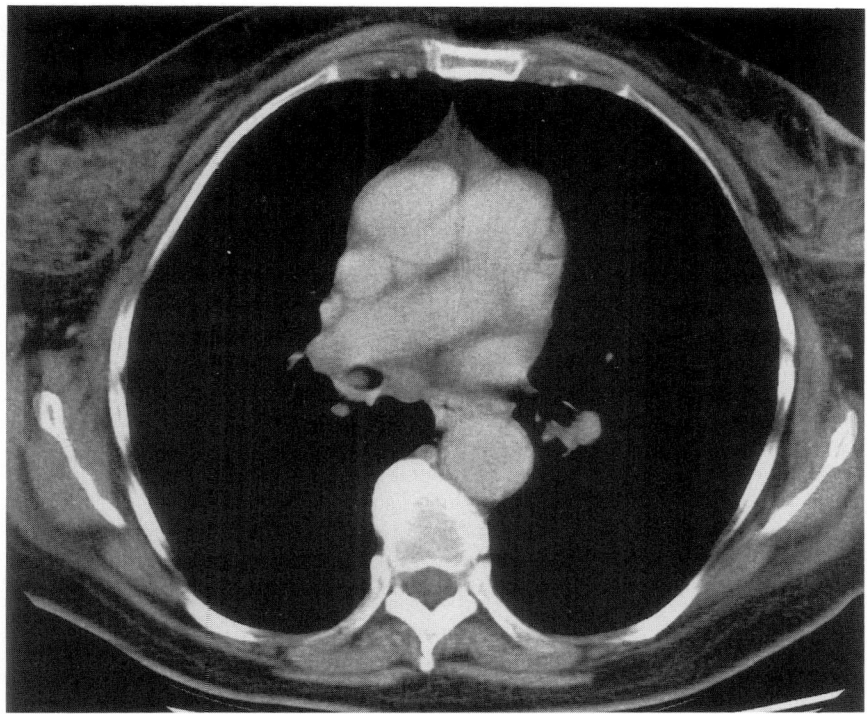

Figure 7 Endobronchial metastasis, malignant melanoma: Computed tomographic image through the midthorax in a 73-year-old patient with melanoma reveals a rounded soft-tissue metastasis (confirmed at bronchoscopy biopsy) in the bronchus intermedius . Also noted is a borderline in size subcarinal lymph node.

alter therapy, or if a new solitary pulmonary nodule is noted, further evaluation with CT and possibly biopsy may be indicated.

Even though surgical palpation consistently finds more nodules (median size 3 mm) than any imaging modality, numerous studies support the greater sensitivity of CT over conventional tomography and plain chest radiography (52–55). The specificity for metastatic disease in the additional nodules detected on CT varies between 45 and 95%, depending on several factors, including the primary tumor type, stage of the disease, and age of the patient (53–55). The highest specificity, 95%, was seen in a study of patients with only osteogenic or soft tissue sarcomas, malignancies that have a great propensity to metastasize to the lungs (55). Another study demonstrated a higher specificity for patients with sarcomas or melanomas (93%) versus carcinomas (77%) (34). The specificity also depends on the age of the patient population studied. The younger the population, the greater the specificity for metastatic disease, presumably because the benign causes of parenchymal opacities, including granulomatous disease, scarring, pulmonary infarcts, and organizing pneumonia are less common in the older population than in children and young adults. Wellner et al. (56) showed that 90% of lesions detected only by CT were metastatic in the 2–30 age range, whereas 67% were metastases in the 31- to 55-year-old group.

In the pediatric population in whom cumulative radiation dose over time is a theoretical factor, low-dose CT scanning in follow-up would have a distinct advantage in lowering radiation exposure and, presumably, the incidence of developing a second, radiation-induced malignancy later in life. In a study of a small group of patients, decreasing the current from 140 to 10 mA did not significantly affect visualization of parenchymal abnormalities (57). Streak artifact was present in the paravertebral regions in two patients, and there was degradation of image quality in the mediastinum (57). Additional studies with a larger cohort of patients with metastatic disease are needed to evaluate the usefulness of this scanning technique in the pediatric population.

Recent studies comparing conventional CT with spiral volumetric (helical) CT scanning demonstrate the superiority of spiral scans; more nodules are detected with this modality, owing to reduced respiratory artifact and slice misregistration (58–60). In the study by Remy-Jardin (59) of 39 patients, 2 patients with a negative conventional CT scan and 3 with a solitary nodule on 10-mm–collimated CT scans had multiple nodules at spiral CT. The mean number of nodules per patient was higher with helical than with conventional CT (18 vs. 12.6) as were the number of nodules smaller than 5 mm. All spiral CT scans were free of the respiratory motion artifact that was noted in 10% of the conventional scans (59). Detection of nodules in the periphery of the lung was thereby facilitated. These data indicate that spiral CT scanning is preferred; particularly when metastatectomy is being contemplated and the detection of additional nodules may alter the surgical approach.

Initial studies evaluating the relative sensitivity of MRI versus CT in the detection of pulmonary nodules supported the greater sensitivity of CT (61,62). Müller et al. (62), in a retrospective review of 25 patients imaged at 0.35 T without cardiac gating or respiratory motion compensation techniques, noted that approximately 15% of nodules between 3 and 10 mm were seen on CT, but were not detected by MRI. Most of these were located at the bases, in the region of greatest motion artifact. In one patient, more nodules close to blood vessels were detected with MRI, presumably easily distinguished by the lack of flow void phenomenon of the metastatic foci (62). In a more recent prospective study (63) of 11 patients imaged at 0.5 T, who underwent pathological confirmation at thoracotomy, the sensitivity of MRI (85%) exceeded that of conventional CT (70%) (63). Specifically, three nodules adjacent to the left ventricle were missed on CT. There were

13 false-positive nodules on MRI sequences and, of these, 46% were located in the perihilar region of the lung. Although the results of this study support the value of MRI, certain limitations remain. Magnetic resonance imaging is inherently poorly suited to detect calcification, a tool in differentiating benign from indeterminate lesions, and the signal characteristics of benign and malignant lesions overlap (64). Further studies are needed comparing the sensitivity of MRI with that of state-of-the-art spiral CT scanning. Additional considerations include the time required to complete the examination and relative ease of interpretation of the two modalities.

In patients with a known ETM and a new solitary pulmonary lesion, imaging with positron emission tomography (PET) with [^{18}F]fluorodeoxyglucose (FDG) may accurately differentiate between a benign and malignant etiology on the basis of increased glucose metabolism in tumor cells (65,66). In a study of 20 patients with an "indeterminate" solitary pulmonary nodule on CT, PET imaging demonstrated hypermetabolism in all 13 patients with a malignant etiology (at least 2 of which were metastatic) (66). Determination of a benign etiology would obviate the need for a more invasive diagnostic procedure (such as percutaneous biopsy) and, therefore, would have a particular role in patients with compromised lung function. However, the limited availability and high cost of the examination currently limit the use of PET scanning in the evaluation of the solitary pulmonary nodule (SPN).

High-resolution CT (HRCT) is the most accurate radiographic tool to diagnose lymphangitic carcinomatosis (LC). The diagnosis may be suggested on the conventional chest radiograph when a reticular or reticulonodular interstitial pattern with thickening of septal lines (Kerley's A and B lines) is detected. The interstitial abnormality may be unilateral or bilateral, diffuse or patchy, in distribution (67). Hilar adenopathy is present in less than 50%, a fact that supports the hypothesis of a bloodborne mechanism for LC versus retrograde extension from diseased hilar nodes (68). In up to 50% of patients with an appropriate clinical presentation and pathologically proved LC, the chest radiograph is normal or equivocal (69). It is in this patient population that HRCT has a particular role by demonstrating subtle features of LC and in guiding bronchoscopic biopsy and bronchoalveolar lavage. Although interstitial abnormality is detected in the vast majority of these patients with conventional 10-mm–collimated scans, thin-section CT more accurately depicts the well-described findings characteristic of LC (Fig. 8), including (1) thickening of the bronchovascular bundles, (2) increase in the number and thickness of visible interlobular septa, (3) nodular or "beaded" thickening of the fissures (68,70,71). Stein et al. (68), in 7 of 12 patients, observed polygonal arcades on HRCT that are felt to represent thickened interlobular septa surrounding secondary lobules seen in cross section (68). All of the foregoing are typically unassociated with significant architectural distortion, a feature that helps distinguish LC from other causes of nodular bronchovascular thickening, such as

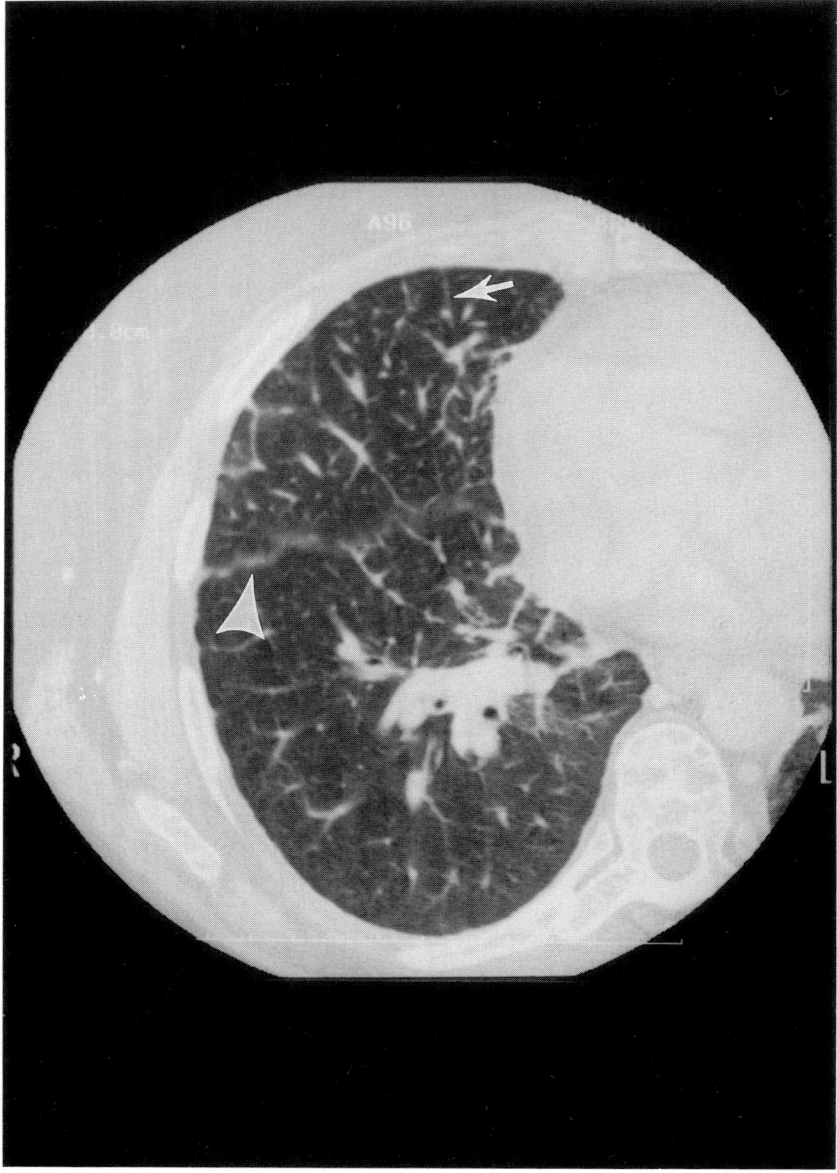

Figure 8 Lymphangitic carcinomatosis, breast carcinoma: Axial CT image through the lower right lung in 46-year-old woman with metastatic breast carcinoma shows "beaded" appearance of major fissure (arrowhead) and thickened interlobular septa (arrow) surrounding secondary pulmonary lobules.

sarcoidosis (71). Both conventional and HRCT underestimate the extent of subpleural lymphangitic tumor.

VI. Summary

A screening posteroanterior and lateral chest radiograph should be obtained in all patients with a known ETM, both at the time of initial diagnosis and in follow-up. If the chest radiograph demonstrates an equivocal finding, additional evaluation with oblique radiographs, fluoroscopy, or CT may be helpful, or if a new "SPN" is identified and the detection of additional nodules will alter therapy, CT is indicated. Further imaging is generally not necessary when multiple nodules are evident.

Routine CT scanning should be reserved for those patients with ETMs having a high propensity to metastasize to the chest, for whom early detection will affect therapy. Computed tomography should also be performed in cases where surgical resection of pulmonary metastases for cure is contemplated. Although all metastatic foci found at surgery may not be visualized, the results of the CT scan may alter the surgical approach (i.e., median sternotomy versus thoracotomy). It may also detect unsuspected involvement of the mediastinum, pleura, or chest wall (72).

Spiral volumetric CT scanning is preferred over conventional scanning, when available, as reduced respiratory motion artifact and slice misregistration results in higher sensitivity for the detection of pulmonary nodules. In the pediatric patient population, preliminary data suggest that low-dose scanning is a satisfactory alternative. High-resolution CT should be used for patients in whom there is clinical suspicion of lymphangitic carcinomatosis.

The role MRI in the evaluation of intrathoracic metastatic disease is not yet well defined. It has been shown that MRI is complementary to CT scanning in assessing the extent of mediastinal disease in patients who are allergic to intravenous contrast material and have known airway involvement (46). Further studies evaluating cost efficacy and sensitivity for state-of-the-art MRI and spiral CT scanning are needed.

References

1. Willis R. Secondary tumors of the lungs. In: The Spread of Tumors in the Human Body. 3rd ed. London: Butterworths & Co, 1973:167–174.
2. Spencer H. Secondary tumors in the lung. In: Pathology of the Lung. Vol. 2. 3rd ed. New York: Pergamon Press, 1977:1085–1099.
3. Crow J, Slavia G, Kreel L. Pulmonary metastasis: a pathologic and radiologic study. Cancer 1981; 47:2595–2602.

4. Gilbert HA, Kagan AR. Metastasis: incidence, detection and evaluation without histologic confirmation. In: Weiss L, ed. Fundamental Aspects of Metastases. Amsterdam: North Holland, 1976.
5. Saegesser F, Besson A, Kofai F. Pulmonary coin lesions and metastases. In: Saegesser F, Pettarol J, eds. Surgical Oncology. Baltimore: Williams & Wilkins, 1970:539–610.
6. McLoud TC, Kalisher L, Stark P, et al. Intrathoracic lymph node metastases from extrathoracic neoplasms. AJR 1978; 131:405–407.
7. Braman SS, Whitcomb ME. Endobronchial metastasis. Arch Intern Med 1975; 135:543–547.
8. Rosenblatt MB, Lisa JR, Trinidad S. Pitfalls in the clinical and histologic diagnosis of bronchogenic carcinoma. Dis Chest 1966; 49:396–404.
9. King DS, Castleman B. Bronchial involvement in metastatic pulmonary malignancy. J Thorac Surg 1943; 12:305–315.
10. Filderman AE, Coppage L, Shaw C, Matthay RA. The biology of pulmonary metastatic disease. Invest Radiol 1990; 25:215–224.
11. Hart IR, Saini A. Biology of tumour metastasis. Lancet 1992; 339:1453–1457.
12. Janower ML, Blennerhassett JB. Lymphangitic spread of metastatic cancer to the lung. Radiology 1971; 101:267–273.
13. Heitzman ER, Markarian B, Baasch BN, et al. Pathways of tumour spread through the lung: radiologic correlations with anatomy and pathology. Radiology 1982; 144:3–14.
14. Rouviere H. Tobias MJ, trans. Lymphatics of the lungs. In: Anatomy of the Human Lymphatic System. Ann Arbor: Edwards Brothers, 1938:113–118.
15. Bross IDK, Blumenson LE. Metastatic sites that produce generalized cancer identification and kinetics of generalizing sites. In: Weiss L, ed. Fundamental Aspects of Metastases. Amsterdam: North Holland, 1976:359–375.
16. Viadara E, Bross IJ, Pickren JQ. Cascade spread of blood borne metastasis in solid and non-solid cancers in humans. In: Weiss L, Gilbert HA, eds. Pulmonary Metastasis. Boston: GK Hall, 1978:143–167.
17. Batson OV. The vertebral vein system. AJR 1957; 78:195–212.
18. Apple JS, Paulson DF, Baber C, Putnam CE. Advanced prostate carcinoma: pulmonary manifestations. Radiology 1985; 154:601–604.
19. Scholten ET, Kreel L. Distribution of lung metastases in the axial plane. Radiol Clin North Am 1977; 46:248–265.
20. Libshitz HI. Pulmonary metastatic disease. In: Freundlich IM, Bragg DG, eds. A Radiologic Approach to Disease of the Chest. Baltimore: Williams & Wilkins, 1991:337–349.
21. Milne ENC, Zerhouii EA. Blood supply of pulmonary metastases. J Thorac Imaging 1987; 2:15–23.
22. Libshitz MI, Baber CE, Hammond CB. The pulmonary metastasis of choriocarcinoma. Obstet Gynecol 1977; 49:412–416.
23. Hirakada K, Naketa H, Haratake J. Appearance of pulmonary metastases on high-resolution CT scans: comparison with histopathologic findings from autopsy specimens. AJR 1993; 161:37–43.

24. Coppage L, Shaw C, Curtis AM. Metastatic disease to the chest in patients with extrathoracic malignancy. J Thorac Imaging 1987; 2:24–37.
25. Dodd GD, Boyle JJ. Excavating pulmonary metastases. AJR 1961; 85:272–293.
26. Charig MJ, Williams MP. Pulmonary lacunae: sequelae of metastases following chemotherapy. Clin Radiol 1990; 42:93–96.
27. Kier R, Godwin JD. Residual cavities of lung metastases following chemotherapy. Comput Radiol 1986; 10:293–296.
28. D'Angio GJ, Iannaccone G. Spontaneous pneumothorax as a complication of pulmonary metastases in malignant tumors of childhood. AJR 1961; 86:1092–1102.
29. Maile CW, Rodan BA, Godwin JD, et al. Calcification in pulmonary metastases. Br J Radiol 1982; 55:108–113.
30. Yousem DM, Scatarige JC, Fishman EK, et al. Low attenuation thoracic metastases in testicular malignancy. AJR 1986; 146:291–293.
31. Glasier CM, Siegel MJ. Multiple pulmonary nodules: unusual manifestation of bleomycin toxicity. AJR 1981; 137:155–156.
32. Libshitz HI, Baber CE, Hammond CB. The pulmonary metastases of choriocarcinoma. Obstet Gynecol 1977; 49:412–416.
33. Libshitz HI. Jing BS, Wallace S, et al. Sterilized metastases: a diagnostic and therapeutic dilemma. AJR 1983; 140:15–19.
34. Peuchot M, Libshitz HI. Pulmonary metastatic disease: radiologic–surgical correlation. Radiology 1987; 164:719–722.
35. Vogelzang NJ, Stenlund R. Residual pulmonary nodules after combination chemotherapy of testicular cancer. Radiology 1983; 146:195–197.
36. Cahan WG, Shah JP, Castro ELB. Benign solitary lung lesions in patients with cancer. Ann Surg 1978; 187:241–244.
37. Williams MP, Husband JE, Heron CW. Intrathoracic manifestations of metastatic testicular seminoma: a comparison of chest radiographic and CT findings. AJR 1987; 149:473–475.
38. Mahon TG, Libshitz HI. Mediastinal metastases of infradiaphragmatic malignancies. Eur J Radiol 1992; 15:130–134.
39. Veronesi V, Cascinellli N, Greco M, et al. Prognosis of breast cancer patients after mastectomy and dissection of internal mammary nodes. Ann Surg 1985; 202:702–707.
40. Scatarige JC, Fishman EK, Zinreich ES, et al. Internal mammary lymphadenopathy in breast carcinoma; CT appraisal of anatomic distribution. Radiology 1988; 167:89–91.
41. Sahn SA. Malignant pleural effusions. Semin Respir Med 1987; 9:43–53.
42. Fracchia AA, Knapper WH, Carey JT, et al. Intrapleural chemotherapy for effusion from metastatic breast carcinoma. Cancer 1970; 26:626–629.
43. Fentiman IS, Millis R, Sexton S, et al. Pleural effusion in breast cancer: a review of 105 cases. Cancer 1981; 47:2087–2092.
44. Sagel SS, Glazer HS. Lung, pleura and chest wall. In: Lee JKT, Sagel SS, Stanley RJ, eds. Computed Body Tomography with MRI Correlation. 2nd ed. New York: Raven Press, 1989:364–366.

45. Adenle AD, Edwards JE. Clinical and pathologic features of metastatic neoplasms of the pericardium. Chest 1982; 81:166–169.
46. Naidich DP. CT/MR correlation in the evaluation of tracheobronchial neoplasia. Radiol Clin North Am 1990; 28:555–571.
47. Woodring JH. Determining the cause of pulmonary atelectasis: a comparison of plain radiography and CT. AJR 1988; 150:757–763.
48. Tobler J, Levitt RG, Glazer HS, et al. Differentiation of proximal bronchogenic carcinoma from post obstructive lobar collapse by magnetic resonance imaging: comparison with computed tomography. Invest Radiol 1987; 22:538–543.
49. Mayr B, Heywang SH, Ingrisch H, et al. Comparison of CT with MR imaging of endobronchial tumors. J Comput Assist Tomogr 1987; 11:43–48.
50. Naidich DP, Lee JJ, Garay SM, et al. Comparison of CT and fiberoptic bronchoscopy in the evaluation of bronchial disease. AJR 1987; 148:1–7.
51. Henschke CI, Davis SD, Auh PR, et al. Detection of bronchial abnormalities: comparison of CT and bronchoscopy. J Comput Assist Tomogr 1987; 11:432–435.
52. Schaner EG, Chang AE, Doppman JL, et al. Comparison of computed tomography and conventional whole lung tomography in detecting pulmonary nodules: a prospective radiologic–pathologic study. AJR 1978; 131:51–54.
53. Muhm JR, Brown LR, Crowe JK, et al. Comparison of whole lung tomography and computed tomography for detecting pulmonary nodules. AJR 1978; 131:981–984.
54. Chang AE, Schaner EG, Conkle DM, et al. Evaluation of computed tomography in the detection of pulmonary metastases. Cancer 1979; 43:913–916.
55. Pass HI, Dwyer A, Makuch R, et al. Detection of pulmonary metastases in patients with osteogenic and soft tissue sarcomas; the superiority of CT scans compared with conventional linear tomograms using dynamic analysis. J Clin Oncol 1985; 3:1261–1265.
56. Wellner LJ, Putnam CE. Imaging of occult pulmonary metastases: state of the art. CA 1986; 36:48–58.
57. Naidich DP, Marshall CH, Gribbin C, et al. Low-dose CT of the lungs: preliminary observations. Radiology 1990; 175:729–731.
58. Costello P, Anderson W, Blume D. Pulmonary nodule: evaluation with spiral volumetric CT. Radiology 1991; 179:875–876.
59. Remy-Jardin M, Remy J, Giraud F, et al. Pulmonary nodules: detection with thick section spiral CT versus conventional CT. Radiology 1993; 187:513–520.
60. Collie DA, Wright AR, Williams JR, et al. Comparison of spiral acquisition computed tomography and conventional tomography in the assessment of pulmonary metastatic disease. Br J Radiol 1994; 67:436–444.
61. Berquist TH, Brown LR, May GR, et al. Magnetic resonance imaging of the chest: a diagnostic comparison with computed tomography and hilar tomography. Magn Reson Imaging 1984; 2:315–327.
62. Muller NL, Gamsu G, Webb WR. Pulmonary nodules: detection using magnetic resonance and computed tomography. Radiology 1985; 155:687–690.
63. Feuerstein IM, Jicha DL, Pass HI, et al. Pulmonary metastases: MR imaging with surgical correlation—a prospective study. Radiology 1992; 182:123–129.
64. Panicek DM. MR imaging for pulmonary metastases? Radiology 1992; 182:10–11.

65. Patz EF, Lowe VJ, Hoffman JM, et al. Focal pulmonary abnormalities: evaluation with F-18 Fluorodeoxyglucose PET scanning. Radiology 1993; 188:487–490.
66. Gupta NC, Frank AR, Dewan NA, et al. Solitary pulmonary nodules: detection of malignancy with PET with 2-(F-18)-fluoro-2-deoxy-D-glucose. Radiology 1992; 184:441–444.
67. Youngberg AD. Unilateral diffuse lung opacity. Radiology 1977; 123:277–281.
68. Stein MG, Mayo J, Muller NL, et al. Pulmonary lymphangitic spread of carcinoma: appearance on CT scans. Radiology 1987; 162:371–375.
69. Trapnell DH. The radiological appearances of lymphangitic carcinomatosa of the lung. Thorax 1964; 19:251–260.
70. Munk PL, Muller NL, Miller RR, et al. Pulmonary lymphangitic carcinomatosis: CT and pathologic findings. Radiology 1988; 166:705–709.
71. Diseases characterized by reticulonodular or nodular opacities. In: Webb WR, Muller NL, Naidich DP, eds. High Resolution CT of the Lung. New York: Raven Press, 1992:71–87.
72. Davis SD. CT evaluation for pulmonary metastases in patients with extrathoracic malignancy. Radiology 1991; 180:1–1.

6

Radiology of Chest Trauma

JOSEPH E. COX
Bowman Gray School of Medicine—Wake Forest University
Winston-Salem, North Carolina

PAUL L. MOLINA
University of North Carolina School of Medicine
Chapel Hill, North Carolina

I. Introduction

Trauma is the leading cause of death in persons 1–35 years of age and is the third most common cause of death overall in the United States (1). Thoracic trauma accounts for 25–33% of all deaths from trauma and contributes to mortality in at least another 25% (2–5). Multisystem trauma is most commonly associated with motor vehicle accidents, and chest injuries play a significant role in 50% of motor vehicle-related deaths.

In recent years, improved triage using telecommunication and expedited transport to regional trauma centers has enhanced survival of major trauma victims (1). The concept of regional trauma centers has evolved over the last 25 years. A report by the National Academy of Sciences in 1966 described accidental death and injury as the "neglected disease of modern society" (6). This report, together with the passage of the National Highway Safety Act and other legislation, led to funding of paramedic training programs and to improvement in hospital trauma care by funding regional trauma care systems (1). All hospitals are now ranked according to their trauma care capabilities. California adopted a three-level system that is also used in other states. Levels I and II require the continuous presence of an emergency department physician, anesthesiologist, and trauma surgeon within the hospital. Level I applies to a teaching hospital, with staff specialists, residents, and research programs. Level I and II trauma centers also require that a board-certified radiologist or senior resident be promptly available at all times. In addition, a technologist qualified in computed tomography (CT), angiography, and general radiography must be in the hospital 24 h/day (7). Both the emergency department and the operating suite must have radiographic equipment available. Level III trauma care most often applies to an institution in a community that lacks hospitals of level I or II capability.

II. Chest Wall Trauma

A. Rib Fractures

Rib fractures occur in approximately 56% of patients with major blunt thoracic trauma (8,9). The fourth through ninth ribs are most frequently fractured (2). As isolated findings, these fractures do not reliably predict underlying visceral injury. However, fractures of the lower ribs (10th through 12th ribs) should raise the possibility of hepatic, splenic, or renal injury, as well as associated intraperitoneal and retroperitoneal hemorrhage. The first three ribs and scapulae are well protected by upper-body musculature. Although fractures of these ribs are not in and of themselves an indication for angiographic assessment (10), they should heighten awareness of injuries to the aorta and great vessels, tracheobronchial tree, and adjacent neurovascular structures (11). Injuries to the aorta and great vessels are discussed in another chapter.

Flail chest is caused by segmental rib fractures involving contiguous ribs, or by multiple rib fractures in combination with a sternal fracture. The presence of a costal hook configuration at the site of rib fracture is a highly suggestive indicator of a flail segment (12). The hook-like configuration of the rib implies significant rotational displacement at a second, invisible fracture site. Flail chest is frequently associated with other serious chest injuries, such as lung contusion, lung laceration, and hemothorax, and is characterized clinically by paradoxical movement of the chest wall during respiration. Paradoxical respiratory motion may not be clinically apparent when the flail segment involves the upper three or four ribs (13). In flail chest, pendelluft ("pendulum air") has been proposed as a cause of respiratory failure (2). *Pendelluft* refers to the contralateral movement of deadspace air from lung on the flail side to lung on the nonflail side. In the absence of severe associated lung injury, however, functional disturbance is unlikely to be significant (5).

Although rib fractures are common in adults with blunt chest trauma, significant intrathoracic injury can be observed in children with no radiographically evident rib fractures (14–16). There are anecdotal reports of children with automobile tire imprints on their chests in the absence of rib fractures (17). The elastic and resilient pediatric rib cage, therefore, may not reflect the severity of chest trauma. Ogden (18) and Smyth (19) have suggested that pediatric rib fractures may be more common than suspected, given the difficulty in observing greenstick-type fractures radiographically. In a child, the presence of healing rib fractures, especially those located posteriorly in the paravertebral region (squeezing-type injury), should raise a suspicion of child abuse, and communication with the referring physician should be documented in the report.

Rib fractures are easily overlooked on chest radiographs, which may demonstrate only 18% of all rib fractures found at autopsy (8). In the acute trauma setting, optimal radiographic technique is often difficult to attain with most single-phase, line-operated portable x-ray machines. In addition, rib fractures are often nondisplaced, obscured by overlying structures, and imaged nontangentially. However, because the treatment of rib fractures is usually conservative, supplementary rib detail films generally are not indicated. A single upright frontal chest film should suffice (20). In a retrospective review of over 1100 cases of chest trauma by Dahner et al. (21), only 17 patients were admitted for reasons exclusively related to rib trauma, and in only 2 of these did oblique views of the ribs provide additional information, and even this was clinically inconsequential. Other reports support these findings (22,23).

The usual treatment for uncomplicated rib fractures is pain control. Relief of pain decreases splinting and improves pulmonary toilet. Strapping of the chest and, rarely, nerve block, may also be employed (20).

Rib fractures are commonly identified in the outpatient setting. Alcoholism is a strong possibility if the patient has multiple healed or healing rib fractures bilaterally. A 16-fold increase in the prevalence of rib fractures and thoracic vertebral fractures has been reported in alcoholic men (24). Chest radiographs may even be helpful in screening for alcoholism (24,25).

Stress fractures of the first and second ribs are associated with activities such as backpacking and surfing. Posterolateral rib stress fractures have been described in amateur golfers (26).

Cough fractures are most common in elderly patients and usually occur in the posterolateral aspects of the lower ribs. These fractures can be induced by a paroxysm of coughing (27) or by conditions that cause a chronic cough, such as postnasal drip (28).

B. Scapular Fractures

With the exception of sternoclavicular dislocations, fractures of the shoulder girdle are usually not of immediate concern in the acute trauma setting. Scapular fractures often remain undiagnosed on initial chest radiographs. Harris and Harris

(29) found that 70% of scapular fractures were overlooked on the initial chest film. They should be actively sought if regional skeletal and soft-tissue injuries are present.

C. Sternoclavicular Joint Dislocations

Anterior sternoclavicular joint dislocations are more common than posterior dislocations, but the latter are more serious, because they can impinge on the adjacent brachiocephalic vessels and trachea (2). Sternoclavicular joint dislocations are easily missed on frontal chest radiographs, but are usually evident clinically and are easily diagnosed with CT.

D. Sternal Fractures

Sternal fractures occur in up to 10% of patients after violent blunt trauma (2) and are most commonly located just inferior to the sternomanubrial junction. These fractures are almost always invisible on frontal chest films, but, if displaced, they can usually be seen on a lateral view. Computed tomography can aid in the detection of retrosternal hematoma, which may result from laceration of the internal mammary vessels by sternal fracture fragments. Computed tomography is also useful in assessing the integrity of the costochondral junctions. Sternal fractures should elicit concern about associated myocardial injury, such as myocardial contusion, which can lead to significant arrhythmias and hemodynamic instability. Mortality rates of 25–45% have been reported in patients with complicated sternal fractures because of concomitant cardiac, aortic, brachiocephalic, bronchial, or head injuries (30).

E. Thoracic Spine Fractures

Thoracic spine fractures account for approximately 25% of all spinal fractures (Fig. 1; 31). They typically result from hyperflexion and axial loading, which are common mechanisms of injury in motor vehicle accidents and in falls from great heights. Most thoracic spine fractures involve the lower thoracic spine (T-9 through T-11 vertebrae), the so-called functional thoracolumbar junction (32,33). The functional thoracolumbar junction refers to a change in the mechanical properties and configuration of articular facets from a "cervical" to a "lumbar" pattern between T-9 and T-11.

Compared with cervical and lumbar levels, the thoracic spinal cord occupies a greater volume of the spinal canal and has a more tenuous blood supply. Consequently, the thoracic spinal cord is very susceptible to injury (32). Only 12% of patients with thoracic spine fracture–dislocations are neurologically intact, substantially fewer than those with lumbar (41%) or cervical spine (26%) fracture–dislocations (32–34). Collimated, centered, and adequately penetrated

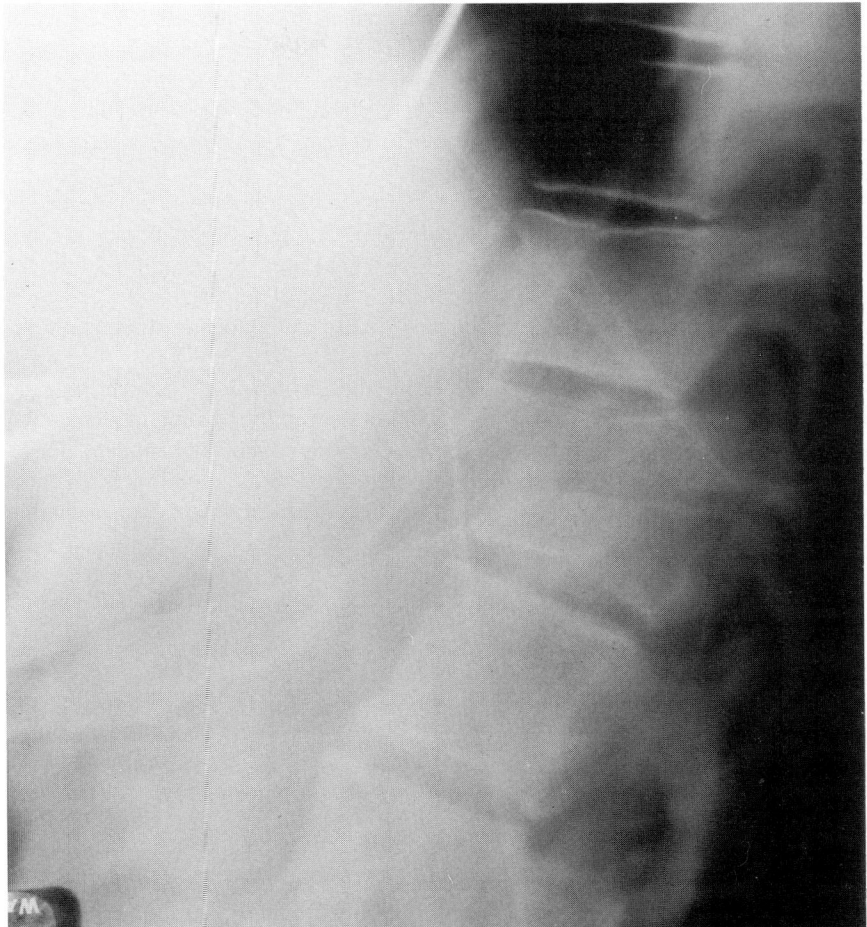

Figure 1 Fracture–subluxation at T11-12 secondary to hyperflexion injury.

frontal and lateral views of the thoracic spine should be part of the initial radiographic evaluation. If the cervicothoracic junction is not visualized on lateral views of the thoracic spine, a swimmer's view should be obtained.

Neurological symptoms or back pain should prompt a careful search for cortical disruption and vertebral displacement on radiographs of the spine. Paraspinal soft-tissue swelling can be very helpful in directing attention to thoracic spine fractures. The "rule of twos" can be helpful in detecting subtle abnormalities (32–35): The interspinous and interpediculate distances of contiguous vertebrae should not vary by more than 2 mm. Also, the vertical distance between pedicles of adjacent vertebrae should not vary by more than 2 mm from contiguous pairs of vertebral bodies above or below. Facet joint width should be less than 2 mm, and the posterior height of a thoracic vertebral body should not exceed its anterior height by more than 2 mm, except at T-11 or T-12, where slightly more anterior wedging can be a normal variant.

Axial computed tomography images of the thoracic spine can be obtained to better evaluate fractures identified on plain film. Computed tomography is more sensitive in demonstrating compromise of the spinal canal by retropulsed fracture fragments. Posterior element fractures and facet joint disruption can be obscured by ribs and soft tissues on plain film, but are usually readily demonstrated on thin-section CT scans.

Magnetic resonance imaging (MRI), with its superior tissue contrast, can identify cord edema and hemorrhage. This is especially helpful in evaluating patients who have spinal cord injuries without radiographic abnormality (SCIWORA; i.e., neurological deficits without conventional radiographic or CT abnormalities; 36). Magnetic resonance imaging is also the most sensitive examination for detecting traumatic disk herniations and spinal epidural hematomas.

III. Pleural Space Injuries

A. Pneumothorax

Potential etiologies of posttraumatic pneumothorax include lung laceration, alveolar rupture, tracheobronchial or esophageal tears, and iatrogenic injury. When a rib fracture is present with a pneumothorax (70% of cases), laceration of the visceral pleura by rib fragments is usually the cause. Thirty percent of pneumothoraces occur without rib fractures. The frequency of pneumothorax in blunt trauma was probably underestimated in early reports. Before the widespread use of CT in the assessment of blunt trauma, it is likely that many pneumothoraces resolved without being recognized clinically. *Occult pneumothorax*, defined as pneumothorax evident by CT, but not by clinical examination or chest radiography, has been reported in numerous studies of patients undergoing CT scanning for blunt trauma (Fig 2; 3,8,37–44). A review of recent literature (3,37,40—44) reveals that of 237 pneumothoraces detected in blunt chest and abdominal trauma, nearly 45% (105/237), were evident only on CT scans. For this reason, images through the lung bases should always be obtained in the CT evaluation of blunt abdominal trauma. Recognition of even a small, occult pneumothorax is sometimes critical, particularly in patients requiring mechanical ventilation or general anesthesia for emergent surgery. In such patients, prophylactic tube thoracostomy is generally recommended to prevent progression to a tension pneumothorax (43,44).

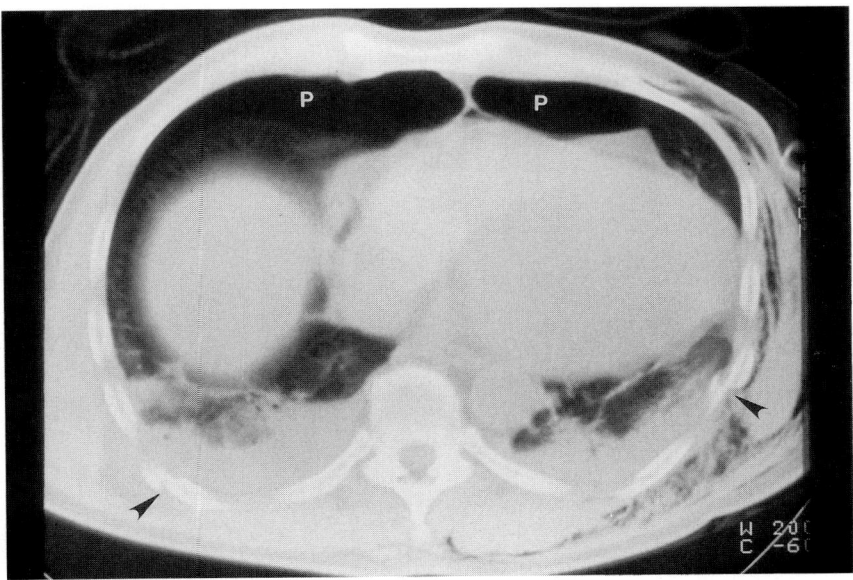

Figure 2 Bilateral "occult" pneumothoraces (P) in a patient with splenic rupture secondary to blunt abdominal trauma. Note bilateral rib fractures (arrowheads) and subcutaneous air in the left chest wall.

The term *tension pneumothorax* deserves further discussion. Mediastinal shift should not be interpreted as evidence of "tension" pneumothorax. Shift of the mediastinum away from the side of a pneumothorax is expected, given the relatively more negative pressure in the contralateral hemithorax. For a closed pneumothorax to increase in volume, the intrapleural pressure must be relatively negative during inspiration, so that air in the lung at atmospheric pressure will flow into the pleural space. If egress of air during expiration is prevented by a check-valve mechanism, the intrapleural pressure will be positive in the latter phases of expiration. Thus, a more correct term would be *expiratory tension pneumothorax* (45). Respiratory failure occurs when increased tension prevents inflation of the normal lung during inspiration. The plain-film assessment of the presence or absence of tension is very unreliable. Tension pneumothorax should be considered a clinical diagnosis characterized by respiratory embarrassment (45). Venous return to the heart is not impeded in a tension pneumothorax because negative intrapleural pressures of up to -70 cmH$_2$O can be generated in the dyspneic patient (46).

Open pneumothorax, which occurs in the presence of a large chest wall defect, can cause a "sucking" chest wound. Inspiration causes outside air to enter the pleural space, counteracting inspired ipsilateral intrapulmonary air. There is mediastinal shift toward the normal side. Expiration then causes pleural air to exit through the chest wound, resulting in mediastinal displacement toward the injured side. This mediastinal flutter, combined with pendelluft (movement of dead-space air from the normal lung into the collapsed lung), can cause rapid respiratory failure (2). An immediate attempt should be made to close the chest wall defect.

Air in an otherwise normal pleural space collects in the most nondependent portion of the hemithorax. On an upright radiograph, pneumothorax is usually readily identified as a visible visceral pleural line over the lung apex. However, a supine position will cause air to collect in the lower anterior pleural space. Signs of pneumothorax on a supine chest radiograph include the deep sulcus sign (increased lucency in the costophrenic angle), sharp hemidiaphragmatic border, double diaphragm sign, sharp mediastinal contour, hyperlucency of the lower hemithorax, and clear visualization of the pericardial fat pads.

B. Pleural Effusion

In the absence of underlying disease, a pleural effusion identified immediately after acute trauma is usually a hemothorax. Hemothoraces occur in approximately 50% of patients with blunt thoracic trauma and are the most common cause of shock after chest trauma (8). Posttraumatic hemothorax can be secondary to intercostal artery laceration, parenchymal lung injury, mediastinal contusion, aortic tears, and iatrogenic causes. Parenchymal lung injuries usually are not associated with excessive bleeding. The low perfusion pressures and rich thromboplastin content of the lung promote hemostasis (30). A massive hemothorax (greater than 1000 ml of blood) should direct attention to central pulmonary vessels, systemic thoracic vessels, or lacerated viscera. Thoracostomy tubes are routinely used to manage hemopneumothoraces, hemothoraces exceeding 500 ml during thoracentesis, hemothoraces producing shock, recurrent hemothoraces after thoracentesis, and hemothoraces in the presence of other injuries that require surgery (8). Thoracostomy tubes placed within a pleural fissure appear to function as effectively as those located elsewhere in the pleural space (47).

In a supine patient, a homogeneous increase in density or "veiling" opacity over the hemithorax, a curvilinear opacity interposed between the ribs and the lung, or an apical pleural cap should suggest a pleural fluid collection (32). Occasionally, even large pleural effusions, particularly if symmetric and bilateral, may not be apparent on supine chest radiographs. Small effusions are usually missed on routine chest radiographs. Of a total of 90 pleural effusions identified by Toombs et al. (42), Rhea et al. (41), and Poole et al. (40), nearly 75% (67/90) could be seen only on CT.

Chylothorax is a pleural effusion having a high lipid content and a characteristic milky appearance. However, not all chylous effusions are milky, and not all milky effusions are truly chylous (45). Chylous pleural fluid may follow injuries of the thorax or neck, with resultant damage to the thoracic duct. Thoracic duct injury occurs most commonly during surgical procedures, but can also be seen in cases of penetrating knife and bullet wounds and blunt trauma. The thoracic duct in the posterior mediastinum crosses the midline from right to left between the fifth and seventh thoracic vertebrae. Crushing injuries of the lower chest, therefore, tend to cause a right-sided chylothorax, and injuries above the left midthorax tend to cause a left-sided chylothorax. Blunt thoracic trauma can also cause bilateral chylothoraces (48). Disruption of the thoracic duct initially causes leakage of chyle into the mediastinum; chylothorax occurs only if the mediastinal pleura is torn by the initial trauma or breaks down under the pressure of mediastinal accumulation (45). Loss of up to 2 L of chyle per day can cause life-threatening dehydration, nutritional deficiencies, and immune system compromise (2). Chylothorax should be considered if several days elapse between the occurrence of chest trauma and the development of pleural effusion. The diagnosis is most easily made by analysis of the triglyceride content of the pleural fluid. Computed tomography may provide indirect evidence of chylous leak by demonstrating low-density fluid collections (49). Lymphangiography is useful in localization of laceration of the thoracic duct, especially in patients with large leaks likely to require surgical intervention (50). In these patients, leaks are seen as collections of contrast medium, outside the confines of normal lymphatic channels, that enlarge over time on serial chest radiographs. Surgical ligation is undertaken if lymphatic drainage persists despite the presence of thoracostomy tube drainage.

A much rarer result of thoracic duct injury is development of a contained pleural or mediastinal lymph collection, or lymphocele. On chest radiographs lymphoceles may appear as focal pleural masses or generalized mediastinal widening (51–53). On CT scans they appear as paraspinal, nonenhancing, water-attenuation masses. Lymphoscintigraphy can be diagnostic if accumulation of activity is demonstrated within the lymphocele.

Infection is second only to neurologic injury as a leading cause of death in severely traumatized patients. Caplan and Hoyt (54) reported that empyema accounts for 11% and pneumonia for 15% of fatal posttraumatic infections. Undrained pleural hemorrhage, occluded thoracostomy tubes, lung abscess, and atelectatic lung in the presence of pneumothorax, all can contribute to empyema formation (55). In addition, studies suggest that both humoral and cellular immunity are decreased after major trauma (56,57).

The plain-film and CT diagnosis of empyema is based on the presence of loculation, air bubbles, and lung consolidation or abscess adjacent to the pleural

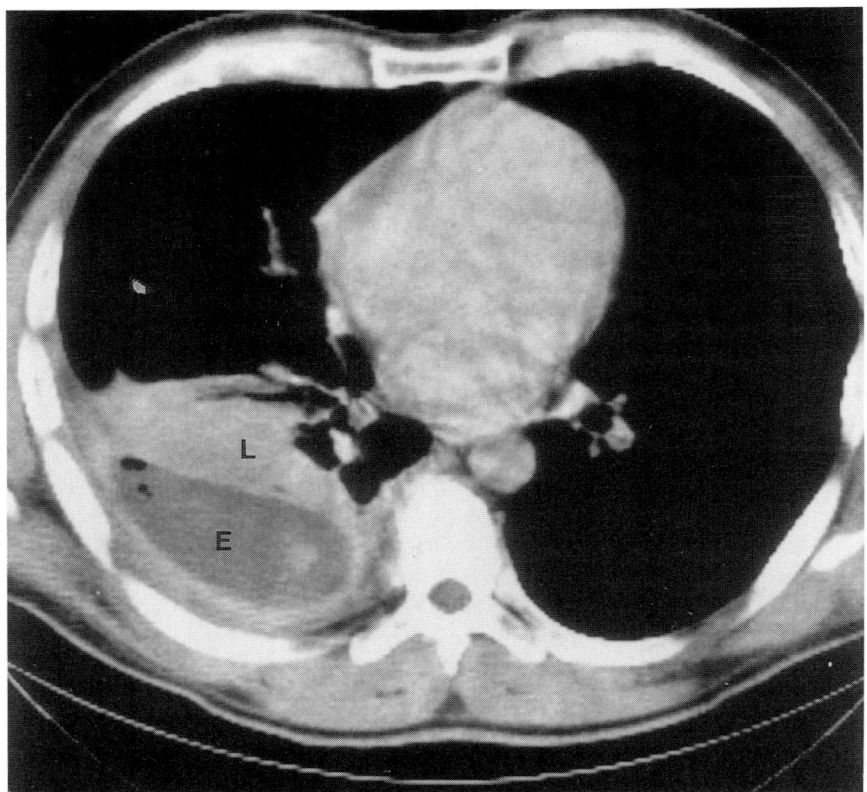

Figure 3 Right posterior–basilar empyema. Thickened pleura defines the borders of the lenticular-shaped empyema (E), which compresses adjacent lung (L). Air bubbles in the pleural space are secondary to bronchopleural fistula.

fluid collection (Fig. 3; 8). Additional CT features of empyema include oval or lenticular shape, obtuse angle with the pleura, compression of adjacent lung, and enhancement of inflamed, separated visceral and parietal pleural surfaces ("split pleura" sign) following intravenous administration of contrast material (58).

Sonographic evaluation of pleural effusion can be performed at the bedside if the patient is too ill to undergo CT. Empyemas usually appear as complex pleural collections with fluid–debris levels and septations. Ultrasound-guided thoracentesis can be very helpful in obtaining samples from small or loculated pleural fluid collections.

IV. Mechanisms of Chest Injury

In the United States, the most common forms of penetrating chest trauma are gunshot wounds and knife injuries. The degree of damage to the lung depends on several characteristics of both the projectile and the tissue through which it passes. The wounding capability of a bullet depends on the efficiency with which energy can be transferred to the tissue. Energy transfer of the projectile is governed by the following formula: kinetic energy = $1/2$ mass $\times$ velocity^2. The ability of a projectile to wound, therefore, increases exponentially with muzzle velocity. High-velocity missiles are those of any size traveling faster than 540 m/sec (1800 ft/sec); this category includes virtually all rifle wounds (except the 0.22 long rifle) (59). Most handgun wounds are low-velocity injuries.

Other determinants of wounding capability include the mass, shape, and orientation of the bullet as it strikes tissue, and whether the bullet deforms or fragments on impact (60). Close-range shotgun wounds are severe because of the large mass of the shot and the intermediate muzzle velocity of these weapons.

The extent to which tissue is injured is determined primarily by its specific gravity and elasticity. The low specific gravity of lung (0.4–0.5) compared with that of skeletal muscle (1.03) and rib (1.11), coupled with its high elastic content, minimize the effects of temporary and permanent cavitation (60,61). A temporary cavity is produced when tissues adjacent to the bullet path are accelerated outward in a radial fashion, injuring structures well beyond the path of the bullet. The diameter of the temporary cavity can be 20–30 times the diameter of the bullet itself (32). Cavitation generates subatmospheric pressures within the body that literally suck dirt and debris into the wound (32). Wound contamination is a much greater problem with high-velocity missiles; wounds from low-velocity missiles are generally clean, unless bowel penetration occurs (59). A permanent cavity is formed as the advancing bullet crushes and tears lung tissue directly in its path; it is this cavity that is shown on radiographs as the bullet track (Fig. 4). Although bullets can pass through lung virtually unimpeded, dense overlying tissue, such as bone or skeletal muscle, absorbs large amounts of kinetic energy, producing extensive damage. However, the dense tissue also decreases the velocity of the bullet and in this way may protect more vital structures from severe injury.

Knives are low-velocity projectiles that injure only tissues directly in their path. Objects impaled in the chest wall should be left in place until they can be removed under direct vision with control of hemorrhage, usually in the operating room (59).

Blunt thoracic trauma is approximately nine times as common as penetrating chest trauma in civilian populations (32). Greene has described three synergistic mechanisms involved in the transfer of kinetic energy to the thorax following blunt trauma: (1) sudden inertial deceleration, (2) spallation, and (3) implosion

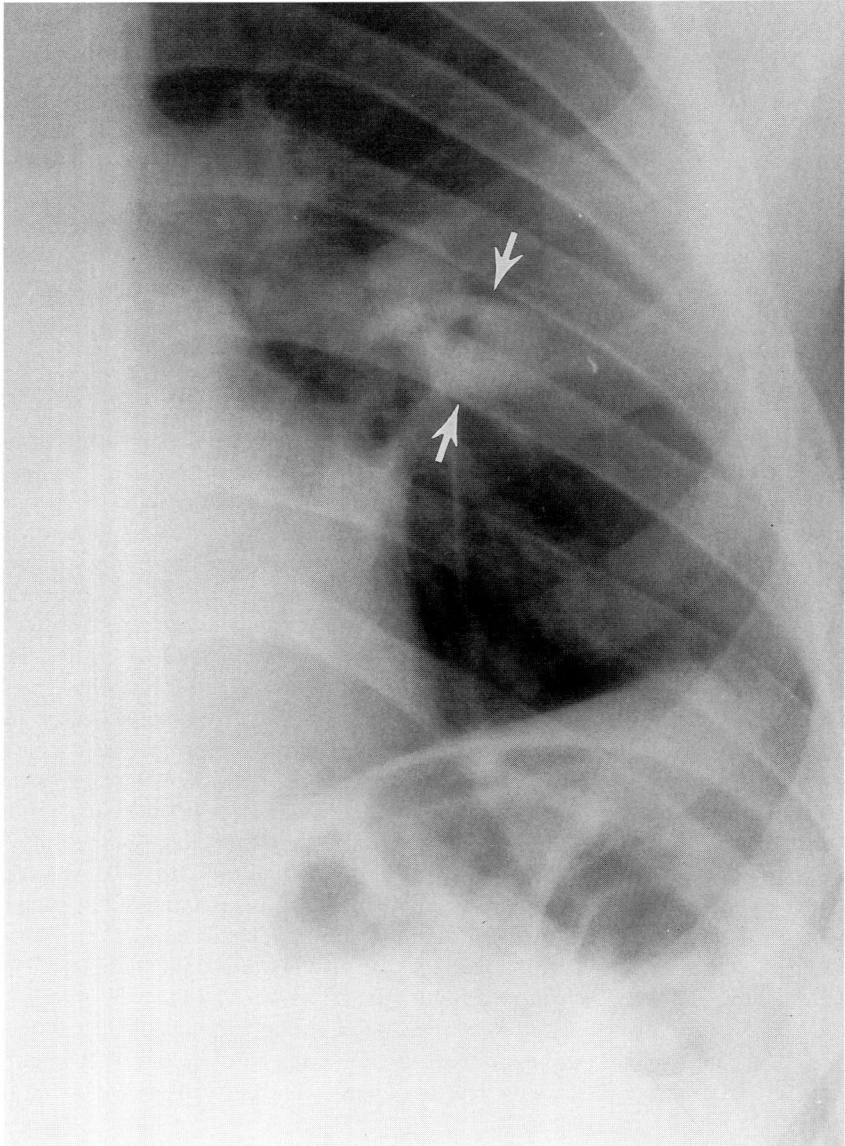

Figure 4 Bullet track in a patient who sustained a gunshot wound to the left chest 2 weeks earlier. The bullet track (arrows), containing mainly hematoma at this time, leaves an air-filled cavity as it resolves. Such cavities, which represent tubular-shaped lacerations, usually resolve completely within a few months.

(5,62). *Sudden inertial deceleration* at the time of impact refers to differential rates of deceleration that thoracic tissues experience according to differences in tissue density. Mobile or elastic structures rotate about points of fixation, resulting in shearing stresses that can, for example, cause gross lacerations at the interface between relatively mobile alveolar tissue and the more fixed bronchovascular network (5,62). Mechanical shearing stresses can also cause aortic or tracheal lacerations. *Spallation* results from partial reflection of a broad kinetic shock wave at gas–fluid interfaces, such as at the alveolocapillary surface. If, for example, the chest wall strikes a steering wheel at high speed, spallation can cause focal disruption of anterior parenchymal lung tissue. *Implosion* is the low-pressure decompressive afterwave causing rebound overexpansion of alveolar gas and disruption of lung tissue (5,62).

The prestress state of a tissue also determines its susceptibility to injury (32). For example, myocardial rupture occurs with significantly greater frequency when anterior chest impact is timed to occur during the peak myocardial stress phase of systole (63).

V. Parenchymal Lung Injuries

A. Laceration

Wagner et al. (64–56) simplified our understanding of parenchymal lung injury. By analyzing CT findings and histopathological specimens, they demonstrated that pulmonary laceration is the primary mechanism of injury in pulmonary contusion, pulmonary hematoma, and pulmonary cyst or pneumatocele (64). From CT findings, mechanism of injury, location of rib fractures, and surgical findings, four types of pulmonary laceration were proposed: compression rupture (type I), compression shear (type II), rib penetration (type III), and adhesion tears (Type IV). Type I lacerations occur when sudden compression of a compliant chest wall causes air-containing lung to rupture. The appearance of type I lacerations on CT is usually that of an intraparenchymal cavity with or without an air–fluid level (Fig. 5). On occasion, type I lacerations may appear as parenchymal air-containing lines extending through the visceral pleura, resulting in a pneumothorax. Type II lacerations occur when compression of the lower chest wall causes a shearing injury as the posteromedial lung is shifted across the vertebral body (15,64). These compression injuries are much more common in children and young adults who have not lost their costal cartilage flexibility. The CT appearance is that of an air-containing cavity or air–fluid level in the paravertebral lung. Type III lacerations appear as peripheral linear radiolucencies situated beneath rib fractures. Type IV lacerations are rare, and occur when lung adjacent to firm pleuroparenchymal scarring is avulsed during violent chest trauma.

The appearance of pulmonary contusions as areas of parenchymal infiltra-

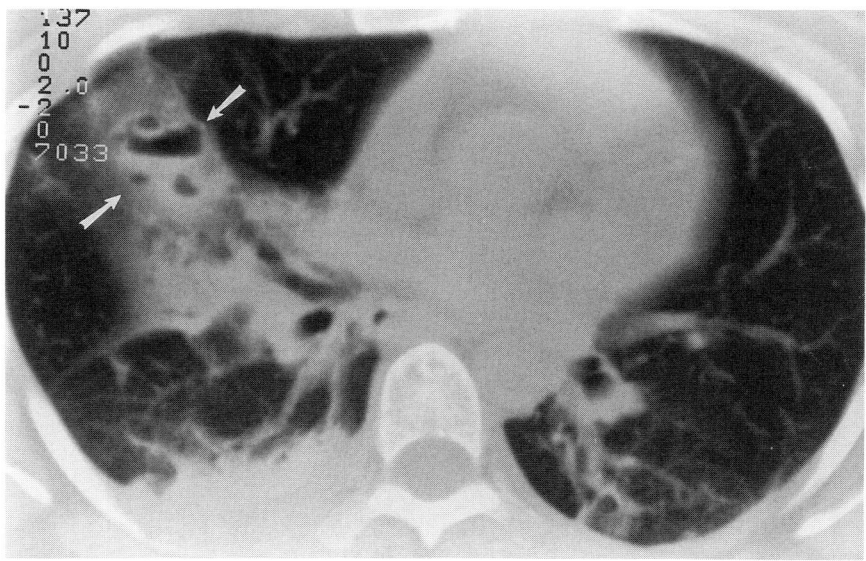

Figure 5 Pulmonary laceration and contusion following blunt thoracic trauma. Note multiple lacerations (arrows), the largest of which contains an air-fluid level. The lacerations were obscured by surrounding contusion on routine chest radiographs.

tion or consolidation on chest radiographs is not completely explained if all types of blunt parenchymal lung injury are ascribed to pulmonary laceration. The radiographic "pulmonary contusion" is likely a laceration surrounded by blood-filled alveoli without significant interstitial injury (66). This idea is contrary to previously held notions that contusion also represents traumatic extravasation of blood and edema fluid into the interstitial compartment of the lung, along with disruption of alveolar–capillary integrity (62,67,68). Wagner et al. (64) found no histological evidence of significant interstitial injury around the laceration itself. Postlaceration spaces may fill with air (pneumatoceles), blood (hematomas), or both (hematopneumatoceles). Their typically ovoid shape is due to elastic recoil in the surrounding intact lung.

The radiographic appearance of pulmonary contusion varies from irregular, patchy areas of airspace opacity to extensive homogeneous consolidation (Fig. 6). Although pulmonary lacerations do not conform to anatomical boundaries, the fact that consolidation is almost always confined by fissures supports the contention that consolidation represents spillover hemorrhage (66). Contusion, or alveo-

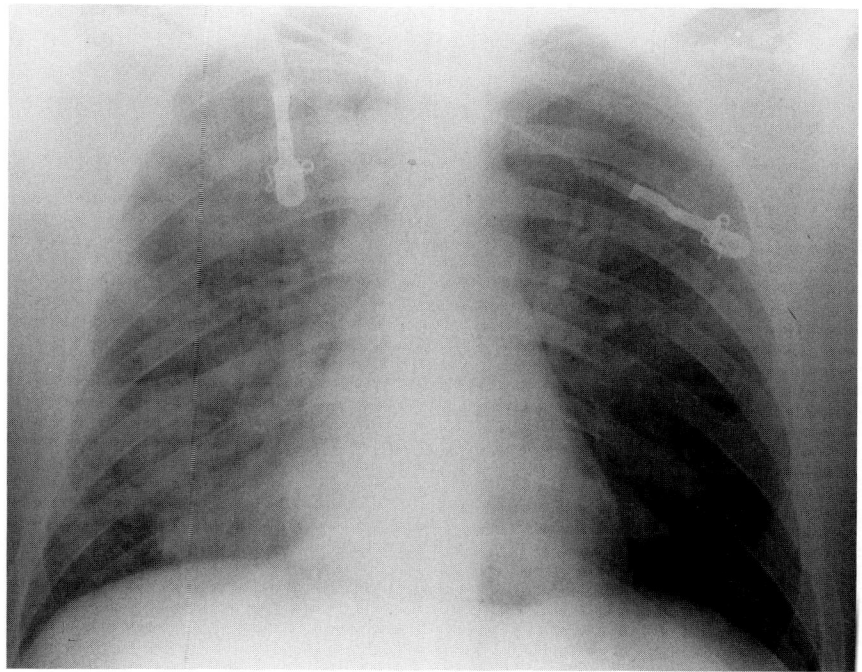

Figure 6 Pulmonary contusion: PA chest radiograph demonstrates diffuse "cloud-like" opacity in the right lung corresponding to extensive parenchymal contusion. Pneumomediastinum is noted along the left heart border.

lar hemorrhage, is an evolving process that may not appear on chest radiographs for up to 6 h (69). Although contusion is usually visible on the admission chest film, the radiographic appearance may considerably underestimate the true extent of lung injury (62,70). Computed tomography is much more sensitive than chest radiography in detecting posttraumatic parenchymal lung abnormalities (64,66,71). Toombs et al. (42) found that for every abnormality seen on chest radiographs after thoracic trauma, four were found on CT scans. In experimentally induced pulmonary contusion, Schild et al. (71) found that CT was 100% sensitive in detecting contusion. On CT, contusion appears as an ill-defined area of hazy ground-glass density or consolidation, usually with a peripheral, nonsegmental distribution. Wagner et al. (66) found that the amount of pulmonary parenchymal injury correlates with ventilation requirements. In a series of 95 patients with chest trauma, they observed that all patients with more than 28% of their total airspace consolidated or lacerated required mechanical ventilation. Lung contusions typically resolve rapidly, improving within 48 h (45,72) and generally clearing in 3–10 days (2,8,45).

Traumatic pneumatoceles or traumatic lung cysts probably result from bursting or shearing of alveolar walls (8,45,73). We prefer the term *pneumatocele*, because there is no epithelial lining; rare excised specimens have shown the "cyst" wall to be composed of fibrous or granulation tissue (45). Stark (2) proposed that the walls consist of compressed alveoli. Pneumatoceles occur mostly in children and young adults, secondary to mechanical ventilation or blunt trauma. They may be masked by surrounding pulmonary contusion and commonly are not recognized for several days (45). Traumatic pneumatoceles frequently develop in a subpleural location, where they may be a source of continual air leak into the pleural space (8). Most appear as ovoid or spherical, thin-walled lucencies, 2–5 cm in diameter. They are often not readily apparent on conventional chest radiographs. If pneumatoceles fill with blood, they may appear as air-filled spaces with fluid levels or as well-circumscribed masses of water density (pulmonary hematomas; 45). Both pneumatoceles and hematomas usually resolve over several weeks, pneumatoceles faster than hematomas. However, a hematoma can remain visible as a circumscribed lung mass for longer than a year and may be mistaken for neoplasm (Fig. 7). If hematomas communicate with a bronchus, they may evacuate themselves with dark, bloody hemoptysis, leaving a cyst that corresponds with the original laceration. Bronchopleural fistulas that connect to postlaceration spaces usually resolve over a 3-month period after mechanical ventilation is discontinued (62).

B. Atelectasis

In the traumatized patient, atelectasis can result from obstruction of bronchial airways by mucous plugs, blood clots, foreign bodies, bronchial compression, or bronchial rupture (2). Compressive atelectasis can occur in patients with hemothorax or pneumothorax. Atelectasis complicates contusion because alveolar hemorrhage deactivates surfactant (74), causing adhesive atelectasis. Atelectatic lung is also prone to infection.

C. Blast Injuries

Blast injuries almost always affect the lungs (75). The abrupt positive and negative pressure changes associated with the shock waves disrupt alveolar–capillary integrity and result in parenchymal lung lacerations, edema, and alveolar hemorrhage. Interstitial emphysema, pneumomediastinum, and pneumothorax are also common. Direct communication between alveoli and blood vessels can lead to air embolism, which is often fatal (76).

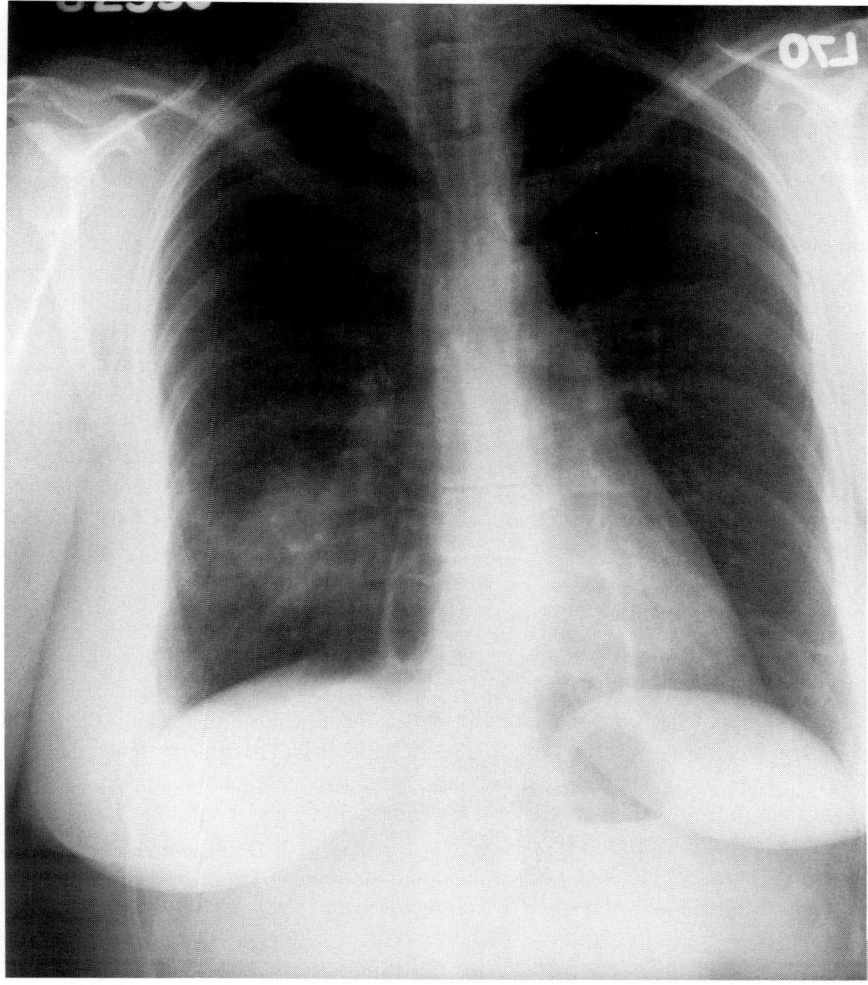

Figure 7 Lung hematoma simulating neoplasm: PA chest radiograph approximately 2 months after a motor vehicle accident demonstrates a well-circumscribed mass in the right lower lobe. The mass resolved slowly on follow-up radiographs.

D. Lung Torsion

Torsion of the lung is an extremely rare sequela of chest trauma, and most often occurs in patients who have undergone prior surgery, usually lobectomy (77). Other reported causes include endobronchial tumors, diaphragmatic hernia, pneumothorax, pneumonia, and needle biopsy of the lung; spontaneous torsion also occurs (77–79). In cases of trauma, the victim is usually a child who has been run over by a car. Traumatic compression of the lower hemithorax is said to cause disruption of the inferior pulmonary ligament and cephalad displacement of the lower lobe. With sudden decompression, the lower lobe reexpands in its new cephalic location, displacing the upper lobe inferiorly (77). Torquing of the hilum may result in hemorrhagic infarction of the lung and abrupt bronchial cut-off, causing atelectasis. The diagnosis is very difficult to make prospectively. Commonly noted is rapid opacification of the torqued lung tissue, which occupies an unusual anatomical position (77,80). Inversion of the normal position and sweep of the pulmonary vascular pattern may signify torsion. If previous films are available, shift in position of a calcified granuloma or pulmonary nodule may be seen. Treatment is surgical reduction of the torsion and removal of the torqued lung if infarction has occurred.

E. Fat Embolism

Skeletal trauma can have indirect effects on the lungs. Although fat embolism is common after trauma, the fat embolism syndrome occurs in only about 3–10% of such patients (46,81). In one series in which the diagnosis of fat embolism was based on the presence of lipiduria, 87.5% of patients had normal chest radiographs (82). Prompt corticosteroid therapy and aggressive ventilatory support have reduced the mortality associated with fat embolism to about 5% (2). The clinical triad consists of central nervous system involvement (confusion, restlessness, delirium, coma), petechial rash, and manifestations of pulmonary involvement (cough, dyspnea, hemoptysis, pyrexia, tachycardia, rales, friction rub) (45). The exact pathogenetic mechanisms of fat embolism syndrome are unclear. Briefly, the mechanical theory proposes that fat emboli from bone marrow enter the lacerated ends of veins and cause pulmonary vascular obstruction. A biochemical theory proposes that released fatty acids, possibly from pulmonary lipases, exert a direct toxic effect on endothelium (83,84). When present, the radiographic appearance is characterized by multifocal alveolar densities attributable to alveolar hemorrhage and edema. The predominantly peripheral distribution and the absence of cardiac enlargement, pleural effusion, or pulmonary venous hypertension are helpful in differentiating this condition from pulmonary edema of cardiac origin (45). The radiographic signs of trauma-related fat embolism are usually not evident for 1–2 days after the traumatic event. This delay is very helpful in distinguishing this entity from lung contusion. Radiographic clearing usually occurs within 2 weeks.

VI. Tracheobronchial Rupture

Tracheobronchial rupture is an infrequent, but serious, complication of blunt chest trauma. It carries an overall mortality rate of approximately 30%, mostly from associated injuries (85,86). Fractures of the upper three ribs are commonly seen. About 90% of tears are in a mainstem bronchus; the remaining 10% are in the trachea within 2 cm of the carina (2). Early diagnosis is important in preventing acute complications of tension pneumothorax, respiratory failure, and airway obstruction (87). Undiagnosed tears may result in tracheal or bronchial stenosis, mediastinal infection, bronchiectasis, and pulmonary fibrosis (86,87).

In approximately 10% of patients, initial radiography is normal, and in the remainder radiologic findings are often nonspecific (88,89). The most common finding is ipsilateral pneumothorax, which occurs in approximately 80% of cases (Fig. 8; 20). The pneumothorax is often large and classically does not respond to chest tube drainage. A check-valve mechanism at the site of the bronchial tear may result in tension pneumothorax.

Other manifestations of air leak at the site of tracheobronchial rupture include pneumomediastinum, deep cervical emphysema, and extensive subcutaneous emphysema (90). However, if the bronchial adventitia remains intact, there may be no associated air leak. Bronchoscopic examination of patients at risk is the only way of making an early diagnosis in these patients (5).

In complete transection of the mainstem bronchus with associated pneumothorax, the lung may fall away from the hilum to a dependent region of the thorax, giving rise to the "falling lung sign" (91). Normally, the lung collapses inwardly toward the hilum when a pneumothorax is present. In patients with bronchial rupture, atelectasis is usually persistent and unresponsive to tracheobronchial suction or physiotherapy (20).

Early radiographic signs of tracheal rupture include overdistension of the endotracheal balloon cuff and orientation of the distal portion of the endotracheal tube to the right of the tracheal air column (87). Computed tomography can diagnose tracheal tears in patients with indwelling endotracheal tubes by demonstrating extraluminal tip position or by showing an overdistended balloon protruding through the tracheal tear into the mediastinum (8). Bronchial rupture has been recognized on CT by abrupt tapering of the injured bronchus, coupled with shift of the mediastinum toward the ipsilateral lung and retraction of the trachea in the opposite direction, indicating their discontinuity (88). Although CT is capable of demonstrating tracheobronchial injury, the standard chest radiograph and appro-

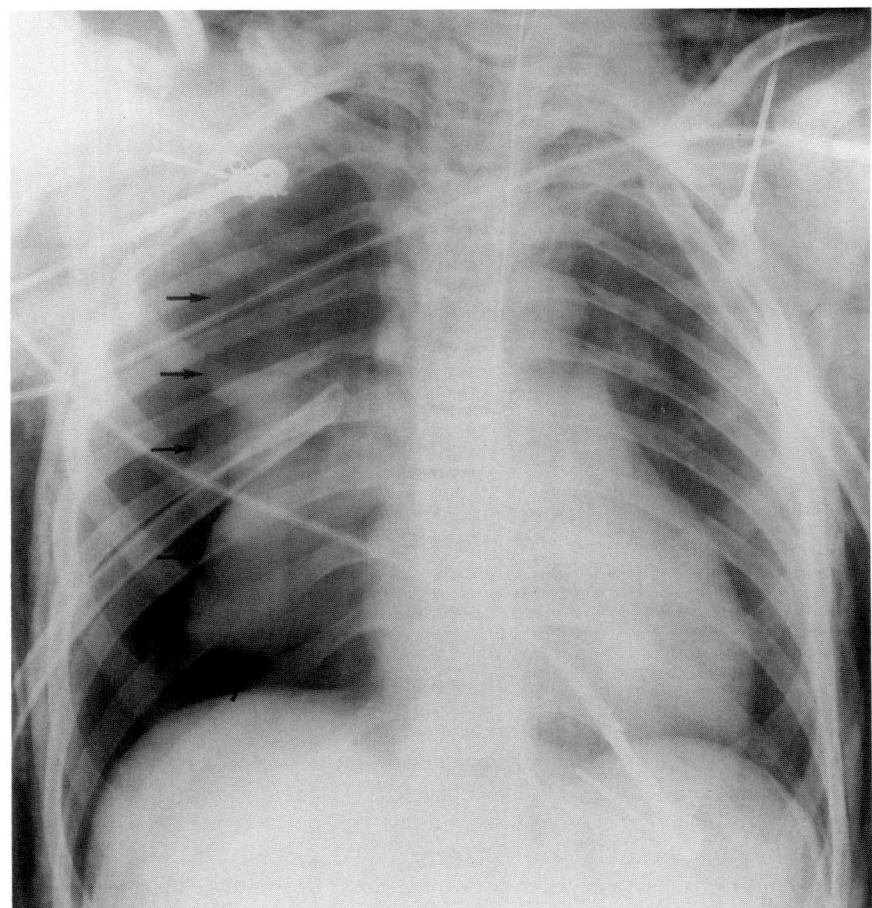

Figure 8 Bronchial tear following blunt trauma: PA chest radiograph following placement of left thoracostomy tube for pneumothorax. The right thoracostomy tube was placed at the scene of the accident because of clinical tension pneumothorax. Extensive mediastinal and deep cervical emphysema is present. Note that the right pneumothorax (arrows) is not responding to chest tube drainage. Multiple bronchoscopies yielded negative results. At autopsy, a tear in the right mainstem bronchus was identified.

priate clinical findings are usually enough to suggest urgent bronchoscopy, which generally is required for definitive diagnosis before surgery.

VII. Esophageal Injury

Esophageal rupture is a rare complication of blunt chest trauma. When it occurs, the cause is sudden elevation of esophageal hydrostatic pressure, presumably from violent ejection of stomach contents when the cricopharyngeal sphincter is closed (20). Penetrating injuries are almost always caused by knife or bullet wounds. Endoscopy accounts for 75–80% of all esophageal perforations (92,93). Other causes of iatrogenic perforation include nasogastric or endotracheal tubes (94), pneumatic dilation balloons (95), Sengstaken–Blakemore tubes (96), and esophageal obturator airways (97). The radiographic findings of traumatic esophageal rupture are generally indistinguishable from those of Boerhaave syndrome and bronchial tear (5,20,98). The majority of esophageal ruptures occur distally because of the lack of supporting mediastinal structures in the lower hemithorax. They also occur more commonly on the left side (99). Distal esophageal ruptures are associated with a pleural effusion or hydropneumothorax in approximately 90% of patients (2,100). Pleural effusion may be a sympathetic reaction secondary to irritation of adjacent mediastinal pleura, or it may be due to direct mediastinal drainage across the ruptured mediastinal pleura. Approximately 75% of hydropneumothoraces occur on the left side, whereas 25% are bilateral, and 5% are on the right (101). Pneumomediastinum, deep cervical emphysema, and mediastinal widening are probably the earliest radiographic findings and occur in approximately 60% of patients who sustain rupture of the esophagus (101). Crescentic gas collections that can form in the diverging mediastinal and pleural facial planes produce the "V sign" of Naclerio (102). Pneumoperitoneum and pneumoretroperitoneum are rarely observed in thoracic esophageal perforations.

If esophageal rupture is suspected clinically or radiographically, the initial esophagogram should be performed with a water-soluble contrast medium, such as Gastrografin. Although barium is radiopaque and has greater adherence to sites of leakage, it may incite an inflammatory reaction in the mediastinum and should be used only if results of the Gastrografin study are negative (103,104). Up to 10% of patients with esophageal perforation have false-negative findings on contrast esophagograms (105). The clinical signs and symptoms of severe chest pain, dyspnea, hypertension, sepsis, and fever may be falsely suggestive of myocardial infarction, acute aortic dissection, or intra-abdominal abnormalities. Angiography or CT may be requested initially. Computed tomographic abnormalities in esophageal perforation include esophageal thickening, periesophageal fluid, extraluminal air, and pleural effusion (106). Identification of extraesophageal air is the most useful finding and is demonstrated on CT with greater sensitivity than on plain chest radiographs. The actual site of perforation may also be visible on CT (106). Acute mediastinitis resulting from virulent organisms in the saliva and leakage of acidic gastric contents is the most lethal complication (98).

VIII. Diaphragmatic Injury

Diaphragmatic rupture occurs in approximately 3% of patients with major blunt thoracoabdominal trauma (42,107). With blunt trauma, most studies report a 70–90% incidence of left hemidiaphragm rupture (108–111), presumably because of the protective effect of the liver on the right hemidiaphragm. Rupture of the right hemidiaphragm may be more common than these series suggest, however, because it is more often clinically inapparent and more difficult to diagnose (112,113). Stab wounds preferentially involve the left hemidiaphragm because 90% of the population is right-handed.

In the immediate posttrauma setting, most diaphragmatic ruptures are not identified radiographically before surgical intervention (114). As proposed by Carter et al. (115), the course of traumatic diaphragmatic hernia can be divided into three phases: (1) acute, (2) latent, and (3) obstructive. The acute phase includes a 2-week period immediately after the trauma. Because diaphragmatic tears are usually not acutely life-threatening, the diagnosis may be missed if nonspecific clinical and radiographic signs are attributed to other processes. In the latent or interval phase, the patient may be asymptomatic or may have nonspecific gastrointestinal or cardiopulmonary symptoms that do not lead to the correct diagnosis. Some patients never progress beyond the latent phase. However, the pressure gradient generated by the negative intrapleural pressure favors progressive lengthening of the rent in the diaphragm and continued herniation of abdominal viscera into the chest (32). The patient enters the obstructive phase of diaphragm rupture if strangulation of intra-abdominal contents occurs. This event usually happens within 3 years after the initial episode of trauma (115). Ball et al. (110) reviewed 42 cases of traumatic rupture of the diaphragm and found that 24% of cases were diagnosed in the early acute phase, 33% were diagnosed during the latent phase, and 43% were not diagnosed until the stage of obstruction.

Chest radiography may be normal in up to 50% of patients with diaphragmatic laceration if there is no herniation of abdominal contents (107,116). Overall, 75–90% of patients with acute diaphragm rupture have abnormal findings on chest radiographs, but only one-third to one-half of these show pathognomonic evidence of diaphragmatic tear, such as bowel loops or a nasogastric tube in the thorax (Fig. 9; 32,111,117,118).

Other radiographic findings include irregularity of the diaphragmatic contour and an elevated lung base, also known as the "pseudodiaphragm effect" (119), or elevation of the apparent left hemidiaphragm. Associated abnormalities

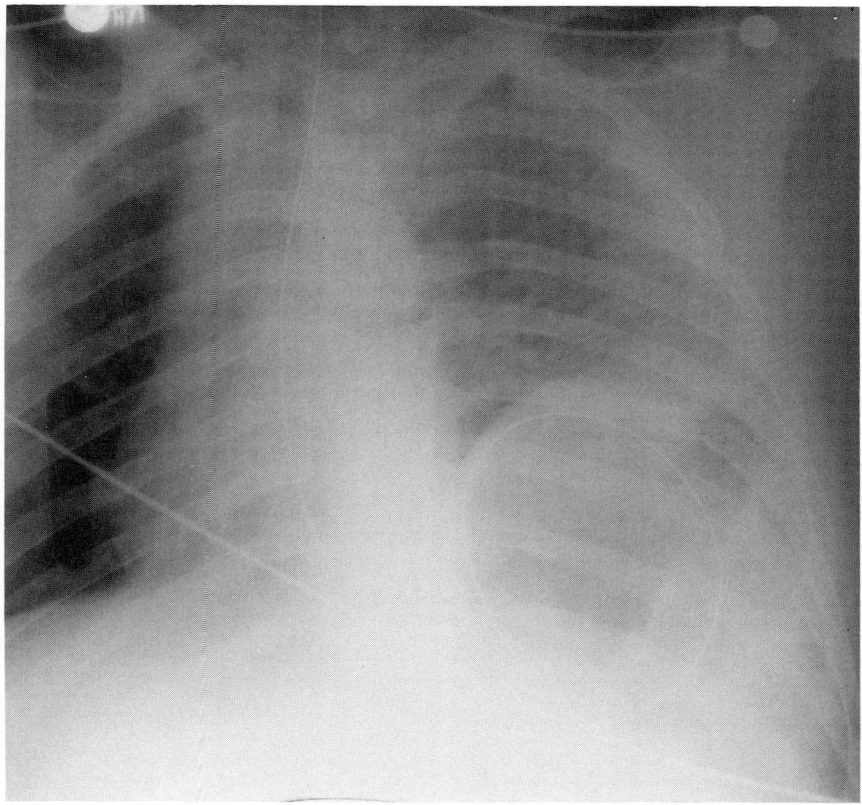

Figure 9 Left hemidiaphragm rupture after motor vehicle accident. The nasogastric tube is coiled in the herniated, intrathoracic stomach.

include pneumothorax, hemothorax, rib fractures, and pulmonary contusion (117). Late strangulation in patients with chronic traumatic diaphragmatic hernia may be heralded by a new unilateral pleural effusion (Fig. 10; 120).

Although diagnosis of diaphragmatic rupture on plain chest films has an unacceptably high false-negative rate, the best or most efficient imaging modality for determining diaphragmatic injury is not clearly defined. Even laparotomy is not 100% sensitive; small rents in the diaphragm are easily missed, especially if they are not meticulously searched for (32). Extraperitoneal lacerations in the region of the bare area of the liver generally are not appreciated at laparotomy.

The usefulness of CT in the diagnosis of traumatic rupture of the diaphragm is somewhat controversial. Some have reported that CT scans rarely show actual

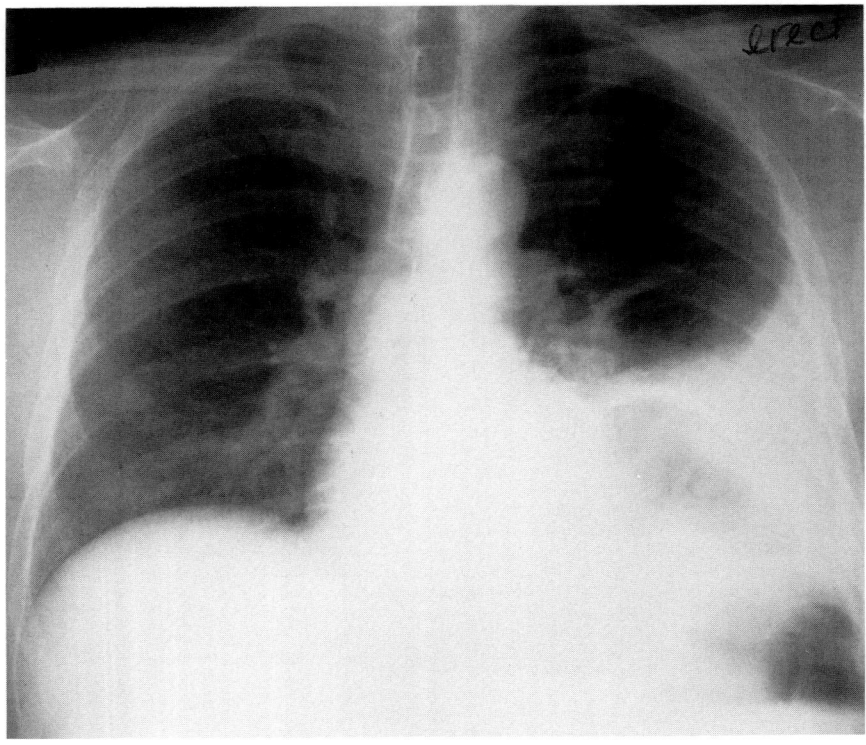

(A)

Figure 10 Delayed presentation of a traumatic diaphragmatic hernia, 5 months after motor vehicle accident. The presence of an ipsilateral pleural effusion is important, because it may indicate strangulation.

lacerations in the diaphragm (32,118). Although the apex of the hemidiaphragm is difficult to detect in the axial plane, defects can be identified posterolaterally or posteromedially where the diaphragm is outlined by lung and subdiaphragmatic fat (117,121,122). Most diaphragmatic tears occur in the posterolateral aspect of the hemidiaphragm and spread in a radial direction (109). Recently, Worthy et al. (109) retrospectively reviewed CT scans in 11 consecutive surgically proved tears of the diaphragm and identified diagnostic findings in 9 patients; these included diaphragmatic discontinuity ($n = 9$), herniation of abdominal contents ($n = 7$), and constriction of the stomach ($n = 3$). Helical scanning and improved coronal and

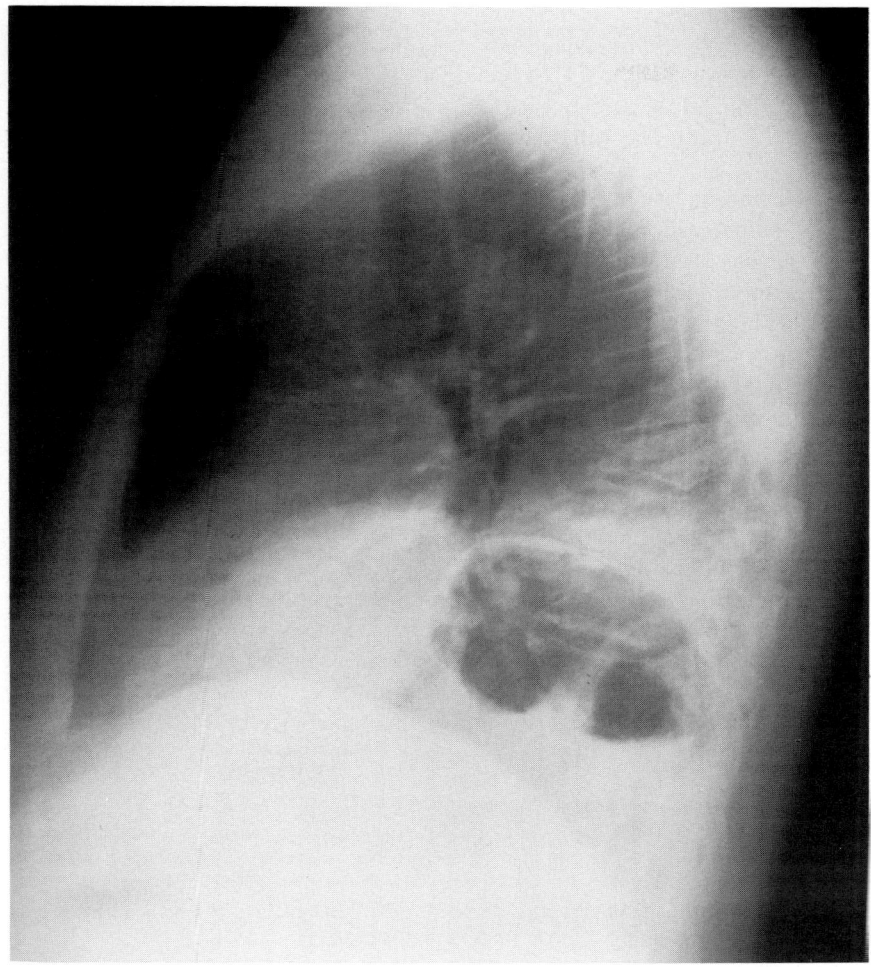

(B)

sagittal reconstruction techniques may improve the sensitivity of CT in diagnosing diaphragmatic injury (123).

Left diaphragmatic rupture most commonly results in gastric or colonic herniation. A delay in diagnosis can be associated with vague gastrointestinal complaints; barium studies are sometimes the first to demonstrate the intrathoracic location of abdominal organs (124).

Nuclear medicine studies can be helpful in detecting intrathoracic splenic or hepatic tissue. In a prospective study of 17 patients with splenic and diaphragmatic injury, Normand et al. (125) found that 18% had evidence of ectopic splenic activity in the left hemithorax with Tc-erythrocyte scintigraphy. On plain radiographs, CT scans, and MRIs, thoracic splenosis typically manifests as pleural masses.

Diagnostic pneumoperitoneography has been used in the past to demonstrate communication between the peritoneal and pleural spaces. However, this technique has been largely discontinued, given the unacceptably high (25–50%) false-negative results and the risk of tension pneumothorax and bowel injury (112–115).

Diaphragmatic contour abnormalities or herniated abdominal contents can be identified with ultrasonography under optimal conditions. However, the presence of gas-filled bowel loops, pneumothorax, subcutaneous emphysema, wound dressings, and excessive subcutaneous fat often preclude an adequate acoustic window into the chest.

Magnetic resonance imaging, with its superior tissue contrast and ability to image in the sagittal and coronal planes, may eventually become the imaging modality of choice in diagnosing diaphragmatic rupture. Currently, the use of sophisticated life-support apparatus is often incompatible with a strong surrounding magnetic field. Also, respiratory and cardiac motion can compromise image quality. The development of MR-compatible life-support devices, together with improved cardiac and respiratory-gating and faster-scanning techniques, may permit a more thorough investigation of the suitability of MRI in diagnosing diaphragm injuries (107,126).

References

1. Baxt WG, Moody P. The impact of a rotorcraft aeromedical emergency care service on trauma mortality. JAMA 1983; 249:3047–3051.
2. Stark P. Radiology of thoracic trauma. Invest Radiol 1990; 25:1265–1275.
3. Wolfman NT, Gilpin JW, Bechtold RE, Meredith JW, Ditesheim JA. Occult pneumothorax in patients with abdominal trauma: CT studies. J Comput Assist Tomogr 1993; 17:56–59.
4. Shorr RM, Crittenden M, Indeck M, Hartunian SL, Rodriguez A. Blunt thoracic trauma: analysis of 515 patients. Ann Surg 1987; 206:200–205.
5. Greene R. Blunt thoracic trauma. In Syllabus: A Categorical Course in Diagnostic Radiology—Chest Radiology. Radiological Society of North America. Oak Brook IL: RSNA Publications, 1992:297–309.
6. Committee on Trauma and Committee on Shock, Division of Medical Sciences, National Research Council. Accidental Death and Disability: The Neglected Disease

of Modern Society. Emergency Health Series A-13. Rockville MD: US Department of Health, Education, and Welfare, 1966.
7. McCort JJ. Caring for the major trauma victim: the role for radiology. Radiology 1987; 163:1–9.
8. Tocino I, Miller MH. Computed tomography in blunt chest trauma. J Thorac Imaging 1987; 2(3):45–59.
9. Dougall AM, Paul ME, Finley RJ, Holliday RL, Coles JC, Duff JH. Chest trauma: current morbidity and mortality. J Trauma 1977; 17:547–552.
10. Fisher RG, Ward RE, Ben-Menachem Y, Mattox KL, Flynn TC. Arteriography and the fractured first rib: too much for too little? AJR 1982; 138:1059–1062.
11. Richardson JD, McElvein RB, Trinkle JK. First rib fracture: a hallmark of severe trauma. Ann Surg 1975; 181:251–254.
12. Jackson A, Fields JM, Wong-You-Chong JJ. The costal hook: an indicator of occult flail segment in chest trauma. Eur J Radiol 1991; 13:69–71.
13. Henry DA. Thoracic trauma: radiologic triage of the chest radiograph. In: Syllabus, Categorical Course on Chest Radiology. American Roentgen Ray Society 1986; Apr: 13–22.
14. Nakayama DK, Ramenofsky ML, Rowe MI. Chest injuries in childhood. Ann Surg 1989; 210:770–775.
15. Eichelberger MR, Randolph JG. Thoracic trauma in children. Surg Clin North Am 1981; 61:1181–1197.
16. Manson D, Babyn PS, Palder S, Bergman K. CT of blunt chest trauma in children. Pediatr Radiol 1993; 23:1–5.
17. Bender TM, Oh KS, Medina JL, Girdany BR. Pediatric chest trauma. J Thorac Imaging 1987; 2(3):60–67.
18. Ogden JA. Chest and pectoral girdle. In: Skeletal Injury in the Child. Philadelphia: Lea & Febiger, 1982.
19. Smyth BT. Chest trauma in children. J Pediatr Surg 1979; 14:41–47.
20. Dee PM. The radiology of chest trauma. Radiol Clin North Am 1992; 30:291–306.
21. Danher J, Eyes BE, Kumar K. Oblique rib views after blunt chest trauma: an unnecessary routine? Br Med J 1984; 289:1271.
22. Thompson BM, Finger W, Tonsfeldt D, et al. Rib radiographs for trauma: useful or wasteful? Ann Emerg Med 1986; 15:261–265.
23. DeLuca SA, Rhea JT, O'Malley TO. Radiographic evaluation of rib fractures. AJR 1982; 138:91–92.
24. Israel Y, Orrego H, Holt S, Macdonald DW, Meema HE. Identification of alcohol abuse: thoracic fractures on routine chest x-rays as indicators of alcoholism. Alcohol Clin Exp Res 1980; 4:420–422.
25. Israel Y, Orrego H, Schmidt W, et al. Trauma in cirrhosis: an indicator of the pattern of alcohol abuse in different societies. Alcohol Clin Exp Res 1991; 15:433–437.
26. Lin HC, Chou CS, Hsu TC. Stress fractures of the ribs in amateur golf players. Chin Med J 1994; 54:33–37.
27. Roberge RJ, Morganstern MJ, Osborn H. Cough fracture of the ribs. Am J Emerg Med 1984; 2:513–517.

28. Sternfeld M, Hay E, Eliraz A. Postnasal drip causing multiple cough fractures. Ann Emerg Med 1992; 21:587.
29. Harris RD, Harris JH Jr. The prevalence and significance of missed scapula fractures in blunt chest trauma. AJR 1988; 151:747–750.
30. Rutherford RB, Campbell DN. Thoracic injuries. In: Zuidema GD, Rutherford RB, Ballinger WF, eds. The Management of Trauma. 4th ed. Philadelphia: WB Saunders, 1985:391–448.
31. Pal JM, Mulder DS, Brown RA, Fleiszer DM. Assessing multiple trauma: is the cervical spine enough? J Trauma 1988; 28:1282–1284.
32. Groskin SA. Selected topics in chest trauma. Radiology 1992; 183:605–617.
33. White A, Paujabi M. Clinical Biomechanics of the Spine. Philadelphia: JB Lippincott, 1978.
34. Meyer PR Jr. Surgery of Spine Trauma. New York: Churchill Livingstone, 1989.
35. Daffner RH. Imaging of Vertebral Trauma. Rockville MD: Aspen Publishers, 1988.
36. Pang D, Pollack IF. Spinal cord injury without radiographic abnormality in children—the SCIWORA syndrome. J Trauma 1989; 29:654–664.
37. Wall SD, Federle MP, Jeffrey RB, Brett CM. CT diagnosis of unsuspected pneumothorax after blunt abdominal trauma. AJR 1983; 141:919–921.
38. Collins JC, Levine G, Waxman K. Occult traumatic pneumothorax: immediate tube thoracostomy versus expectant management. Am Surg 1992; 58:743–746.
39. McGonigal MD, Schwab CW, Kauder DR, Miller WT, Grumbach K. Supplemental emergent chest computed tomography in the management of blunt torso trauma. J Trauma 1990; 30:1431–1434.
40. Poole GV, Morgan DB, Cranston PE, Muakkassa FF, Griswold JA. Computed tomography in the management of blunt thoracic trauma. J Trauma 1993; 35:296–300.
41. Rhea JT, Novelline RA, Lawrason J, Sacknoff R, Oser A. The frequency and significance of thoracic injuries detected on abdominal CT scans of multiple trauma patients. J Trauma 1989; 29:502–506.
42. Toombs BD, Sandler CM, Lester RG. Computed tomography of chest trauma. Radiology 1981; 140:733–738.
43. Bridges KG, Welch G, Silver M, Schinco MA, Esposito B. CT detection of occult pneumothorax in multiple trauma patients. J Emerg Med 1993; 11:179–186.
44. Tocino IM, Miller MH, Frederick PR, Bahr AL, Thomas F. CT detection of occult pneumothorax in head trauma. AJR 1984; 143:987–990.
45. Fraser RG, Paré JAP, Paré PD, Fraser RG, Genereux GP, eds. Diagnosis of Diseases of the Chest. 3rd ed. Philadelphia: WB Saunders, 1988.
46. Stark P, Jacobson F. Radiology of thoracic trauma. Curr Opin Radiol 1992; 4:87–93.
47. Curtin JJ, Goodman LR, Quebbeman EJ, Haasler GB. Thoracostomy tubes after acute chest injury: relationship between location in a pleural fissure and function. AJR 1994; 163:1339–1342.
48. Brook MP, Dupree DW. Bilateral traumatic chylothorax. Ann Emerg Med 1988; 17:69–72.
49. Watanabe AT, Jeffrey RB Jr. CT diagnosis of traumatic rupture of the cisterna chyli. J Comput Assist Tomogr 1987; 11:175–176.

50. Sachs PB, Zelch MG, Rice TW, Geisinger MA, Risius B, Lammert GK. Diagnosis and localization of laceration of the thoracic duct: usefulness of lymphangiography and CT. AJR 1991; 157:703–705.
51. Hom M, Jolles H. Traumatic mediastinal lymphocele mimicking other thoracic injuries: case report. J Thorac Imaging 1992; 7(3):78–80.
52. Ellis MC, Gordon L, Gobien RP, Cooper JF, Vujic I. Traumatic lymphocele: demonstration by lymphoscintigraphy with modified ^{99m}Tc sulfur colloid. AJR 1983; 140:973–974.
53. Perusse KR, McAdams HP, Earls JP, Peller PJ. General case of the day. Posttraumatic thoracic lymphocele. Radiographics 1994; 14:192–195.
54. Caplan ES, Hoyt N. Infection surveillance and control in the severely traumatized patient. Am J Med 1981; 70:638–640.
55. Villalba M, Lucas CE, Ledgerwood AM, Asfaw I. The etiology of post-traumatic empyema and the role of decortication. J Trauma 1979; 19:414–420.
56. Munster AM. Immunologic response of trauma and burns: an overview. Am J Med 1984; 76(3A):142–145.
57. Lundy J, Ford CM. Surgery, trauma and immune suppression: evolving the mechanism. Ann Surg 1983; 197:434–438.
58. Stark DD, Federle MP, Goodman PC, Podrasky AE, Webb WR. Differentiating lung abscess and empyema: radiography and computed tomography. AJR 1983; 141:163–167.
59. Mattox KL, Allen MK. Penetrating wounds of the thorax. Injury 1986; 17:313–317.
60. George PY, Goodman P. Radiographic appearance of bullet tracks in the lung. AJR 1992; 159:967–970.
61. DeMuth WE Jr. High velocity bullet wounds of the thorax. Am J Surg 1968; 115:616–625.
62. Greene R. Lung alterations in thoracic trauma. J Thorac Imaging 1987; 2(3):1–11.
63. Gurdjiam ES, Lange WA, Patrick LM, Thomas LM. Impact Injury and Crash Protection. Springfield IL: Charles C Thomas, 1970.
64. Wagner RB, Crawford WO Jr, Schimpf PP. Classification of parenchymal injuries of the lung. Radiology 1988; 167:77–82.
65. Wagner RB, Crawford WO Jr, Schimpf PP, Jamieson PM, Rao KCVG. Quantitation and pattern of parenchymal lung injury in blunt chest trauma: diagnostic and therapeutic implications. J Comput Tomogr 1988; 12:270–281.
66. Wagner RB, Jamieson PM. Pulmonary contusion: evaluation and classification by computed tomography. Surg Clin North Am 1989; 69:31–40.
67. Shackford SR. Blunt chest trauma: the intensivist's perspective. J Intensive Care Med 1986; 1:125–136.
68. Williams JR, Stembridge VA. Pulmonary contusion secondary to nonpenetrating chest trauma. AJR 1964; 91:284–290.
69. Goodman LR, Putman CE. The S.I.C.U. chest radiograph after massive blunt trauma. Radiol Clin North Am 1981; 19:111–123.
70. Erickson DR, Shinozaki T, Beekman E, Davis JH. Relationship of arterial blood gases and pulmonary radiographs to the degree of pulmonary damage in experimental pulmonary contusion. J Trauma 1971; 11:689–693.

71. Schild HH, Strunk H, Weber W, et al. Pulmonary contusion: CT vs plain radiograms. J Comput Assist Tomogr 1989; 13:417–420.
72. Reynolds J, Davis JT. Injuries of the chest wall, pleura, pericardium, lungs, bronchi and esophagus. Radiol Clin North Am 1966; 4:383–401.
73. Black WC, Gouse JC, Williamson BRJ, Newman BM. Computed tomography of traumatic lung cyst: case report. J Comput Tomogr 1986; 10:33–35.
74. Kerns SR, Gay SB. CT of blunt chest trauma. AJR 1990; 154:55–60.
75. Coppel DL. Blast injuries of the lung. Br J Surg 1976; 63:735–737.
76. Adler OB, Rosenberger A. Blast injuries. Acta Radiol 1988; 29:1–5.
77. Moser ES Jr, Proto AV. Lung torsion: case report and literature review. Radiology 1987; 162:639–643.
78. Huang T-Y, Cho S-R. Torsion of the lung without trauma. Radiology 1979; 132:25–26.
79. Graham RJ, Heyd RL, Raval VA, Barrett TF. Lung torsion after percutaneous needle biopsy of lung. AJR 1992; 159:35–37.
80. Felson B. Lung torsion: radiographic findings in nine cases. Radiology 1987; 162:631–638.
81. Feldman F, Ellis K, Green WM. The fat embolism syndrome. Radiology 1975; 114:535–542.
82. Glas WW, Grekin TD, Musselman MM. Fat embolism. Am J Surg 1953; 85:363–368.
83. Peltier LF. Fat embolism. III. The toxic properties of neutral fat and free fatty acids. Surgery 1956; 40:665–670.
84. Jones JG, Minty BD, Beeley JM, Royston D, Crow J, Grossman RF. Pulmonary epithelial permeability is immediately increased after embolisation with oleic acid but not with neutral fat. Thorax 1982; 37:169–174.
85. Guest JL Jr, Anderson JN. Major airway injury in closed chest trauma. Chest 1977; 72:63–66.
86. Burke JF. Early diagnosis of traumatic rupture of the bronchus. JAMA 1962; 181:682–686.
87. Rollins RJ, Tocino I. Early radiographic signs of tracheal rupture. AJR 1987; 148:695–698.
88. Weir IH, Müller NL, Connell DG. CT diagnosis of bronchial rupture. J Comput Assist Tomogr 1988; 12:1035–1036.
89. Unger JM, Schuchmann GG, Grossman JE, Pellett JR. Tears of the trachea and main bronchi caused by blunt trauma: radiologic findings. AJR 1989; 153:1175–1180.
90. Palder SB, Shandling B, Manson D. Rupture of the thoracic trachea following blunt trauma: diagnosis by CAT scan. J Pediatr Surg 1991; 26:1320–1322.
91. Oh KS, Fleischner FG, Wyman SM. Characteristic pulmonary finding in traumatic complete transection of a main-stem bronchus. Radiology 1969; 92:371–372.
92. Berry BE, Ochsner JL. Perforation of the esophagus: a 30 year review. J Thorac Cardiovasc Surg 1973; 65:1–7.
93. Love L, Berkow AE. Trauma to the esophagus. Gastrointest Radiol 1978; 2:305–321.
94. Ghahremani GG, Turner MA, Port RB. Iatrogenic intubation injuries of the upper gastrointestinal tract in adults. Gastrointest Radiol 1980; 5:1–10.

95. Zegel HG, Kressel HY, Levine GM, Rosato EF. Delayed esophageal perforation after pneumatic dilatation for the treatment of achalasia. Gastrointest Radiol 1979; 4:219–221.
96. Rubin SA, Winsett MZ, Diner WC. Intrathoracic gastric balloon: radiographic recognition of esophageal perforation. Gastrointest Radiol 1982; 7:311–313.
97. Scholl DG, Tsai SH. Esophageal perforation following the use of the esophageal obturator airway. Radiology 1977; 122:315–316.
98. Worman LW, Hurley JD, Pemberton AH, Narodick BG. Rupture of the esophagus from external blunt trauma. Arch Surg 1962; 85:333–338.
99. Rogers LF, Puig AW, Dooley BN, Cuello L. Diagnostic considerations in mediastinal emphysema: a pathophysiologic–roentgenologic approach to Boerhaave's syndrome and spontaneous pneumomediastinum. AJR 1972; 115:495–511.
100. Priviteri CA, Gay BB Jr. Spontaneous rupture of the esophagus: with report of five cases. Radiology 1951; 57:48–57.
101. Levine MS, ed. Radiology of the Esophagus. Philadelphia: WB Saunders, 1989.
102. Naclerio EA. The "V sign" in the diagnosis of spontaneous rupture of the esophagus (an early roentgen clue). Am J Surg 1957; 93:291–298.
103. Dodds WJ, Stewart ET, Vlymen WJ. Appropriate contrast media for evaluation of esophageal disruption. Radiology 1982; 144:439–441.
104. Foley MJ, Ghahremani GG, Rogers LF. Reappraisal of contrast media used to detect upper gastrointestinal perforations: comparison of ionic water-soluble media with barium sulfate. Radiology 1982; 144:231–237.
105. Bladergroen MR, Lowe JE, Postlethwait RW. Diagnosis and recommended management of esophageal perforation and rupture. Ann Thorac Surg 1986; 42:235–239.
106. White CS, Templeton PA, Attar S. Esophageal perforation: CT findings. AJR 1993; 160:767–770.
107. Mirvis SE. Imaging confirms diagnosis in multitrauma victims. Diagn Imaging 1989; 11:226–235, 337, 357.
108. Rodriguez-Morales G, Rodriguez A, Shatney CH. Acute rupture of the diaphragm in blunt trauma: analysis of 60 patients. J Trauma 1986; 26:438–444.
109. Worthy SA, Kang EY, Hartman TE, Kwong JS, Mayo JR, Müller NL. Diaphragmatic rupture: CT findings in 11 patients. Radiology 1995; 194:885–888.
110. Ball T, McCrory R, Smith JO, Clements JL Jr. Traumatic diaphragmatic hernia: errors in diagnosis. AJR 1982; 138:633–637.
111. Gelman R, Mirvis SE, Gens D. Diaphragmatic rupture due to blunt trauma: sensitivity of plain chest radiographs. AJR 1991; 156:51–57.
112. Estrera AS, Platt MR, Mills LJ. Traumatic injuries of the diaphragm. Chest 1979; 75:306–313.
113. Estrera AS, Landay MJ, McClelland RN. Blunt traumatic rupture of the right hemidiaphragm: experience in 12 patients. Ann Thorac Surg 1985; 39:525–530.
114. Morgan AS, Flancbaum L, Esposito T, Cox EF. Blunt injury to the diaphragm: an analysis of 44 patients. J Trauma 1986; 26:565–568.
115. Carter BN, Giuseffi J, Felson B. Traumatic diaphragmatic hernia. AJR 1951; 65:56–71.
116. Beal SL, McKennan M. Blunt diaphragm rupture: a morbid injury. Arch Surg 1988; 123:828–832.

117. Holland DG, Quint LE. Traumatic rupture of the diaphragm without visceral herniation: CT diagnosis. AJR 1991; 157:17–18.
118. Voeller GR, Reisser JR, Fabian TC, Kudsk K, Mangiante EC. Blunt diaphragm injuries: a five-year experience. Am Surg 1990; 56:28–31.
119. Fataar S, Schulman A. Diagnosis of diaphragmatic tears. Br J Radiol 1979; 52:375–381.
120. Aronchick JM, Epstein DM, Gefter WB, Miller WT. Chronic traumatic diaphragmatic hernia: the significance of pleural effusion. Radiology 1988; 168:675–678.
121. Demos TC, Solomon C, Posniak HV, Flisak MJ. Computed tomography in traumatic defects of the diaphragm. Clin Imaging 1989; 13:62–67.
122. Heiberg E, Wolverson MK, Hurd RN, Jagannadharao B, Sundaram M. CT recognition of traumatic rupture of the diaphragm. AJR 1980; 135:369–372.
123. Brink JA, Heiken JP, Semenkovich J, Teefey SA, McClennan BL, Sagel SS. Abnormalities of the diaphragm and adjacent structures: findings on multiplanar spiral CT scans. AJR 1994; 163: 307–310.
124. Cruz CJ, Minagi H. Large-bowel obstruction resulting from traumatic diaphragmatic hernia: imaging findings in four cases. AJR 1994; 162:843–845.
125. Normand J-P, Rioux M, Dumont M, Bouchard G, Letourneau L. Thoracic splenosis after blunt trauma: frequency and imaging findings. AJR 1993; 161:739–741.
126. Mirvis SE, Keramati B, Buckman R, Rodriguez A. MR imaging of traumatic diaphragmatic rupture. J Comput Assist Tomogr 1988; 12:147–149.

7

Radiology of Thoracic Surgical Complications

ROBERT D. TARVER
Indiana University School of Medicine,
 Wishard Memorial Hospital
Indianapolis, Indiana

**LYNN S. BRODERICK and
DEWEY J. CONCES, JR.**
Indiana University School of Medicine,
 University Hospital
Indianapolis, Indiana

I. Introduction

The rapid escalation in the number and complexity of thoracic surgical procedures in the recent past has been astonishing. Moreover, the complexity of the operations has increased as surgery has been made safer for all patients and especially for those considered to be at high risk. The average age of the population has increased significantly and the number of thoracic surgical procedures performed in the elderly has risen accordingly. The improved methods for diagnostic accuracy, the intensive preoperative preparation of high-risk patients, the success of surgical procedures generally have been widely noted. Significant improvements in perioperative and postoperative care have very likely been the primary features assuring the success of thoracic procedures. With the increasing number of operations, the diagnosis and treatment of complications of thoracic procedures have also become of increasing significance: David C. Sabiston, Jr. (1).

Radiology has improved along with thoracic surgery and now plays an important part in diagnosing postoperative complications. In years past, the portable chest radiograph was the only tool available to the radiologist to detect postoperative complications. Currently, computed tomography (CT) and bedside ultrasound have had the greatest influence in diagnosing postoperative complications of thoracic surgery. Computed tomography allows cross-sectional visualization of the thorax and is very effective in displaying and localizing anatomical and pathological deformities of the chest wall, alterations of soft-tissue structures, and the anatomy of the mediastinum and pleural spaces (2). Ultrasound gives the radiologist the capability of imaging the pleural space at the bedside, allowing diagnostic and therapeutic pleural aspirations and drainages. Other radiographic techniques, including esophography, angiography, and nuclear medicine studies, offer a wide range of imaging capabilities to detect postoperative complications. Magnetic resonance imaging (MRI), with its unique abilities to detect moving blood, to image in several planes, and to detect inflammation, is being used to image postoperative thoracic surgery complications. Imaging capabilities have managed to keep pace with the ever-changing and enlarging number of thoracic surgery procedures.

II. General Problems

A. Airway Obstruction

Airway obstruction can occur at any time during the postoperative period. Malposition of the endotracheal tube in the right mainstem bronchus is a common cause of left lung collapse and right upper lobe obstruction. Daily radiographs and the monitoring of breath sounds can reduce this complication. Mucous plugs within the endotracheal tube or the bronchi can also lead to atelectasis (Fig. 1). Hemoptysis may be a clue to the etiology of airway obstruction caused by clotted blood. Postintubation edema of the airway and vocal cords can cause partial or complete airway obstruction. Tracheal granulation tissue can lead to airway narrowing after prolonged intubation or tracheostomy.

B. Aspiration of Gastric Contents

Aspiration of gastric contents can occur in the postoperative period. The risk can be minimized by decreasing the gastric volumes and increasing the gastric pH. The radiologic findings of aspiration are alveolar opacities in the dependent portions of the lungs, usually the superior and posterior segments of the lower lobes and the posterior segments of the upper lobes. The radiographic findings, which can mimic pulmonary edema, may be nonspecific and may take several hours to develop. The diagnosis must rest on the clinical scenario, combined with the radiographic findings.

C. Laryngeal and Tracheal Injuries

Injury to the larynx and trachea can occur anytime during intubation and throughout the course of intubation. Laceration of the larynx or trachea is uncommon and is manifested radiographically as pneumomediastinum or air within the soft

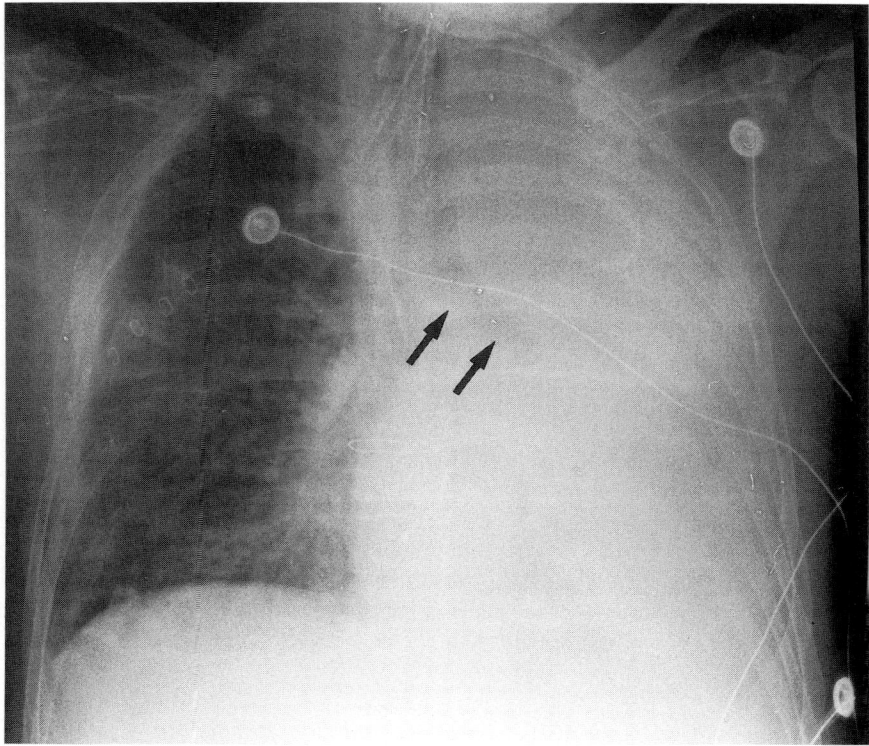

Figure 1 Mucous plugging of the bronchi: One-day status-post right lung wedge resection the patient developed shortness of breath. A chest radiograph demonstrated total opacification of the left lung. The left mainstem bronchus can be seen entering the left lung (arrows). At bronchoscopy, several mucous plugs were removed from the left bronchi.

tissues of the neck. Such complications are more common when the patient is intubated in the field. Postintubation narrowing of the trachea can occur and is usually due to granuloma formation (Fig. 2). This complication is more common in women owing to their smaller airway and thin mucoperichondrium.

D. Barotrauma

Barotrauma caused by mechanical ventilation can cause pneumothorax or pneumomediastinum. As peak inspiratory pressures rise and positive end-expiratory pressure (PEEP) is used, the incidence of pneumothorax and pneumomediastinum increases. Both are easily diagnosed on portable chest radiographs. When the

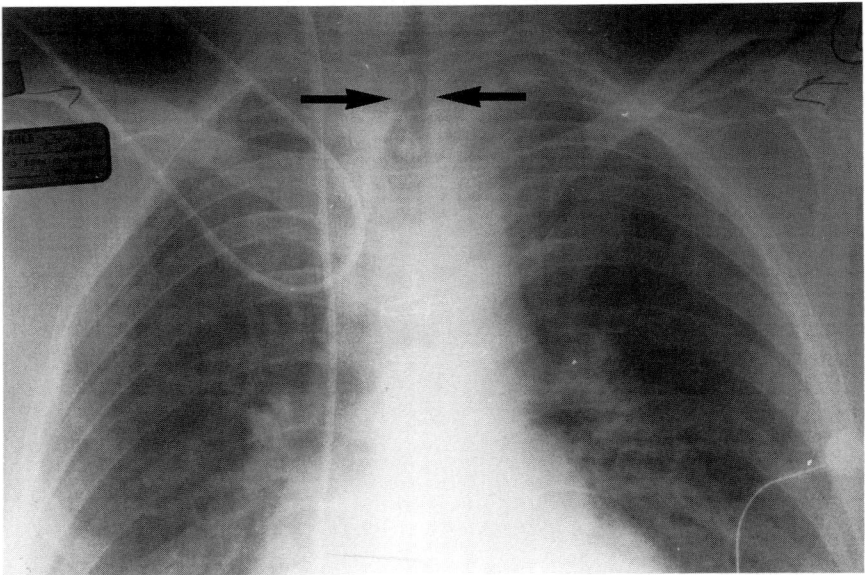

Figure 2 Tracheal stenosis: The patient is status-post tracheostomy. Chest radiograph shows narrowing of the trachea (arrows) at the prior tracheostomy site.

patient is supine, and if the lungs are stiff, as in adult respiratory distress syndrome (ARDS), the pneumothorax is not always in the typical apical location. In these patients, the air may collect anteriorly and inferiorly within the thorax, creating a lucency in the lateral costophrenic recess, the so-called deep sulcus sign. Air may also collect in a subpulmonic location or medial to the lung, simulating a pneumomediastinum. Pneumomediastinum is manifested by linear lucencies adjacent to the mediastinum and heart, and may extend into the neck. A pneumomediastinum can be differentiated from a medial pneumothorax by obtaining a lateral decubitus radiograph. Air in the pleural space usually will rise to the nondependent position, whereas air in the mediastinum will not move.

E. Central Venous Cannulation

Numerous complications can occur during the placement of central venous catheters and pulmonary artery catheters. The overall complication rate ranges from 0.4% to 11% (3). Most minor complications occur because of inadvertent malposition of the catheters (Fig. 3). Central venous catheters are properly positioned with the tip in the superior vena cava. Misplaced catheters usually are within the right atrium, the coronary sinus, or may pass into a smaller venous branch, such as

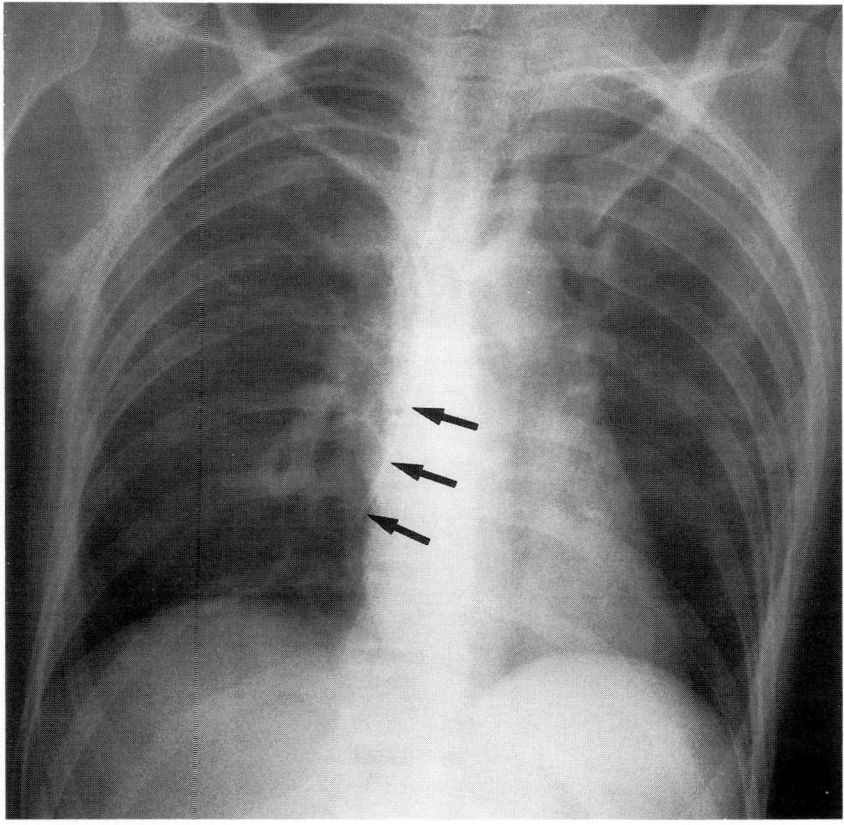

Figure 3 Catheter misplacement: A central venous catheter was placed. On the postplacement chest radiograph the tip of the catheter is seen to lie outside of the vascular structures (arrows).

the contralateral brachiocephalic vein, the internal mammary vein, or the ipsilateral internal jugular vein. Inadvertent cannulation of the subclavian arteries usually causes no significant complication other than an occasional, usually self-limited, mediastinal hematoma. Hematomas caused by inadvertent subclavian artery catheterization or puncture are the second most common complication of central venous access insertion. Small lacerations of the mediastinal veins can cause similar problems. The hematomas are easily visualized on a portable chest radiograph as a new mediastinal mass, usually in the superior mediastinum. Rarely, massive bleeding occurs, requiring chest tube drainage or surgical intervention. Catheters can also be incorrectly placed into the pleural space, resulting in a pneumothorax (Fig. 4). Pneumothorax is the most common major complication of placement of central venous catheters, with a reported incidence of 6%, and it accounts for over 50% of all complications (3). Unrecognized malpositioned central catheters can result in infusion of fluids into the pericardium, mediastinum, or pleural space. Prevention of catheter malpositions relies on experience. Checking the postplacement radiograph for proper catheter position and recognizing the abnormal position of the catheter is important to prevent further complications of misplaced catheters.

F. Pulmonary Artery Catheterization

In a large series of postoperative patients, the incidence of serious complications following Swan–Ganz catheter placement was 3% (4). The risks can be classified

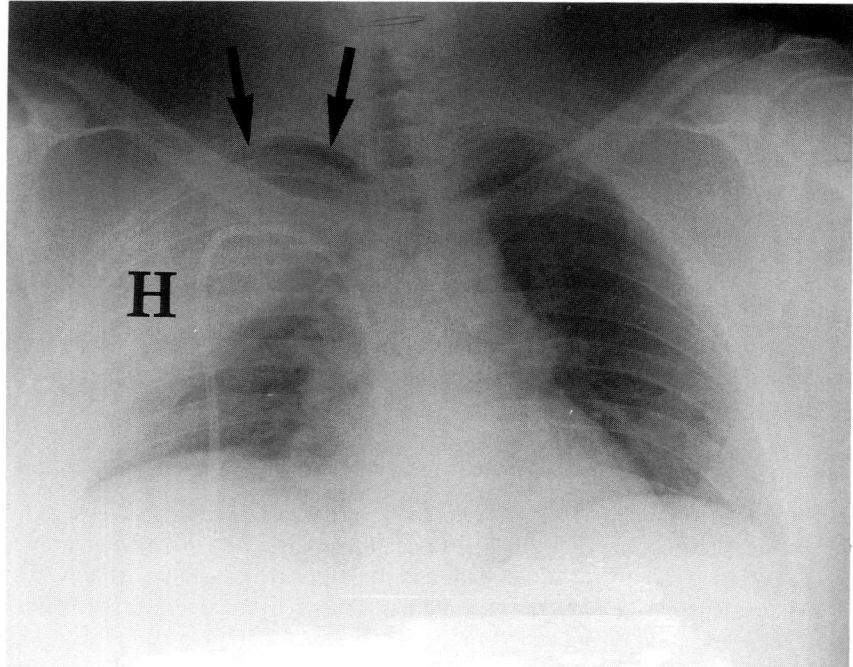

Figure 4 Central line complication: The patient has a hemothorax and a pneumothorax after the placement of a central venous catheter. The hemothorax is the large opacity in the right upper thorax (H) and the pneumothorax is the lucency above (arrows).

into those that occur during placement and those related to the prolonged use of the catheter. Pneumothorax occurs less than 0.5% of the time and is easily detected on the postplacement chest radiograph. Inadvertent arterial puncture is less common with the internal jugular approach (1.5%) than with the subclavian approach (4.5%). Arterial puncture does not usually cause any adverse sequelae, although rarely, a hemothorax may develop. Mediastinal widening owing to hematoma can be identified on follow-up chest radiographs even in cases of uncomplicated venous puncture. Swan–Ganz catheters may come to rest in abnormal positions, such as the inferior vena cava, the opposite subclavian or internal jugular vein, the coronary sinus, or in a distal branch of the pulmonary artery. Peripheral placement of the catheter in the pulmonary artery can cause a pulmonary infarction. Prompt recognition of the abnormal course of the catheter on the chest radiograph can allow the catheter to be quickly readjusted. Prolonged use of a Swan–Ganz catheter can lead to thrombosis or infection. Thrombosis of the great veins can be detected with CT or contrast venography. Rarely, distal peripheral pulmonary artery perforation can occur. Radiographically, the resulting hemorrhage is manifested as alveolar filling in the lung surrounding the catheter tip.

G. Tube Thoracostomy

Tube thoracostomy is a common procedure. Complication rates are near 1% in trauma patients and include diaphragmatic, lung, and liver lacerations (3). Lung laceration is a complication that occurs more commonly in patients with pleural adhesions or in patients with "stiff" lungs, as found in patients with ARDS (Fig. 5). Malpositioning the chest tube in the subcutaneous tissues is common (Fig. 6). Oblique radiographs are helpful in demonstrating its subcutaneous position. Kinking of the chest tube within the subcutaneous tissue may cause the tube to malfunction and can be demonstrated on the plain radiographs. Reexpansion pulmonary edema can result from the rapid reexpansion of a long-standing pleural effusion or pneumothorax. Efforts should be made to slowly reexpand such a lung to avoid this complication, which is readily identified on a chest radiograph. Failure of the chest tube to evacuate the fluid or air may be due to the malposition of the tube within the pleural space. Tubes within the fissures may not function properly, and if the tube is not situated within the pleural fluid or pneumothorax, these collections will not drain properly. Radiographs usually offer an explanation for the malfunctioning tubes, but occasionally, a CT scan may be needed to reveal the cause of the malfunction (5,6).

H. Intra-aortic Counterpulsation Balloon

The intra-aortic counterpulsation balloon (IAB) is used postoperatively to assist the left ventricle. It is positioned in the descending thoracic aorta, usually by a common femoral artery approach. The balloon, synchronized with the patient's

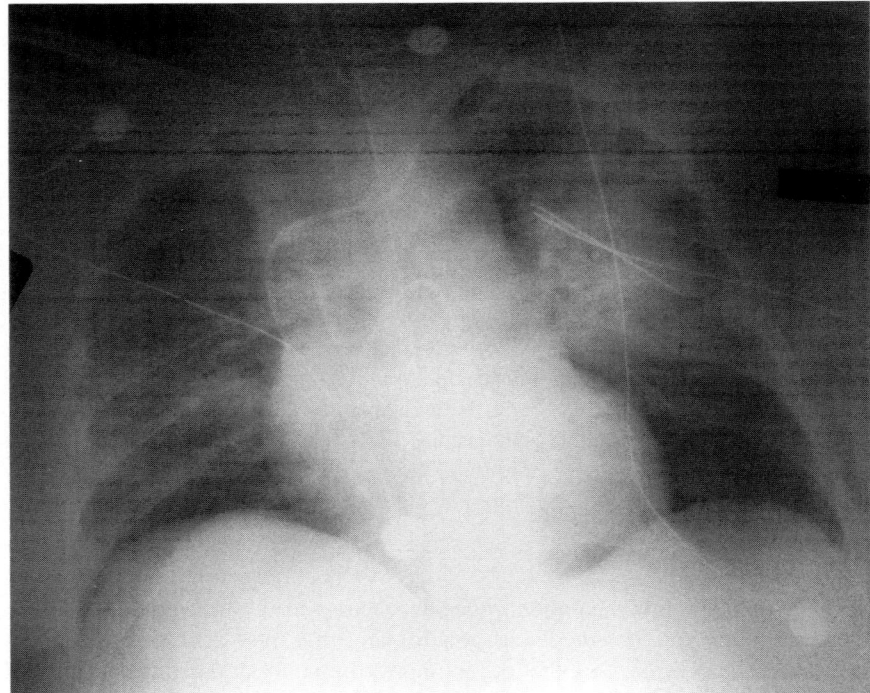

Figure 5 Lung laceration following chest tube placement: Immediately after the placement of a left pleural drain, the patient developed hemoptysis and a new alveolar opacity developed on the chest radiograph. The patient died of unrelated causes and the autopsy demonstrated a laceration in the left lung with surrounding hematoma.

electrocardiogram, is inflated during diastole, which causes an increase in systemic perfusion and aortic root pressure. Proper positioning in the descending aorta is the most important role radiology has to play in the evaluation of these devices. The metallic marker on the cephalad end of the IAB should be in the descending aorta, 1–2 cm distal to the takeoff of the left subclavian artery. If the balloon is advanced too far into the left subclavian artery or other arch vessels the vessel can be temporarily occluded. If the balloon is too low, intermittent occlusion of the visceral arteries and renal arteries can occur. Aortic dissection is a rare, less than 1%, complication that can occur during placement of the IAB (7,8).

I. Pacemakers

Pacemakers are used for various cardiac arrhythmias. There are numerous types that include both temporary and permanent pacemakers. Permanent pacemakers are placed transvenously through the subclavian vein with fluoroscopic guidance. Temporary pacemakers can be placed through the subclavian or transjugular approach. As with any subclavian venous approach, the complications of pneumothorax and mediastinal hematoma exist. Malposition of the pacemaker tip can occur and must be recognized. The tip should lie within the right ventricle. Placement within the coronary sinus or other coronary vein should be recognized on the initial radiograph and corrected. Lateral radiographs will demonstrate the posterior location of a pacer tip in the coronary sinus or venous branch of the coronary sinus rather than the proper anterior position in the right ventricle. Perforation of the right ventricle occurs in fewer than 1% of cases (9). It is often recognized clinically and rarely causes problems. Radiographically, in perforation, the pacemaker tip can be seen to deviate from its normal course and can be demonstrated to lie outside of the myocardium by CT. Occasionally, radiographs are required to investigate for a fracture of the pacer wire, which appears as a discontinuity in the course of the wire. Disruption of the insulation on the wire cannot be visualized on radiographs, since it is not radiopaque.

III. Aortic Surgery

Hemorrhage is an important cause of early morbidity and mortality following operations on the thoracic aorta. The incidence of death from hemorrhage varies, but ranges from 5 to 10%. Hemorrhage usually occurs at suture lines and through porous grafts (10).

Acute respiratory failure is a serious complication of thoracic aorta operations, especially in patients in whom cardiopulmonary bypass is used. It occurs in 3–5% of patients. The chest radiographs are often initially normal, but diffuse alveolar infiltrates subsequently develop that can lead to ARDS (10).

Pseudoaneurysms at the anastomotic suture line can develop after aortic surgery. They occur most commonly in patients who have undergone composite graft replacement of the ascending aorta with reanastomosis of the coronaries. Scans with CT or MRI may be needed to detect these pseudoaneurysms (10).

Aneurysms can develop in patients after the repair of a dissection, an aortic aneurysm, or in patients with Marfan's syndrome, where progressive dilatation of the native aorta can occur above or below the graft. In patients who have undergone an ascending aortic dissection repair, persistence of the dissection in the descending aorta may require reoperation and repair (10).

IV. Coronary Artery Bypass Surgery

Complications of elective bypass surgery are steadily decreasing, but the overall operative risks are increasing, as more cases are done emergently and on more complicated patients. Recognition of the radiographic findings of postoperative

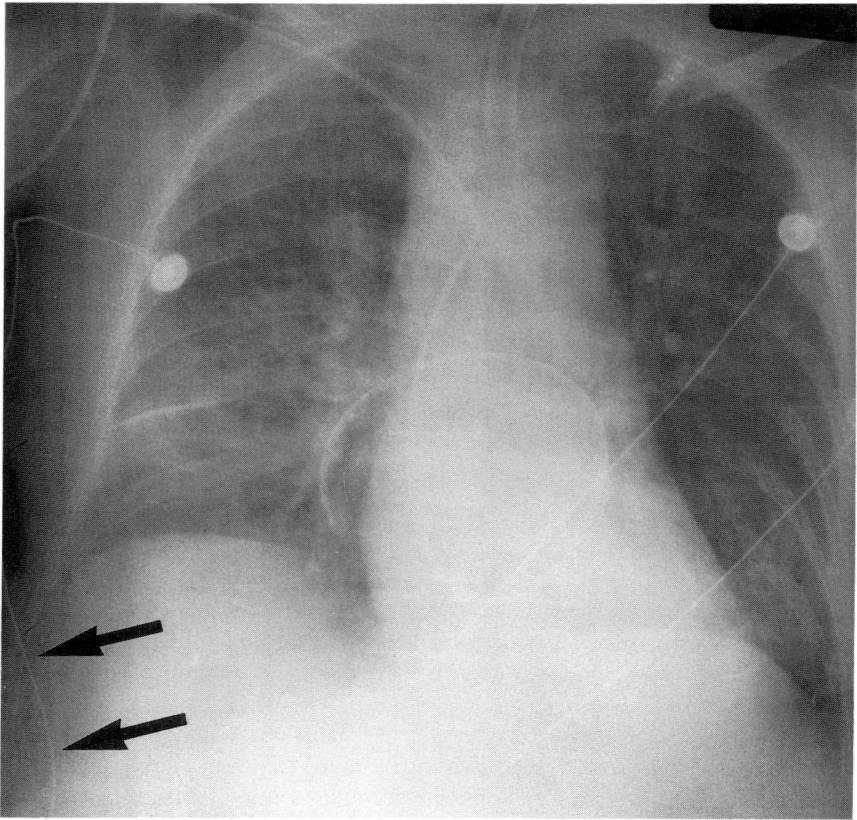

(a)

Figure 6 Intraperitoneal chest tube placement: (a) Chest radiograph obtained for right chest tube placement. The tube is seen passing through the upper abdomen (arrows). The tube was removed and successfully placed in the right pleural space. (b) A CT of the upper abdomen shows a liver laceration (arrows) caused by the misplaced chest tube.

complications, therefore, is of paramount importance in keeping the morbidity low (11).

Postoperative bleeding is almost always an indication for reoperation, and careful examination of serial postoperative chest radiographs along with clinical signs may give an early indication that hemorrhage is occurring. Mediastinal hematoma will be manifest as an increasing density or widening of the mediastinal contour (Fig. 7).

Respiratory complications, including atelectasis and pulmonary edema, can

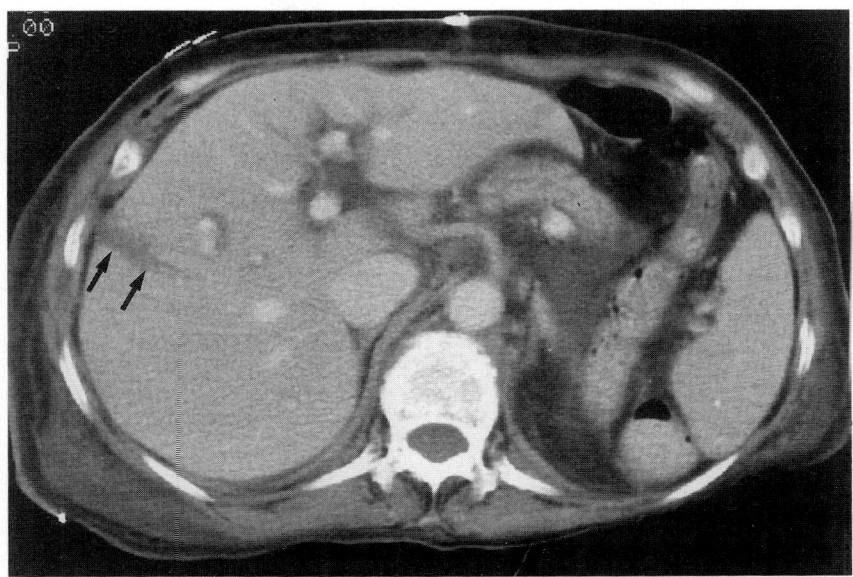

(b)

clearly be recognized on postoperative chest radiographs. Prolonged ventilation is necessary in less than 5% of patients and is due to several interrelated problems. ARDS or pneumonia may develop as the need for prolonged ventilation continues.

Diaphragmatic paralysis following heart surgery can be asymptomatic or can require prolonged mechanical ventilation. The exact incidence is underestimated, because patients are frequently asymptomatic. Clinical symptoms are characterized by recurrent episodes of respiratory failure within the first few weeks after surgery. Phrenic nerve injury is rare (1.5%), but may occur if pericardial ice slush is used without an insulating pad, or if there is direct surgical trauma. Diaphragmatic paralysis is suspected when the chest radiograph demonstrates elevation of the left hemidiaphragm. The diagnosis is confirmed with fluoroscopy. The affected diaphragm will have paradoxical motion when the patient sniffs. Many patients will have left lower lobe atelectasis and effusions that may make the left hemidiaphragm appear elevated. With time, up to 2 weeks, the atelectasis and effusions resolve and the diaphragm appears normal once again (12).

A. Postcardiotomy Mediastinitis

The diagnosis of postcardiotomy mediastinitis is often difficult to make with accuracy and may have grave consequences (13). The mortality rate for mediastinal infection after sternotomy is 27%, and it is 50% if diffuse mediastinitis is

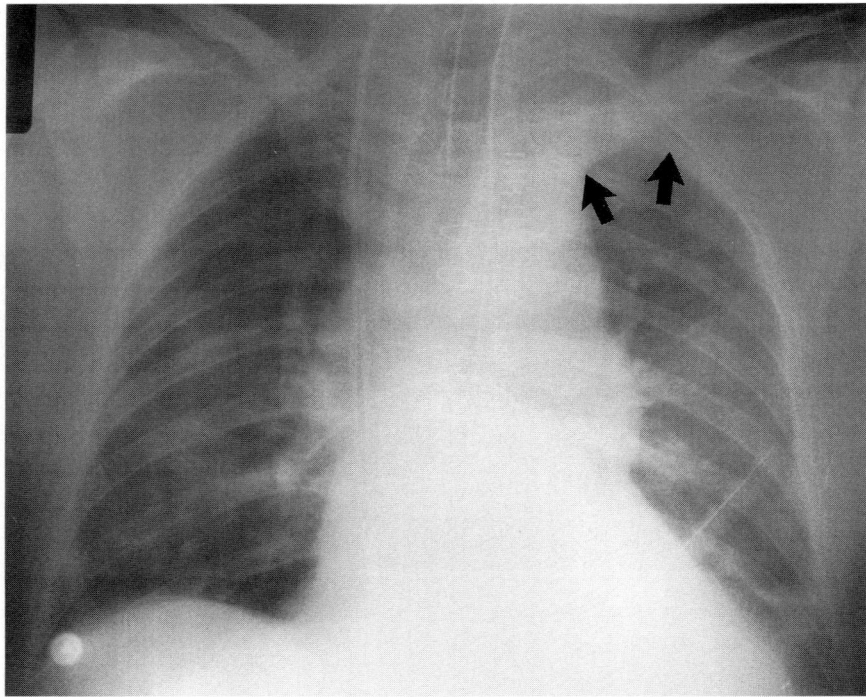

Figure 7 Mediastinal hematoma: Postoperative chest radiograph of a patient 1 day after coronary artery bypass grafting. Radiograph shows new widening of the mediastinum and a left apical cap (arrows). At reexploration a hematoma from a leaking graft was evacuated.

present. Obesity, diabetes mellitus, respiratory failure, and prolonged operative time, all are risk factors for developing mediastinitis. Motion between the sternal fragments and purulent drainage often signal the presence of an infection. Both sternal motion and purulent drainage can occur without mediastinitis, but mediastinitis should be suggested by the presence of either. Radiographs can show widening of the sternotomy, with or without the presence of infection. Scans with CT and MRI are often helpful in detecting postcardiotomy infections, but normal postoperative changes can cause confusion (Fig. 8) (14,15). Normally, there are small fluid collections, air collections, small bony fragments, and hematomas in the anterior mediastinum for 2–3 weeks postoperatively. Therefore, mediastinitis can be difficult to diagnose. Obliteration of mediastinal fat planes and diffuse soft-tissue infiltration, with or without gas collections, are suggestive. Abscesses are usually of low density and contain air (Fig. 9). Needle aspiration under CT guid-

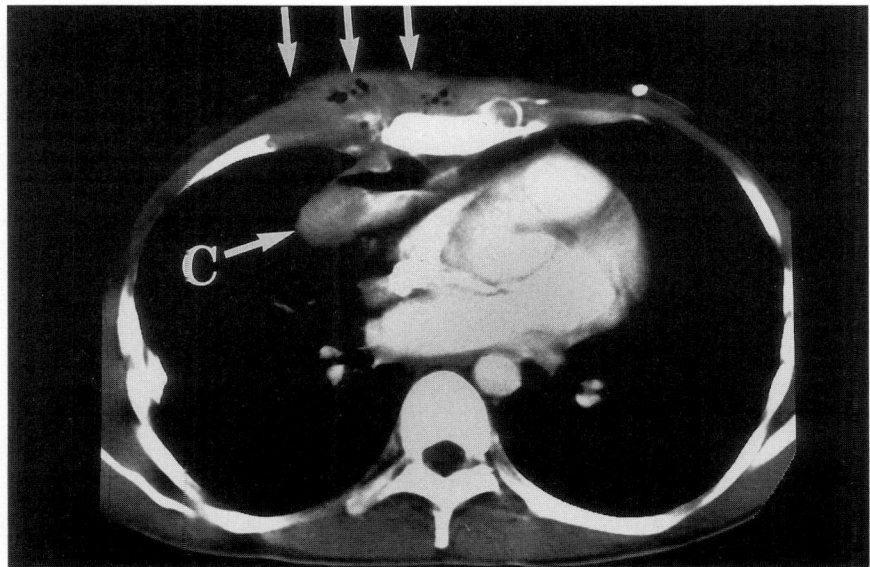

Figure 8 Chest wall abscess: The patient is several weeks out from a tracheoesophageal fistula repair and developed pain and tenderness in the midsternum. The CT scan demonstrates fluid and air surrounding the sternum (arrows). Drainage of the collection demonstrated infection. Note the retrosternal colonic interposition (C).

ance may aid in making the diagnosis of mediastinitis. Sternal osteomyelitis can be difficult to differentiate from normal postoperative changes until frank bone destruction, severe demineralization, and dehiscence occur. Treatment includes antibiotics, debridement, irrigation, and drainage. If this is not successful, plastic reconstruction may be needed.

B. Infected Thoracotomy

Because of the excellent blood supply to the thoracic wall and the immunological competence of the pleural space, infection of the chest wall following thoracotomy incisions is infrequent. The overall infection rate is between 0.5 and 2% for infection involving any structures of the chest wall or pleural space. Emergency thoracotomy carries a slightly higher rate of infection, approximately 5% (16). Although uncommon, the consequences can be quite serious. Most wound infections are apparent clinically at the surgical site. However, the total extent of infections and the presence of drainable fluid collections can all be imaged with CT scanning.

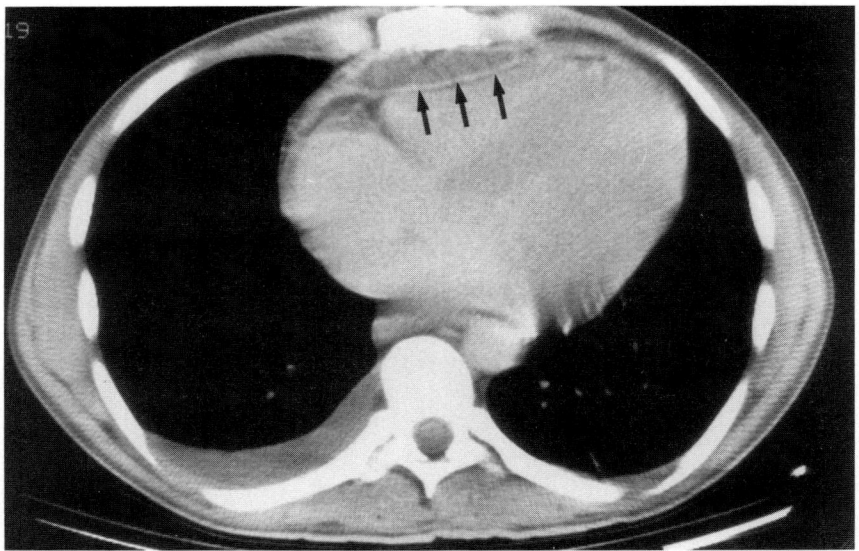

Figure 9 Mediastinal abscess: Patient is status-poststernotomy and developed a fever and chest pain several weeks after the operation. A CT scan demonstrates a retrosternal fluid collection without air bubbles (arrows). Needle aspiration, drainage, and culture proved the collection to be infected.

C. Herniations

Small subxiphoid hernias are common after sternotomy, but are rare following thoracotomy. Small hernias are of no consequence, although larger ones need repair. Herniation of the lung through a thoracotomy site can be diagnosed with physical examination and confirmed with tangential inspiratory radiographs or CT (17).

V. Pulmonary Resection Complications

The incidence of major complications and death after pulmonary resection has steadily declined since the inception of thoracic surgery. Mortality following pneumonectomy is currently approximately 7%, and the causes of death are most commonly pneumonia, myocardial infarction, pulmonary embolus, or a complication of a bronchopleural fistula (18). Morbidity following lobectomy or pneumonectomy can be minimized by quick recognition of complications both clinically and radiographically (Fig. 10).

A. Cardiac Herniation

Cardiac herniation following an intrapericardial pneumonectomy is rare. Cardiac herniation carries a 50% mortality, even if it is recognized and correction undertaken. Unrecognized cardiac herniation has a 100% mortality (19). Cardiac herniation is the result of a breach in the fibrous pericardium. Displacement of the heart through a right pericardial opening results in a 90–180° rotation, with the cardiac apex pointing laterally and posteriorly into the right hemithorax. Left and right herniation occur with equal frequency. The heart is mechanically displaced through, and entrapped by, the pericardial defect, effectively angulating and obstructing the superior and inferior vena cava, pulmonary arteries, and the aorta.

Clinically, the patients will have acute cardiac collapse and jugular venous distention. Herniation usually occurs at the conclusion of the operation, or in the immediate postoperative period. The precipitating event is usually a change in patient position, coughing, or positive-pressure ventilation. Firm pericardial adhesions that form by 3 weeks after an operation, effectively eliminate the risk of late herniation. Radiographically a right-sided herniation is unmistakable. The cardiac apex projects laterally, touching the chest wall, or is wedged into the posterior costophrenic sulcus. In contrast, a left cardiac herniation is less recognizable. The heart appears more horizontally oriented along the left hemidiaphragm. A left-sided herniation may not be appreciated without a lateral radiograph to show the posterior displacement of the heart (20,21). Often there is not time to obtain a radiograph, and the patient is taken for reoperation on clinical grounds alone. Placing the patient onto the side of the pneumonectomy may relieve symptoms. Immediate reoperation with the placement of a patch to prevent recurrence is required to save the patient's life.

B. Lobar Torsion and Gangrene

Lobar torsion is the twisting of a lobe of the lung on its vascular pedicle (22). Although uncommon, it occurs most frequently to the right middle lobe after a right upper lobectomy. Untreated lobar torsion will progress to infarction and gangrene. Pulmonary gangrene (hemorrhagic infarction), which is the most serious sequela of torsion, generally results from the associated pulmonary venous obstruction. The mortality rate is high, at 16%. Predisposing factors to torsion include a long, free lobar pedicle, especially when accompanied by a complete fissure; other factors include release or absence of the inferior pulmonary ligament, an airless lobe, pneumothorax, and pleural effusion. If the minor fissure is

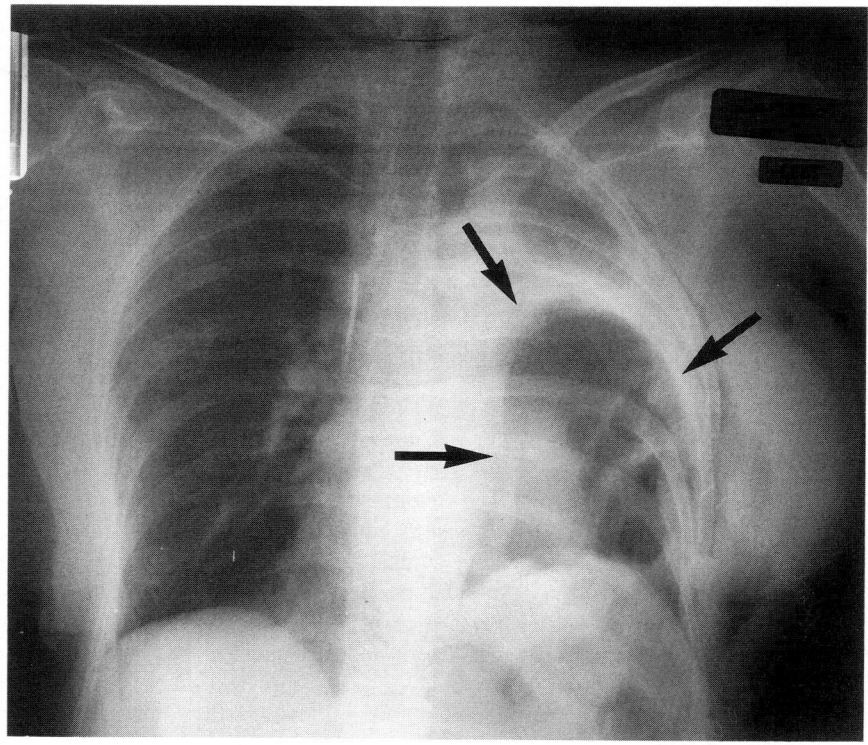

(a)

Figure 10 Stomach herniation: Two days after a left pneumonectomy for lung cancer the patient experienced left chest pain. (a) A chest radiograph shows a new air collection in the lower left hemithorax (arrows). (b) An upper gastrointestinal examination shows a portion of the stomach herniated through a small hole in the diaphragm into the postpneumonectomy space (arrows). The diaphragmatic defect was repaired.

complete, the right middle lobe can twist 180° on its bronchovascular pedicle. Postlobectomy torsion has also been reported in other lobes.

Additionally torsion has been reported in blunt chest trauma. The right middle lobe can be sutured to the remaining upper or lower lobe if the minor fissure is complete in a effort to prevent the possibility of lobar torsion. Radiographs play an important role in diagnosing lobar torsion (23,24). Early consolidation of a lobe with absent breath sounds may indicate the presence of lobar torsion. Hilar displacement, bronchial cutoff, an enlarged lobar consolidation, and unusual positioning of lobar consolidation or suture lines may also suggest lobar torsion.

Radiology of Thoracic Surgical Complications

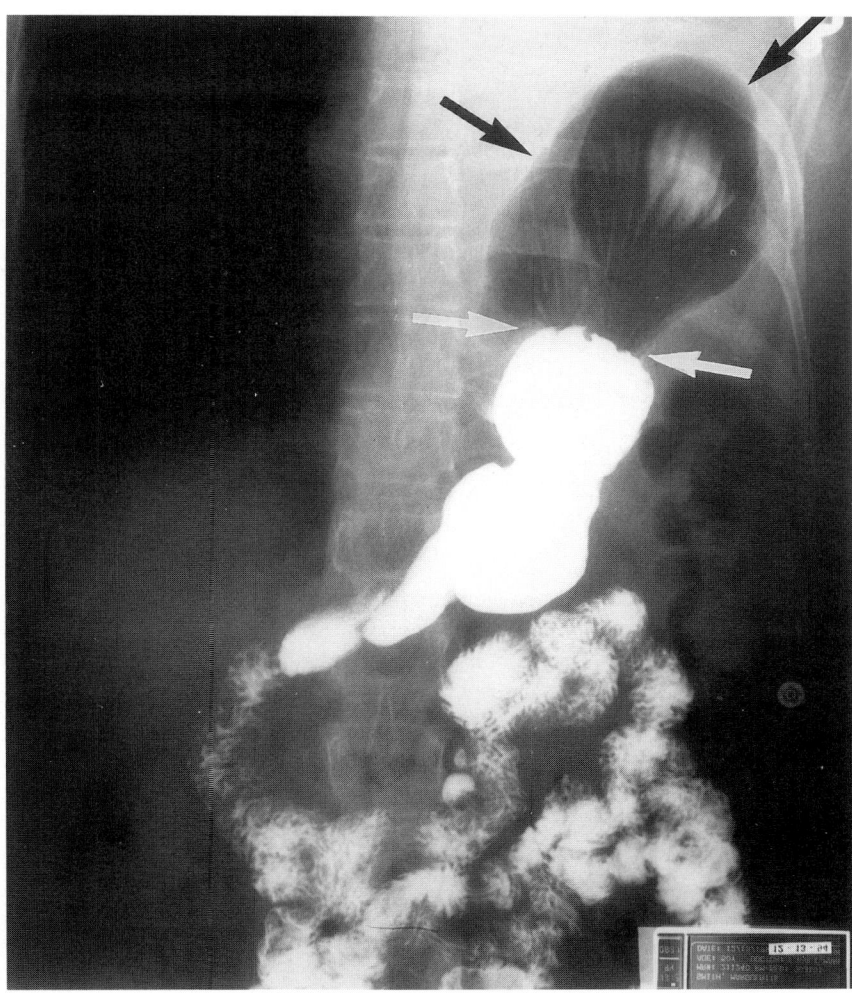

(b)

The differential diagnosis includes atelectasis, hemothorax, and pulmonary lobar hemorrhage.

C. Atelectasis

Atelectasis or collapse is the most common postoperative complication following thoracotomy. The incidence varies from 10 to 70%, with significant atelectasis affecting between 20 and 30% of patients (25). Atelectasis is multifactorial with mucous plugging of airways, shallow breathing, pleural fluid, postoperative pain, and splinting, all contributing to volume loss. The consequences are great as the patient may be hypoxic as a result of the atelectasis, and collapsed lobes are predisposed to infection. Radiographically, atelectasis may vary from plate-like atelectasis to segmental and lobar areas of collapse. On a properly exposed radiograph in a patient taking a good breath, the diagnosis is easily made. However, the diagnosis can be difficult to make in the patient with low lung volumes, or if the radiograph is underexposed. In addition, the differentiation of atelectasis from an area of pneumonia with associated atelectasis is difficult.

D. Bronchopleural Fistula

Bronchopleural fistula is defined as a communication of the bronchial tree with the pleural space. Bronchopleural fistula is one of the most dreaded complications that can occur after pulmonary surgery. The fistulas can occur in association with trauma, lung abscess, or empyema, but most are associated with previous pulmonary surgery. Air leaks following pulmonary resection are common. If an air leak is large enough that it prevents full expansion of the residual lung, or if it persists for a prolonged period, it represents a significant clinical problem and is termed bronchopleural fistula. Postresection bronchopleural fistulas are most frequently associated with empyema, although they can occur in its absence (25,26).

Bronchopleural fistulas usually develop 7–15 days following surgery (Fig. 11). The current rate of bronchopleural fistula following thoracotomy for lung cancer is 2.5%; 6% after pneumonectomy, and 1.4% after lobectomy. Mortality may reach 50% in postpneumonectomy lung cancer patients who develop a bronchopleural fistula. The fistula may be manifest by a persistent and moderate air leak, despite adequate chest tube placement. If chest tubes are removed, the fistula can present as hydropneumothorax.

In postpneumonectomy patients, bronchopleural fistulas are suspected when the fluid level in the postoperative thorax decreases, instead of its expected gradual increase (Fig. 12). However, a small drop in the fluid level of less than 2 cm is often seen in an uncomplicated pneumonectomy (27). Most postpneumonectomy pleural spaces are completely filled with fluid after an average of 3.9 months (range of 3 weeks to 7 months). If a bronchopleural fistula occurs, the remaining lung may demonstrate a new alveolar infiltrate as the fluid spills into the

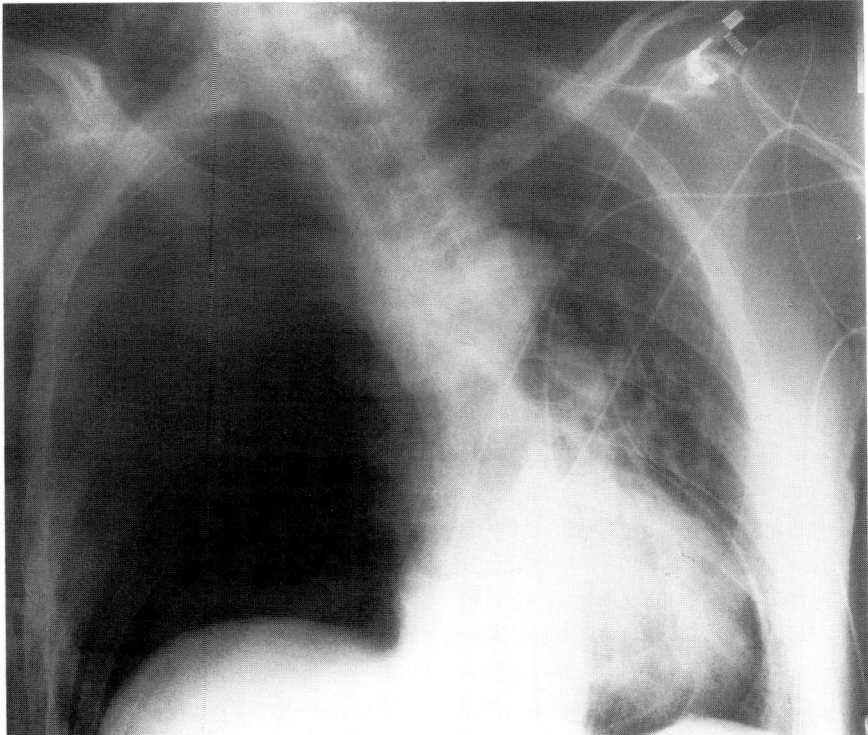

Figure 11 Tension pneumothorax: The patient underwent a right pneumonectomy and became suddenly short of breath on the second postoperative day. A chest radiograph demonstrates marked shift of the mediastinum to the left, with an increased size of the right hemithorax. At reexploration a leak at the bronchial stump was repaired.

bronchi. In a normal postpneumonectomy chest radiograph, the trachea is bowed toward the operative side. If a fistula develops, the trachea may assume a midline position.

The patient may describe a change in the pattern of coughing, or the sudden onset of paroxysms of unrelenting cough. Immediate bronchoscopy should be performed to confirm the diagnosis and the size of the leak, although small leaks may be difficult to visualize. Thin-section contiguous CT scans may also confirm the diagnosis and help locate the fistula site (Fig. 13). Treatment options include oversewing the stump, shortening the stump and oversewing it, as well as various

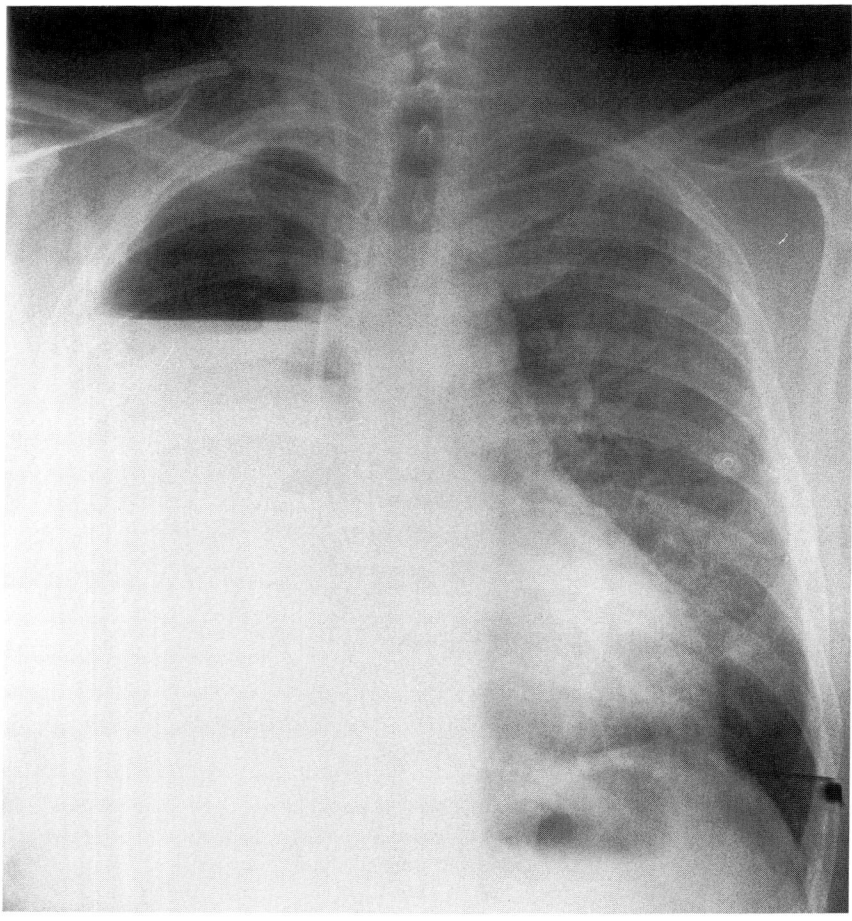

(a)

Figure 12 Bronchopleural fistula: Patient is status-post right pneumonectomy and experienced a new productive cough. (a) Previous radiograph demonstrated the expected increase in the right pleural effusion. (b) Current chest radiograph demonstrates a decrease in the air–fluid level within the pleural space, indicative of a bronchopleural fistula. The fistula resolved with conservative treatment.

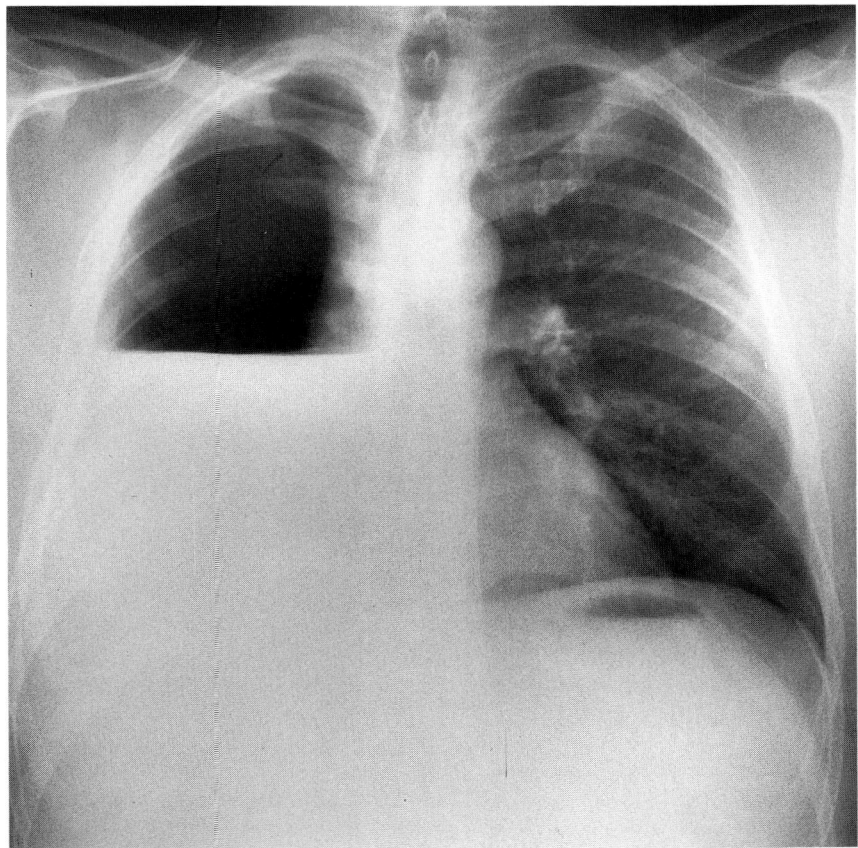

(b)

wrapping procedures that take normal vascularized pedicles of tissue and place them around the leak.

E. Persistent Pleural Spaces

Unresolved air or fluid collections within the postoperative thorax present several problems (28). This problem usually occurs when the remaining lung cannot expand enough to fill the new space. The unresolved space may fill with fluid that can become infected or prevent the complete expansion of the remaining lung. Persistent pleural fluid collections can also be a cause of persistent pleural drain-

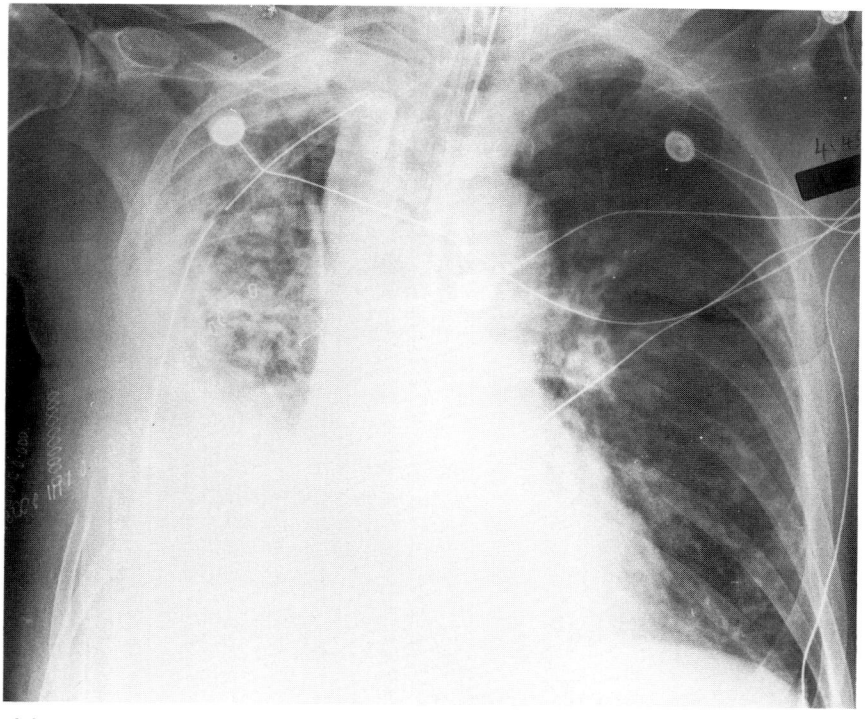

(a)

Figure 13 Broncho-cutaneous fistula: The patient is status-postlobectomy. (a) Initial radiograph shows a right pleural drain and airspace disease in the remaining right lobes. (b) The patient suddenly developed subcutaneous emphysema on the right (S). (c) A CT scan demonstrates a bronchocutaneous fistula (arrow).

age. A CT scan is an excellent imaging method to evaluate air or fluid collections within the postoperative thorax (29,30).

After pneumonectomy, air in the surgically incised hemithorax is gradually reabsorbed and replaced with fluid, with a net volume loss of the hemithorax. Thus, the trachea and mediastinum gradually shift toward the surgical side. In the immediate postoperative period, a shift away from the surgical side indicates an abnormal accumulation of air or fluid on the surgical side, most often as a result of a bronchopleural fistula, hemorrhage, or empyema. Immediate postoperative shift away from the side operated on can also result from atelectasis of the remaining lung (27).

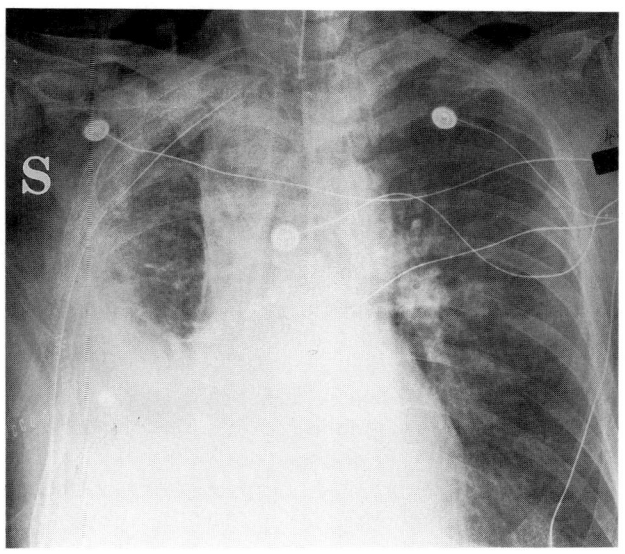

(b)

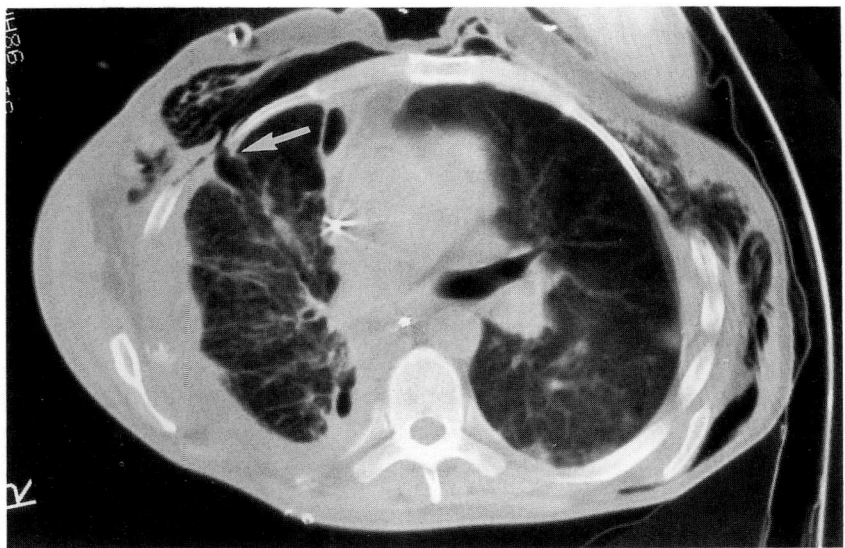

(c)

F. Empyema

An *empyema* is a collection of pus within the hemithorax. The diagnosis is based on a positive Gram stain or culture of fluid obtained from the pleural space. A postoperative empyema is most likely to occur if the pleural space is not completely drained and serosanguineous fluid is allowed to accumulate. When these predisposing factors exist, a high index of suspicion must be present to achieve early diagnosis and successful management. If suspected, thoracentesis is performed and cultures obtained.

Empyema after a lung resection has decreased in frequency with improvements in surgical technique and judicious use of antibiotics. In modern series, the incidence of empyema ranges from 2.2 to 8% after pneumonectomy and 0.6 to 5.6% after lobectomy, and usually occurs within the first few weeks after surgery. The chest radiograph frequently demonstrates a fluid collection within the hemithorax. Unexplained air within the fluid collection is very suggestive of infection (28).

Serial chest radiographs may demonstrate rapid accumulation of fluid within the pleural space in postlobectomy patients. In postpneumonectomy patients, empyema may be difficult to detect because the hemithorax normally fills with fluid. In postpneumonectomy patients, empyema is often associated with a bronchopleural fistula. Empyema is treated with chest tube drainage and antibiotics. Smaller tubes placed with radiographic guidance are often adequate. Streptokinase instillation may speed the clearing of the fluid and debris.

G. Hemothorax

Radiology usually does not play a role in the detection of postoperative bleeding after thoracic surgical procedures. The chest tubes are checked frequently for the amount and color of the drainage and serial hematocrits are checked. Usually, bleeding of more than 1 L within the first 24 h requires surgical reexploration. The incidence of hemothorax necessitating reoperation is 2.8%. Hemorrhage after pulmonary resection usually arises from an extrapulmonary site, most commonly an intercostal artery (28). Occasionally, the bleeding occurs in a site not in communication with the chest tube, or the chest tube is malfunctioning. In these instances, the development of a large hematoma can be detected on chest radiographs. A CT scan may demonstrate the hematoma as a high-density fluid collection, much denser than water.

H. Postthoracotomy Pulmonary Infections

Pulmonary infection is probably the most common postthoracotomy complication (31). The incidence of bacterial pneumonia following thoracic surgery has been estimated to be as high as 40%. Pneumonia in postthoracotomy patients is almost invariably bacterial in origin. Gram-negative organisms tend to predominate. In postoperative patients, it may be very difficult to differentiate postoperative fluid, atelectasis, and pneumonia. It is often the combination of clinical findings and radiographic abnormalities that lead to treatment for pneumonia. In ventilated patients the diagnosis is even more difficult, and bronchoalveolar lavage or protected specimen brushings are needed to confirm the diagnosis of pneumonia.

Aspiration is a common cause of pneumonia in recently extubated postthoracotomy patients. Gram-negative organisms are usually cultured in aspiration pneumonia. The radiographic findings in aspiration pneumonia are nonspecific. However, if the patient is suspected of aspirating and the infiltrates are in a dependent segments of the lung, the diagnosis can be entertained. Aspiration of acidic gastric contents (Mendelson's syndrome) results in a chemical pneumonitis. Theoretically, this syndrome should not require antibiotics for treatment because the gastric contents are sterile.

I. Postpneumonectomy Pulmonary Edema

Postpneumonectomy pulmonary edema is uncommon. When it occurs, it is usually seen following a right pneumonectomy. The diagnosis is one of exclusion. Chest radiographs show a diffuse alveolar infiltrate without clinical evidence of cardiac failure, pneumonitis, sepsis, or aspiration. The onset is insidious. After 12–36 uneventful postoperative hours the patient becomes dyspneic, and the chest radiograph shows rapidly worsening alveolar infiltrates. The etiology of this syndrome is unclear, but three risk factors have been identified: right pneumonectomy, large perioperative fluid load, and high urine output. Treatment is supportive (32).

J. Postpneumonectomy Syndrome

Postpneumonectomy syndrome is a rare, delayed complication, usually affecting young patients following a right pneumonectomy. It involves herniation of the mediastinum, heart, and contralateral lung into the postpneumonectomy pleural space (Fig. 14). Obstruction of the contralateral mainstem bronchus occurs as these structures cross the midline and stretch across the vertebral column and descending aorta. Signs and symptoms include progressive dyspnea, stridor, recurrent pulmonary infections, and respiratory arrest. The diagnosis is usually established by chest radiographs that demonstrate a marked mediastinal shift to the pneumonectomy side with hyperinflation of the remaining lung. A CT scan will also demonstrate the findings, including the bronchial compression. Treatment often involves surgical repositioning of the mediastinum (33,34).

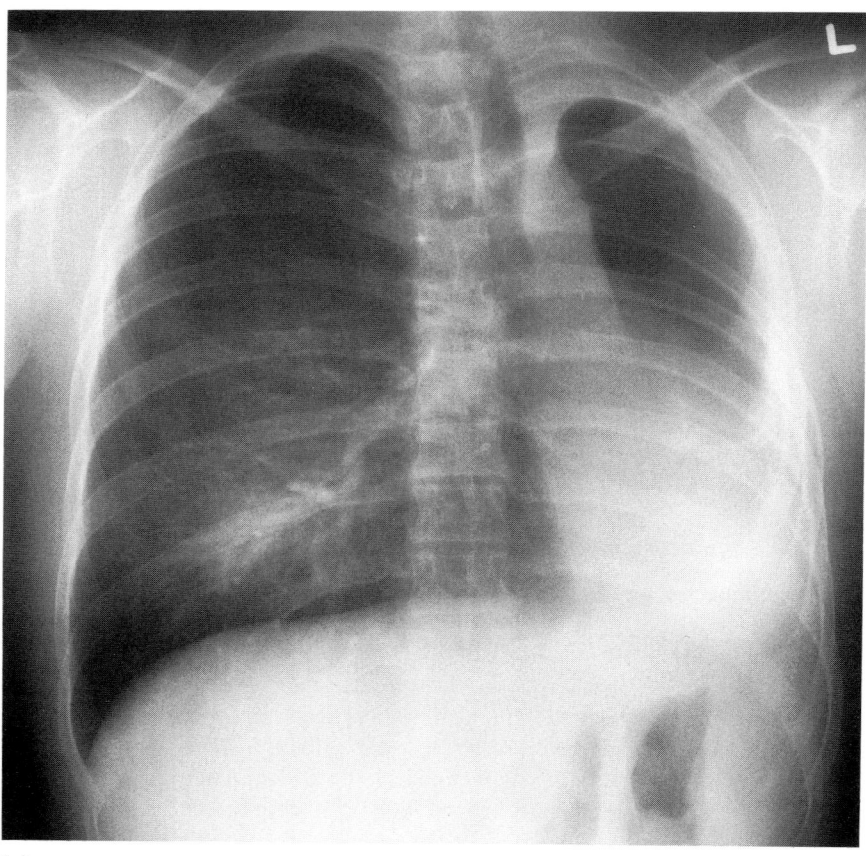

(a)

Figure 14 Mediastinal shift: The patient is several months status-post a left pneumonectomy. The mediastinum is shifted far to the left seen on (a) chest radiograph and (b) CT.

K. Complications of One-Lung Ventilation

One-lung ventilation during surgery allows procedures to be done thoracoscopically, and improves the surgical access for upper lobectomy. Postoperative radiographs may show residual atelectasis or minimal edema in the collapsed lung (Fig. 15). Similar radiographic findings can be seen in patients operated on in the lateral decubitus position. The lung that was in the dependent position during the procedure often has more retained secretions, residual edema, and atelectasis, which are reflected on the postoperative chest radiograph. Selective intubation of

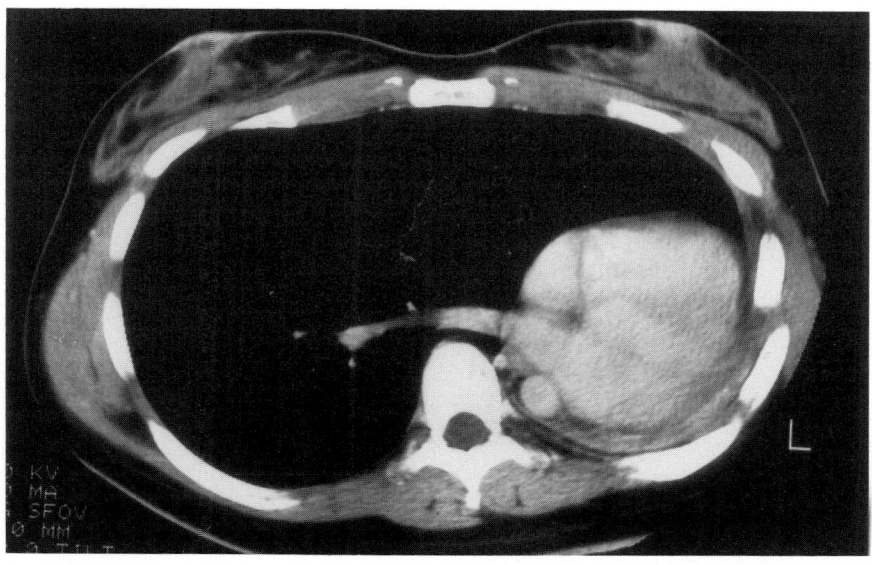

(b)

the left mainstem bronchus may occlude the left upper lobe bronchus. Thus, left upper lobe collapse may be seen on radiographs obtained in the operating room.

VI. Esophageal Surgery

A. Esophageal and Hiatal Hernia Surgery

Anastomotic leaks or perforation of the esophagus can occur following esophageal and hiatal hernia surgery. The development of a fever, chest pain, or new pleural effusion may herald the development of a leak or an unrecognized perforation. Examination of the esophagus with water-soluble contrast is an important tool in making the diagnosis, as endoscopy may not see small tears. The dreaded complication of an esophageal leak is the development of mediastinitis. Small leaks are managed conservatively with antibiotics and suction, whereas larger leaks often result in emergent reoperation (Fig. 16) (35,36).

Recurrent herniation can occur after hiatal hernia repair. It occurs in the immediate postoperative period owing to breakdown of the sutures, or it can occur much later, perhaps as a continuation of the processes that led to the development of the hiatal hernia in the first place. The postoperative chest radiograph can easily identify the recurrent hernia as a mass in the retrocardiac region. Contrast esopha-

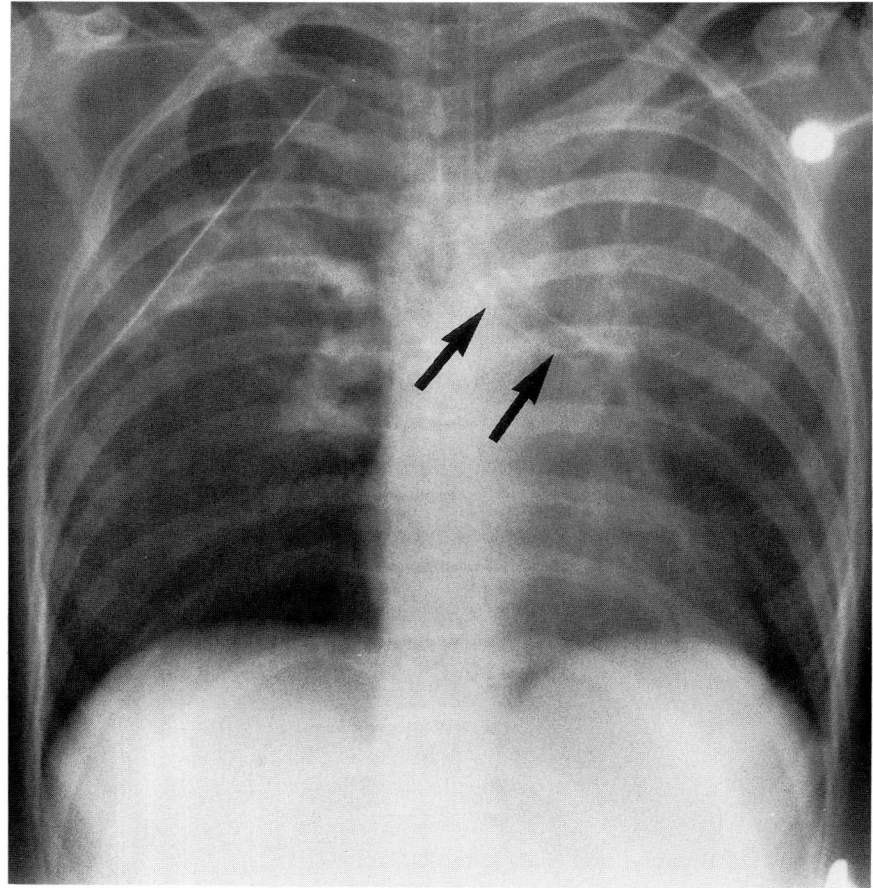

Figure 15 Left upper lobe collapse: The patient underwent partial right lung resection. Following selective intubation of the left mainstem bronchus the endotracheal tube (arrows) passed beyond the left upper lobe bronchus, resulting in its occlusion. The left upper lobe collapse appears as a vague increased density over the left upper hemithorax.

gograms clearly depict the recurrent hiatal hernia. Reflux can recur if the sutures are disrupted and the repair loses its integrity. Barium esophagogram can demonstrate the reflux. Dysphagia may occur if the repair is too tight. This may also be seen on an esophagogram. A postoperative paraesophageal herniation of the stomach may occur as well. Small leaks can develop in the distal esophagus in the immediate postoperative period, as well as later in the recovery period, usually after dilation of a postoperative stricture. An esophagogram is the imaging procedure of choice. Water-soluble contrast is initially used, followed by barium if no leak is seen. If a postoperative abscess is suspected, CT of the chest and upper abdomen with oral and intravenous contrast is better able to detect the presence and extent of the abscess (35,36).

B. Esophageal Perforation and Rupture

Esophageal perforation and rupture are life-threatening injuries that require prompt imaging and surgical intervention. Dilation of strictures is a common cause of iatrogenic esophageal perforation. Symptoms of new dysphagia and chest pain often lead to imaging of the esophagus to detect a perforation. A chest radiograph is obtained initially to detect the presence of a pneumomediastinum, a common finding in esophageal perforation. An esophagogram with water-soluble contrast is obtained next to determine the site and extent of the perforation. Barium may be used if the water-soluble esophagogram fails to detect a perforation, as barium is able to demonstrate very small abnormalities not seen with the less dense water-soluble contrast. A CT scan of the mediastinum can detect the complications of perforation, such as a fluid collection and abscess formation (37).

Esophageal rupture, or Boerhaave's syndrome, has a much more dramatic presentation, with pneumomediastinum, hydropneumothorax, mediastinal widening, and air–fluid levels. Imaging is identical with that for perforation, and postoperative imaging is usually used to determine the integrity of the esophagus and to detect accompanying abscess or fluid collection (37).

VII. Complications of Mediastinal Tumor Surgery

The preoperative accuracy in the diagnosis of mediastinal masses has improved dramatically in the last decade with the availability of CT imaging and preoperative needle biopsy. With more precise preoperative diagnoses and the use of adjuvant chemotherapy and radiotherapy, improved long-term results in the treatment of mediastinal masses and tumors have been achieved.

As in other surgical treatments in the chest, postoperative bleeding and infection are the primary complications of the surgery. Hemorrhage is more frequent after resection of vascular mediastinal tumors, such as pheochromocytoma, hemangioma, and the highly vascular Castleman's tumor. Infectious complications are infrequent, occurring in less than 1% of patients undergoing surgery for mediastinal masses at one institution. Immunocompromised patients or patients whose mediastinal mass or cyst is secondarily infected are at a higher risk to develop postoperative infections (38,39).

Follow-up chest radiographs and CT scans can identify most cases of significant bleeding and infection. Postoperative chest radiographs and fluoros-

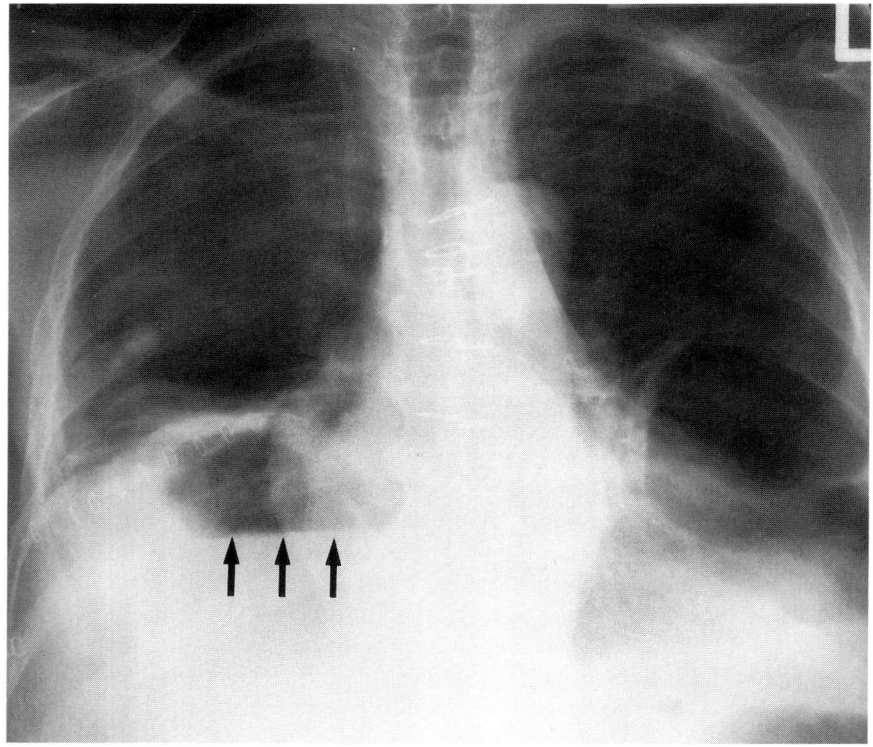

(a)

Figure 16 Subdiaphragmatic abscess after a gastrectomy and esophagojejunostomy: (a) Chest radiograph shows an air–fluid collection in the right lower hemithorax (arrows). (b) A CT scan demonstrates a subdiaphragmatic air–fluid collection in the right upper quadrant (arrows) (L, liver). At drainage this proved to be an abscess, and no bowel leak was demonstrated.

copy can identify patients in whom the phrenic nerve has been injured during mediastinal surgery. The nerve may be injured inadvertently or may be sacrificed during the removal of a mass. If the nerve has been injured, but not severed, function may return within 6–8 weeks. Chylothorax may occur after mediastinal surgery. The course of the thoracic duct and its tributaries is variable and can be interrupted during surgery for a mediastinal mass. Postoperative chest radiographs demonstrate a pleural effusion, which, when sampled, meets the criteria for chyle. A CT scan after a lymphangiogram may demonstrate the site of the chyle leakage

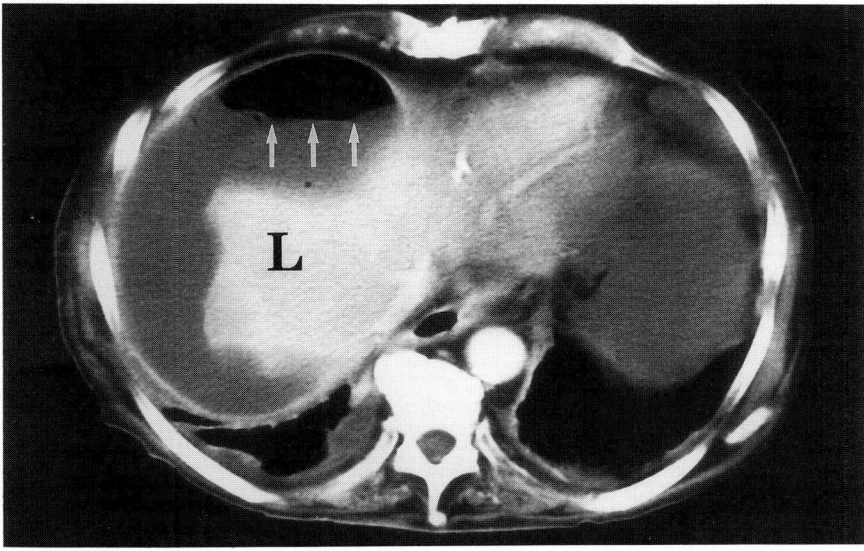

(b)

and aid in planning an operative procedure. Another important role that imaging, particularly CT scanning, plays in this group of patients is the detection of residual disease. The detection of residual tumor is often of paramount importance in determining future clinical therapy (38,39).

VIII. Thoracic Transplant Surgery

A. Cardiac Transplantation

Cardiac transplantation offers a life-saving option for patients with end-stage cardiac disease. The patient's cardiac failure is often traded for a new set of problems, owing to the complications of rejection and infection. Often the balance between rejection and infection is a precarious one, as increasing the antirejection drugs causes the patient's own immunodefenses to weaken. Radiology does not play a major role in detecting rejection, other than the detection of cardiac failure. Use of MRI has not proved to be accurate in detecting rejection (40,41).

The role that radiology plays in the detection of infection is great. Numerous infections occur in cardiac transplant patients. The types of infections vary in relation to the time after surgery and the doses of immunosuppressive therapy (42). Over 70% of transplant patients develop a severe infection, and infection is the primary cause of death in over 10% of cardiac transplant patients. Bacteria are the most frequent pathogens, but over a third of the infections are caused by viruses, fungi, and protozoans. In 40% of the infections, the organisms are opportunistic. Infections in the first 6 weeks are equally likely to be bacterial or viral. Severe viral infections are often seen in the first and sixth months following transplantation. Severe fungal infections are most common in the first 2 months. Protozoal infections appear after 1 month and peak in the third to sixth month. The clinical course of the patient and the radiographic finding can be combined with the knowledge of when certain types of infections are likely to occur. This knowledge can narrow the realm of possible infectious agents so that a reasonable treatment plan can be instituted until cultures or stains of material obtained by lavage or biopsy yield an answer.

B. Lung Transplantation

The increased survival of patients undergoing lung transplantation has depended on improved surgical techniques, immunosuppressive therapy, and the rapid identification of complications. The role that radiology plays is to detect pulmonary opacities that may signal rejection or infection. The first few days after a lung transplant can be associated with various pulmonary complications, including reperfusion edema, acute rejection, pneumothorax, and pneumonia (41,43).

Transplant edema is an almost universal finding in patients during the first 3 days after lung transplantation. Reperfusion pulmonary edema is the accumulation of extravascular lung water in the early posttransplant period. It is a self-limited phenomenon that has been generally less severe with improved donor lung preservation methods. Chest radiographs show edema in the transplanted lung. Management is supportive, with mechanical ventilation, diuretics, and fluid restriction. Spontaneous resolution or improvement usually occurs within 36–72 h (44,45).

Acute rejection is usually diagnosed, based on a combination of signs, symptoms, laboratory and radiological findings, along with the patient's response to increased immunosuppression once infection has been excluded (46). Acute rejection usually occurs within the first 2 weeks. There is usually an acute deterioration in the patient's clinical status. The chest radiograph may initially be normal, but will develop perihilar or diffuse alveolar infiltrates in the transplanted lung. Other radiographic findings include, new or increasing pleural effusions, thickening of septal lines, peribronchial cuffing, and airspace disease, without increase in cardiac size. Unfortunately, these findings may be compatible with bacterial pneumonias, and cytomegalovirus, herpes simplex, or *Pneumocystis carinii* infections. Bronchoscopy is usually performed, and if no organisms are seen, the patient is treated for rejection. If rejection was the cause of the deterioration, the treatment usually results in a dramatic improvement in the patient's condition. Ventilation and perfusion lung scanning can also aid in the diagnosis of acute rejection. Decreased flow to the transplanted lung is seen with acute rejection. High-resolution CT scanning has demonstrated ground-glass opacities in as many as 65% of patients during acute rejection episodes (47).

The diagnosis of chronic rejection is mostly based upon the patient's complaints of malaise, slowly worsening dyspnea, and deteriorating pulmonary function, combined with the results of transbronchial lung biopsy and lavage. Obliterative bronchiolitis is known to affect approximately 50% of heart–lung patients and is felt to be due to chronic rejection. The incidence is less in lung transplantation alone (30%) (46). The syndrome typically begins from 6 months to 2 years after transplantation. Initial symptoms are dyspnea and productive cough, progressing to hypoxia and hyperventilation. The most striking histological abnormality is the filling of terminal and respiratory bronchioles, alveolar ducts, and adjacent airspaces with plugs of loose connective tissue. The disease is characterized by patchy panlobular obliteration of distal bronchioles. Early chest radiographs may demonstrate peribronchial cuffing and diffuse interstitial infiltrates. Other radiographic findings include both increased and decreased lung volumes, central and peripheral bronchiectasis, localized airspace disease, segmental atelectasis, thin linear irregularities, areas of increased opacity, pleural thickening, and diminished peripheral lung markings. A CT scan is more sensitive in detecting these abnormalities, including the detection of bronchiectasis and air trapping (41,46).

Infection is the leading cause of morbidity and mortality in recipients of lung or heart–lung transplantations. It is at least twice as common in these groups than in heart or liver transplant patients. Most of the reported infections are bacterial (65%), but viral and fungal infections are more lethal. Life-threatening infections usually occur in the lung graft, but infection elsewhere or extrapulmonary dissemination of lung infection also contributes to significant morbidity and mortality (45).

A combination of atypical clinical presentations and nonspecific radiographic patterns makes diagnosis of opportunistic infections difficult. Sputum culture has a very low diagnostic yield in these patients. Bronchoscopy with lavage and brushings is the most important initial diagnostic procedure to evaluate unexplained pulmonary infiltrates detected on a chest radiograph. Transtracheal and transthoracic fine-needle aspiration biopsies have also had diagnostic success in transplant patients. Common opportunistic infections include those caused by *Listeria, Legionella, Nocardia, Mycobacterium, Aspergillus, Candida, Coccidioides, Cryptococcus,* phycomycosis, cytomegalovirus, herpes simplex, varicella–zoster, *Toxoplasma gondii,* and *Pneumocystis carinii.* Because radiographic findings seen with these infections in transplant patients are often nonspecific, a diagnostic procedure is often required to confirm the diagnosis.

Bacterial infections occur in lung transplant patients during the first 4–8

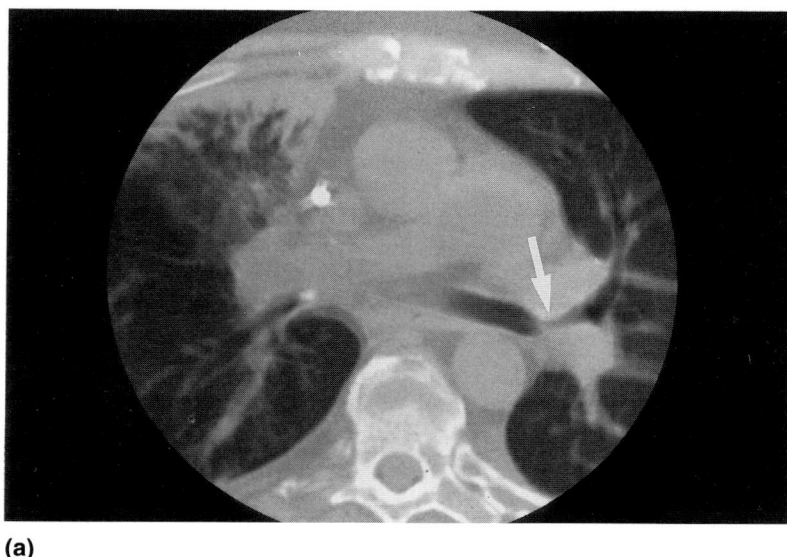

(a)

Figure 17 Stent placement in a posttransplant bronchial stenosis: (a) A CT scan demonstrating narrowing of the left mainstem bronchus (arrow). (b) Fluoroscopic spot film of the balloon expanding the metallic stent within the bronchus. Note the narrow waist at the site of maximum stenosis (arrows). (c) Postdilation film showing the patent bronchus and stent (arrows).

weeks posttransplantation. Three-fourths of the bacterial pneumonias are caused by gram-negative rods, with *Pseudomonas aeruginosa*, *Serratia marcescens*, and *Enterobacter* predominating.

The significant viral pathogens for lung and heart–lung transplant recipients include herpesvirus I and II, herpes zoster virus, Epstein-Barr virus, and cytomegalovirus. Of these, the cause of greatest morbidity and mortality and the focus of the greatest interest is cytomegalovirus (CMV). Infection with CMV most commonly occurs between 1 and 4 months posttransplantation, the period of most intense immunosuppression. The clinical manifestations in symptomatic cases are variable, ranging from a mild flu-like syndrome, to a fulminant picture of disseminated disease with severe pneumonia. Radiographically there are minimal to moderate interstitial and alveolar infiltrates. Posttransplant herpes simplex infections have been greatly reduced by acyclovir prophylaxis. Herpes pneumonia is most common early in the posttransplantation period and presents with focal or diffuse infiltrates. Mortality is often due to a bacterial or fungal superinfection. Varicella–zoster pulmonary infections are usually accompanied by skin lesions as

Radiology of Thoracic Surgical Complications

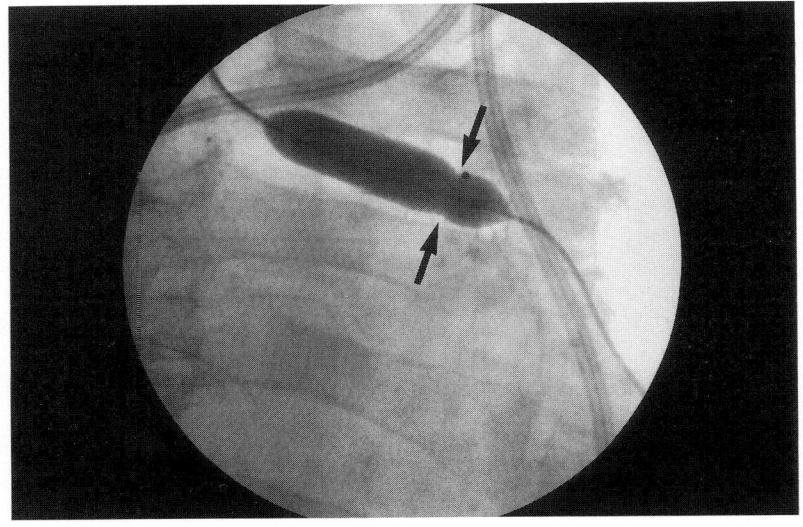

(b)

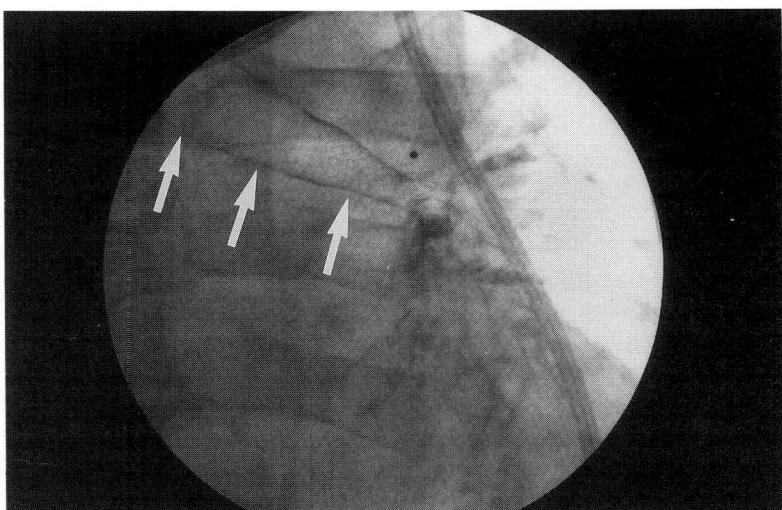

(c)

well, giving an important clue to the cause of the pneumonia. Epstein-Barr virus infection usually occurs in the first 3 months posttransplantation. The radiographic manifestations of all the viral infections are nonspecific.

Fungal infections in transplant patients occur in 3–15% of heart and heart–lung transplants. Fungal infections that infect transplant recipients can be considered in the following categories: (1) the mycoses with geographic distribution such as *Histoplasma capsulatum*, *Coccidioides immitis*, and *Blastomyces dermatitidis*; and (2) the ubiquitous organisms, such as *Candida* species, *Aspergillus* species, and *Cryptococcus neoformans*. Pulmonary aspergillosis in the immunocompromised host can present either as a progressive indolent pneumonia or as an acute fulminant infection. The timing of infection can be highly variable, and symptoms are often indistinguishable from bacterial pneumonia. The other fungal infections in these hosts often have no distinguishable radiographic features to set them apart from each other.

Pneumocystis carinii pneumonia is an important late cause of morbidity and mortality in immunosuppressed organ transplant recipients. It occurs in 1–10% of heart transplant recipients and more frequently in heart–lung transplant patients. Radiographically, diffuse perihilar alveolar and interstitial infiltrates are common, but the chest film may be normal.

Airway complications thwarted the initial attempts at successful lung transplantation (48). Following isolated lung transplantation, early bronchial viability must rely exclusively on retrograde flow from the pulmonary circulation to the bronchial circulation. Necrosis and subsequent dehiscence of the bronchial anastomosis were responsible for the death of many patients who survived the first few weeks posttransplant. Extrabronchial air collections are a radiologic manifestation of anastomotic dehiscence. However, the majority of airway complications are first noted on bronchoscopy. Often routine bronchoscopy is performed at specified intervals. Immediately postoperatively the anastomosis usually has a pink and healthy appearance. At 1 week the donor mucosa typically appears inflamed and friable. It is common to note a ring of whitish slough at the anastomosis. If symptoms of stridor or wheeze develop, bronchoscopy may show a late stricture or bronchomalacia. Posttransplant CT, especially spiral CT with reconstructions, can routinely identify these strictures. A small partial dehiscence can cause an air leak into the mediastinum which is also easily identified on CT. Bronchial strictures and bronchomalacia can be stented with plastic stents or with expandable metallic stents placed with bronchoscopic and fluoroscopic guidance (Fig. 17) (49).

References

1. Wolfe WG. Complications in Thoracic Surgery. St Louis: Mosby Year Book, 1992:ix.

2. Snow N, Bergin KT, Horrigan TP. Thoracic CT scanning in critically ill patients. Chest 1990; 97:1467–1470.
3. Bolling SF. The management of complications of venous access monitoring and chest tubes. In Waldhausen JA, Orringer MB, eds. Complications in Cardiothoracic Surgery. St Louis: Mosby Year Book, 1991:29–38.
4. Purut CM, Smith PK. Complications of pulmonary artery catheterization. In Wolfe WG, ed. Complications in Thoracic Surgery. St Louis: Mosby Year Book, 1992: 282–287.
5. Baldt MM, Bankier AA, Germann PS, Poschl GP, Skrbensky GT, Herlod CJ. Complications after emergency tube thoracostomy: assessment with CT. Radiology 1995; 195:539–543.
6. Stark DD, Federle MP, Goodman PC. CT and radiographic assessment of tube thoracostomy. AJR 1983; 141:253–258.
7. Landay MJ, Mootz AR, Estrera AS. Apparatus seen on chest radiographs after cardiac surgery in adults. Radiology 1990:174:477–482.
8. Richenbacher WE, Pierce WS. Management of complications of intraaortic balloon counterpulsation. In: Waldhausen JA, Orringer MB, eds. Complications in Cardiothoracic Surgery. St Louis: Mosby Year Book, 1991:97–102.
9. Luck JC, Pae WE. Pacemaker complications. In: Waldhausen JA, Orringer MB, eds. Complications in Cardiothoracic Surgery. St Louis: Mosby Year Book, 1991:114–124.
10. Kouchoukos NT, Wareing TH. Management of complications of aortic surgery. In: Waldhauser JA, Orringer MB, eds. Complications in Cardiothoracic Surgery. St Louis: Mosby Year Book, 1991:224–236.
11. Mahfood SS, Higgins TL, Loop FD. Management of complications related to coronary bypass surgery. In: Waldhausen JA, Orringer MB, eds. Complications in Cardiothoracic Surgery. St Louis: Mosby Year Book, 1991:265–280.
12. Sivak ED. Management of ventilator dependency following heart surgery. Semin Thorac Cardiovasc Surg 1991; 3:53–62.
13. Craver JM, Rand RP, Bostwick J III, Hatcher CR Jr. Management of postcardiotomy mediastinitis. In: Waldhausen JA, Orringer MB, eds. Complications in Cardiothoracic Surgery. St Louis: Mosby Year Book, 1991:125–131.
14. Templeton PA, Fishman EK. CT evaluation of poststernotomy complications. AJR 1992; 159:45–50.
15. Randall PA, Trasolini NC, Kohman LJ, et al. MR imaging in the evaluation of the chest after uncomplicated median sternotomy. Radiographics 1993; 13:329–340.
16. Douglas JM. Complications related to patient positioning, thoracic incisions, and chest tube placements. In: Wolfe WG, ed. Complications in Thoracic Surgery. St Louis: Mosby Year Book, 1992:76–87.
17. DiMarco AF, Oca O, Renston JP. Lung herniation. Chest 1995; 107:877–879.
18. Busch E, Verazin G, Antkowaik JG, Driscoll D, Takita H. Pulmonary complications in patients undergoing thoracotomy for lung carcinoma. Chest 1994; 105:760–766.
19. Mathisen DJ, Wain JC Jr. Cardiac complications following pulmonary resection. Chest Surg Clin North Am 1992; 2:793–802.
20. Gurney JW, Arnold S, Goodman LR. Impending cardiac herniation:the snow cone sign. Radiology 1986; 161:653–655.

21. Brady MB, Brogdon BG. Cardiac herniation and volvulus: radiographic findings. Radiology 1986; 161:657–658.
22. Wagner RB, Nesbitt JC. Pulmonary torsion and gangrene. Chest Surg Clin North Am 1992; 2:839–852.
23. Munk PL, Vellet AD, Zwirewich C. Torsion of the upper lobe of the lung after surgery: findings on pulmonary angiography. AJR 1991; 157:471–472.
24. Chan MCK, Scott JM, Mercer CD, Conlan AA. Intraoperative whole-lung torsion producing pulmonary venous infarction. Ann Thorac Surg 1994; 57:1330–1331.
25. Piccione W Jr, Faber LP. Management of complications related to pulmonary resection. In: Waldhausen JA, Orringer MB, eds. Complications in Cardiothoracic Surgery. St Louis: Mosby Year Book, 1991:336–353.
26. Allen MS, Deschamps C, Trastek VF, Pairolero PC. Bronchopleural fistula. Chest Surg Clin North Am 1992; 2:823–837.
27. Wechsler RJ, Goodman LR. Mediastinal position and air–fluid height after pneumonectomy: the effect of the respiratory cycle. AJR 1985; 145:1173–1176.
28. Duhaylongsod FG, Wolfe WG. Complications of pulmonary resection. In: Wolfe WG, ed. Complications in Thoracic Surgery. St Louis: Mosby Year Book, 1992:105–127.
29. Heater K, Revzani L, Rubin JM. CT evaluation of empyema in the postpneumonectomy space. AJR 1985; 145:39–40.
30. Biondetti PR, Fiore D, Sartori F, Cologanato A, Ravasini R, Romani S. Evaluation of the post-pneumonectomy space by computed tomography. JCAT 1982; 6:238–242.
31. Nelson ME, Moran JF. Post-thoracotomy pulmonary infections. In: Wolfe WG, ed. Complications in Thoracic Surgery. St Louis: Mosby Year Book, 1992:146–152.
32. Deschamps C, Pairolero PC, Allen MS, Trastek VF. Postpneumonectomy pulmonary edema. Chest Surg Clin North Am 1992; 2:785–791.
33. Shepard JO, Grillo HC, McCloud TC, Dedrick CG, Spizarny DL. Right-pneumonectomy syndrome: radiological findings and CT correlation. Radiology 1986; 161:661–664.
34. Trastek VF, Pairolero PC, Allen MS, Deschamps C. Unusual complications of pulmonary resection. Chest Surg Clin North Am 1992; 2:853–860.
35. Orringer MB. Complications of esophageal resection and reconstruction. In: Waldhausen JA, Orringer MB, eds. Complications in Cardiothoracic Surgery. St Louis: Mosby Year Book, 1991:354–369.
36. Orringer MB.Complications of hiatus hernia surgery. In: Waldhausen JA, Orringer MB, eds. Complications in Cardiothoracic Surgery. St Louis: Mosby Year Book, 1991:370–386.
37. Tedder M, Lowe JE. Esophageal perforation and rupture. In: Wolfe WG, ed. Complications in Thoracic Surgery. St Louis: Mosby Year Book, 1992:233–243.
38. Oldham HN Jr. Complications of surgical treatment of mediastinal tumors. In: Waldhausen JA, Orringer MB, eds. Complications in Cardiothoracic Surgery. St Louis: Mosby Year Book, 1991:404–412.
39. Davis RD, Oldham HN Jr. Complications occurring during mediastinal surgery. In: Wolfe WG, ed. Complications in Thoracic Surgery. St Louis: Mosby Year Book, 1992:253–263.
40. Bahnson HT, Hardesty RL, Griffith BP, Armitage JM, Kormos RL. Management of

complications related to cardiac transplantation. In: Waldhausen JA, Orringer MB, eds. Complications in Cardiothoracic Surgery. St Louis: Mosby Year Book, 1991: 425–433.
41. Casale AS, Reitz BA. Management of complications in transplantation: heart–lung. In: Waldhausen JA, Orringer MB, eds. Complications in Cardiothoracic Surgery. St Louis: Mosby Year Book, 1991:434–443.
42. Kramer MR, Marshall SE, Starnes VA, Gamberg P, Amitia Z, Theodore J. Infectious complications in heart-lung transplantation. Arch Intern Med 1993:153:2010–2016.
43. O'Donovan PB. Imaging the complications of lung transplantation. Radiographics 1993; 13:787–796.
44. Anderson DC, Glazer HS, Semenkovich JW, et al. Lung transplant edema: chest radiography after lung transplantation—the first 10 days. Radiology 1995; 195:275–281.
45. DeHoyos A, Maurer JR. Complications following lung transplantation. Semin Thorac Cardiovasc Surg 1992; 4:132–146.
46. Kirby TJ, Metha A, Rice TW, Gephardt GN. Diagnosis and management of acute and chronic lung rejection. Semin Thorac Cardiovasc Surg 1992; 4:126–131.
47. Loubeyre P, Revel D, Delignette A, Loire R, Mornex J. High-resolution computed tomographic findings associated with histologically diagnosed acute lung rejection in heart–lung transplant recipients. Chest 1995; 107:132–138.
48. Ramirez J, Patterson GA. Airway complications after lung transplantation. Semin Thorac Cardiovasc Surg 1992; 4:147–153.
49. Quint LE, Whyte RI, Kazerooni EA. Stenosis of the central airways: evaluation by using helical CT with multiplanar reconstructions. Radiology 1995; 194:871–877.

8

High-Resolution Computed Tomography of Chronic Infiltrative Lung Disease

THOMAS E. HARTMAN

Mayo Clinic and Mayo Foundation
Rochester, Minnesota

I. Introduction

There are over 150 pulmonary diseases that cause chronic infiltrative lung disease (CILD). However, over 90% of the causes of CILD can be accounted for by the diseases in Table 1 (1). These diseases will be the focus of this chapter. Additional chronic lung diseases that are primarily related to the airways, such as bronchiolitis obliterans and bronchiolitis obliterans organizing pneumonia (BOOP) will be discussed in a later chapter.

In the evaluation of chronic infiltrative lung disease, high-resolution computed tomography (HRCT) is currently the best imaging modality available to depict the morphological features of pulmonary parenchymal disease. It is superior to the chest radiograph in the prediction of specific diagnoses in patients with CILD (2,3). Additionally, HRCT may demonstrate abnormalities that are undetected by the chest radiograph. In some patients, the findings on HRCT are diagnostic and can obviate biopsy. In patients for whom HRCT cannot provide a definitive diagnosis, it can provide helpful information about the potential type of biopsy (i.e., transbronchial vs. thoracoscopic or open-lung biopsy) and optimal location for biopsy.

In the evaluation of CILD on HRCT, there are several patterns of abnor-

Table 1 Chronic Infiltrate Lung Diseases[a]

UIP
   Idiopathic pulmonary fibrosis (IPF)
   Collagen vascular associated interstitial lung disease
      Scleroderma
      Rheumatoid arthritis
Asbestosis
Sarcoidosis
Silicosis
Coal workers pneumoconiosis
Pulmonary Langerhans cell histiocytosis
Lymphangiomyomatosis
Extrinsic allergic alveolitis
Alveolar proteinosis
Chronic eosinophilic pneumonia
Bronchiolitis obliterans
Bronchiolitis obliterans with organizing pneumonia
Respiratory bronchiolitis-associated interstitial lung disease
Desquamative interstitial pneumonitis (DIP)
Bronchioloalveolar carcinoma
Lymphoma
Berylliosis
Talcosis

[a]Italics designate diseases covered in this chapter.

malities that can be identified (Table 2). Although any particular chronic infiltrative lung disease may demonstrate several of the patterns, the predominant pattern of abnormality coupled with the distribution of the abnormalities can often allow a specific diagnosis (2–6).

II. Usual Interstitial Pneumonia

Usual interstitial pneumonia (UIP) is the underlying pathological abnormality in idiopathic pulmonary fibrosis (IPF) and in the interstitial lung diseases associated with collagen vascular diseases. The most common collagen vascular diseases that have associated development of interstitial lung disease are rheumatoid arthritis and scleroderma.

    The most common HRCT findings in UIP are irregular lines of attenuation and honeycombing (7–11). The irregular lines of attenuation are often associated with architectural distortion and indicate the presence of pulmonary fibrosis. As

Table 2 Patterns of Abnormalities on High-Resolution CT

Conglomerate mass: irregular mass formed by coalescence of interstitial granulomas—has associated architectural distortion and paracicatricial emphysema
Consolidation: areas of increased attenuation that obscure underlying vascular structures
Ground-glass attenuation: areas of increased attenuation that do not obscure underlying vascular structures
Honeycombing: small (2 to 10-mm) cystic airspaces with well-defined walls seen in end-stage fibrosis—cysts are often subpleural in location
Interlobular septa: define the structural borders of the secondary pulmonary lobule—contain pulmonary veins and lymphatics
Irregular lines of attenuation: linear areas of increased attenuation that do not conform to the boundaries of a secondary pulmonary lobule
Parabronchovasular: located adjacent to the bronchovascular bundles
Traction bronchiectasis/bronchiolectasis: dilation of the airway secondary to fibrosis in the adjacent lung

the disease progresses, areas of traction bronchiectasis and bronchiolectasis develop, with the eventual formation of honeycombing.

Usual interstitial pneumonia has a characteristic subpleural and basilar distribution of the findings, which enables distinction of UIP from other causes of pulmonary fibrosis (Fig. 1). Areas of ground-glass attenuation can also be seen on images of patients with UIP; however, this is not usually the predominant finding. If areas of ground-glass attenuation with a subpleural and basilar distribution are the predominant finding, the possibility of desquamative interstitial pneumonitis should be considered (12,13).

In the past, it was thought that the areas of ground-glass attenuation seen in UIP could indicate potentially reversible disease (14–16). However, although areas of ground-glass attenuation may be potentially reversible, they represent active disease and often progress to fibrosis, despite treatment (17,18).

Because UIP is the common pathological entity in IPF and the interstitial lung diseases associated with collagen vascular diseases, it is reasonable to expect that these would all have similar appearances on HRCT (20–23). This is indeed true, and clinical history with appropriate laboratory studies is necessary to discriminate among the causes.

Regardless of the underlying disease processes associated with UIP, when the HRCT appearance is characteristic, confirmation by open-lung biopsy or video-assisted thoracoscopic biopsy is unnecessary (24). However, if the HRCT appearance is atypical and the diagnosis remains in question, HRCT can provide guidance for video-assisted thoracoscopic or open-lung biopsy (8). Areas that show honeycombing on HRCT should be avoided, because these will show only

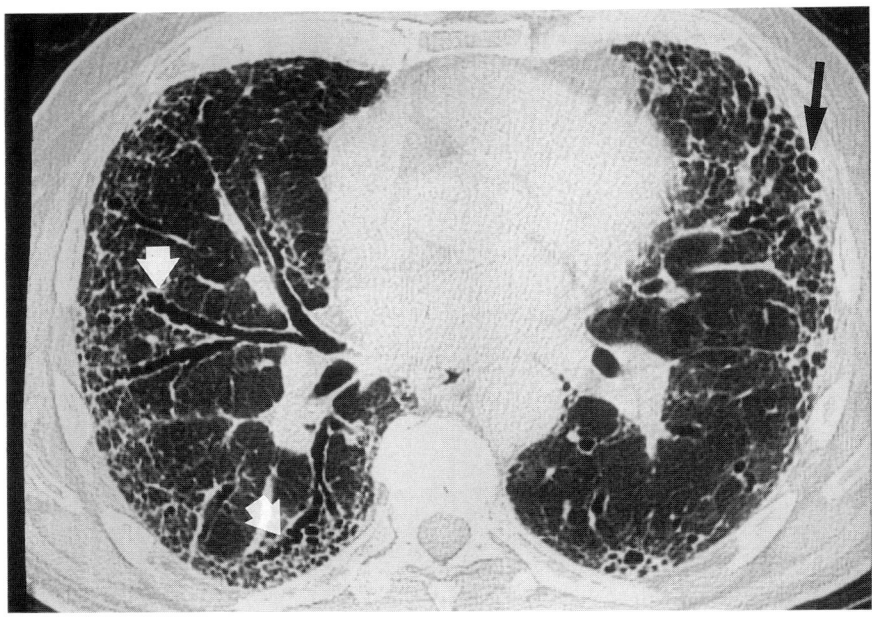

Figure 1 High-resolution CT of 71-year-old man with idiopathic pulmonary fibrosis: Irregular lines of attenuation and honeycombing (black arrow) are seen in a subpleural distribution bilaterally. Traction bronchiectasis can be seen involving bronchi in the right middle and right lower lobes (white arrows).

nonspecific histological findings of end-stage lung disease. Ideally, areas of ground-glass attenuation or irregular linear opacities with little associated architectural distortion should be targeted for biopsy.

III. Asbestosis

Asbestosis is the interstitial pulmonary fibrosis caused by asbestos exposures. The chest radiograph, in combination with the appropriate clinical and functional findings in the setting of previous asbestos exposure, is usually sufficient for the diagnosis. However, HRCT is more sensitive than the chest radiograph in detecting mild cases of asbestosis (25).

Asbestosis, similar to UIP, is characterized on HRCT by irregular lines of attenuation that often progress to honeycombing. Areas of ground-glass attenuation may also be seen. The irregular lines of attenuation and honeycombing in asbestosis have a basilar and subpleural predominance similar to the findings seen in UIP (26–30). However, in most cases of asbestosis there are associated pleural plaques that allow accurate differentiation of asbestosis from idiopathic pulmonary fibrosis (Fig. 2).

IV. Sarcoidosis

Sarcoidosis is a systemic disease characterized by noncaseating granulomas. In pulmonary involvement by sarcoidosis, the granulomas are distributed along the lymphatics. On HRCT, the granulomas are seen as nodules along the bronchovascular bundles, the interlobular septa, and the visceral pleura (31–35). Characteristically, the nodules are most numerous along the perihilar bronchovascular bundles (Fig. 3). In the majority of cases, these nodules will also have a predominate upper lung distribution. As the disease progresses, the nodules may coalesce, leading to the formation of conglomerate masses. The masses usually develop in the upper lungs, followed by retraction of the masses toward the hila secondary to associated pulmonary fibrosis (36–38; Fig. 4). The retraction of the masses leads to paracicatricial emphysematous changes in the upper lungs. Bilateral hilar and mediastinal adenopathy is present in most cases on HRCT, and the nodes may calcify.

V. Silicosis and Coal Workers Pneumoconiosis

Silicosis and coal workers pneumoconiosis (CWP) are chronic lung diseases caused by inhalation of silica or coal mine dust respectively. Although distinct disease entities, they are indistinguishable radiographically. However, in the appropriate clinical setting, the chest radiograph is usually sufficient for diagnosis and staging. In simple silicosis or CWP all the nodules seen on the radiograph are smaller than 10 mm. Complicated silicosis or CWP occurs when the nodules exceed 10 mm. These larger nodules are called conglomerate masses, or progressive massive fibrosis (PMF). These areas have associated fibrosis and paracicatricial emphysematous changes. These findings are responsible for the functional changes seen in patients with complicated silicosis and CWP. Although the chest radiograph is the standard for diagnosing conglomerate masses and PMF, HRCT is more sensitive (39–41).

On HRCT, simple silicosis and CWP are characterized by multiple bilateral pulmonary nodules. Similar to sarcoidosis, these nodules may have an upper lung predominance; however, the distinctive parabronchovascular distribution of sarcoidosis is not present in silicosis or CWP. Additionally, the nodules in silicosis and CWP are often more prominent in the posterior aspects of the upper lungs (39–42; Fig. 5). In patients with silicosis and CWP, the small nodules in the subpleural lung may coalesce, an appearance that has been termed *pleural pseu-*

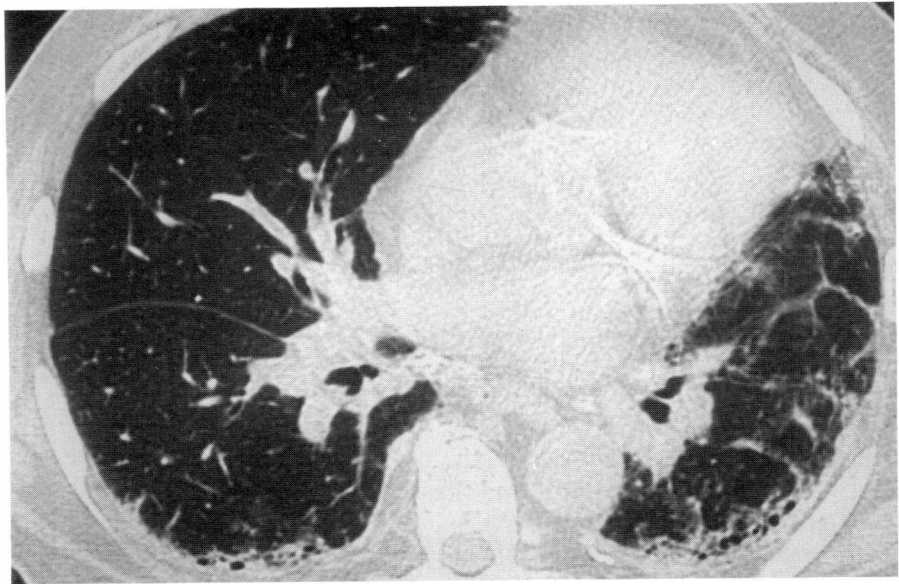

Figure 2 High-resolution CT of 66-year-old man with asbestosis: (a) Lung windows show irregular lines of attenuation and honeycombing in a subpleural distribution, most marked posteriorly. (b) Soft tissue windows show bilateral pleural plaques (arrows), some of which are calcified. The presence of pleural plaques allow confident differentiation of asbestosis from UIP.

HRCT of Chronic Infiltrative Lung Disease

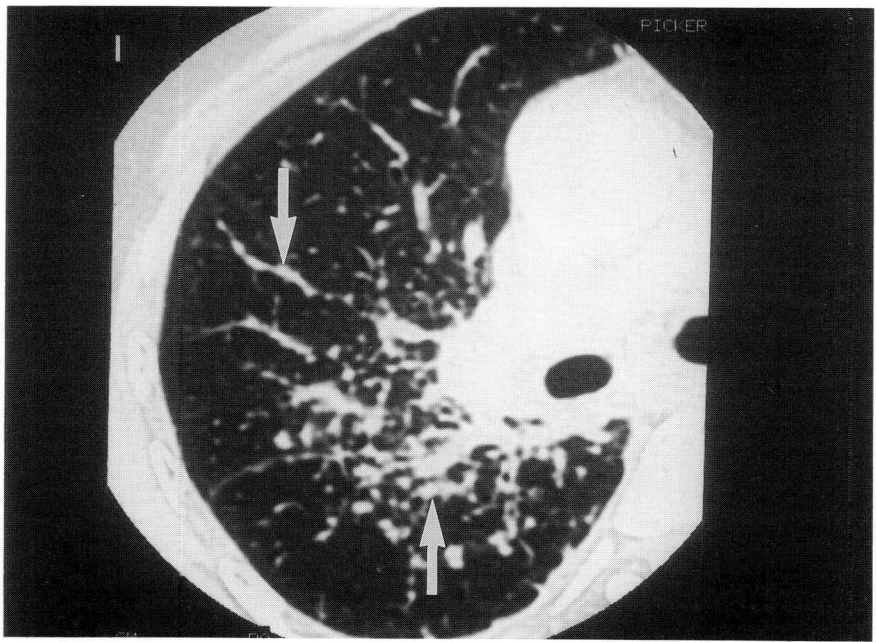

Figure 3 High-resolution CT targeted to the right lung in a 68-year-old woman: There is irregular nodular thickening along the bronchovascular bundles, most marked in the perihilar region (arrows). Also, note the subpleural nodules.

doplaques (39). When present, pleural pseudoplaques can be a helpful differentiating feature from sarcoidosis.

With disease progression, these nodules coalesce to form conglomerate masses or areas of progressive massive fibrosis (PMF), with associated fibrosis and paracicatricial emphysematous changes (39–42). The masses occur most commonly in the upper lungs, with retraction toward the hila (Fig. 6). Mediastinal and hilar adenopathy is also present, and the nodes frequently calcify.

VI. Pulmonary Langerhans Cell Histiocytosis

Pulmonary Langerhans cell histiocytosis has also been known as eosinophilic granuloma and histiocytosis X. Pulmonary Langerhans cell histiocytosis occurs most commonly in patients in the third to fifth decades of life. Over 90% of the patients are smokers (43), and up to 20% present with spontaneous pneumothorax (44).

The appearance of pulmonary Langerhans cell histiocytosis on HRCT varies, depending on the stage of the disease. Early in the course of the disease, the

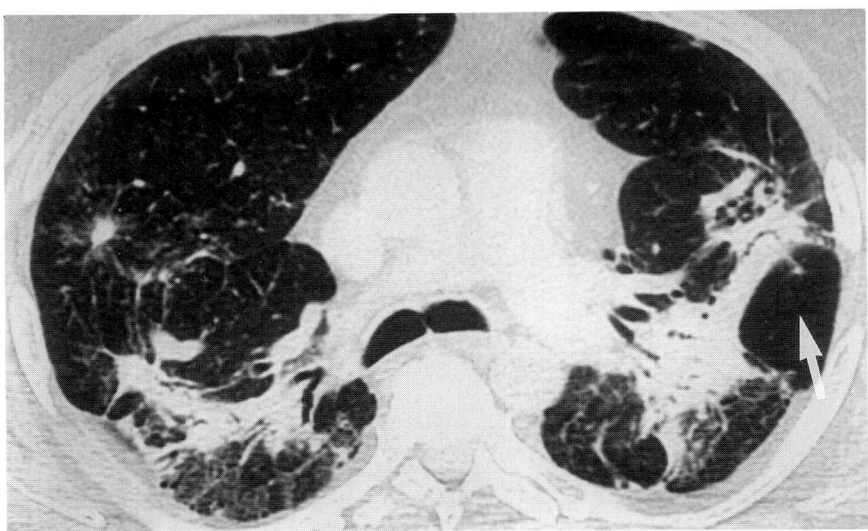

Figure 4 High-resolution CT of a 53-year-old man with end-stage sarcoidosis: Conglomerate masses are seen in the perhilar regions bilaterally. These caused marked distortion of the underlying lung architecture. Paracicatricial emphysematous changes can be seen in the left lung laterally (arrow).

HRCT findings are characterized by multiple nodules that have an upper lung predominance and spare the lung bases. This upper lung distribution is similar to sarcoid and silicosis; however, there are differentiating features. The nodules in Langerhans cell histiocytosis are in a random distribution. In addition to the nodules, in most cases of Langerhans cell histiocytosis, there are cystic spaces with thin, well-defined walls that can be seen even in the earliest stages of the disease (43–46; Fig. 7). Thin-walled cysts are distinctly unusual in sarcoidosis or silicosis. Additionally, adenopathy in association with Langerhans cell histiocytosis is distinctly unusual, whereas it is commonly seen in sarcoidosis or silicosis.

As the disease progresses, the cystic spaces become more numerous and the nodules decrease (43–46). In end-stage histiocystosis, there may be only diffuse cysts without nodules present. The cysts may coalesce to form larger, irregular cystic spaces within the lungs. However, similar to the early stages of the disease, there will be relative sparing of the lung bases (Fig. 8).

The exact cause of the cystic spaces is controversial. In the past, it has been postulated that the cysts represented cavitation of the nodules or a check-valve bronchiolar obstruction resulting in dilation of the distal airways (43–46). However, more recent studies suggest that the cysts probably represent paracicatricial

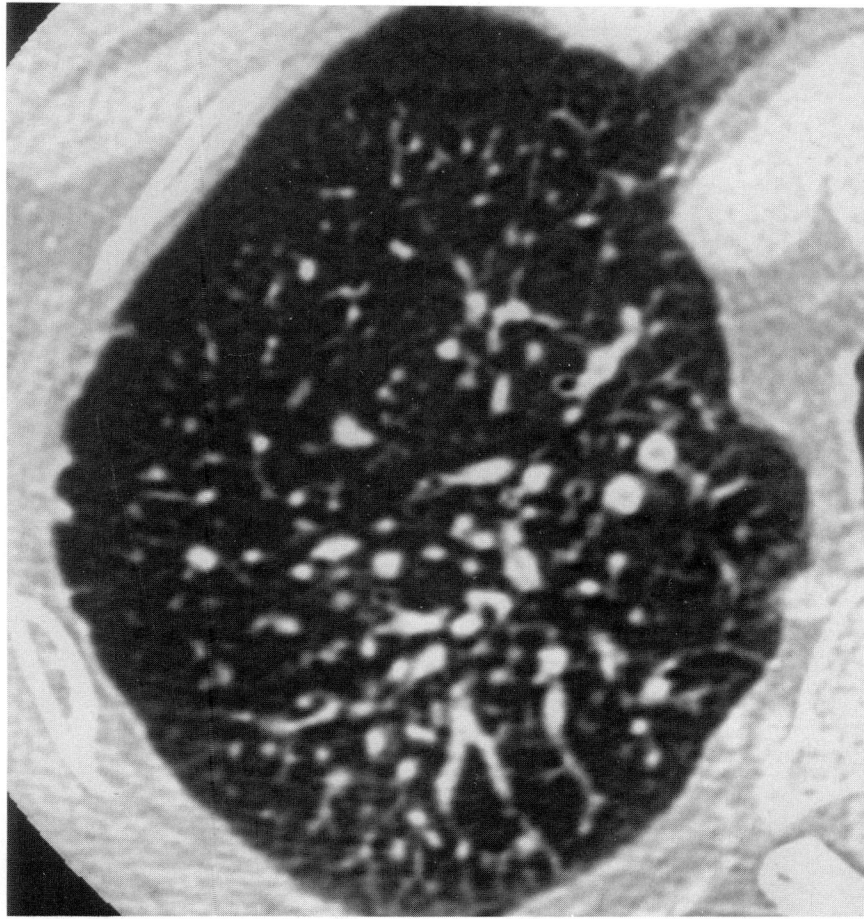

Figure 5 High-resolution CT targeted to the right lung in a 67-year-old man with simple silicosis: Multiple small pulmonary nodules are seen in the right upper lung. Most of the nodules are located in the posterior half of the right upper lobe.

emphysematous changes in the lung surrounding the bronchiolar inflammation (47).

VII. Lymphangiomyomatosis

Lymphangiomyomatosis (LAM) is characterized by progressive proliferation of smooth muscle in the pulmonary lymphatics, vessels, alveolar septa, and in the

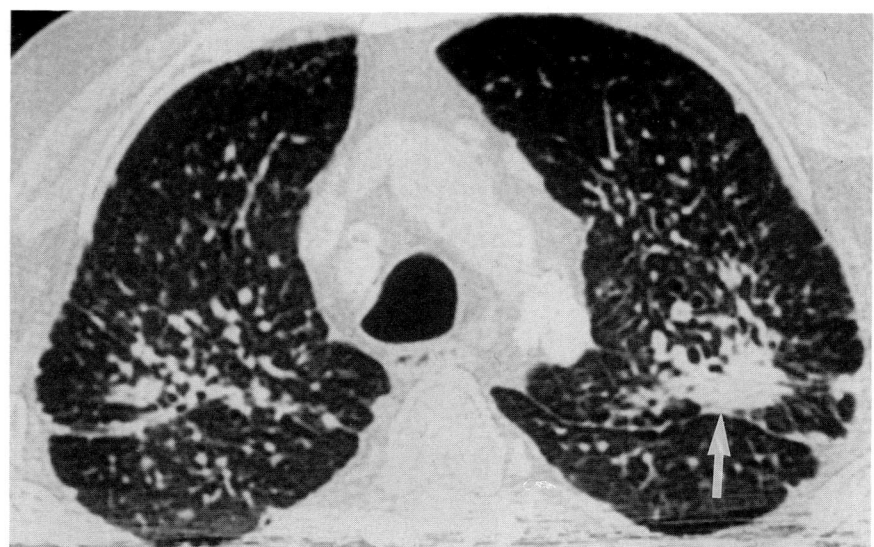

Figure 6 High-resolution CT of a 63-year-old man with complicated silicosis: There are multiple bilateral pulmonary nodules. Additionally, there is a conglomerate mass in the left upper lobe adjacent to the major fissure (arrow). The architectural distortion caused by the conglomerate mass causes anterior displacement of the major fissure.

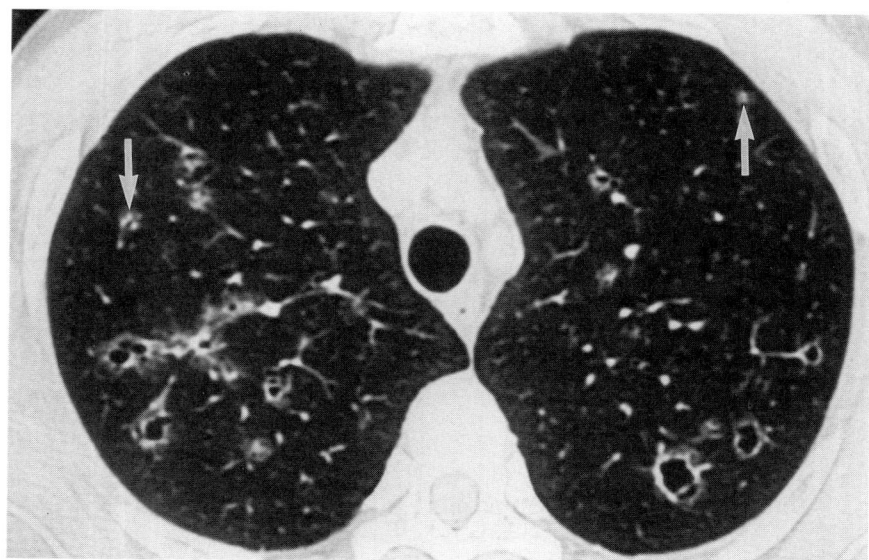

Figure 7 High-resolution CT of a 33-year-old woman with pulmonary Langerhans cell histiocytosis: Several nodules are seen in both lungs (arrows). In addition, there are multiple cystic spaces with well-defined walls. On lower images the lung bases were spared.

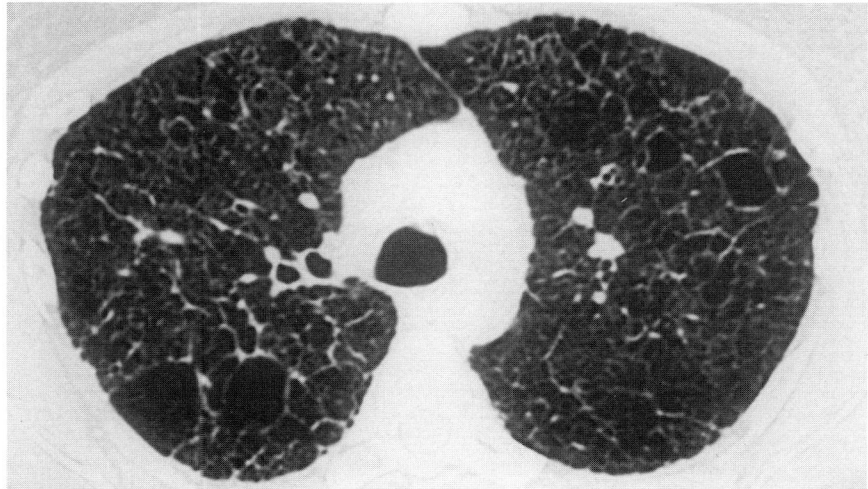

Figure 8 High-resolution CT of a 48-year-old man with end-stage pulmonary Langerhans cell histiocytosis: There are extensive thin-walled cysts throughout both lungs. At this stage there are no pulmonary nodules visible; however, on lower images the lung bases were again sparred.

walls of the bronchi and bronchioles. It occurs exclusively in women, usually of childbearing age. Approximately 60% develop pleural effusions, and 40% develop spontaneous pneumothorax (48–52).

The characteristic HRCT finding in LAM is the presence of diffuse, thin-walled cysts (48–52). Unlike Langerhan's cell histiocytosis, the cysts in the lymphangiomyomatosis involve the bases with relatively uniform involvement throughout the lungs (Fig. 9). This diffuse distribution of the cysts is the key differentiating feature of LAM from pulmonary Langerhans cell histiocytosis on HRCT. The cysts in LAM also tend to be more uniform than in histiocytosis. Additionally, the lung parenchyma between the cystic spaces in LAM is normal, whereas in histiocytosis small nodules may be seen.

VIII. Extrinsic Allergic Alveolitis

Extrinsic allergic alveolitis (EAA) or hypersensitivity pneumonitis is an allergic reaction of the lungs caused by inhalation of organic antigens. It can be subdivided into acute, subacute, and chronic stages. In its subacute form, EAA is characterized on HRCT by patchy bilateral areas of ground-glass attenuation throughout the lungs (53–56). In some regions these may resolve into numerous tiny, poorly defined nodular areas of ground-glass attenuation (Fig. 10). In the subacute phase, these findings on HRCT can be diagnostic.

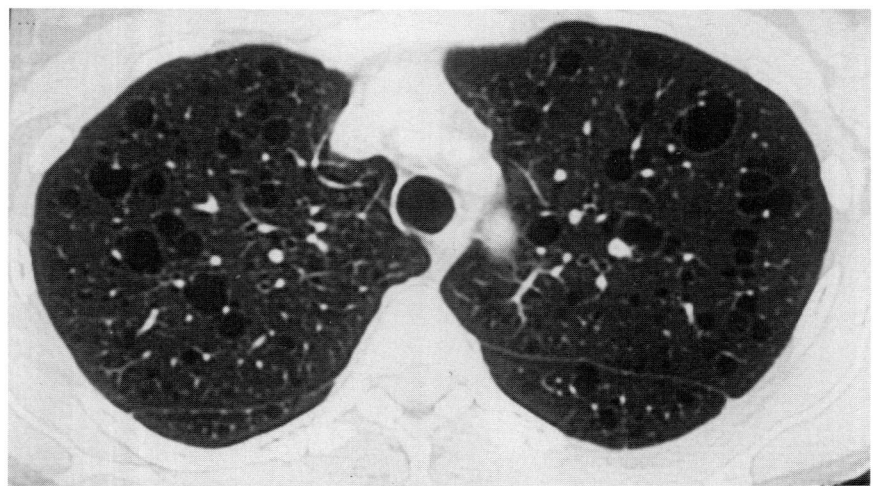

Figure 9 High-resolution CT of a 47-year-old woman with lymphangiomyomatosis: There are bilateral thin-walled cystic spaces. The intervening lung is normal, without evidence of pulmonary nodules. These cystic spaces were present diffusely throughout the lungs, including involvement of the lung bases.

In chronic extrinsic allergic alveolitis, fibrosis predominates. On HRCT, this is seen as irregular lines of attenuation, with associated architectural distortion. These tend to predominate in the midlungs and may have a subpleural distribution (57,58; Fig. 11). There may also be associated honeycombing and traction bronchiectasis. Although the midlung predominance of these findings is most suggestive of chronic EAA, it can be difficult to distinguish chronic EAA from UIP, and a biopsy is often necessary to make the diagnosis (59).

IX. Alveolar Proteinosis

Alveolar proteinosis is characterized on HRCT by bilateral, predominantly perihilar, areas of ground-glass attenuation that spare the apices and costophrenic angles. Typically, there is a sharp demarcation between the areas of ground-glass attenuation and normal parenchyma (58,59). An additional finding that may be present in cases of alveolar proteinosis is smooth interlobular septal thickening (Fig. 12). Interlobular septal thickening, when present, is seen only in the areas with ground-glass attenuation, an appearance that has been described as resembling "crazy paving." Crazy paving can be seen in a variety of diseases; however, in the setting of chronic infiltrative lung disease, crazy paving in a perihilar distribution is characteristic of alveolar proteinosis.

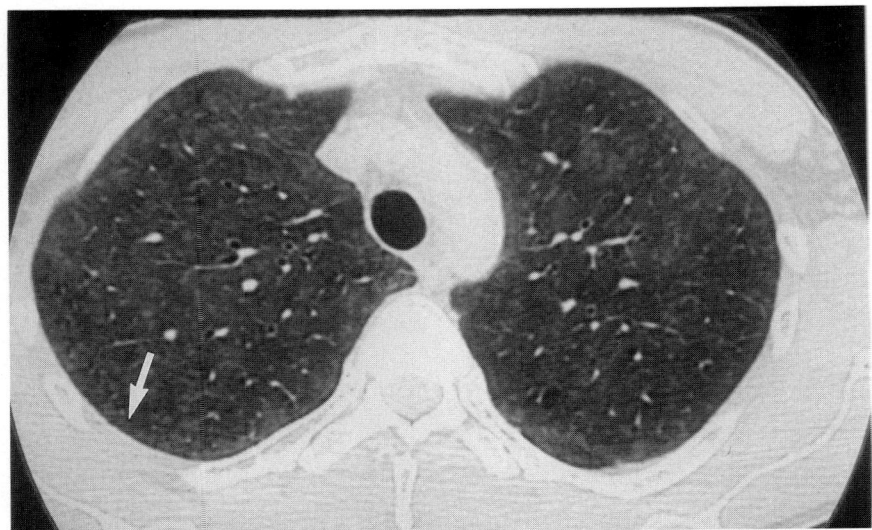

Figure 10 High-resolution CT of a 49-year-old woman with subacute extrinsic allergic alveolitis: Patchy areas of ground-glass attenuation are seen in both lungs. In the right upper lobe posteriorly, several poorly defined nodular areas of ground-glass attenuation can be appreciated (arrow).

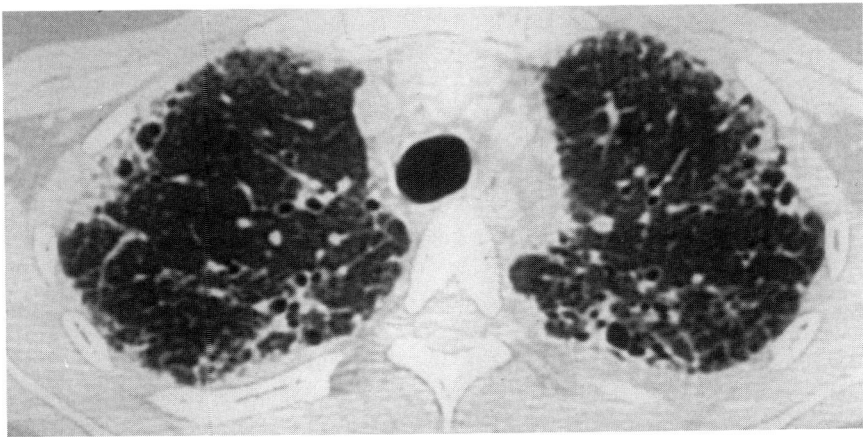

Figure 11 High-resolution CT of a 48-year-old woman with chronic extrinsic allergic alveolitis: Irregular lines of attenuation are seen in the subpleural lung bilaterally. These were most marked in the midlung, with relatively less in involvement of the lung bases.

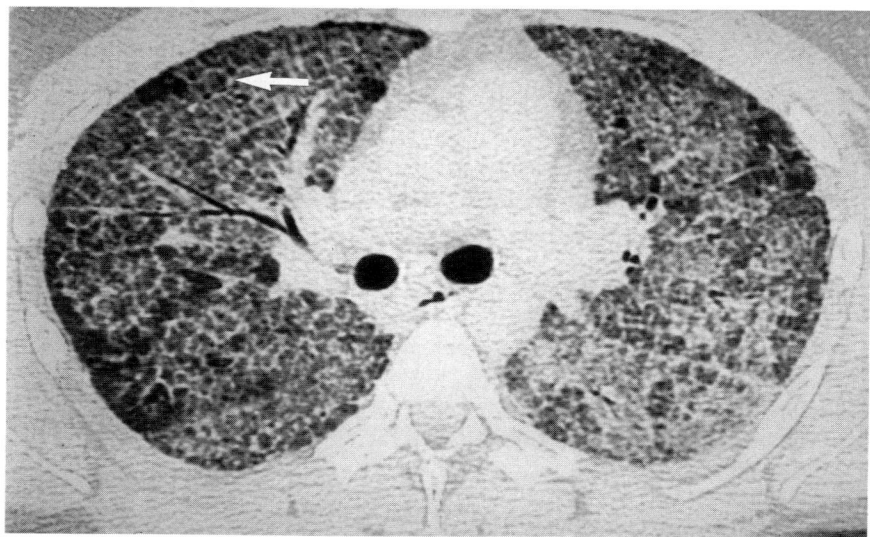

Figure 12 High-resolution CT of a 28-year-old man with alveolar proteinosis: There are diffuse bilateral areas of ground-glass attenuation. Within the areas of ground-glass attenuation, several lines of attenuation can be seen that represent thickened septa. This is most easily appreciated in the right upper lobe where the polygonal shape of the secondary pulmonary lobule can be seen owing to the interlobular septal thickening (arrow). This combination of areas of ground-glass attenuation and interlobular septal thickening is referred to as crazy paving.

X. Lymphangitic Carcinomatosis

Pulmonary lymphangitic carcinomatosis is characterized by tumor growth along the lymphatics of the lung. The most common malignancies to develop lymphangitic metastases are breast, lung, stomach, colon, and pancreas.

The characteristic HRCT finding in lymphangitic carcinomatosis is nodular interlobular septal thickening (62,63; Fig. 13). The interlobular septal thickening is most often bilateral and symmetric, with a basilar predominance, but in cases of lung or breast carcinoma may be unilateral. Irregular nodular thickening of the bronchovascular bundles is also commonly seen. Lymphangitic carcinomatosis may also present with smooth interlobular septal thickening, and in these cases, may be difficult to distinguish from pulmonary edema.

XI. Chronic Eosinophilic Pneumonia

Chronic eosinophilic pneumonia (CEP) is characterized by eosinophilic infiltration of the lungs. In most patients, there is associated peripheral eosinophilia. On

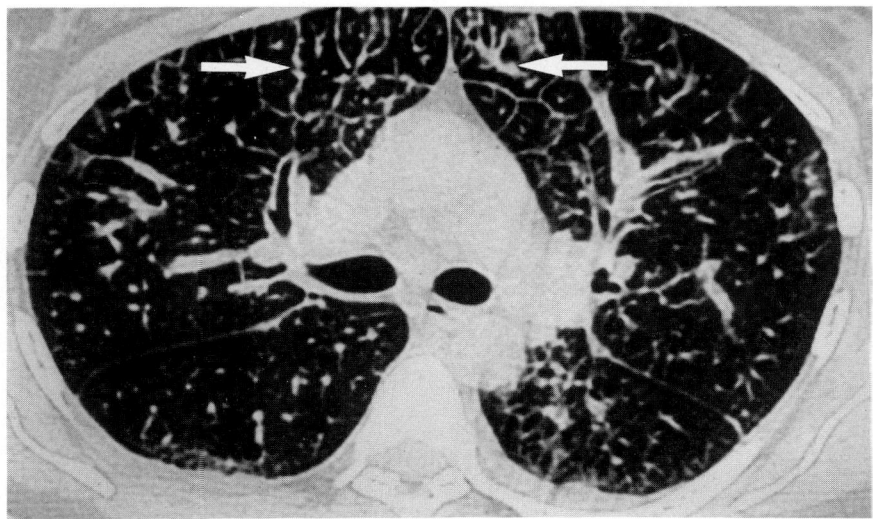

Figure 13 High-resolution CT of a 46-year-old woman with lymphangitic metastases from vaginal carcinoma: Interlobular septal thickening can be seen bilaterally, most marked in the anterior lung. Interlobular septal thickening creates the polygonal patterns that are the borders of the secondary pulmonary lobule. There is some nodularity of the interlobular septal thickening (arrows).

the chest radiograph, the classic appearance of CEP is peripheral airspace consolidation. The combination of blood eosinophilia and peripheral infiltrates on the chest radiograph are often sufficient to suggest the diagnosis. Rapid resolution with steroid therapy is corroborating evidence. However, the blood eosinophilia may be transient, and the radiograph may not show the classic peripheral distribution in up to 50% of patients (64). In these cases, HRCT may be helpful in the diagnosis.

Because of the ability of CT to take transverse images through the chest, the peripheral distribution of the consolidation is more easily appreciated than on the chest radiograph. As with the chest radiograph, CEP is characterized on HRCT by peripheral consolidation (65). This peripheral distribution is seen on HRCT even when it is not apparent on the radiograph. In most cases the consolidation is also most marked in the mid- and upper lungs (Fig. 14).

XII. Conclusion

High-resolution CT can show several patterns of abnormality in the chronic infiltrative lung diseases, and each disease can manifest several of the patterns.

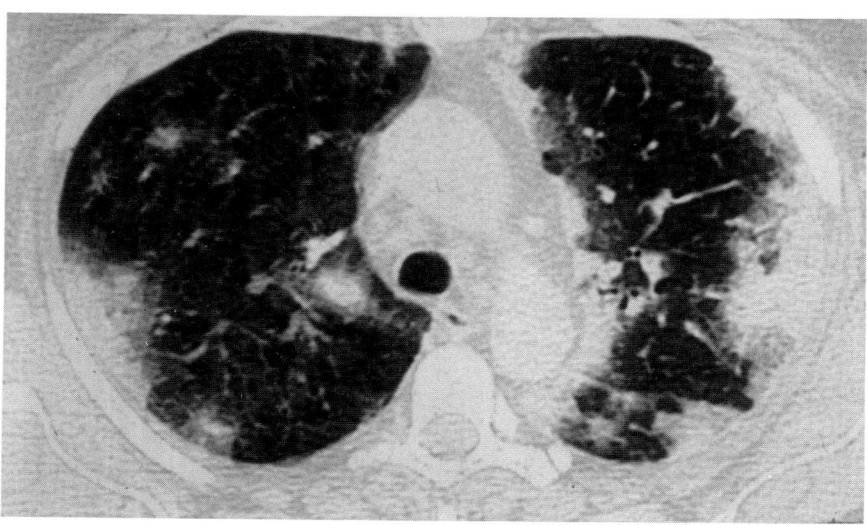

Figure 14 High-resolution CT of a 51-year-old man with chronic eosinophilic pneumonia: Consolidation is seen in a subpleural distribution in both lungs. These findings were more marked in the upper lungs in this patient.

Table 3 Diagnosis of Chronic Infiltrative Lung Disease with HRCT

Predominant pattern	Distribution	Diagnostic possibilities	Additional findings
Irregular lines c̄/s̄ honeycombing	Subpleural, basilar	UIP	
	Subpleural, basilar	Asbestosis	Pleural plaques
Nodules	Upper lung, parabronchovascular	Sarcoidosis	
	Upper lung, posterior	Silicosis/CWP Sarcoidosis	Pleural pseudoplaques
Ground-glass	Patchy, diffuse	EAA	
	Subpleural, basilar	DIP	
	Perihilar	Alveolar proteinosis	Interlobular septal thickening
Cysts	Upper lung, bases spared	Langerhans cell histiocytosis	Nodules
	Diffuse, bases involved	LAM	
Nodular interlobular septal thickening	Basilar symmetric or unilateral	Lymphangitic carcinomatosis	
Consolidation	Subpleural, upper lung	Chronic eosinophilic pneumonia	

However, with knowledge of the predominate pattern and distribution of the findings for the specific diseases, it is often possible to arrive at a confident diagnosis in the evaluation of chronic infiltrative lung diseases using HRCT (Table 3).

References

1. McLoud TC, Carrington CB, Gaensler EA. Diffuse infiltrative lung disease: a new scheme for description. Radiology 1983; 149:353–363.
2. Mathieson JR, Mayo JR, Staples CA, Müller NL. Chronic diffuse infiltrative lung disease: comparison of diagnostic accuracy of CT and chest radiography. Radiology 1989; 171:111–116.
3. Bergin CJ, Coblentz CL, Chiles C, Bell DY, Castellino RA. Chronic lung diseases: specific diagnosis by using CT. AJR 1989; 152:1183–1188.
4. Müller NL, Miller RR. Computed tomography of chronic diffuse infiltrative lung disease: Part I. Am Rev Respir Dis 1990; 142:1206–1215.
5. Müller NL, Miller RR. Computed tomography of chronic diffuse infiltrative lung disease: Part II. Am Rev Respir Dis 1990; 142:1440–1448.
6. Swensen SJ, Aughenbaugh GL, Douglas WW, Myers JL. High-resolution CT of the lungs: findings in various pulmonary diseases. AJR 1992; 158:971–979.
7. Müller NL. Differential diagnosis of chronic diffuse infiltrative lung disease on high-resolution computed tomography. Semin Roentgenol 1991; 26:132–142.
8. Müller NL, Miller RR, Webb WR, Evans KG, Ostrow DN. Fibrosing alveolitis: CT–pathologic correlation. Radiology 1986; 160:585–588.
9. Staples CA, Müller NL, Bedal S, Abboud R, Ostrow D, Miller RR. Usual interstitial pneumonia; correlation of CT with clinical, functional, and radiologic findings. Radiology 1987; 162:377–381.
10. Müller NL, Staples CA, Miller RR, Bedal S, Thurlbeck WM, Ostrow DN. Disease activity in idiopathic pulmonary fibrosis: CT and pathologic correlation. Radiology 1987; 165:731–734.
11. Nishimura K, Kitaishi M, Izumi T, Nagai S, Kanaoka M, Itoh H. Usual interstitial pneumonia: histologic correlation with high-resolution CT. Radiology 1992; 182:337–342.
12. Vedal S, Welsh EV, Miller RR, Müller NL. Desquamative interstitial pneumonia: computed tomographic findings before and after treatment with corticosteroids. Chest 1988; 93:215–217.
13. Hartman TE, Primack SL, Swensen SJ, Hansell D, McGuiness G, Müller NL. Desquamative interstitial pneumonia: thin-section CT findings in twenty-two patients. Radiology 1993; 187:787–790.
14. Lee JN, Im JG, Ahn JM, Kim YM, Han MC. Fibrosing alveolitis: prognostic implication of ground glass attenuation at high-resolution CT. Radiology 1992; 184:451–454.
15. Wells AU, Rubens MB, duBois RM, Hansell DM. Serial CT in fibrosing alveolitis: prognostic significance of the initial pattern. AJR 1993; 161:1159–1165.
16. Remy-Jardin M, Giraud F, Remy J, Copin MC, Gosselin B, Duhamel A. Importance

of ground glass attenuation in chronic diffuse infiltrative lung disease: pathologic–CT correlation. Radiology 1993; 189:693–698.
17. Terriff BA, Kwan SY, Chan-Yeung MM, Müller NL. Fibrosing alveolitis: chest radiography and CT as predictors of clinical and functional impairment at follow-up in twenty-six patients. Radiology 1992; 184:445–449.
18. Akira M, Sakatani M, Ueda E. Idiopathic pulmonary fibrosis: progression of honeycombing at thin-section CT. Radiology 1993; 189:687–691.
19. Wells AU, Hansell BM, Rubens MB, Cullinan P, Black CM, duBois RM. The predictive value of appearances on thin-section computed tomography and fibrosing alveolitis. Am Rev Respir Dis 1993; 148:1076–1082.
20. Fujii M, Adachi S, Shimizu T, Hirota S, Sako M, Kono M. Interstitial lung disease in rheumatoid arthritis: assessment with high-resolution computed tomography. J Thorac Imaging 1993; 8:54–62.
21. Remy-Jardin M, Remy J, Cortet B, Mauri F, Delcambre B. Lung changes in rheumatoid arthritis: CT findings. Radiology 1994; 193:375–382.
22. Wells AU, Hansell DM, Corrin B, Harrison NK, Goldstraw P, Black CM, duBois RM. High-resolution computed tomography as a predictor of lung histology in systemic sclerosis. Thorax 1992; 47:508–512.
23. Remy-Jardin M, Remy J, Wallaert B, Bataille D, Hatron P-Y. Pulmonary involvement in progressive systemic sclerosis: sequential evaluation with CT pulmonary function tests and broncho-alveolar lavage. Radiology 1993; 188:499–506.
24. Tong KT, Wells AU, Rubens MB, Kirk JME, duBois RM, Hansell DM. Accuracy of the typical computed tomographic appearances of fibrosing alveolitis. Thorax 1993; 48:334–338.
25. Friedman AC, Fiel SB, Fisher MS, Radecki PD, Lev-Toaff AF, Caroline DF. Asbestos related pleural disease and asbestosis: a comparison of CT and chest radiography. AJR 1988; 150:269–275.
26. Akira M, Yoko-Yama K, Yamamoto S, et al. Early asbestosis: evaluation with high-resolution CT. Radiology 1991; 178:409–416.
27. Aberle DR, Gamsu G, Ray CS. High-resolution CT of benign asbestos related diseases: clinical and radiographic correlation. AJR 1988; 151:883–891.
28. Aberle DR, Gamsu G, Ray CS, et al. Asbestos related pleural and parenchymal fibrosis: detection with high-resolution CT. Radiology 1988; 166:729–734.
29. McLoud TC. The use of CT in the examination of asbestos exposed persons. Radiology 1988; 169:862–863.
30. Yoshimura H, Hatakeyama M, Otsuji H, et al. Pulmonary asbestosis: CT study of subpleural curvilinear shadow. Radiology 1986; 158:653–658.
31. Müller NL, Kulling P, Miller RR. The CT findings of pulmonary sarcoidosis: analysis of twenty-five patients. AJR 1989; 152:1179–1182.
32. Bergin CJ, Bell BY, Coblentz CL, Chiles C, Gamsu G, MacIntyre NR, Coleman RE, Putman CE. Sarcoidosis: correlation of pulmonary parenchymal pattern at CT with results of pulmonary function tests. Radiology 1989; 171:619–624.
33. Brauner MW, Grenier P, Mompoint D, Lenoir S, deCrémoux H. Pulmonary sarcoidosis: evaluation with high-resolution CT. Radiology 1989; 172:467–471.

34. Lynch DA, Webb WR, Gamsu G, Stulbarg M, Golden J. Computed tomography in pulmonary sarcoidosis. J Comput Assist Tomogr 1989; 13:405–410.
35. Nishimara K, Ioto H, Kitaishi M, Nagai S, Izumi T. Pulmonary sarcoidosis: correlation of CT and histopathologic findings. Radiology 1993; 189:105–109.
36. Brauner MW, Lenoir S, Grenier P, Cluzel P, Battesti J-P, Valeyre D. Pulmonary sarcoidosis: CT assessment of lesion reversibility. Radiology 1992; 182:349–354.
37. Remy-Jardin M, Giraud F, Remy J, Wattinne L, Wallaert B, Duhamel A. Pulmonary sarcoidosis: role of CT in the evaluation of disease activity and functional impairment and in prognosis assessment. Radiology 1994; 191:675–680.
38. Murdoch J, Müller NL. Pulmonary sarcoidosis: changes on follow-up CT examination. AJR 1992; 159:473–477.
39. Remy-Jardin M, Remy J, Farre I, Marquette CH. Computed tomographic evaluation of silicosis in coal workers pneumoconioses. Radiol Clin North Am 1992; 30:1155–1176.
40. Remy-Jardin M, Degreef JM, Beuscart R, Boisin C, Remy J. Coal workers pneumoconioses: CT assessment in exposed workers in correlation with radiographic findings. Radiology 1990; 177:363–371.
41. Bégin R, Bergeron D, Samson L, Boctor M, Cantin A. CT assessment of silicosis in exposed workers. AJR 1987; 148:509–514.
42. Bergin CJ, Müller NL, Bedal S, Chan-Yeung M. CT in silicosis: correlation with plain films and pulmonary function tests. AJR 1987; 146:477–483.
43. Kulwiec, Lynch EL, Lynch DA, Aguayo SM, Schwartz MI, King PE Jr. Imaging of pulmonary histiocytosis X. Radiographics 1992; 12:515–526.
44. Naidich DP. High-resolution computed tomography of cystic lung disease. Semin Roentgenol 1991; 26:151–174.
45. Moore ADA, Godwin JD, Müller NL, et al. Pulmonary histiocytosis X: comparison of radiographic and CT findings. Radiology 1989; 172:249–254.
46. Brauner MW, Grenier P, Mouelhi MM, Mompoint D, Lenoir S. Pulmonary histiocytosis X: evaluation with high-resolution CT. Radiology 1989; 172:255–258.
47. Colby T, Lombard C. Histiocytosis X in the lung. Hum Pathol 1983; 14:847–856.
48. Templeton PA, McLoud TC, Müller NL, Shepard JO, Moore EH. Pulmonary lymphangioleiomyomatosis: CT and pathologic findings. J Comput Assist Tomogr 1989; 13:54–57.
49. Müller NL, Chiles C, Kullnig P. Pulmonary lymphangiomyomatosis: correlation of CT with radiographic and functional findings. Radiology 1990; 175:335–339.
50. Rappaport DC, Weisborg GL, Herman SJ, Chamberlain DW. Pulmonary lymphangioleiomyomatosis: high-resolution CT findings in four cases. AJR 1989; 152:961–964.
51. Sherrier RH, Chiles C, Roggli V. Pulmonary lymphoangioleiomyomatosis: CT findings. AJR 1989; 153:937–940.
52. Lenoir S, Grenier P, Brauner MW, Frija J, Remy-Jardin M, Revel V, Cordier J-F. Pulmonary lymphangiomyomatosis and tuberous sclerosis: comparison of radiographic and thin-section CT findings. Radiology 1990; 175:329–334.
53. Silver SF, Müller NL, Miller RR, Lefcoe MS. Hypersensitivity pneumonitis: evaluation with CT. Radiology 1989; 173:441–445.

54. Lynch DA, Rose CS, Way D, King TE Jr. Hypersensitivity pneumonitis: sensitivity of high-resolution CT in a population-based study. AJR 1992; 159:469–472.
55. Hansell DM, Moskovic E. High-resolution computed tomography and extrinsic allergic alveolitis. Clin Radiol 1991; 43:8–12.
56. Akira M, Kita N, Higashihara T, Sakatani M, Kozuka T. Summer type hypersensitivity pneumonitis: comparison of high-resolution CT and plain radiographic findings. AJR 1992; 158:1223–1228.
57. Adler BD, Padley SPG, Müller NL, Remy-Jardin M, Remy J. Chronic hypersensitivity pneumonitis: high-resolution CT in radiographic features in sixteen patients. Radiology 1992; 185:91–95.
58. Buschman DL, Gamsu G, Waldron JA Jr, Klein JS, King TE Jr. Chronic hypersensitivity pneumonitis: use of CT in diagnosis. AJR 1992; 159:957–960.
59. Lynch DA, Newell JD, Logan PM, King TE, Müller NL. Can CT distinguish hypersensitivity pneumonitis from idiopathic pulmonary fibrosis? AJR 1995 165:807–811.
60. Godwin JD, Müller NL, Takasugi JE. Pulmonary alveolar proteinosis: CT findings. Radiology 1988; 169:609–613.
61. Murch CR, Carr DH. Computed tomography appearances of pulmonary alveolar proteinosis. Clin Radiol 1989; 40:240–243.
62. Stein MG, Mayo J, Müller NL, Aberle DR, Webb WR, Gamsu G. Pulmonary lymphangitic spread of carcinoma: apparent on CT scans. Radiology 1987; 162:371–375.
63. Munk PA, Müller NL, Miller RR, Ostrow DN. Pulmonary lymphangitic carcinomatosis: CT and pathologic findings. Radiology 1988; 166:705–709.
64. Jederlinic PJ, Sicilian L, Gaensler EA. Chronic eosinophilic pneumonia: a report of 19 cases and review of the literature. Medicine 1988; 67:154–162.
65. Mayo JR, Müller NL, Road J, Sisler J, Lillington G. Chronic eosinophilic pneumonia: CT findings in six cases. AJR 1989; 153:727–730.

9

Pulmonary Hemorrhage

STEVEN L. PRIMACK
Oregon Health Sciences University
Portland, Oregon

I. Introduction

Numerous diseases may lead to pulmonary hemorrhage. The most common clinical manifestation is hemoptysis. Although chest radiography is the first imaging procedure performed in patients with hemoptysis, computed tomography (CT) may be helpful, particularly in patients with focal pulmonary hemorrhage. Currently, magnetic resonance imaging (MRI) plays a very limited role in the assessment of those patients.

This chapter will first review the imaging techniques that may be used in the assessment of patients with hemoptysis, and then will review the various causes of focal and diffuse hemorrhage.

II. Imaging Techniques

A. Chest Radiography

The conventional posteroanterior (PA) and lateral chest radiograph is usually the first procedure in a patient with pulmonary hemorrhage. Ideally, the PA and lateral radiographs are obtained with high kilovoltage (kV) technique (110–140 kVp). A high kilovoltage technique permits improved visualization of the trachea and major bronchi for identification of an endobronchial lesion as the cause of hemorrhage. However, patients with significant pulmonary hemorrhage are often too unstable for a PA and lateral radiograph, and a portable anteroposterior (AP) chest radiograph is then obtained. The portable radiograph uses a lower kilovoltage, with less penetration and, therefore, the airway is are usually not as well delineated.

Distinction between focal and diffuse pulmonary hemorrhage can usually be ascertained from the radiographic findings. In patients with focal pulmonary hemorrhage, the chest radiograph demonstrates a localized abnormality in approximately 60% of cases (1,2). Consolidation, atelectasis, mass, and cavitation are the most common radiographic findings of focal pulmonary hemorrhage. The radiograph is normal or shows a nonlocalizing abnormality in 40% of cases of focal pulmonary hemorrhage. In patients with normal or nonlocalizing chest radiographs, a specific cause is established bronchoscopically in fewer than 20% of cases (3,4). However, when the chest radiograph showed a localizing abnormality, a specific etiology for hemoptysis was identified in 35 of 87 (40%) cases (3). The usual radiographic finding in a patient with hemoptysis and diffuse pulmonary hemorrhage is bilateral airspace consolidation. Occasionally, localized pulmonary hemorrhage with diffuse aspiration of blood can mimic diffuse pulmonary hemorrhage.

B. Computed Tomography

Several studies have demonstrated that computed tomography (CT), particularly high-resolution computed tomography (HRCT), can be useful in assessment of patients with hemoptysis. The HRCT consists of thin sections (1- to 2-mm collimation) optimized by using an edge-enhancing ("bone") algorithm. The role of CT is most clearly defined in patients with focal pulmonary hemorrhage. High-resolution CT is the imaging modality of choice for the evaluation of suspected bronchiectasis (1,5,6). The sensitivity of HRCT in the detection of bronchiectasis is approximately 95%, compared with 60% for conventional (8- to 10-mm collimation) scans (1,6) because of less volume averaging and improved resolution. Use of CT often identifies unsuspected abnormalities in patients with normal or nonlocalizing chest radiographs (7). In patients in whom the radiograph is localizing, CT is usually indicated for assessment of the tumor and for mediastinal staging. Findings at CT also guide the decision to proceed with bronchoscopy, biopsy of enlarged mediastinal lymph nodes, or transthoracic needle aspiration with fluoroscopic or CT guidance.

In a recent prospective study of 57 consecutive patients with hemoptysis, McGuinness et al. (5) found that the overall diagnostic yield of HRCT was 61%, compared with 43% for bronchoscopy. High-resolution CT may allow a specific diagnosis, such as bronchiectasis, and obviate bronchoscopy in a number of patients, or may guide bronchoscopy in others.

The optimal CT scan technique for the assessment of bronchiectasis consists of HRCT scans performed through the chest at 10-mm intervals. This technique, however, may miss focal tumors between sections. Therefore, in the assessment of patients with hemoptysis, it is recommended that HRCT scans be combined with thicker sections obtained contiguously. The most commonly recommended technique for the assessment of patients with hemoptysis and without evidence of a focal lung lesion on the chest radiograph consists of HRCT scans at 10-mm intervals through the chest, plus contiguous 5-mm sections obtained through the region of the pulmonary hila to assess for the presence of central endobronchial lesions. In patients with focal abnormalities on the chest radiograph, contiguous 10-mm–collimation CT scans through the chest are recommended.

C. Magnetic Resonance Imaging

Currently, magnetic resonance imaging (MRI) has little role in the evaluation of patients with hemoptysis. MRI shows the airway as a signal void, compared with the soft tissues of the surrounding mediastinum. However, MRI has no advantage over CT in evaluation of the airways, and it is clearly inferior in the assessment of pulmonary parenchyma. Although MRI has been anecdotally used to confirm hemorrhage (8,9), it is of limited use in most clinical settings of focal or diffuse pulmonary hemorrhage.

III. Focal Pulmonary Hemorrhage

In patients with hemoptysis, the source of bleeding is usually from the bronchial wall. Bronchial vessels are usually involved, although occasionally bleeding originates from a pulmonary artery branch. The vast majority of patients presenting with hemoptysis have a focal abnormality. The most common diagnoses are bronchitis, carcinoma, and bronchiectasis (Fig. 1; 10). Other etiologies of focal pulmonary hemorrhage include pulmonary infarction and infection, particularly tuberculosis. However, many times no specific cause is found. In a study of 196 patients, Poe et al. (4) found that 86 (44%) patients had bronchitis and 65 (33%) had no definitive diagnosis. Peters et al. (3) found that none of the 26 patients with hemoptysis and a normal chest radiograph had a specific diagnosis at bronchoscopy. However, in this same study 34/87 (40%) patients with a localizing chest radiograph had a specific diagnosis at bronchoscopy. Other studies have also shown that bronchoscopy is more frequently diagnostic if the chest radiograph shows a focal abnormality (11–13).

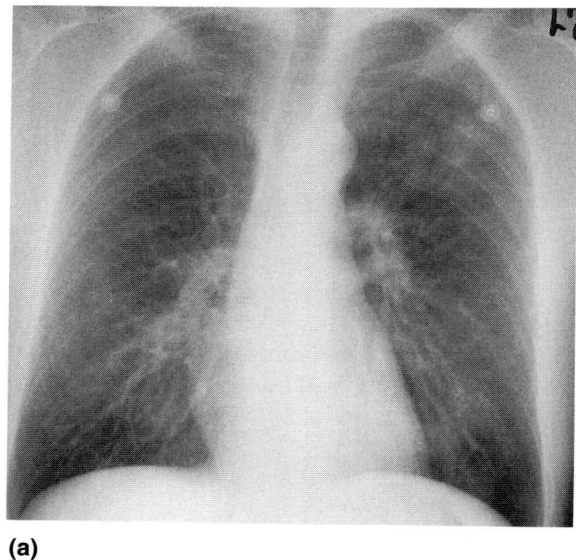

(a)

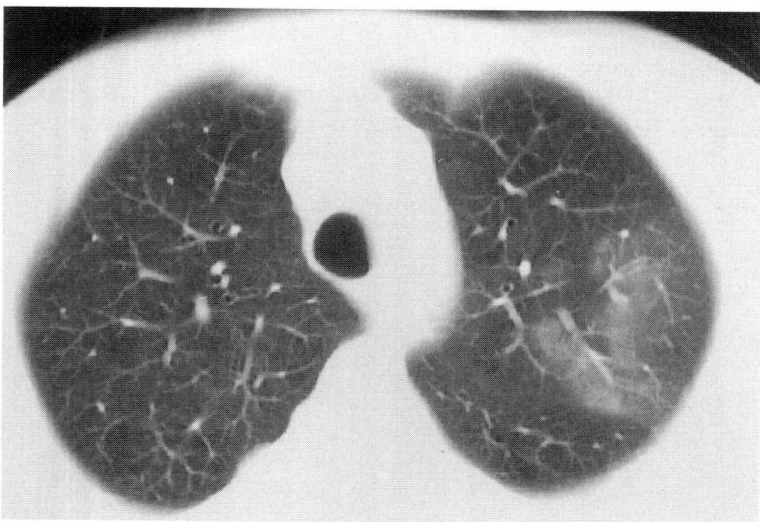

(b)

Figure 1 A 49-year-old man with hemoptysis caused by bronchitis: (a) Chest radiograph shows patchy opacification in the left upper lobe; (b) CT scan demonstrates a patchy area of ground-glass attenuation in the left upper lobe. No focal mass or bronchiectasis was present. The ground-glass attenuation represents pulmonary hemorrhage.

A. Bronchogenic Carcinoma

Hemoptysis is present in up to 50% of patients with bronchogenic carcinoma (14). However, in clinical practice, lung cancer accounts for a small percentage of cases with hemoptysis, being present in approximately 6% of patients (5,10,12). The chest radiograph will usually be abnormal in patients with bronchogenic carcinoma and hemoptysis. Hemoptysis is more commonly seen in central tumors, with the radiographic findings consisting of a central mass or postobstructive atelectasis (Fig. 2). A cavitated mass may also be seen. Occasionally, the chest radiograph may be normal when there is a small endobronchial tumor. These small endobronchial tumors, however, are detected on CT (Fig. 3). The margins and

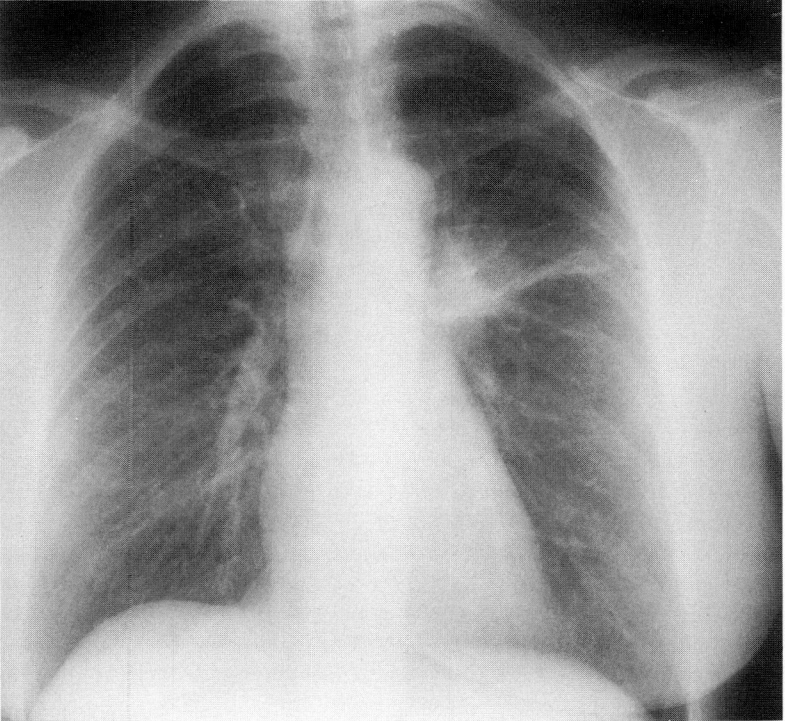

Figure 2 A 51-year-old woman with bronchogenic carcinoma: Chest radiograph demonstrates a left perihilar mass with postobstructive atelectasis. Diagnosis of large-cell carcinoma was obtained at bronchoscopy.

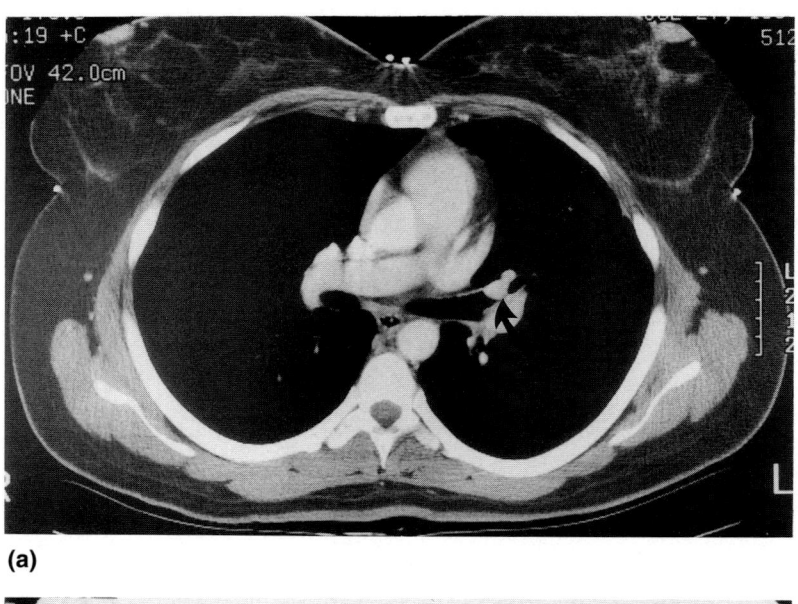

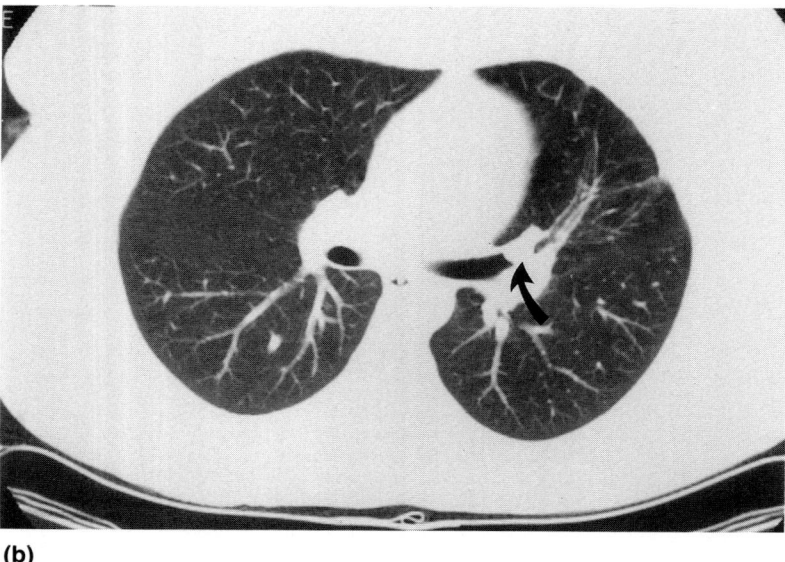

Figure 3 A 38-year-old woman with hemoptysis: Chest radiograph (not shown) was normal. 5-mm–thick CT scan filmed at (a) mediastinal and (b) lung windows demonstrates a 1-cm endobronchial mass (arrow) in the left upper lobe bronchus. An endobronchial carcinoid tumor was diagnosed at bronchoscopy, and a subsequent left upper lobectomy was performed.

B. Bronchiectasis

Bronchiectasis is defined as irreversible dilation of bronchi, usually with associated thickening of bronchial walls. Bronchiectasis most commonly occurs as a result of previous airway infection. Cough with purulent sputum production is the most common clinical presentation. Hemoptysis is present in approximately 50% of older patients (15).

The chest radiograph is of limited value in the diagnosis of bronchiectasis. Nonspecific findings, such as increased interstitial markings or atelectasis, may be present. In a few cases, parallel lines representing bronchial walls of a dilated bronchus, or ring opacities caused by dilated airways with thickened walls are present. If the dilated airways are filled with secretions, these result in the "finger-in-glove" appearance. Bronchiectasis usually involves the lung bases, lingula, or right middle lobe.

A more definitive study than radiography is usually necessary to diagnose bronchiectasis. In most institutions, CT has replaced bronchography for the evaluation of bronchiectasis. High-resolution CT with slice thickness of 1–2 mm is required for accurate diagnosis of bronchiectasis. Volume averaging with thicker 10-mm sections results in a low sensitivity for detecting bronchiectasis involving small-diameter peripheral airways. The CT diagnosis of bronchiectasis depends on the identification of dilated bronchi. When viewed in cross section, a dilated bronchus will be larger than the adjacent pulmonary artery and result in a "signet ring" appearance (Fig. 4). When a dilated bronchus is in the plane of section a "tramline" appearance will result. Additionally, bronchi seen within 1 cm of the pleural surface are considered dilated. In a patient with acute bleeding caused by bronchiectasis, ground-glass attenuation or consolidation representing hemorrhage may be the predominant abnormality on HRCT (Fig. 5).

Bronchiectasis has been divided into three types according to the severity of bronchiectasis. With cylindrical bronchiectasis, there is mild bronchial dilation, and the bronchial outline is smooth and regular. Varicose bronchiectasis is characterized by a "beaded" appearance, with alternating areas of dilation and constriction (Fig. 6). Saccular or cystic bronchiectasis is the most severe form of bronchiectasis, with the formation of cystic spaces (Fig. 7). A potential pitfall in the diagnosis of bronchiectasis is "reversible bronchiectasis," which may be seen with pneumonia. Bronchial dilation normally occurs with pneumonia, and this dilation may last for 4–6 months. Therefore, in patients with a history of pneumonia, bronchiectasis, which is by definition irreversible, should not be diagnosed until 6 months following a pneumonia.

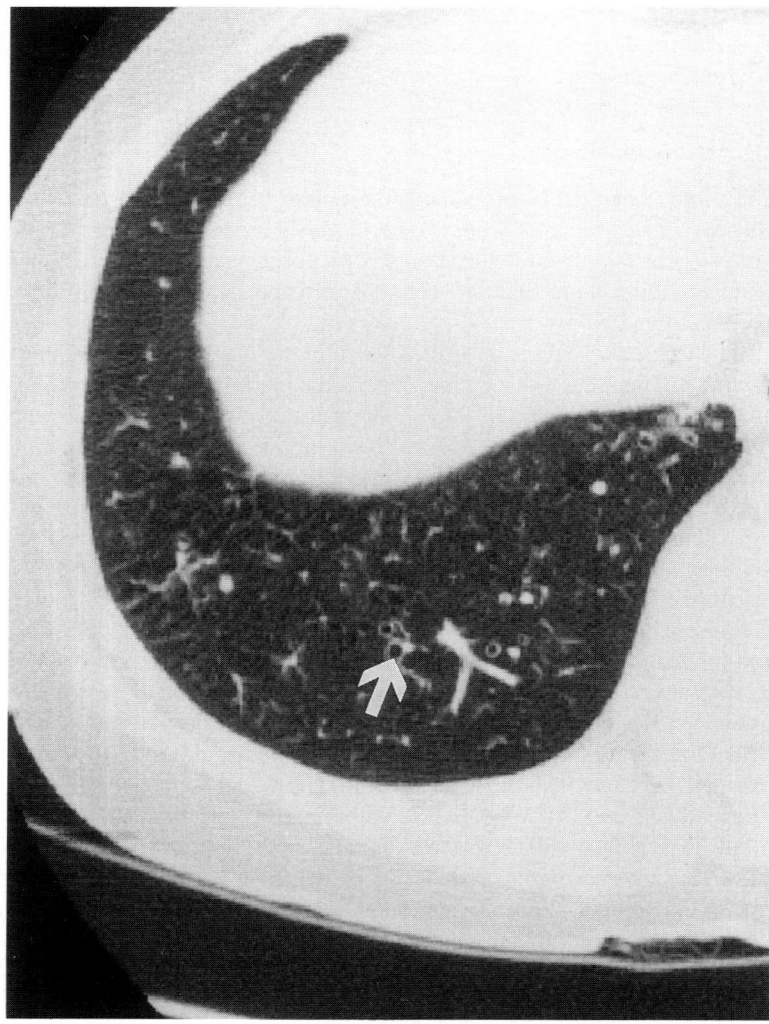

Figure 4 Mild cylindrical bronchiectasis: Targeted HRCT scan of the right lung base shows a dilated bronchus (arrow) that is larger than the adjacent pulmonary artery (arrowhead) resulting in a signet-ring appearance.

C. Infection

Pulmonary infection, particularly tuberculosis, is a relatively uncommon cause of hemoptysis. Although the presenting symptoms of patients with tuberculosis are usually nonspecific, consisting of fatigue and weight loss, 10% of patients with tuberculosis present with hemoptysis. Hemoptysis is most commonly seen in reactivation tuberculosis. Reactivation tuberculosis typically involves the apical and posterior segments of the upper lobes, but involves the lower lobes in approximately 10% of cases (16). Radiographic findings of reactivation tuberculosis include ill-defined nodules, areas of patchy or confluent airspace consolidation, and cavities. A calcified granuloma, indicative of previous tuberculosis, can be seen in more than 50% of patients with reactivation tuberculosis (17). The characteristic finding on CT is the presence of micronodules in a centrilobular distribution, indicating bronchogenic spread of tuberculosis (Fig. 8; 18–20). Consolidation and cavitation are also commonly seen. Interlobular septal thickening is present in 30–50% of cases (18–20).

Bacterial pneumonia, either gram-positive or gram-negative, also may result in focal pulmonary hemorrhage. Pneumococcal and klebsiella pneumonia typically result in lobar airspace consolidation (Fig. 9). Aspiration pneumonia caused by anaerobic organisms or gram-negative bacteria causes areas of patchy airspace consolidation in the dependent portions of the lungs. Bronchopneumonia, such as staphylococcal pneumonia, may lead to pulmonary hemorrhage. Radiographic findings typically include patchy segmental consolidation, often with associated atelectasis. Air bronchograms are rare, and several lobes are frequently involved.

IV. Diffuse Pulmonary Hemorrhage

Diffuse pulmonary hemorrhage (DPH) has several defining clinical, pathological, and radiologic features (21–23). The classic clinical presentation consists of iron-deficiency anemia and hemoptysis. The most common symptoms are cough and dyspnea. Although usually present, hemoptysis may be absent, even with pulmonary hemorrhage severe enough to cause a drop in hematocrit (21). The radiographic findings are nonspecific and consist of bilateral airspace consolidation in a perihilar or basilar distribution. However, the radiograph may be atypical, with focal or asymmetric bilateral areas of consolidation (24).

Histologically, the unifying features of diffuse pulmonary hemorrhage are the presence of recent hemorrhage in alveolar spaces and hemosiderin-laden macrophages in alveolar spaces and interstitium.

There are many causes of diffuse pulmonary hemorrhage, and the differential diagnosis depends on whether the patient is immunocompetent or immunocompromised (Table 1).

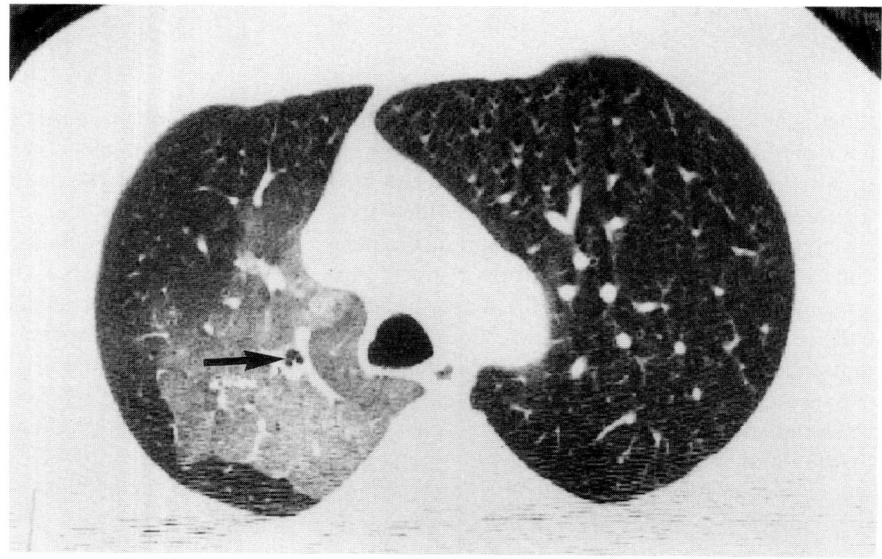

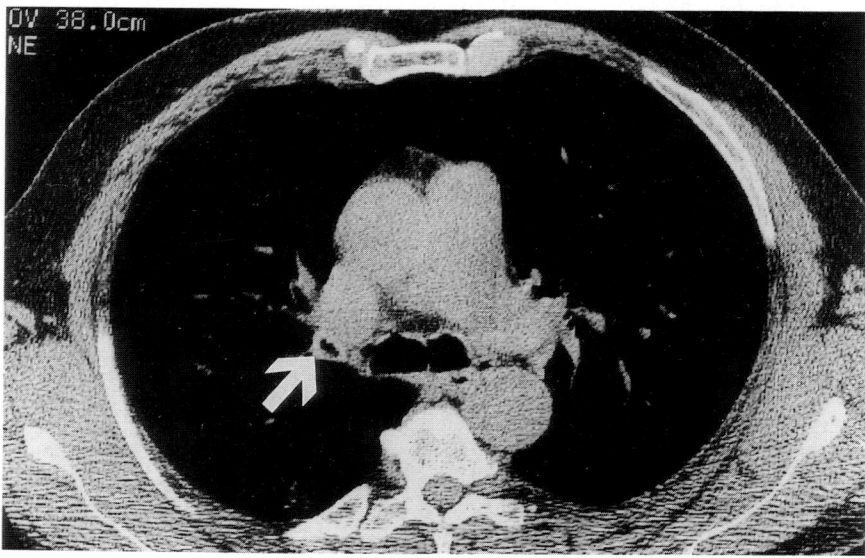

Figure 5 A 54-year-old man with severe hemoptysis: (a) An HRCT scan at the level of the aortic arch shows confluent ground-glass attenuation in the right upper lobe. Note the dilated bronchus (arrow). (b) Mediastinal window at the level of the carina demonstrates bronchial wall thickening of the right upper lobe bronchus (arrow). Right upper lobectomy was performed for intractable hemorrhage and showed bronchiectasis.

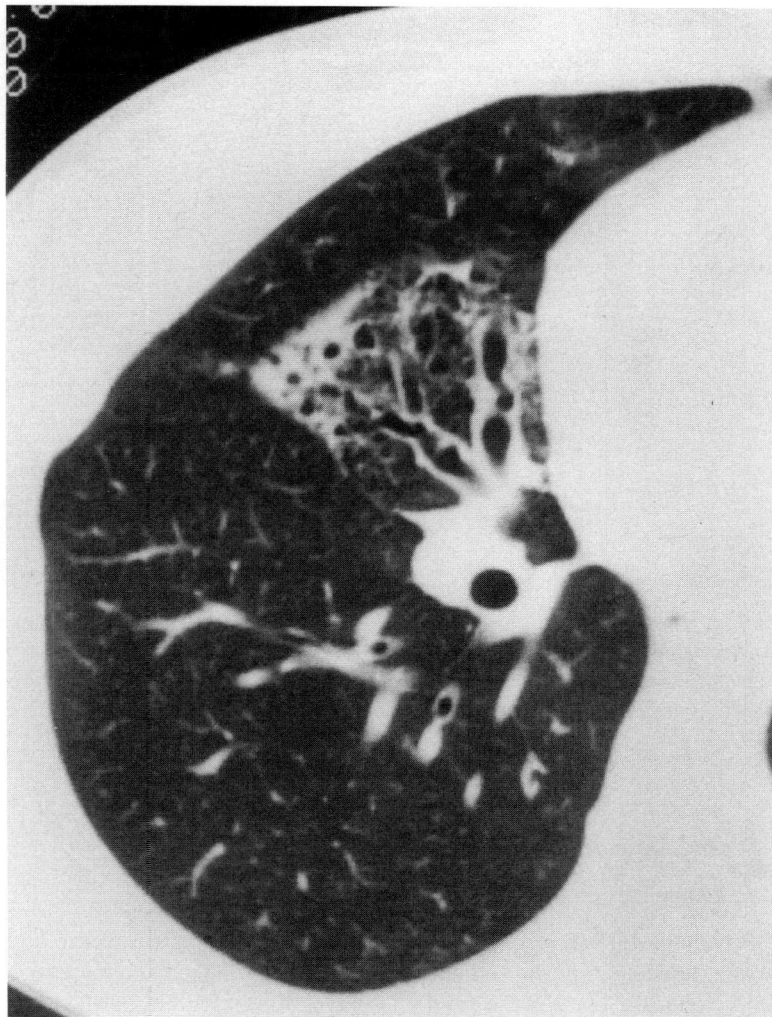

Figure 6 Varicose bronchiectasis: Targeted HRCT scan of the right lung demonstrates dilated bronchi, with areas of constriction in the right middle lobe.

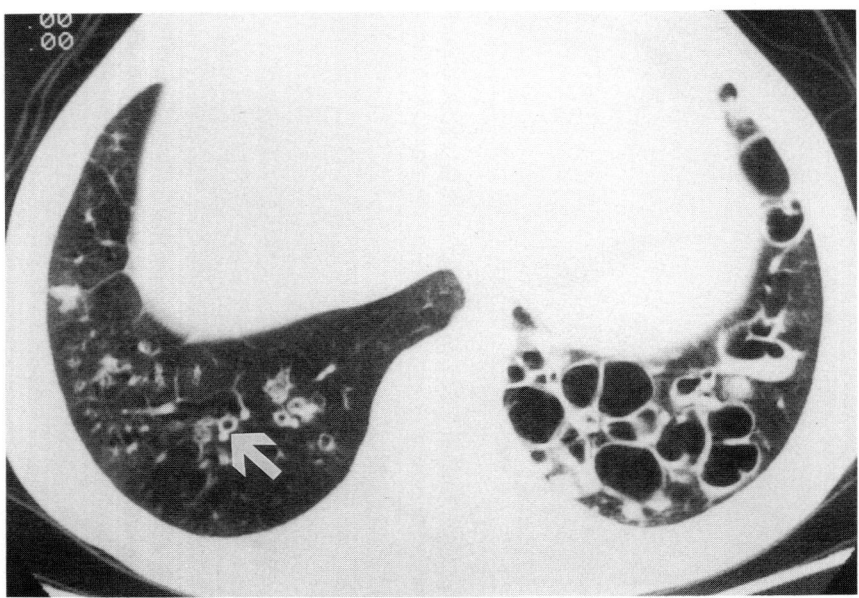

Figure 7 Cystic bronchiectasis: An HRCT scan at the lung bases shows multiple cystic spaces in the left lower lobe, representing markedly dilated bronchi (cystic bronchiectasis). Also note the presence of the signet-ring sign (arrow) at the right lung base, indicating mild cylindrical bronchiectasis in the right lower lobe.

A. In Immunocompetent Patients

Antiglomerular Basement Membrane Disease

In 1919 Goodpasture (25) reported a patient with hemoptysis 6 weeks after an attack of influenza. Autopsy demonstrated diffuse pulmonary hemorrhage and glomerulonephritis. In 1958 the eponym Goodpasture's syndrome was first used to describe the combination of diffuse pulmonary hemorrhage and glomerulonephritis (26). Many patients with this syndrome have since been found to have antibodies against their glomerular basement membrane, and the condition was renamed antiglomerular basement membrane disease (AGBMD). Diffuse pulmonary hemorrhage, glomerulonephritis, and circulating antiglomerular basement membrane antibodies are the three necessary components of AGBMD.

This disorder usually occurs in young adult men. The clinical presentation of AGBMD usually consists of cough, mild hemoptysis, progressive dyspnea, and anemia. Although most patients present with pulmonary symptoms, most also

Table 1 Classification of Diffuse Pulmonary Hemorrhage

I. Immunocompetent patients
   A. Antiglomerular basement membrane disease
   B. Collagen vascular autoimmune diseases
      1. Systemic lupus erythematosus
      2. Wegener's granulomatosis
      3. Other
   C. Not apparently immunologically mediated
      1. Idiopathic pulmonary hemosiderosis
      2. Blood dyscrasias
      3. Drug reactions
      4. Tumors
II. Immunocompromised patients
   A. Associated with infection
   B. Idiopathic
   C. Tumors

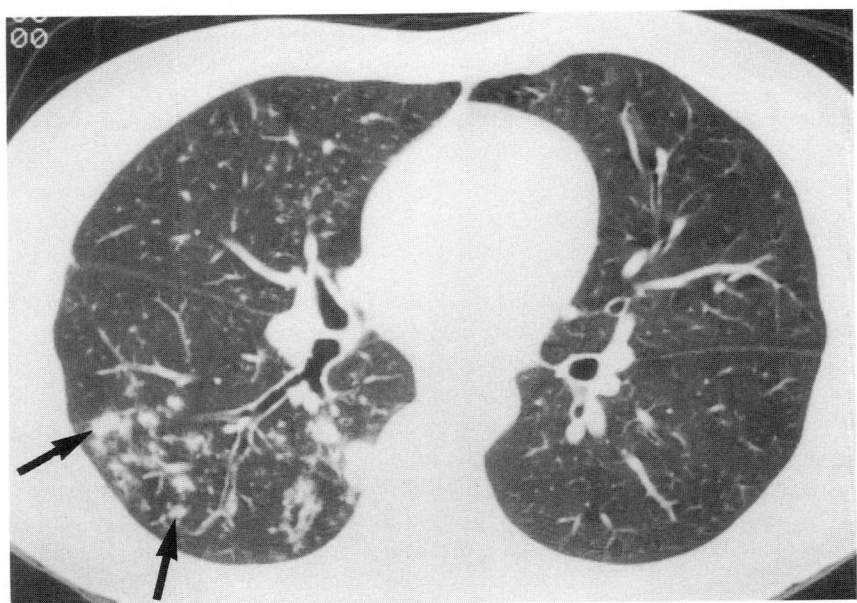

Figure 8 Pulmonary tuberculosis: An HRCT scan demonstrates multiple centrilobular nodules in the superior segment of the right lower lobe (arrows).

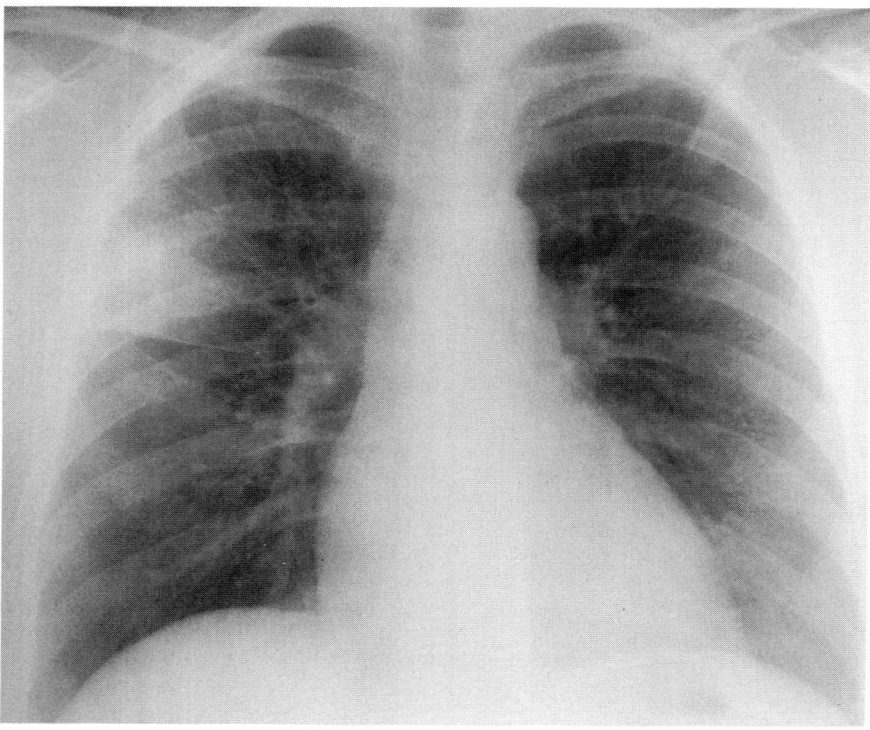

Figure 9 Pneumococcal pneumonia in a 33-year-old woman with hemoptysis: Chest radiograph shows airspace consolidation in the right upper lobe.

have laboratory evidence of renal disease at the time of presentation, including microscopic hematuria, proteinuria, and elevated serum creatinine levels.

The radiographic appearance of AGBMD is that of diffuse airspace consolidation that is usually bilateral and symmetric and often has a perihilar predominance (24,27; Fig. 10). The consolidation usually resolves within 2–3 days and is replaced by reticular opacities and interlobular septal thickening (27).

A few patients have a normal chest radiograph, despite the presence of extensive pulmonary hemorrhage. In a series of 39 patients, Bowley et al. (24) found the radiograph to be normal in 7 (18%). Computed tomography scanning is usually not necessary, but shows airspace consolidation or areas of ground-glass attenuation, with relative sparing of the lung periphery (Fig. 11).

The diagnosis of AGBMD is established by detecting antiglomerular base-

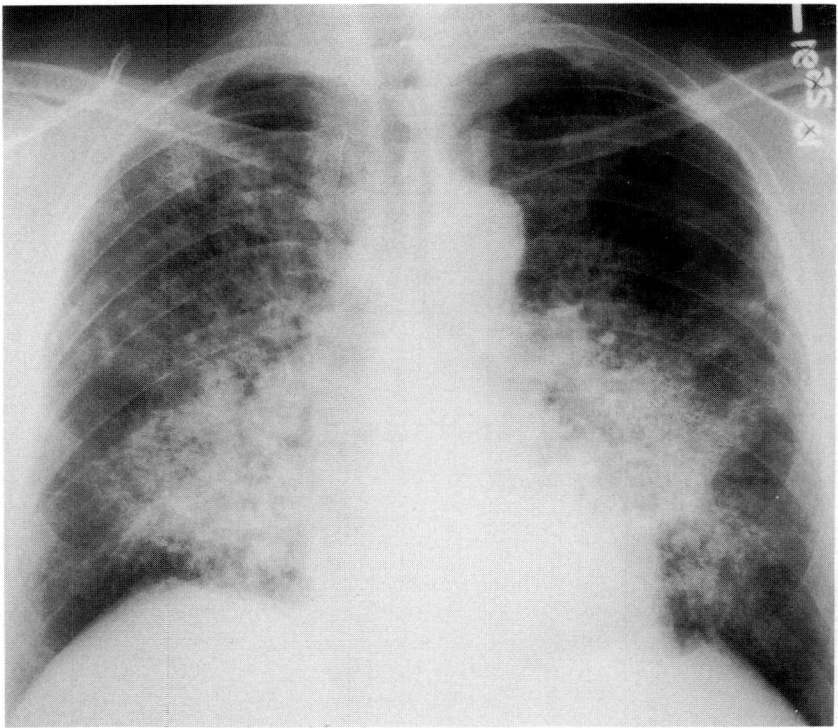

Figure 10 A 50-year-old man with diffuse pulmonary hemorrhage caused by anti-glomerular basement membrane disease: Chest radiograph demonstrates bilateral airspace consolidation with a perihilar predominance.

ment membrane antibodies, and radioimmunoassay can detect these antibodies in the serum in over 90% of patients (21). Demonstration by immunofluorescence of linear deposition of IgG on glomerular basement membranes in renal biopsy specimens can also establish the diagnosis (21,23). Lung biopsy is seldom performed in cases of suspected AGBMD. Linear deposition of immunoglobulin is found along alveolar basement membranes. Open-lung biopsy specimens typically demonstrate intra-alveolar hemorrhage and hemosiderin deposition. However, the distribution is patchy, and autofluorescence of lung tissue makes interpretation of lung biopsies more difficult than interpretation of renal biopsies. AGBMD usually has a fulminant course if untreated, but remissions in both renal and pulmonary disease can occur if treated early (28).

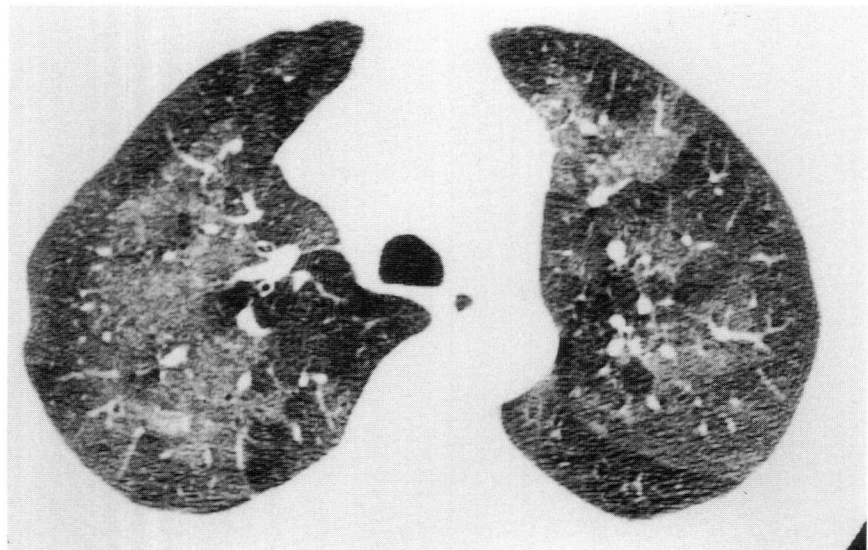

Figure 11 Antiglomerular basement membrane disease in a 45-year-old woman: An HRCT scan at the level of the tracheal carina demonstrates patchy bilateral areas of ground-glass attenuation, with relative sparing of the subpleural lung regions.

Associated with Collagen Vascular or Autoimmune Disease

Diffuse pulmonary hemorrhage may occur in association with many collagen vascular diseases. This complication is most commonly seen in patients with systemic lupus erythematosus (SLE) and Wegener's granulomatosis and less commonly in patients with rheumatoid arthritis, mixed connective tissue disease, or systemic necrotizing vasculitis (29–31).

Most patients with DPH in association with SLE have an established diagnosis of multisystem SLE before diffuse DPH occurs. Rarely, this condition occurs in SLE and results in rapidly progressive respiratory failure and hemoptysis, which is often massive. The chest radiograph in cases of DPH associated with SLE usually demonstrates bilateral areas of airspace consolidation.

Patients with Wegener's granulomatosis usually present with sinusitis, rhinitis, and cough. Hemoptysis is common and may be massive. Renal manifestations, including hematuria, proteinuria, and renal failure, eventually develop in most patients with Wegener's granulomatosis, but they are not common at presentation (29,32–34). The radiographic findings of diffuse pulmonary hemorrhage associated with Wegener's granulomatosis consist of bilateral airspace consolidation. Multiple pulmonary nodules that frequently cavitate are the most common radiographic findings of patients with Wegener's granulomatosis without DPH. Papiris et al. (35) described the CT findings in two patients with diffuse pulmonary hemorrhage associated with Wegener's granulomatosis. The predominant finding in both of these patients was the presence of diffuse consolidation. Additionally, nodules in a peribronchovascular distribution were demonstrated on CT. The CT scan may demonstrate areas of ground-glass attenuation in the setting of a normal chest radiograph.

B. Not Immunologically Mediated

Idiopathic Pulmonary Hemosiderosis

Idiopathic pulmonary hemosiderosis (IPH) is a disorder of unknown etiology, characterized by diffuse pulmonary hemorrhage without glomerulonephritis or immune complex serological abnormalities. It most commonly occurs in children younger than 10 years old, but may also be seen in the late teens and twenties. Although there is an equal sex incidence in children, in adults IPH occurs more commonly in men (36,37). Occasionally, it is associated with celiac disease (38) or IgA gammopathy (39). Patients with IPH usually present with hemoptysis, which is often recurrent. Dyspnea, cyanosis, and anemia are common. The disease is usually chronic with recurrences and spontaneous remissions occurring over many years.

The radiographic findings of IPH in children and adults are identical (36,40). The chest radiograph typically shows areas of airspace consolidation or ground-glass opacities (Fig. 12). There is usually a perihilar or lower lung zone predominance (36). The areas of consolidation usually clear within 3 days of presentation, being replaced by a reticular pattern. The reticular opacities will often initially resolve, but may progress to fibrosis following multiple recurrences.

The CT findings of four patients with IPH have been described (41). Findings in the subacute phase included diffuse nodules and patchy areas of ground-glass attenuation. Two of these patients were also scanned during an exacerbation, and CT demonstrated diffuse areas of ground-glass attenuation, presumably representing active bleeding. The MRI findings of a 2.5 year-old boy with IPH have been described (9). The T_1-weighted images showed diffusely increased parenchymal signal intensity. The T_2-weighted images demonstrated markedly reduced signal intensity owing to the paramagnetic properties of hemosiderin. Edema fluid or pneumonia should cause increased signal on T_2-weighted images. In this case, the noninvasive presumptive diagnosis allowed initiation of therapy before the diagnosis was confirmed with open lung biopsy.

Most patients with IPH develop pulmonary fibrosis within 5 years of presentation (40). Corticosteroid and immunosuppressive therapy can be used, but the efficacy of treatment has been difficult to assess because of the occurrence of

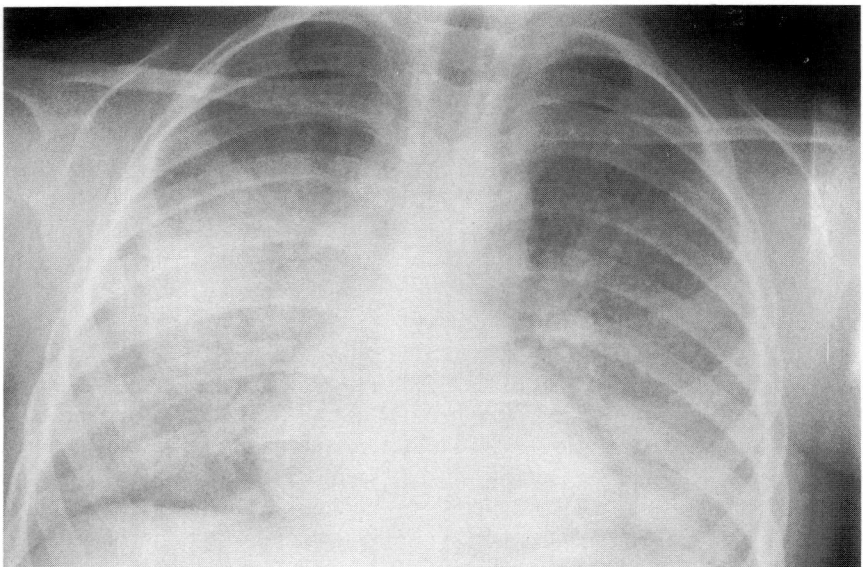

Figure 12 A 4-year-old girl with idiopathic pulmonary hemosiderosis: Chest radiograph demonstrates bilateral hazy airspace opacities with a perihilar and lower lung zone predominance.

spontaneous remissions. In some of the cases of IPH associated with celiac disease, both diseases improved when the patients were placed on a gluten-free diet (38,41).

Other Nonimmunologically Mediated Causes

Diffuse pulmonary hemorrhage has been described only rarely as a complication of anticoagulants, such as warfarin, despite their frequent use (42,43). Radiographic findings are similar to other causes of diffuse pulmonary hemorrhage. Rapid clearing occurs following cessation or reduction of anticoagulant therapy (42). A group of rodenticides has a method of action identical with warfarin and a much longer duration of action. Diffuse pulmonary hemorrhage following ingestion of rat poison has recently been described (44). Diffuse pulmonary hemorrhage is a rare manifestation of penicillamine toxicity, usually occurring in patients receiving relatively high doses (21). Inhalation of trimellitic anhydride or related acid anhydrides which are used in the manufacture of plastics and paints, has been reported to cause DPH (21,45,46). Reactions to these drugs are thought to be immunologically mediated (22). Diffuse pulmonary hemorrhage is an infrequently reported complication following lymphography (47,48) that is thought to be due to direct pulmonary capillary damage by embolized ethiodized oil (Ethiodol). Diffuse pulmonary hemorrhage has also been reported as a direct toxic or possibly hypersensitivity reaction to cocaine (49).

Diffuse pulmonary hemorrhage occurs in approximately 14% of patients with disseminated intravascular coagulation (DIC) and is frequently the cause of death (50). Diffuse pulmonary hemorrhage as a complication of thrombotic thrombocytopenic purpura has also been described (51). Angiosarcoma, both primary and metastatic to the lung, has been described, presenting as diffuse pulmonary hemorrhage (52,53).

C. In Immunocompromised Patients

Some degree of diffuse pulmonary hemorrhage is common among immunocompromised patients, particularly in patients with leukemia (54,55), in patients within the first month following bone marrow transplantation (56), and in cardiac transplant patients (57).

Although thrombocytopenia or a coagulopathy are usually present, a coexisting abnormality seems to be necessary for the development of DPH. Most commonly, coexisting fungal, bacterial, or viral pneumonia is found. No associated pathogens are found in the minority of cases (54,58–60). In these cases of idiopathic DPH, damage induced by radiation or chemotherapy may have predisposed to the disorder (61).

The earliest radiographic manifestation of DPH in immunocompromised patients is the presence of fine reticular opacities (58,62). There is usually a mid- and lower lung zone predominance. The radiographic findings can rapidly progress to diffuse bilateral airspace consolidation. Although clearing can occur with treatment of the underlying causes, DPH in an immunocompromised patient is often a terminal even (56,58). In addition to the findings of DPH, radiologic changes suggestive of associated infection may be found in these patients.

Although angioinvasive aspergillosis usually causes focal pulmonary hemorrhage, it may also present with DPH. Pathologically, angioinvasive aspergillosis is characterized by vascular invasion and thrombosis, leading to hemorrhagic infarction. Radiographic findings consist of subsegmental, segmental, or lobar consolidation. Nodules may also be present. A CT scan permits early recognition of angioinvasive pulmonary aspergillosis by the presence of nodules with a surrounding halo of ground-glass attenuation (Fig. 13; 63). The halo of ground-glass attenuation has been shown pathologically to represent hemorrhagic necrosis. Although the halo sign is most commonly seen in patients with angioinvasive pulmonary aspergillosis, it may also be seen with candidiasis, cytomegalovirus, and herpes simplex viral pneumonia (64).

Candidal pneumonia is characterized pathologically by the presence of

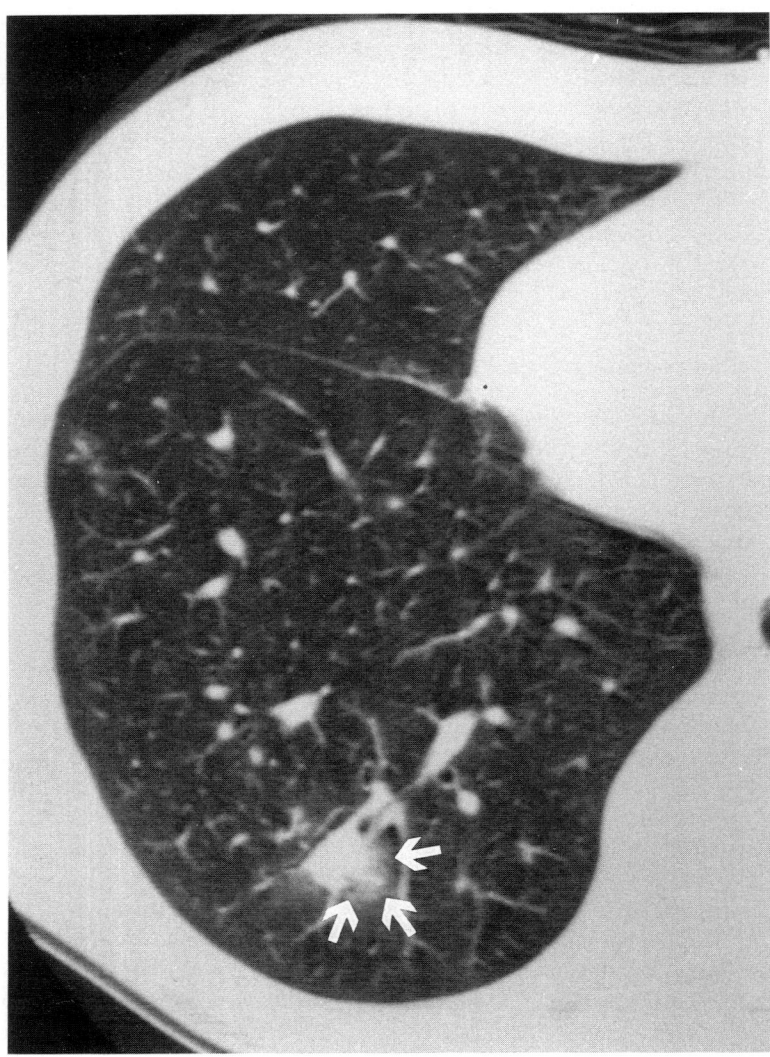

Figure 13 Invasive aspergillosis in a 38-year-old man with leukemia: Targeted HRCT of the right lung demonstrates a nodule in the right lower lobe, with a surrounding halo of ground-glass attenuation (arrows).

multiple small abscesses, occasionally associated with diffuse pulmonary hemorrhage. The chest radiographic appearance consists of patchy airspace consolidation (65) or a diffuse miliary pattern (66). The most common CT finding in patients with candidal pneumonia is the presence of 3- to 10-mm–diameter nodules (67). Halos of ground-glass attenuation surrounding the nodules, presumably caused by hemorrhage, are seen in most cases (67).

Cytomegaloviral pneumonia is most commonly sene in solid organ and bone marrow transplant patients. Pathologically, it is characterized by the presence of randomly distributed hemorrhagic nodules. The radiographic findings consist of diffuse reticulation or airspace consolidation. The most common pattern on CT in CMV pneumonia is of multiple, small nodules, with associated areas of ground-glass attenuation (67).

In patients who are immunocompromised by human immunodeficiency virus (HIV) infection, hemoptysis and DPH may be found as a complication of Kaposi's sarcoma (68). Most patients with pulmonary Kaposi's sarcoma also have cutaneous lesions (69). The radiologic features of Kaposi's sarcoma include bilateral, poorly defined, nodular opacities, and interstitial and airspace infiltrates

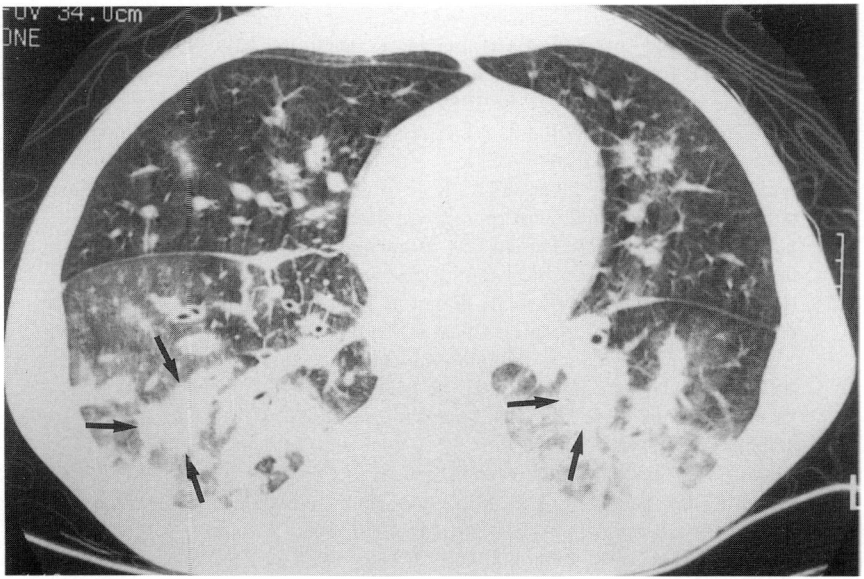

Figure 14 Kaposi's sarcoma in a 35-year-old man with AIDS: An HRCT scan demonstrates irregular nodular thickening of the bronchovascular bundles (arrows). Note associated ground-glass opacities in the right lower lobe that are due to hemorrhage.

(70). On CT the nodules and areas of consolidation are most marked in the perihilar regions and have a peribronchial and perivascular distribution (Fig. 14; 70–72). The nodules have irregular margins, and are often associated with ground-glass attenuation, which is likely due to hemorrhage.

References

1. Naidich DP, Funt S, Ettenger NA, et al. Hemoptysis: CT–bronchoscopic correlations in 58 cases. Radiology 1990; 177:357–362.
2. Set PAK, Flower CDR, Smith IE, et al. Hemoptysis: comparative study of the role of CT and fiberoptic bronchoscopy. Radiology 1993; 189:677–680.
3. Peters J, McClung HC, Teague RB. Evaluation of hemoptysis in patients with a normal chest roentgenogram. West J Med 1984; 141:624–627.
4. Poe RH, Israel RH, Marin MG, et al. Utility of fiberoptic bronchoscopy in patients with hemoptysis and a nonlocalizing chest roentgenogram. Chest 1988; 92:70–75.
5. McGuinness G, Beacher JR, Harkin TJ, et al. Hemoptysis: prospective high-resolution CT/bronchoscopic correlation. Chest 1994; 105:1155–1162.
6. Grenier P, Maurice F, Musset D, et al. Bronchiectasis: assessment by thin-section CT. Radiology 1986; 161:95–99.
7. Millar AB, Boothroyd AE, Edwards D, et al. The role of computed tomography (CT) in the investigation of unexplained haemoptysis. Respir Med 1992; 86:39–44.
8. Hsu BY, Edwards DK III, Trambert MA. Pulmonary hemorrhage complicating systemic lupus erythematosus: role of MR imaging in diagnosis. AJR 1992; 158:519–520.
9. Rubin GD, Edwards DK III, Reicher MA, et al. Diagnosis of pulmonary hemosiderosis by MR imaging. AJR 1989; 152:573–574.
10. Santiago S, Tobias J, Williams AJ. A reappraisal of the causes of hemoptysis. Arch Intern Med 1991; 151:2449–2551.
11. Jackson CV, Savage PJ, Quinn DL. Role of fiberoptic bronchoscopy in patients with hemoptysis and normal chest roentgenograms. Chest 1985; 87:142–144.
12. Lederle FA, Nichol KL, Parenti CM. Bronchoscopy to evaluate hemoptysis in older men with nonsuspicious chest roentgenograms. Chest 1989; 95:1043–1047.
13. Rath GS, Schaff JT, Snider GL. Flexible fiberoptic bronchoscopy techniques and review of 100 bronchoscopies. Chest 1973; 63:389–693.
14. Santiago SM, Lehrman S, Williams AJ. Bronchoscopy in patients with hemoptysis and normal chest roentgenograms. Br J Dis Chest 1987; 81:186–190.
15. Fraser RG, Paré JAP, Paré PD. Diagnosis of Diseases of the Chest. 3d ed. Philadelphia: WB Sanders, 1989.
16. Berger HW, Granda MG. Lower lung field tuberculosis. Chest 1974; 65:522–526.
17. Woodring JH, Vandiviere HM, Fried AM, et al. Update: the radiographic features of pulmonary tuberculosis. AJR 1986; 146:497–506.
18. Ikezoe J, Takeuchi N, Johkoh T, et al. CT appearance of pulmonary tuberculosis in diabetic and immunocompromised patients: comparison with patients who had no underlying disease. AJR 1992; 159:1175–1179.

19. Im J, Itoh H, Shim Y, et al. Pulmonary tuberculosis: CT findings—early active disease and sequential change with antituberculous therapy. Radiology 1993; 186:563–660.
20. Primack SL, Logan PM, Hartman TE, et al. Pulmonary tuberculosis and *Mycobacterium avium-intracelluare*: a comparison of CT findings. Radiology 1995; 194: 413–447.
21. Leatherman JW, Davies SF, Hoidal JR. Alveolar hemorrhage syndromes: diffuse microvascular lung hemorrhage in immune and idiopathic disorders. Medicine 1984; 63:343–361.
22. Albelda SM, Gefter WB, Epstein DM, et al. Diffuse pulmonary hemorrhage: a review and classification. Radiology 1985; 154:289–297.
23. Bradley JD. The pulmonary hemorrhage syndromes. Clin Chest Med 1982; 3: 593–605.
24. Bowley NB, Steiner RE, Chin WS. The chest x-ray in antiglomerular basement membrane antibody disease (Goodpasture's syndrome). Clin Radiol 1979; 30: 419–429.
25. Goodpasture EW. The significance of certain pulmonary lesions in relation to the etiology of influenza. Am J Med Sci 1919; 158:863–870.
26. Stanton MC, Tange JD. Goodpasture's syndrome (pulmonary hemorrhage associated with glomerulonephritis). Aust Ann Med 1958; 7:132–144.
27. Sybers RG, Sybers JL, Dickie HA, et al. Roentgenographic aspects of hemorrhagic pulmonary–renal disease (Goodpasture's syndrome). AJR 1965; 94:674–680.
28. Case records of the Massachusetts General Hospital 16-1993. N Engl J Med 1993: 328:1183–1190.
29. Travis WD, Colby TV, Lombard C, et al. A clinicopathologic study of 34 cases of diffuse pulmonary hemorrhage with lung biopsy confirmation. Am J Surg Pathol 1990; 14:1112–1125.
30. Imoto EM, Lombard CM, Sachs DPL. Pulmonary capillaritis and hemorrhage: a clue to the diagnosis of systemic necrotizing vasculitis. Chest 1989; 96:927–928.
31. Ognibene AJ, Dito WR. Rheumatoid disease with unusual pulmonary manifestations. Arch Intern Med 1965; 116:567–572.
32. Cordier JF, Valeyre D, Guillevin L, et al. Pulmonary Wegener granulomatosis: a clinical and imaging study of 77 cases. Chest 1990; 97:906–912.
33. Myers JL, Katzenstein AL. Wegener's granulomatosis presenting with massive pulmonary hemorrhage and capillaritis. Am J Surg Pathol 1987; 11:895–898.
34. Travis WD, Carpenter HA, Lie JT. Diffuse pulmonary hemorrhage: an uncommon manifestation of Wegener's granulomatosis. Am J Surg Pathol 1987; 11:702–708.
35. Papiris SA, Manoussakis MN, Drosos AA, et al. Imaging of thoracic Wegener's granulomatosis: the computed topographic appearance. Am J Med 1992; 93:529–536.
36. Bronson SM. Idiopathic pulmonary hemosiderosis in adults. Report of a case and review of the literature. AJR 1960; 83:260–273.
37. Bruwer AJ, Kennedy RLJ, Edwards JE. Recurrent pulmonary hemorrhage with hemosiderosis: so-called idiopathic pulmonary hemosiderosis. AJR 1956; 76:98–107.

38. Pacheco A, Casanova C, Fogne L, et al. Long-term clinical follow-up of adult idiopathic pulmonary hemosiderosis and celiac disease. Chest 1991; 99:1525–1526.
39. Case records of the Massachusetts General Hospital, 30-1988. N Engl J Med 1988; 319:227–237.
40. Soergel KH, Sommers SC. Idiopathic pulmonary hemosiderosis and related syndromes. Am J Med 1962; 32:499–511.
41. Cheah FK, Sheppard MN, Hansell DM. Computed tomography of diffuse pulmonary hemorrhage with pathological correlation. Clin Radiol 1993; 48:89–93.
42. Finley TN, Aronow A, Cosentino AM, et al. Occult pulmonary hemorrhage in anticoagulated patients. Am Rev Respir Dis 1975; 112:23–29.
43. Brown OL, Garvey JM, Stern CA. Diffuse intrapulmonary hemorrhage caused by Coumadin intoxication. Chest 1965; 48:525–526.
44. Barnett VT, Bergmann F, Humphrey H, et al. Diffuse alveolar hemorrhage secondary to superwarfarin ingestion. Chest 1992; 102:1301–1302.
45. Herbert FA, Orford R. Pulmonary hemorrhage and edema due to inhalation of resins containing trimellitic anhydride. Chest 1979; 76:546–551.
46. Kaplan V, Baur X, Czuppon A, et al. Pulmonary hemorrhage due to inhalation of vapor containing pyromellitic dianhydride. Chest 1993; 104:644–645.
47. Marglin SI, Castellino RA. Severe pulmonary hemorrhage following lymphography. Cancer 1979; 43:482–483.
48. Tapper DP, Taylor JR. Diffuse pulmonary infiltrates following lymphography. Chest 1989; 96:915–916.
49. Murray RJ, Albin RJ, Mergner W, et al. Diffuse alveolar hemorrhage temporally related to cocaine smoking. Chest 1988; 93:427–429.
50. Robboy SJ, Minna JD, Colman RW, et al. Pulmonary hemorrhage syndrome as a manifestation of disseminated intravascular coagulation: analysis of ten cases. Chest 1973; 63:718–721.
51. Martinez AJ, Maltby JD, Hurst DJ. Thrombotic thrombocytopenic purpura seen as pulmonary hemorrhage. Arch Intern Med 1983; 143:1818–1820.
52. Patel AM, Ryu JH. Metastatic angiosarcoma and pulmonary hemorrhage. Am Rev Respir Dis 1991; 143(suppl):A63.
53. Segal SL, Lenchner GS, Cichelli AV, et al. Angiosarcoma presenting as diffuse alveolar hemorrhage. Chest 1988; 94:214–216.
54. Kahn FW, Jones JM, England DM. Diagnosis of pulmonary hemorrhage in the immunocompromised host. Am Rev Respir Dis 1987; 136:155–160.
55. Hildebrand FL, Rosenow EC, Habermann TM, et al. Pulmonary complications of leukemia. Chest 1990; 98:1233–1239.
56. Robbins RA, Linder J, Stahl MG, et al. Diffuse alveolar hemorrhage in autologous bone marrow transplant recipients. Am J Med 1989; 87:511–518.
57. deLassence A, Beaune J, Fleury J, et al. Diagnostic criteria for alveolar hemorrhage in immunocompromised hosts. Am Rev Respir Dis 1993; 147(suppl):A83.
58. Witte RJ, Gurney JW, Robbins RA, et al. Diffuse pulmonary alveolar hemorrhage after bone marrow transplantation: radiographic findings in 39 patients. AJR 1991; 157:461–464.

59. Smith LJ, Katzenstein AL. Pathogenesis of massive pulmonary hemorrhage in acute leukemia. Arch Intern Med 1982; 142:2149–2152.
60. Tenholder MF, Hooper RG. Pulmonary hemorrhage in the immunocompromised host—an elusive reality [abstr]. Am Rev Respir Dis 1980; 121(suppl):198.
61. Sisson JH, Thompson AB, Anderson JR, et al. Airway inflammation predicts diffuse alveolar hemorrhage during bone marrow transplantation in patients with Hodgkin disease. Am Rev Respir Dis 1992; 146:439–443.
62. Maile CW, Moore AV, Ulreich S, et al. Chest radiographic–pathologic correlation in adult leukemic patients. Invest Radiol 1983; 18:495–499.
63. Kuhlman JE, Fishman EK, Siegelman SS. Invasive pulmonary aspergillosis in acute leukemia: characteristic findings on CT, the CT halo sign, and the role of CT in early diagnosis. Radiology 1985; 157:611–614.
64. Primack SL, Hartman TE, Lee KS, et al. Pulmonary nodules and the CT halo sign. Radiology 1994; 190:513–515.
65. Buff SJ, McLelland R, Gallis HA, et al. *Candida albicans* pneumonia: radiographic appearance. AJR 1982; 138:645–648.
66. Pagani JJ, Libshitz HI. Opportunistic fungal pneumonias in cancer patients. AJR 1981; 137:1033–1039.
67. Janzen DL, Padley SPG, Adler BD, et al. Acute pulmonary complications in immunocompromised non-AIDS patients: comparison of diagnostic accuracy of CT and chest radiography. Clin Radiol 1993; 47:159–165.
68. Ognibene FP, Shelhamer JH. Kaposi's sarcoma. Clin Chest Med 1988; 9:459–465.
69. Nash G, Fligiel S. Kaposi's sarcoma presenting as pulmonary disease in the acquired immunodeficiency syndrome. Hum Pathol 1984; 15:999–1001.
70. Naidich DP, McGuinness G. Pulmonary manifestations of AIDS: CT and radiographic correlations. Radiol Clin North Am 1991; 29:999–1017.
71. Wolff SD, Kuhlman JE, Fishman EK. Thoracic Kaposi sarcoma in AIDS: CT findings. J Comput Assist Tomogr 1993; 17:60–62.
72. Hartman TE, Primack SL, Müller NL, et al. Diagnosis of thoracic complications in AIDS: accuracy of CT. AJR 1994; 162:547–553.

10

Diseases of the Airways

S. MELANIE GREAVES and DENISE R. ABERLE

UCLA School of Medicine
Los Angeles, California

I. Introduction

Diseases of the airways include diverse conditions, ranging from focal tracheobronchial neoplasms to inflammatory bronchiolitis. Recent advances in imaging technology have greatly improved our ability to noninvasively diagnose and characterize these conditions. This chapter will provide an overview of contemporary imaging techniques for the investigation of common airway problems confronting the practicing pulmonologist. Because of its cross-sectional perspective, high contrast, and high spatial resolution, computed tomography (CT) is a central component of the radiology of airways diseases and will be the focus of this chapter. Four major categories of airways abnormalities are addressed, including (1) focal or central airway lesions, (2) bronchiectasis, (3) small airways disease, and (4) physiological imaging. The role of imaging in the evaluation of hemoptysis is also individually considered.

II. Focal or Central Lesions

A. Technical Considerations

With contemporary CT technique, the proximal five to seven generations of airways are normally directly visible, beginning with the trachea and continuing to the level of the subsegmental or slightly higher-order bronchi. In the absence of disease, the smaller airway generations, including the terminal and respiratory bronchioles, are below the limits of macroscopic resolution, even with high-resolution CT (HRCT) technique. The macroscopic (central) airways are a common site for both inflammatory and neoplastic diseases. Although projectional chest radiographs allow the diagnosis of some airway lesions, many tracheobronchial abnormalities are not readily appreciated on conventional chest radiographs. Computed tomography has become the principal advanced-imaging modality for the investigation of focal or central airways pathology and has largely replaced conventional tomography at most institutions.

The use of CT for the assessment of focal or central airway disease requires a clear understanding of the conditions in question, meticulous attention to technique, and an appreciation of the limitations of cross-sectional imaging. Because most segmental airways are less than 5 mm in diameter, optimal technique requires the use of thinner collimation ranging from 1 to 5 mm thickness, to maximize spatial resolution. By using these guidelines, most segmental and subsegmental airways are identifiable on CT (2–5). For most routine thoracic applications, contiguous axial images of 5-mm collimation are acquired through the hila, corresponding to the most concentrated central airway anatomy; wider collimation may be used for imaging the upper and lower thorax. The examination may then be tailored with additional 1- to 1.5-mm–thick sections obtained through areas of suspected abnormality. The decision to use intravenous contrast is guided by the clinical history and by chest radiographic findings. Intravenous contrast is particularly helpful when investigating hilar or juxtamediastinal masses, as it enables the differentiation of masses or adenopathy from adjacent hilar vessels (6).

Traditional incremental axial CT is obtained during suspended breath-holding and requires that the patient breath-hold for sequential axial images. Between scans, the patient is allowed to breathe normally while the table advances to the next scanning position. Slight variations in the depth of breath-hold can result in respiratory misregistration, in which axial levels are missed during scanning. This may result in the failure to visualize small tracheobronchial lesions, even when using high-resolution technique. Helical CT is a recent technical advance, introduced in 1989, in which scanning occurs continuously as the patient passes through the x-ray gantry. Scan times range from less than 10 sec to over 30 sec, during which a continuous volume of image data is acquired in a single breath-hold. The image data is acquired as a helix; interpolation algorithms are applied to generate axial image data. Helical CT technique offers several advantages over traditional incremental axial CT. First, because a volume of lung is imaged in a single breath-hold, respiratory misregistration artifacts are eliminated. Second, the volume data set can be used to generate arbitrary or overlapping image data sets from which high-quality three-dimensional and multiplanar reformations can be produced. Finally, it is usually possible to scan during smaller time intervals using less contrast and to better synchronize image acquisition with peak time of contrast enhancement, improving the quality of the images (7,8).

B. Focal Tracheobronchial Lesions

The most common primary neoplasms to affect the central bronchi are bronchogenic carcinoma, bronchial carcinoid, endobronchial hamartoma, and lymphoma. The tracheobronchial tree is also a common site for metastatic disease from extrathoracic primary neoplasms, most commonly of breast, renal cell, melanoma, or colorectal origins. The chest radiograph is the first radiographic investigation in patients with suspected focal tracheobronchial neoplasms, but may be surprisingly unremarkable, even with central lesions of moderate size. Patients often present with cough or hemoptysis and, in advanced cases, may exhibit stridor, focal wheezing, or other complications of airway occlusion. Fiberoptic bronchoscopy (FOB) provides direct visualization of the tracheobronchial tree and offers a means of tissue diagnosis. However, CT offers several advantages that make it complementary to FOB in the evaluation of patients with focal airway disease.

Several studies have compared CT and FOB in the evaluation of focal bronchial disease. Although most of these published studies used incremental CT of varying spatial resolution, the results suggest complementary roles. In 1987, Naidich and colleagues (9) performed a retrospective comparison of FOB and CT with varying slice collimation of 1.5, 5, and 10 mm. The CT scans accurately identified 88 (90%) of 98 lesions seen bronchoscopically; diagnostic accuracy was greater for mainstem and lobar lesions (93%) than for segmental bronchial lesions (73%). Most misdiagnoses were secondary to observer error; in only one case was the abnormality missed because of nonvisualization of the involved bronchus by CT. A second study comparing FOB with CT scans of 4- and 8-mm CT collimation in 143 patients corroborated these findings and concluded that CT is a reliable method for demonstrating bronchial tumor (Fig. 1; 10).

With CT, airway anatomy is accessible even when beyond the reach of the bronchoscope within bronchi distal to occlusions. Similarly, CT provides a topographic assessment of extraluminal disease, such as the extension of tumor into adjacent structures and the presence of adenopathy (Figs. 2 and 3). This cross-sectional perspective is important for staging cancers and for guiding the bronchoscopic biopsy of extraluminal neoplasms. In addition, the extraluminal extent

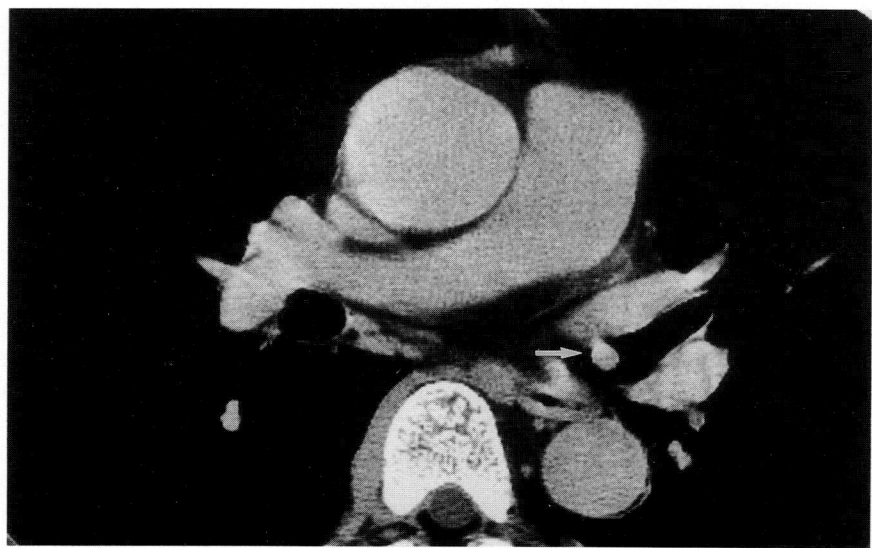

Figure 1 A 48-year-old man with a history of renal cell carcinoma: On CT at the level of the left hilum there is a focal endobronchial lesion of the distal left mainstem bronchus (arrow). This proved to be a benign bronchial hamartoma of the bronchus that was successfully resected with bronchoscopic laser photoresection.

of neoplasms influences the management of patients under consideration for palliative laser photoresection; tumors with large extraluminal components are poor candidates for laser photoresection. The CT bronchus sign in which a third- to fifth-order bronchus directly enters a peripheral neoplasm improves the yield the bronchoscopic biopsy of peripheral neoplasms (Fig. 4; 11,12). Those lesions not associated with a CT bronchus will usually have a low yield of tissue with FOB and are more amenable to percutaneous or thoracoscopic biopsy.

A CT scan is not without limitations. First, CT does not reliably distinguish benign from malignant disease. Second, lesions within airways coursing obliquely relative to the scan plane are less well characterized on incremental axial CT. This limitation is likely to be overcome with contemporary high-resolution helical acquisition, but no large-scale studies have yet been reported. Finally, CT may underestimate the degree of proximal submucosal extent of tumor. Therefore, aggressive bronchoscopic staging is required in patients with central neoplasm in whom curative bronchoplastic procedures are a consideration (Fig. 5).

Because of exquisite contrast resolution, CT is the diagnostic modality of choice in patients with broncholithiasis. Calcified peribronchial or bronchopulmonary lymph nodes that have eroded into the adjacent bronchial lumen may be a cause of persistent cough or hemoptysis and have been associated with occult fever caused by postobstructive atelectasis and pneumonitis. These broncholiths may be extremely difficult to document with fiberoptic bronchoscopy because the greater component of the lesion is extraluminal. Use of FOB may identify a suspected submucosal irregularity; but focal biopsies often yield only nonspecific inflammatory material. A CT scan is exquisitely sensitive to the presence of calcification, can reliably demonstrate both the endo- and peribronchial components, and provides an accurate assessment of associated complications of bronchial obstruction. In some instances, CT provides a definitive diagnosis of broncholithiasis in patients with chronic unexplained symptoms (14).

C. Diffuse Tracheobronchial Lesions

Diffuse tracheobronchial narrowing has been described with various inflammatory diseases, including sarcoidosis, Wegener's granulomatosis, amyloidosis, relapsing polychondritis, and tracheobronchopathia osteochondroplastica (15,16). Certain malignant lesions, such as lymphoma, diffuse submucosal spread of malignancy, and Kaposi's sarcoma, are also associated with diffuse tracheobronchial narrowing. A CT scan is an elegant means of assessing the extent, distribution, and severity of tracheobronchial wall thickening and luminal narrowing (Fig. 6). In conditions such as tracheobronchopathia osteochondroplastica or amyloidosis, in which calcification (or ossification) is a conspicuous feature of the disease, CT may be the diagnostic procedure of choice.

III. Bronchiectasis

Bronchiectasis is defined as irreversible dilation of the bronchial tree and should not be confused with the transient reversible dilation of bronchi associated with acute inflammatory disease. Chest radiographic abnormalities, such as bronchial wall thickening, bronchial dilation, mucous plugging and volume loss, suggest the diagnosis of bronchiectasis in severe cases. However, patients with milder disease frequently have nonspecific or normal chest radiographs. Although bronchography has historically been considered the gold standard in the diagnosis of bronchiectasis, CT has become the diagnostic procedure of choice.

The earliest descriptions of CT for this application used 10-mm collimation (17); not surprisingly, when compared with bronchography, CT was insufficiently sensitive to diagnose mild bronchiectasis. With high-resolution technique, scan collimation is limited to 1–5 mm, and images are reconstructed using small fields of view and high spatial frequency algorithms that maximize spatial resolution and fine bronchopulmonary detail. With these modifications, airways as small as 1–2 mm in diameter can be resolved. In 1986, Grenier and colleagues prospec-

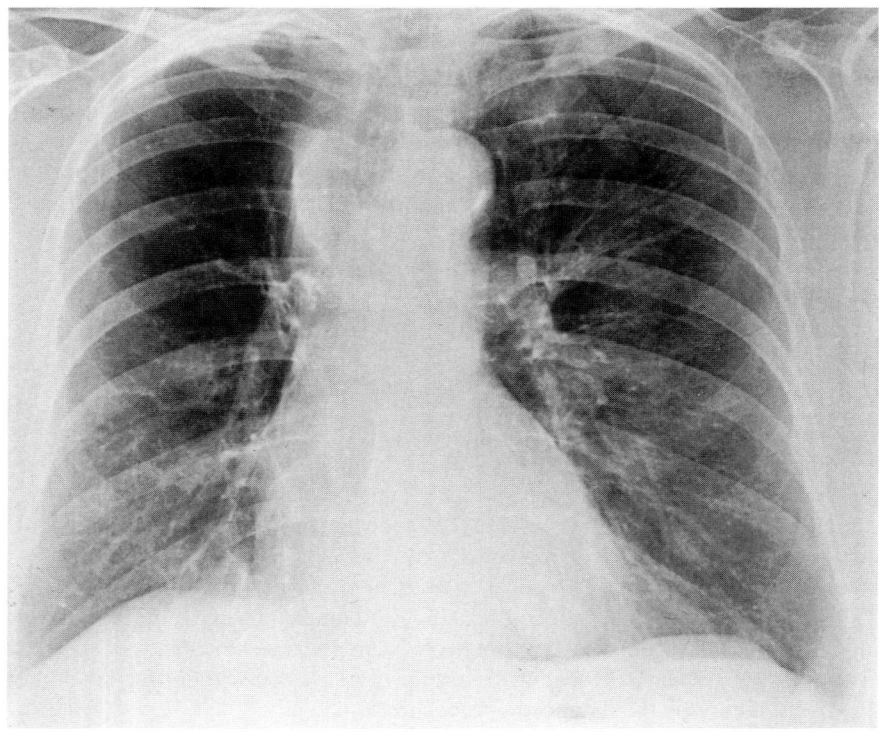

(a)

Figure 2 A 68-year-old woman with persistent cough and wheezing: (a) The frontal chest radiograph demonstrates volume loss in the right upper thorax with superior retraction of the right hilum. There is a prominent right paratracheal opacity, of which a component represents complete right upper lobe collapse. (b) On CT scan with intravenous contrast enhancement, there is extensive mass in the medial right upper lobe extending into the right lateral and posterior tracheal regions (arrows). (c) At a slightly lower level, there is severe narrowing of the right mainstem bronchus. Obliteration of the right upper lobe bronchus has resulted in complete right upper lobe collapse. This was a poorly differentiated adenocarcinoma at biopsy. Because of distal tracheal involvement and the CT identification of liver metastasis (not shown), the patient was not resectable and underwent thoracic radiation and systemic chemotherapy.

Diseases of the Airways

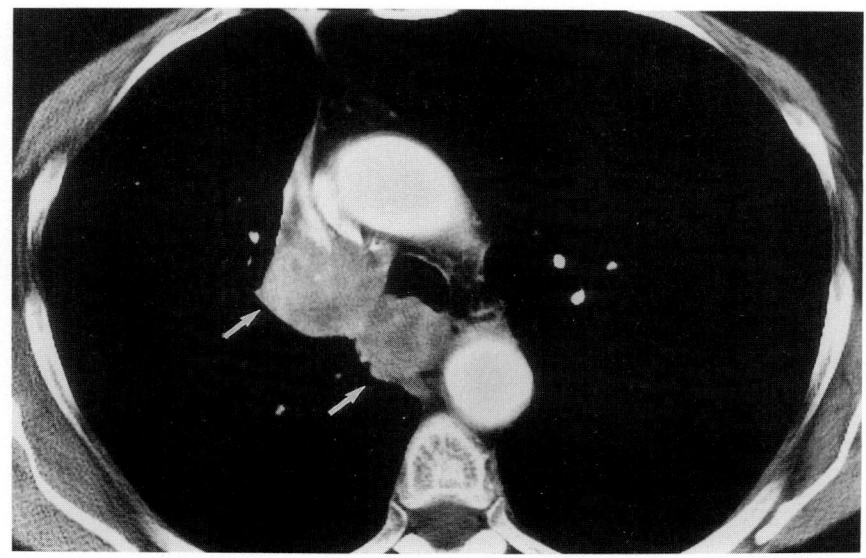
(b)

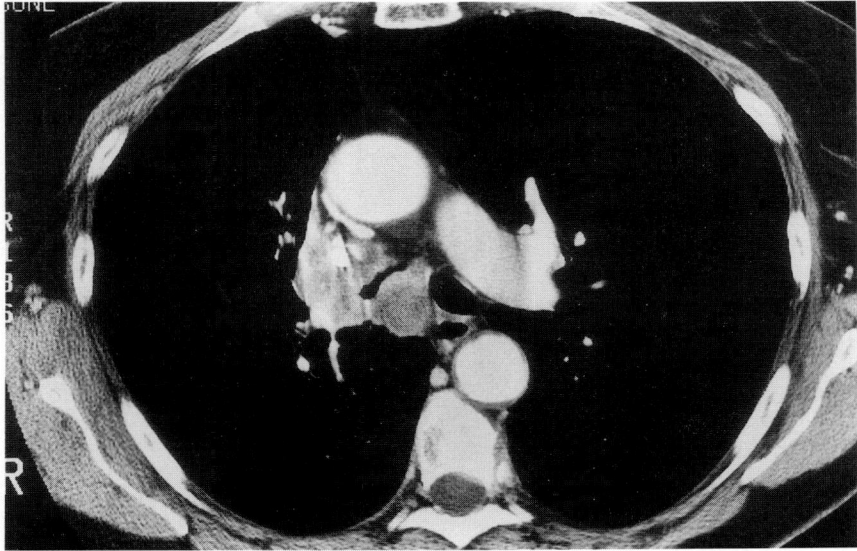
(c)

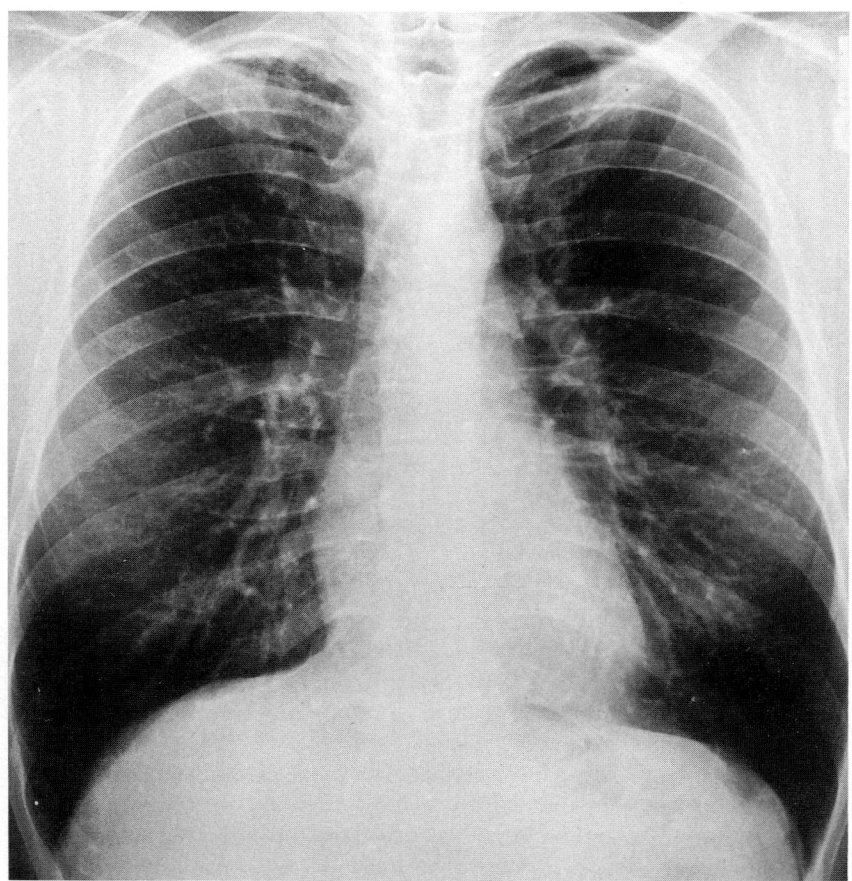

(a)

Figure 3 A 63-year-old man, with a history of metastatic disease to a cervical lymph node 5 years earlier, presenting with hemoptysis: (a) The frontal chest radiograph shows narrowing of the trachea at the thoracic inlet. (b) On helical CT, there is circumferential narrowing of the trachea, with an eccentric mass along the right posterolateral wall. Small necrotic lymph nodes are present bilaterally in the lateral paratracheal regions (arrows). (c) A coronal reformation demonstrates the primary tumor and its cephalocaudal extent. At surgery, this was a squamous cell carcinoma of the trachea; nodal sampling yielded local metastatic adenopathy.

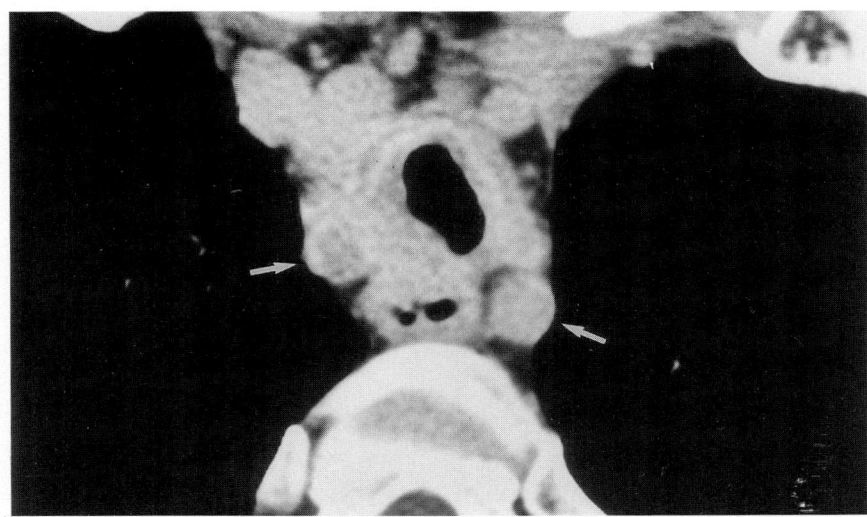
(b)

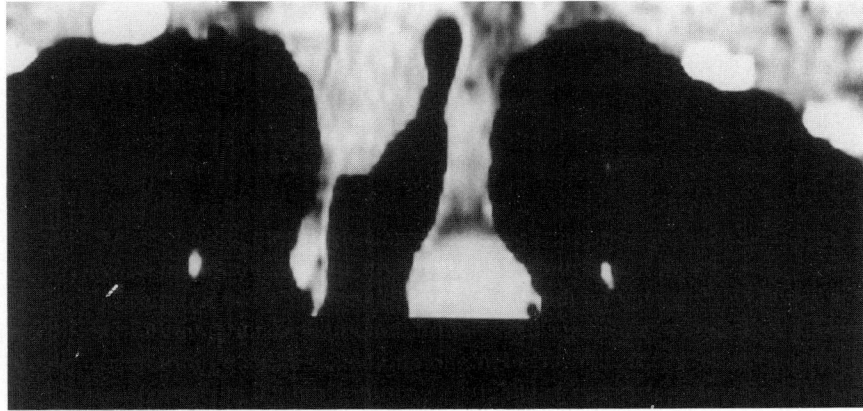
(c)

tively compared HRCT to bronchography in 44 lungs. Relative to bronchography, HRCT had a sensitivity of 96% and a specificity of 93% (18). Joharjy and colleagues used slightly thicker scan collimation at 5-mm increments and observed 97% concordance between CT and bronchography (19). Current image quality is such that only mild cylindrical bronchiectasis may be misdiagnosed, and false-positive diagnoses are rare. At most institutions, bronchography is reserved

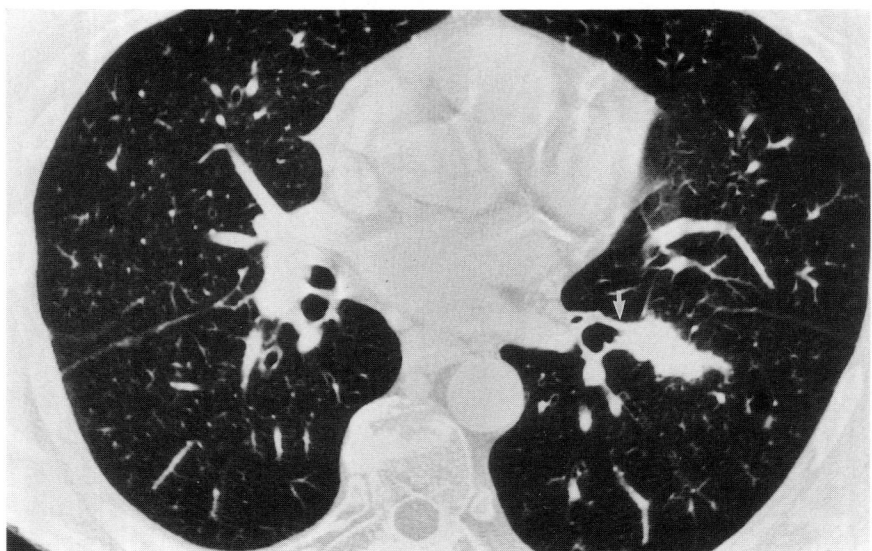

Figure 4 A 72-year-old man who smokes with prior history of head and neck neoplasm and a mass on chest radiographs: On CT, a 3-cm diameter mass is observed in the proximal anterior basal subsegment of the left lower lobe. There is a CT bronchus sign, with the subsegmental bronchus entering the proximal margin of the mass (arrow). A successful biopsy of the mass was taken by bronchoscopic approach.

for the exceptional patient anticipating surgical management in which HRCT has documented segmental or unilateral involvement. Motion artifacts resulting from either respiratory or vascular pulsation are the most common pitfalls in the CT diagnosis of bronchiectasis. Cardiac pulsation may produce double images of pulmonary vessels, resulting in a pseudotramtrack; this artifact is most commonly observed in the lingula and dependent lower lobes, and it is often minimized with reduced image acquisition times of 1 sec or less or with repositioning of the patient, such that the lung and airways in question are nondependent relative to the heart.

The CT findings of bronchiectasis include bronchial wall thickening and bronchial dilation. These observations are largely subjective because there are no absolute criteria for defining normal bronchial wall thickness or diameter. As a rough guide, the diameter of a bronchus should be similar to that of its adjacent pulmonary artery branch (20); small variations in this ratio must be interpreted with caution (21). In cylindrical bronchiectasis, the bronchus is typically much larger than the accompanying artery and appears as a signet ring in airways oriented perpendicular to the scan plane and as tramtracks in airways oriented within the scan plane. Bronchiectasis is also suggested if bronchi fail to taper normally as they approach the lung periphery. On HRCT, normal bronchi are not visible in the peripheral one-third of the lung; bronchiectatic airways are commonly observed in the lung periphery owing to associated bronchial wall thickening, peribronchiolar fibrosis, and bronchial dilation (22). With more advanced bronchiectasis, the abnormal bronchi appear beaded along their length, a finding that has been descriptively termed *string of pearls*.

Bronchiectasis may be of varying severity within an individual patient. Severe bronchiectasis results in clusters of multiple cystic lesions (Fig. 7), frequently containing air–fluid levels or retained secretions. Mucus-filled bronchi appear as broad linear or branching opacities when oriented along the scan plane. When oriented perpendicular to the scan plane, they appear as nodular or oval-shaped masses and may be misinterpreted as a pulmonary nodule. The diagnosis of mucous plugging is supported if these tubular structures are observed at successive axial levels and do not enhance following contrast administration. Focal bronchiectasis, particularly if associated with mucous plugging, should prompt a careful evaluation of the subtending proximal airway anatomy to exclude a benign or malignant bronchial stenosis.

A. Hemoptysis

Hemoptysis is an important, but nonlocalizing, symptom that requires thorough investigation. Studies in the United States suggest that most cases of hemoptysis result from bronchogenic carcinoma, bronchiectasis, or infection. Unfortunately, the etiology is indeterminant in up to 50% of cases and poses a considerable challenge to diagnosis (23). Fiberoptic bronchoscopy has traditionally been considered to be the primary diagnostic modality and is most likely to be diagnostic if the chest radiograph shows hilar or mediastinal mass, atelectasis, or a discrete parenchymal mass (24). In patients with central endobronchial disease, definite bronchoscopic diagnoses are achieved in over 95% of cases. Moreover, bronchoscopy is useful in localizing bleeding sites, removing blood clots or other bronchial debris, and in providing a mechanism for histological sampling.

The diagnostic yield of FOB in patients with hemoptysis and normal or nonlocalizing chest radiographs is much lower (25,26). In one study published by Poe et al. (25), the diagnostic yield of bronchoscopy in patients with hemoptysis and a nonlocalizing chest radiograph was only 23% if bronchitis was excluded; among all patients with nonlocalizing chest radiographs, only 6% had bronchogenic carcinoma (25). Several investigators contend that, in patients with hemoptysis and nonlocalizing chest radiographs, FOB should be reserved for only those individuals with risk factors for bronchogenic carcinoma, such as male gender, age older than 40–50, and significant smoking history, or for patients

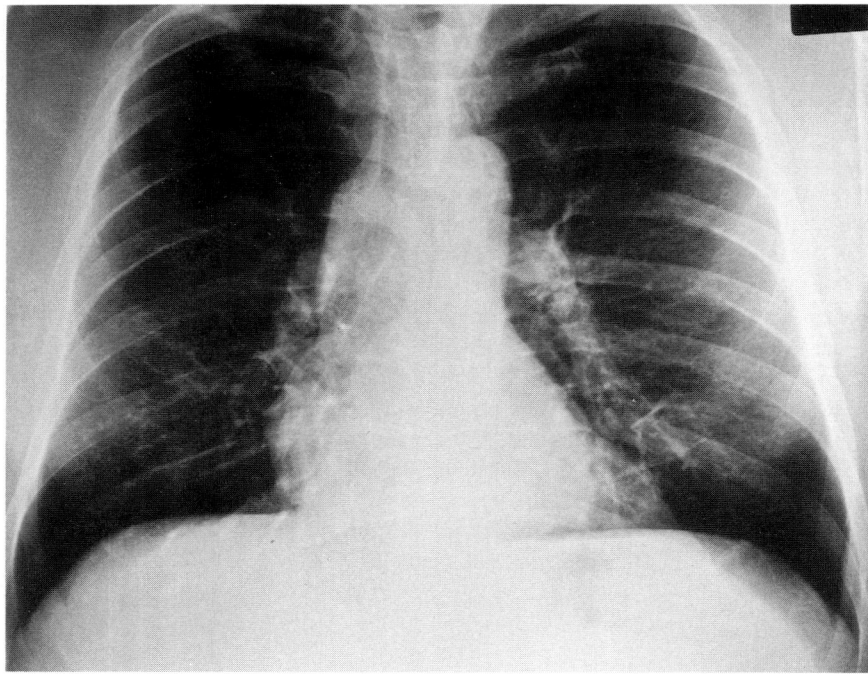

(a)

Figure 5 A 59-year-old man, with a history of wheezing and sputum cytologic studies indicative of squamous cell carcinoma: (a) Frontal chest radiograph is normal. (b) On CT, there is moderate thickening of the wall of the left upper lobe bronchus (arrows), which extends into the upper lobe segmental bronchi. At lower levels (not shown), subtle bronchial wall thickening of the left lower lobe bronchus was also present. At thoracotomy, histological sampling was obtained to determine the proximal and distal extent of submucosal neoplasm. The patient underwent successful sleeve lobectomy of the left upper lobe and end-to-end anastomosis of the left lower lobe and mainstem bronchi.

with hemoptysis of certain duration or severity (23,25,26). These studies suggest that using combinations of risk factors or clinically significant hemoptysis will identify those patients with bronchogenic carcinomas who will benefit from bronchoscopy as well as those patients who can be safely followed.

Several recent studies support the role of CT in the preliminary investigation of patients with hemoptysis (23,24,27). A CT scan may identify a cause for the hemoptysis, such as bronchiectasis, that will obviate bronchoscopy or may guide

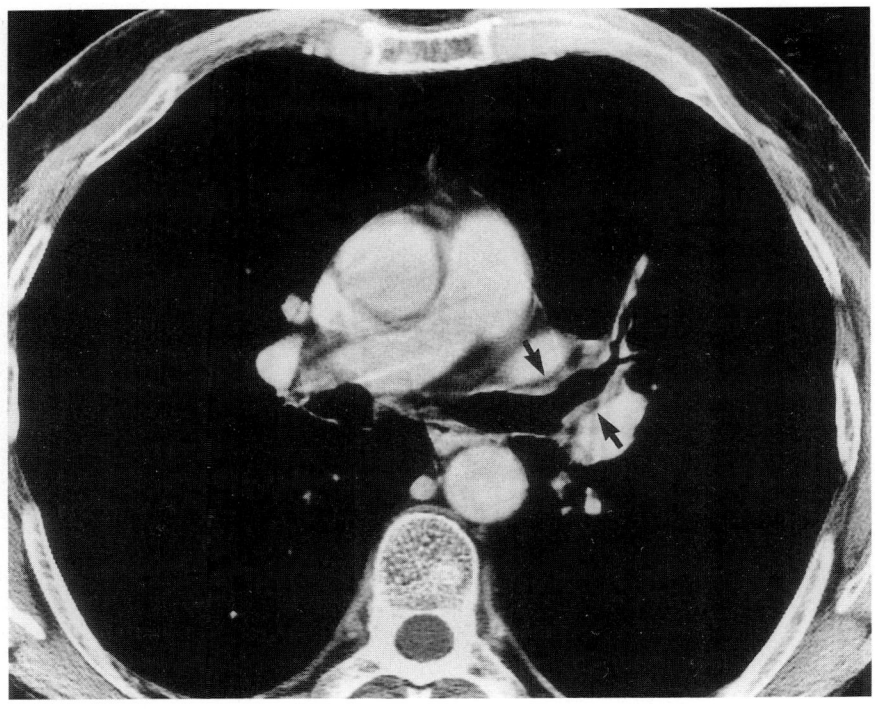

(b)

the bronchoscopist to a focal lesion. Naidich and co-workers (24) retrospectively compared incremental CT with FOB in 58 patients presenting with hemoptysis. In this study, CT identified focal lesions in 18 (31%) of the patients, of which malignancy was histologically confirmed in 17 patients. The CT scan was particularly valuable in patients who had a normal or nonlocalizing chest radiograph, diagnosing bronchiectasis in 35% of these patients. Set and colleagues (27) prospectively compared FOB and CT in 91 patients presenting with hemoptysis. The CT scans demonstrated all 27 tumors seen at bronchoscopy as well as an additional 7 neoplasms, of which 5 were beyond bronchoscopic range. Only 5% of patients with a normal chest radiograph had bronchogenic carcinoma, and all were detected by both CT and FOB. All 17 cases of bronchiectasis were diagnosed solely by CT. The CT scan did not demonstrate early mucosal abnormalities, such as bronchitis and squamous metaplasia. Because of respiratory misregistration, a benign papilloma was missed. Recently, McGuiness and colleagues (23) confirmed the value of CT in hemoptysis in a prospective study of 57 patients

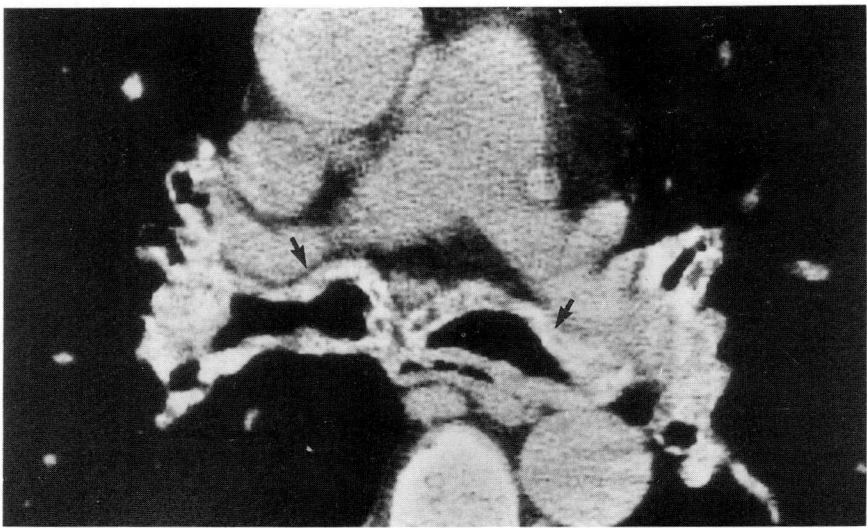

Figure 6 A 65-year-old woman with tracheobronchial amyloidosis: An axial CT section at the carinal bifurcation shows diffuse bronchial wall thickening of the mainstem bronchi (arrows) with associated calcifications. On CT, these changes were observed in the lobar and segmental airways.

comparing CT and bronchoscopy. Use of CT prospectively identified all tumors and suggested the correct diagnosis in 50% of patients with a nondiagnostic FOB.

These studies were all based on incremental CT technique. Because the most likely causes of hemoptysis in the general population are bronchiectasis and bronchogenic carcinoma, the CT technique should be optimized for the detection of these lesions. Naidich et al. (24) suggest the following protocol in patients with nonlocalizing chest radiographs: The upper and lower thorax are imaged with 1.5-mm collimation at 10-mm intervals, and the central (hilar) anatomy is imaged with contiguous 5-mm collimation. This preserves spatial resolution for the detection of subtle bronchiectasis throughout the lung, yet reduces the possibility of missing focal lesions in the central tracheobronchial tree owing to undersampling (24). With helical CT, it may be possible to image the central airway anatomy to the segmental level using narrow collimation in a single breath-hold. This should further improve the CT diagnosis of small focal lesions by the elimination of respiratory misregistration and by providing for overlapping axial reconstructions of the central tracheobronchial tree so that adequate sampling is achieved.

Diseases of the Airways

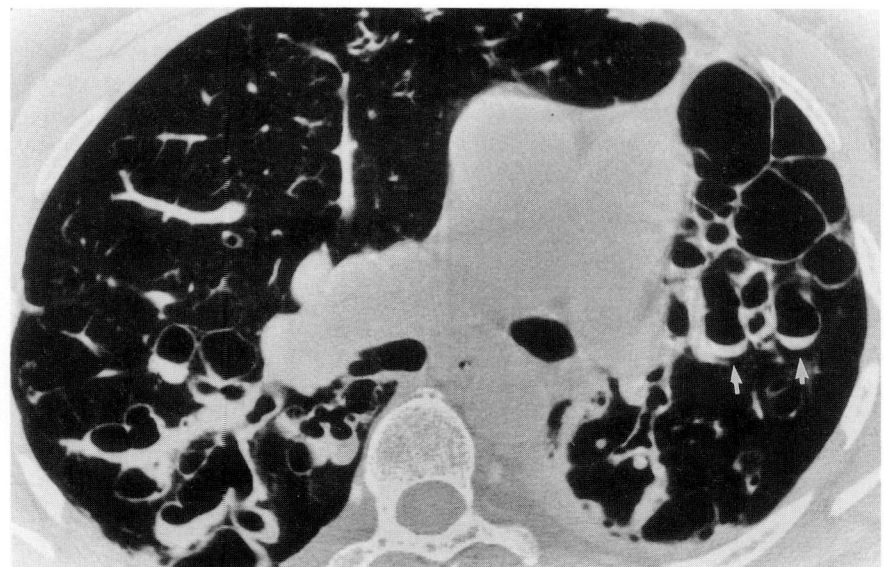

Figure 7 A 49-year-old woman with severe long-standing cystic bronchiectasis: On CT, there are markedly dilated bronchi bilaterally. The bronchiectatic airways appear as clusters of cysts. Air–fluid levels are present in some of the diseased bronchi (arrows).

IV. Small Airways

A. Anatomical Considerations

The small airways are classified as those airways 2 mm or smaller in diameter and include the terminal and respiratory bronchioles. The terminal (membranous) bronchioles are conducting airways having a maximum diameter of approximately 0.6 mm and represent the 8th–14th orders of airway branching. The terminal bronchioles lack cartilage but have a lining of epithelial cells. Respiratory bronchioles are the transitional structures between conducting airways and gas-exchanging parenchyma. They are characterized by outpouchings, representing alveolar structures, and lead to alveolar ducts and sacs.

The secondary pulmonary lobule is the basic anatomical unit of lung structure and measures approximately 1–2.5 cm in maximal diameter. The secondary lobule is subtended by three to five terminal bronchioles, which arborize from the center of the lobule with their accompanying pulmonary arterial branches. The lobule is marginated by connective tissue septa, the interlobular septa, containing venules and lymphatics. Normally, because of the extremely high contrast of aerated lung, intrapulmonary structures as small as 0.2 mm can be resolved with HRCT (1 to 1.5-mm collimation). The intralobular pulmonary arteries measure approximately 0.7 mm in diameter and are normally visible as Y-shaped branching or dot-like structures within the central portion of the secondary lobule. Although intralobular bronchi have a diameter similar to the accompanying arterioles, their visibility is determined primarily by bronchiolar wall thickness, which at 0.1 mm is below the limits of resolution with HRCT.

Diseases of the small airways effect morphological abnormalities that render the bronchioles visible on HRCT. Peribronchiolar and endobronchiolar inflammation or fibrosis are depicted on HRCT as small, irregular centrilobular nobules, with an average diameter of approximately 1 mm. Bronchiolar wall thickening and the presence of sections within the bronchiole result in centrilobular nodular and branching structures, likened to the appearance of a "tree in bud." Bronchiolectasis without mucous plugging will also increase the visibility of air-filled centrilobular bronchioles (28,29).

B. Panbronchiolitis

Diffuse panbronchiolitis has received increasing attention as a distinct sinobronchial entity, characterized by chronic sinusitis and bronchial inflammation. Rare among the white population, this syndrome is comparable in incidence with that of emphysema in Japan and appears to have a genetic basis. Chest radiographs demonstrate micronodular or reticulonodular opacities, tramlines, and hyperinflation. Akira and colleagues (30) described the HRCT features in 20 patients, which consist of distinctive centrilobular nodules and branching structures, the tree-in-bud appearance. These morphological features correlate with cellular infiltration of the walls of the respiratory bronchioles, secondary ectasia of the proximal terminal bronchioles, and bronchiolar sections. Heterogeneous lung attenuation as well as abnormalities of the larger airways, such as bronchial wall thickening and dilation, have also been observed.

The identification of tree-in-bud opacities usually indicates mucous plugging or intercurrent infection with *Pseudomonas* or *Haemophilus* organisms. Other diseases associated with intrabronchiolar secretions can result in the tree-in-bud appearance, including cystic fibrosis (31), congenital immunodeficiency states, ciliary dysmotility syndromes, and endobronchial dissemination of bacteria or mycobacteria (Fig. 8; 32).

C. Proliferative Bronchiolitis

The term *bronchiolitis obliterans* has been used to describe a heterogeneous group of diseases that result in inflammation and fibrosis of the small airways. These lesions may be classified according to etiology; however, a histopathological

Diseases of the Airways

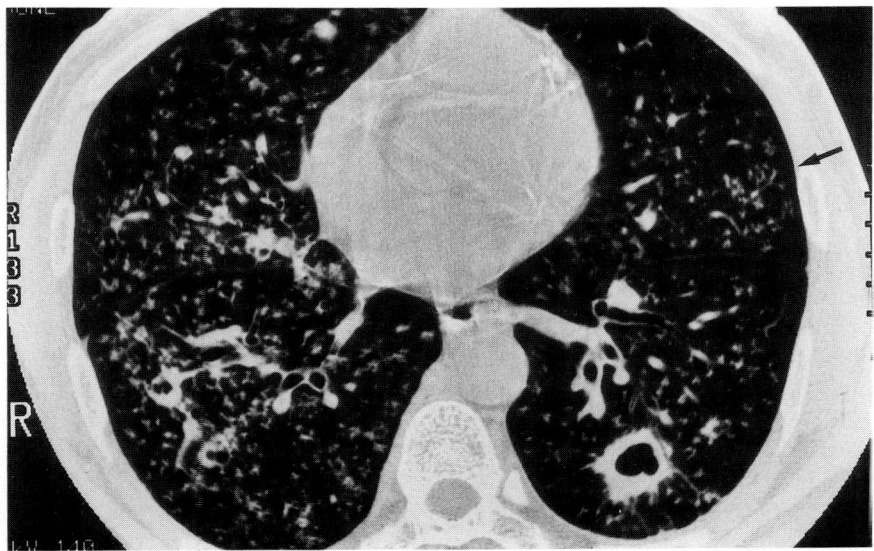

Figure 8 Acute tuberculous bronchiolitis in a 60-year-old diabetic man with intermittent cough. On HRCT, there is diffuse micronodularity and a discrete cavity in the left lower lobe. The mucous-filled small bronchioles have a distinctive tree-in-bud appearance (arrow) that is typically seen with bronchiolar infection or secretions. Bronchogenous dissemination of infection presumably originated from the cavity.

classification into proliferative bronchiolitis and constrictive bronchiolitis appears to be most useful, because this correlates best with the radiographic and functional manifestations of the syndromes. Although the causes of both forms of bronchiolitis are similar, the pathological and radiologic features of these two groups of diseases are very different (33,34). Moreover, patients with proliferative bronchiolitis more often respond to corticosteroid therapy, whereas those with constrictive bronchiolitis may exhibit progressive, inexorable respiratory insufficiency.

Proliferative bronchiolitis is characterized by organizing granulation tissue filling the bronchiolar lumen and represents a nonspecific reparative reaction to injury. When the disease process extends outward into the peribronchiolar alveolar spaces, it is known as cryptogenic organizing pneumonia (also called bronchiolitis obliterans organizing pneumonia, or BOOP). Although many cases are idiopathic, cryptogenic organizing pneumonia is also secondary to a variety of insults, including collagen vascular disorders, inhaled or systemic toxins, or chronic infection (33). Patients typically present with a short history of cough and shortness of breath; pulmonary function tests reveal a predominantly restrictive defect associated with a decreased diffusing capacity. Findings on chest radiographs and CT are usually those of bilateral patchy ground-glass or airspace consolidations that are predominantly peripheral, predominantly peribronchovascular, or a combination of the two (35). These foci of consolidation may be migratory (36); well-defined or poorly defined nodules have also been described (36).

D. Constrictive Bronchiolitis

Constrictive bronchiolitis is much less common than proliferative bronchiolitis and is primarily a lesion of terminal bronchioles. Histological findings range from mild inflammation to concentric fibrosis leading to bronchiolar obliteration (38). Although constrictive bronchiolitis may be idiopathic, it is also associated with heart–lung, lung, and bone marrow transplantation, as well as many of the syndromes associated with proliferative bronchiolitis, including collagen vascular disorders (particularly rheumatoid arthritis), previous viral infection, and toxic fume inhalation. Pulmonary function tests typically indicate severe airflow obstruction. The reported radiologic findings are varied. Patients with pure constrictive bronchiolitis may exhibit normal or increased lung volumes on chest radiographs. Attenuation of midlung and peripheral vessels has been described (39). Both CT and HRCT typically demonstrate alternating regions of abnormal decreased and increased lung attenuation. This finding has been termed *mosaic perfusion*, or *mosaic oligemia*, and appears to result from hypoxic vasoconstriction within an area of air-trapping or poorly ventilated lung. The affected lung appears on CT as a region of abnormally low lung attenuation; areas of normal or slightly increased lung attenuation reflect the redistribution of perfusion to unaffected lobules (40). Heterogeneous lung attenuation has also been described in patients with occlusive pulmonary vascular disease (chronic pulmonary emboli). Constrictive bronchiolitis as the etiology of mosaic oligemia can be suggested in the appropriate clinical setting or when the mosaic oligemia is accompanied by other bronchial abnormalities on HRCT (Fig. 9; 41,42).

Constrictive bronchiolitis obliterans affects up to 50% of heart–lung transplant recipients and is presumed to be related to graft rejection; in patients following bone marrow transplantation, it is a feature of graft-versus-host disease (Fig. 10). Both constrictive and proliferative forms of bronchiolitis have been described in transplant patients (38), and the diagnosis may be complicated by concurrent infection. Radiographic findings may be nonspecific and range from nodules to diffuse airspace disease (43). Many patients exhibit dilation of the visible airways, which is often more conspicuous than mosaic oligemia or other abnormalities referable to the small airways (44,45).

Patients who have viral infections in childhood may develop constrictive bronchiolitis obliterans in the form of unilateral hyperlucent lung (Swyer-James

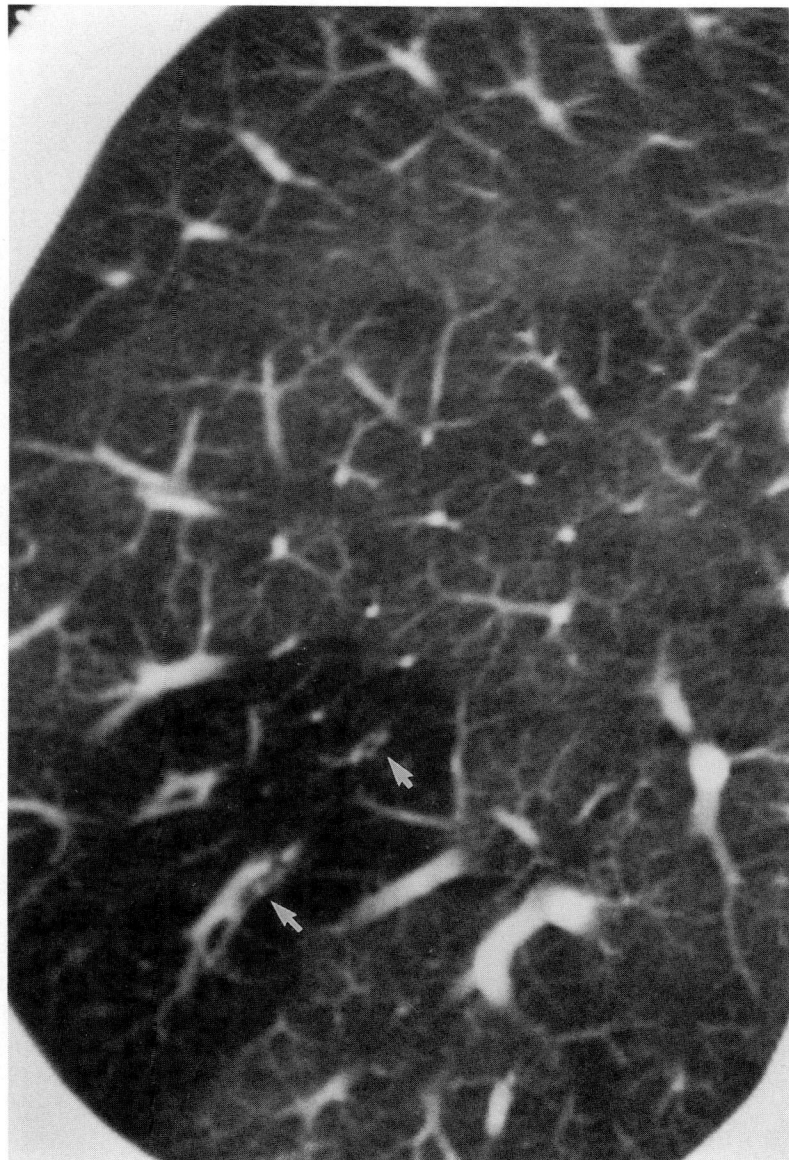

Figure 9 Focal oligemia in the right lower lobe, appearing as a geometric region of abnormal low lung attenuation: The diagnosis is suggested by the associated changes of cylindrical bronchiectasis of the subtending airways (arrows). Mosaic oligemia may be the primary manifestation of constrictive bronchiolitis.

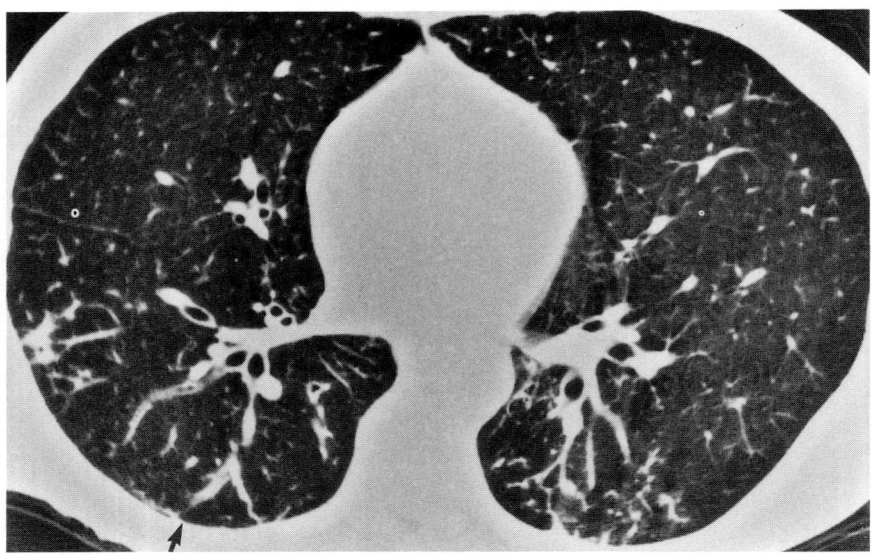

Figure 10 Constrictive bronchiolitis in the context of bone marrow transplant, with graft-versus-host disease: On CT there is moderate, multifocal peribronchial thickening, bronchiectasis (arrow), and peribronchial nodularity.

syndrome). This syndrome is typically asymmetric in distribution and preferentially affects the left lung. Chest radiographs may demonstrate a decrease in volume of the affected lung with associated decreases in the size and number of pulmonary vessels. Expiratory images will document air-trapping. With CT, several additional features of this disease are visible, including decreased lung attenuation, loss of the normal anterior–posterior lung attenuation gradient, decreased pulmonary arterial caliber within the affected lung, and bronchiectasis (46). It is also known from cross-sectional imaging that this syndrome is not purely unilateral; the contralateral lung will also exhibit fewer, but similar, findings. Because CT can precisely demonstrate the extent of bronchiectasis and location of air-trapping, it has replaced radionuclide ventilation–perfusion imaging as the primary imaging modality for the diagnosis of Swyer-James syndrome (34).

E. Respiratory (Smoker's) Bronchiolitis

Respiratory bronchiolitis is an inflammatory lesion of the respiratory bronchioles found in the lungs of many cigarette smokers. Pathologically, the lesion consists of macrophages within the respiratory bronchioles and surrounding alveoli, ectatic bronchioles with thickened walls, and epithelial metaplasia. These cigarette smoke-induced abnormalities are now presumed to be associated with the development of chronic obstructive pulmonary disease (COPD), particularly chronic bronchitis and emphysema (47). Virtually all patients are current heavy cigarette smokers and may present with cough, dyspnea, interstitial patterns, or "dirty lungs" on chest radiographs, and restrictive or mixed restrictive–obstructive patterns on spirometry.

Several HRCT abnormalities have been described in cigarette smokers and correlated with pulmonary function tests (48,49). Remy-Jardin and colleagues demonstrated that parenchymal micronodules, ground-glass attenuation, and emphysema were statistically more prevalent in smokers than in nonsmokers (49). The study groups all had normal pulmonary function tests, but the presence of bronchial wall thickening and emphysema were associated with a decreasing forced expiratory volume in 1 sec (FEV_1). Their data suggest that parenchymal abnormalities are visible on HRCT in asymptomatic smokers with normal chest radiographs and pulmonary function tests.

V. Functional Imaging

The role of HRCT has traditionally been limited to the morphological demonstration of static large and small airway abnormalities. Contemporary CT technology includes not only incremental CT, with individual image acquisition times of 1 sec or less, but also continuous helical volume acquisition and ciné (electron beam) CT, in which sequential images are acquired within several milliseconds, effectively achieving real-time CT. The temporal and spatial resolution achievable with current CT technology makes it possible to explore respiratory function by structural analysis. In contrast with pulmonary function tests, which provide global measures of lung function, functional HRCT affords a cross-sectional perspective, making possible the *regional* assessment and localization of physiological changes affecting the pulmonary airways and vasculature.

Computed tomography has been used to explore dynamic airway changes in various pulmonary conditions, including asthma and emphysema, following specific physiological maneuvers, and after pharmacological interventions. With CT, quantitative changes in the caliber of the airways, pulmonary vasculature, and thoracic diameters can be directly measured under differing physiological conditions. In addition, by referencing image acquisition to specific lung volumes, changes in the attenuation of lung provide an indirect index of air-trapping, akin to mosaic oligemia.

When using CT as a physiological tool, meticulous attention to technique is absolutely critical. First, it is important to ensure that identical anatomical regions are evaluated in the control and modified states. Currently anatomical landmarks of the fine lung structure are used to ensure comparability between imaging

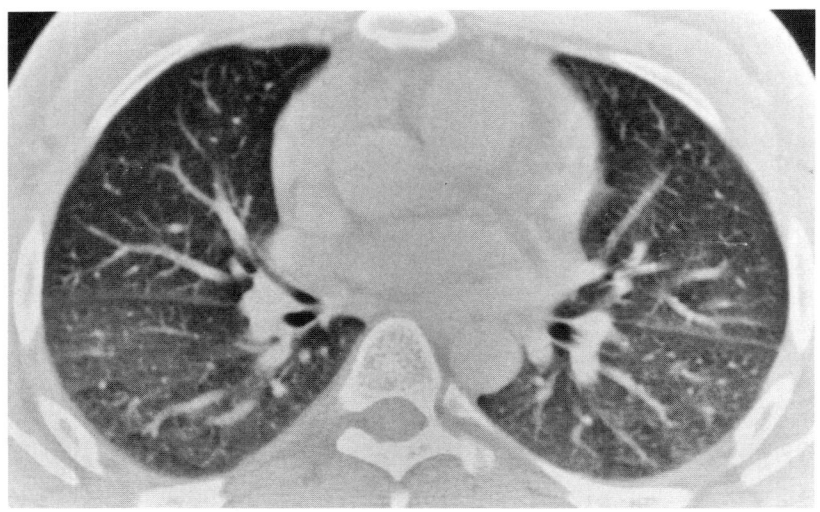

(a)

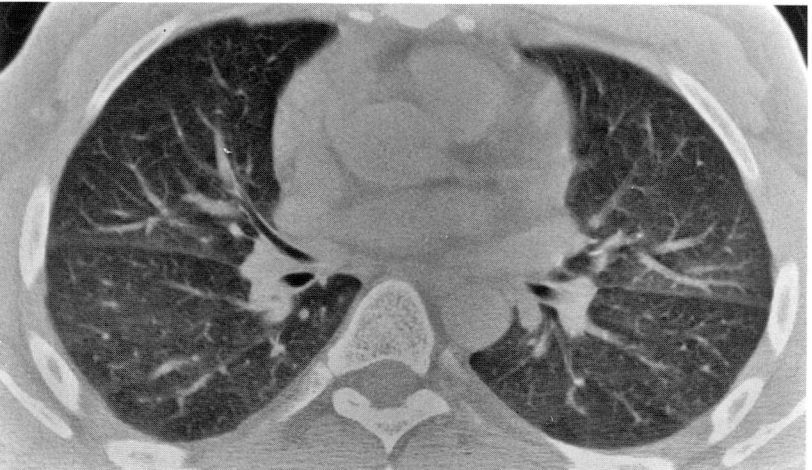

(b)

Figure 11 Computed tomographic images through like anatomical regions in a normal subject during suspended residual volume (RV) at (a) baseline and (b) after methacholine challenge: (a) During suspended RV, there is a relatively uniform, increasing gradient of lung attenuation in going from the nondependent to the dependent lung. (b) Following methacholine administration, this pattern of lung attenuation is stable.

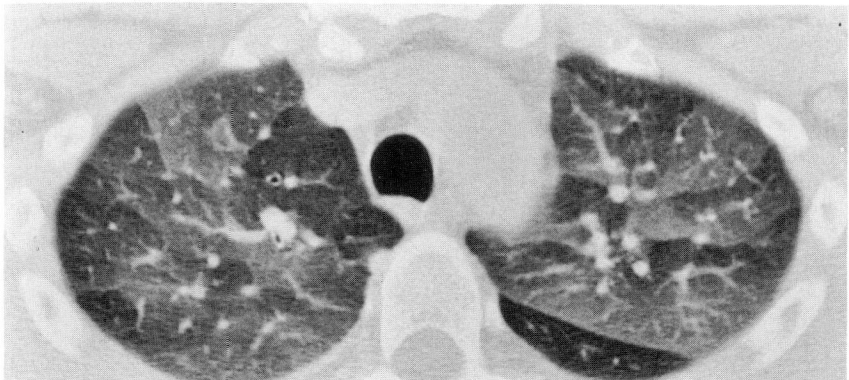

(a)

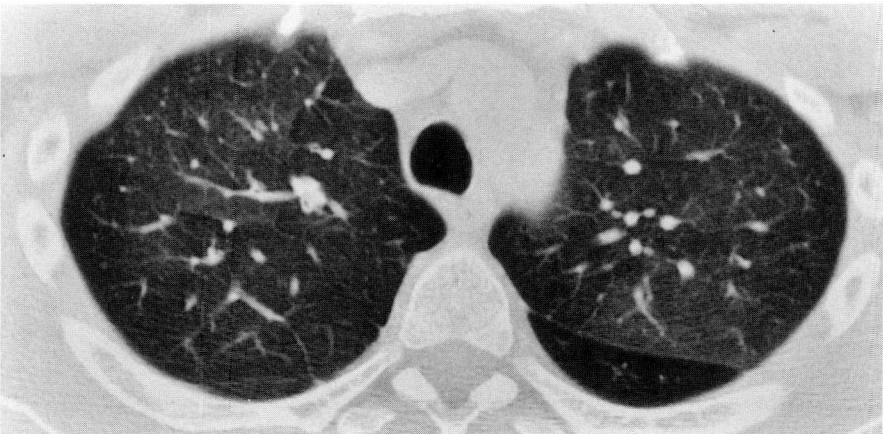

(b)

Figure 12 Computed tomographic images taken through like anatomical regions in a mild asthmatic during suspended residual volume (RV) at (a) baseline and (b) after methacholine challenge: (a) At baseline, the asthmatic demonstrates a distinctive pattern of mosaic oligemia. This was observed despite normal baseline spirometry. (b) After methacholine administration, lung attenuation remains slightly heterogeneous, but is abnormally low. This correlated with significant expiratory airflow obstruction on spirometry.

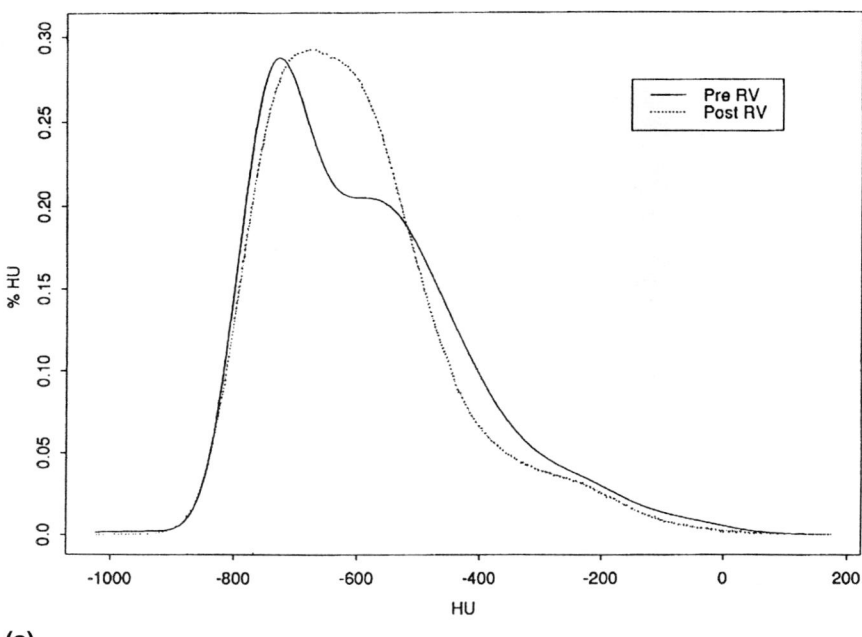

(a)

Figure 13 Frequency distribution curves of lung attenuation for the right lung axial sections in the (a) normal subject and (b) mild asthmatic (see Figs. 11 and 12), corresponding to suspended RV at baseline and after methacholine administration: (a) In the normal subject, the frequency distribution of lung attenuation is roughly stable following methacholine challenge. (b) In the asthmatic subject, there is a distinctive leftward shift of the curve (to low lung attenuation) coincident with significant airflow obstruction.

sequences, although three-dimensional reconstructions of the bronchovascular tree may permit more precise localization and volumetric measurements in the near future. Second, all structural information is heavily influenced by the state of lung inflation, which should be precisely referenced to spirometry between physiological sequences. A number of investigators have addressed these issues in various ways, including the use of respiratory-gating devices, such as spirometers or respitrace devices operating on the principal of impedance conductance that allow the subject to achieve reproducible lung volumes between image sequences. Helical volume acquisition CT overcomes some of the potential problems associated with respiratory misregistration, because all images are acquired during a single breath-hold. From this single-volume data set, axial images can be reconstructed at arbitrary and overlapping levels to optimize the anatomical repro-

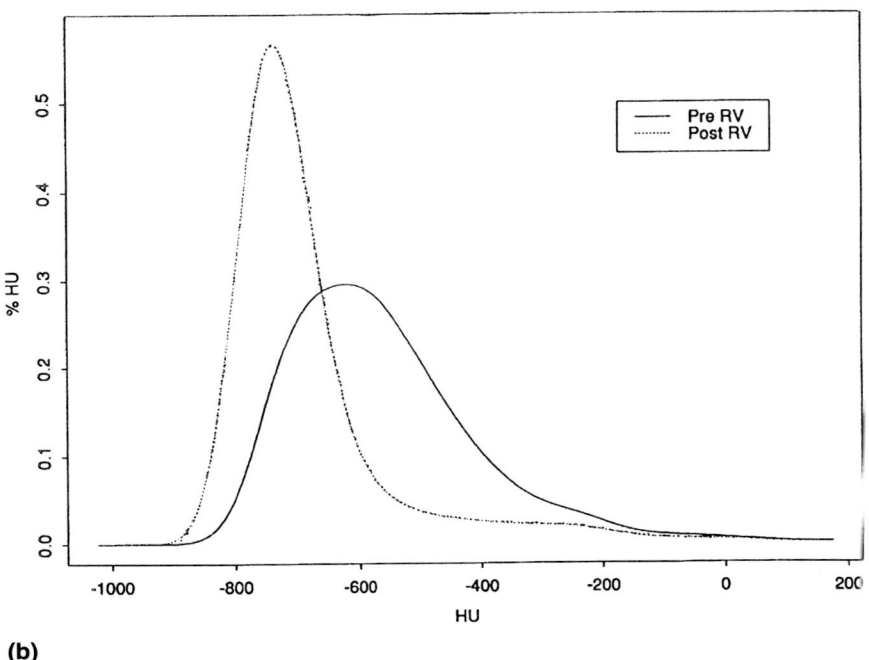

(b)

ducibility between image sequences (or physiological conditions). Finally, advanced image-processing techniques enable the reliable measurement of diameters, areas, volumes, and parameters of lung attenuation.

Although considerable research has been done in animal models (52–55), several investigators have begun to explore functional-imaging applications in human subjects. Different investigators have observed that with decreasing lung volume, normal lung increases in attenuation in a consistent and linear manner. On CT, the normal density of lung averages −700 to −800 Hounsfield units (HU) on deep inspiration. By using electron beam CT, mean lung attenuation in normal subjects increases by roughly 200 HU during a forced expiratory maneuver (56). Although, normally, lung attenuation increases most dramatically in the dependent lung parenchyma, the absolute attenuation of lung varies in different patients and in different regions of lung.

In patients with airflow obstruction caused by airway disease, expiratory air-trapping is reflected by abnormal lung lucency during exhalation (56). These lung attenuation changes correlate with spirometric abnormalities in patients with asthma. In a study comparing 18 nonsmoking asthmatics and 22 normal subjects,

Newman et al. (57) observed significant correlations between expiratory lung attenuation, as measured by mean pixel index (the percentage of lung pixels below -900 HU), and measures of FEV_1, residual volume (RV), and functional residual capacity (FRC).

More recently, Goldin et al. (58) studied 12 mild asthmatics and 5 normal subjects in whom spirometry and helical HRCT were performed at baseline and following a standardized methacholine challenge test. Imaging was performed at both suspended FRC and RV using a respitrace to reproduce lung volumes. Like anatomical regions between the physiological sequences were analyzed for changes in bronchial area and lung attenuation. At baseline, spirometry was normal in both asthmatic and normal subjects; however, differences in lung attenuation between FRC and RV images were statistically significant between the two groups.

Following methacholine challenge, normal subjects showed less than 10% decreases in FEV_1, and asthmatics experienced 20–36% decreases in FEV_1. This was associated with decreases in mean bronchial area of 12 and 36% in the normal and asthmatic groups, respectively, although these differences were significant only for the smallest visible airways.

Indices of lung attenuation for the whole lung were similar in the normal and asthmatic subjects at baseline. However, following methacholine challenge, lung attenuation in normal subjects remained unchanged (Fig. 11), but significantly decreased in asthmatic subjects (Fig. 12). These differences were reflected by significant airflow obstruction on spirometry and leftward shifts of the frequency distribution curves of lung attenuation (Fig. 13; 58). Decreased lung attenuation appears to represent air-trapping and may be the morphological correlate of small-airways closure. In this experimental setting, helical HRCT has been a sensitive measure of airway hyperreactivity and can capture both the bronchoconstrictive responses of the visible airways as well as the degree and distribution of air-trapping in affected individuals.

These preliminary investigations are extremely promising and underscore the potential of contemporary imaging to provide information not otherwise accessible in vivo. Many of these principles are now being applied to address other contemporary issues in respiratory physiology: the characterization of pulmonary function abnormalities in postoperative lung transplant patients, the functional assessment of emphysema patients under consideration for lung reduction surgery, and the effects of new drugs for the treatment of chronic obstructive pulmonary disease. The integration of pulmonary function and imaging equipment, combined with volume acquisition CT technology and refinements in advanced image processing will allow us to interrogate the cardiopulmonary systems and to extract information that is currently unprecedented in human physiology.

References

1. Kwong JS, Adler BD, Padley SPG, Müller NL. Diagnosis of diseases of the trachea and main bronchi: chest radiography versus CT. AJR 1993; 161:519–522.
2. Osborne D, Vock P, Godwin JD, Silverman PM. CT identification of bronchopulmonary segments: 50 normal subjects. AJR 1982; 142:47–52.
3. Lee KS, Bae WK, Lee BH, Kim IY, Choi EW, Lee BH. Bronchovascular anatomy of the upper lobes: evaluation with thin section CT. Radiology 1991; 181:765–772.
4. Naidich DP, Zinn WL, Ettenger NA, McCauley DI, Garray SM. Basilar segmental bronchi: thin section CT evaluation. Radiology 1988; 169:11–16.
5. Lee K, Im-J-G, Bae WK, et al. CT anatomy of the lingular segmental bronchi. J Comput Assist Tomogr 1991; 15:86–91.
6. Webb WR, Gamsu G, Speckman JM. Computed tomography of the pulmonary hilum in patients with bronchogenic carcinoma. J Comput Assist Tomogr 1983; 7:219–225.
7. Mogavero Newmark G, Conces DJ, Kopecky KK. Spiral CT evaluation of the trachea and bronchi. J Comput Assist Tomogr 1994; 18:552–554.
8. Heiken JP, Brink JA, Vannier MW. Spiral (helical) CT. Radiology 1993; 189: 647–656.
9. Naidich DP, Lee JJ, Garay SM, McCauley DI, Aranda CP, Boyd AD. Comparison of CT and fiberoptic bronchoscopy in the evaluation of bronchial disease. AJR 1987; 148:1–7.
10. Mayr B, Ingrisch H, Haussinger K, Huber RM, Sunder-Plassmann L. Tumors of the bronchi: role of evaluation with CT. Radiology 1989; 172:647–652.
11. Naidich DP, Sussman R, Kutcher WL, Aranda CP, Garay SM, Ettinger NA. Solitary pulmonary nodules. CT–bronchoscopic correlation. Chest 1988; 93:595–598.
12. Gaeta M, Pandolfo I, Volta S, Russi EG, Bartiromo G, Girone G, La Spad Barone M, Casablanca G, Minutoli A. Bronchus sign on CT in peripheral carcinoma of the lung: value in predicting results of transbronchial biopsy. AJR 1991; 157:1181–1185.
13. Gaeta M, Russi EV, La Spada, Barone M, Casablanca G, Pandolfo I. Small bronchogenic carcinomas presenting as solitary pulmonary nodules. Bioptic approach guided by the CT-positive bronchus sign. Chest 1992; 102:1167–1170.
14. Conces DJ, Tarver RD, Vix VA. Broncholithiasis: CT features in 15 patients. AJR 1991; 157:249–253.
15. Lenique F, Brauner MW, Grenier P, Battesti JP, Loiseau A, Valeyre D. CT assessment of bronchi in sarcoidosis: endoscopic and pathologic correlations. Radiology 1995; 194:419–423.
16. Kwong JS, Müller NL, Miller RR. Diseases of the trachea and mainstem bronchi: correlation of CT with pathologic findings. Radiographics 1992; 12:645–657.
17. Müller NL, Bergin CJ, Ostrow DN, Nichols DM. Role of computed tomography in the recognition of bronchiectasis. AJR 1984; 143:971–976.
18. Grenier P, Maurice F, Musset D, Menu Y, Nahum H. Bronchiectasis: assessment by thin section CT. Radiology 1986; 161:95–99.
19. Joharjy IA, Bashi SA, Adbullah AK. Value of medium-thickness CT in the diagnosis of bronchiectasis. AJR 1987; 149:1133.

20. Naidich DP, McCauley DI, Khoury NF, Stitik FP, Siegelman SS. Computed tomography of bronchiectasis. J Comput Assist Tomogr 1982; 6:437–444.
21. Lynch DA, Newell JD, Tschomper BA, Cink TM, Newman LS, Bethel R. Uncomplicated asthma in adults: comparison of CT appearance of the lungs in asthmatic and healthy subjects. Radiology 1993; 188:829–833.
22. Webb WR. High-resolution computed tomography of obstructive lung disease. Radiol Clin North Am 1994; 32:745–757.
23. McGuiness G, Beacher JR, Harkin TJ, Garay SM, Rom WN, Naidich DP. Hemoptysis: prospective high-resolution CT bronchoscopic correlation. Chest 1994; 105:1155–1162.
24. Naidich DP, Funt SF, Ettinger NA, Aranda C. Hemoptysis: CT–bronchoscopic correlations in 58 cases. Radiology 1990; 177:357–362.
25. Poe RH, Israel RH, Marin MG, Ortiz CR, Dale RC, Wahl GW, Kallay MC, Greenblatt DG. Utility of fiberoptic bronchoscopy in patients with hemoptysis and a nonlocalizing chest roentgenogram. Chest 1988; 93:70–75.
26. Jackson CV, Savage PJ, Quinn DL. Role of fiberoptic bronchoscopy in patients with hemoptysis and a normal chest roentgenogram. Chest 1985; 87:142–144.
27. Set PAK, Flower CDR, Smith IE, Cahn AP, Twentyman OP, Shneerson JM. Hemoptysis: comparative study of the role of CT and fiberoptic bronchoscopy. Radiology 1993; 189:677–680.
28. Nishimura K, Kitaichi M, Izumi T, Itoh H. Diffuse panbronchiolitis: correlation of high-resolution CT and pathologic findings. Radiology 1992; 184:779–785.
29. Gruden JF, Webb WR, Warnock M. Centrilobular opacities in the lung on high-resolution CT: diagnostic considerations and pathologic correlation. AJR 1994; 162:569–574.
30. Akira M, Kitatani F, Lee YS, Kita N, Yamamoto S, Higashihara T, Morimoto S, Ikezoe J, Kozuka T. Diffuse panbronchiolitis: evaluation with high-resolution CT. Radiology 1988; 168:433–438.
31. Lynch DA, Brasch RC, Hardy KA, Webb WR. Pediatric pulmonary disease: assessment with high-resolution ultrafast CT. Radiology 1990; 176:243–248.
32. Im J, Itoh H, Shim Y, Lee JH, Ahn J, Han MC, Noma S. Pulmonary tuberculosis: CT findings—early active disease and sequential change with antituberculous therapy. Radiology 1993; 186:653–660.
33. Myers JL, Colby TV. Pathologic manifestations of bronchiolitis, constrictive bronchiolitis, cryptogenic organizing pneumonia and diffuse panbronchiolitis. Clin Chest Med 1993; 14:611–622.
34. Lynch DA. Imaging of small airways diseases. Clin Chest Med 1993; 14:623–634.
35. Lee KS, Kullnig P, Hartman TE, Müller NL. Cryptogenic organizing pneumonia: CT findings in 43 patients. AJR 1994; 162:543–546.
36. Nishimura K, Itoh H. High-resolution computed tomographic features of bronchiolitis obliterans organizing pneumonia. Chest 1992; 102(suppl):26S–31S.
37. Bouchardy LM, Kuhlman JE, Ball WC, Hruban RH, Askin FB, Siegelman SS. CT findings in bronchiolitis obliterans organizing pneumonia (BOOP) with radiographic, clinical and histologic correlation. J Comput Assist Tomogr 1993; 17:352–357.

38. Colby TV, Myers JL. Clinical and histologic spectrum of bronchiolitis obliterans, including bronchiolitis obliterans organizing pneumonia. Semin Respir Med 1992; 13:119–133.
39. Breatnach E, Keer I. The radiology of cryptogenic obliterative bronchiolitis. Clin Radiol 1982; 33:657–661.
40. Sweatman MC, Millar AB, Strickland B, Turner-Warwick M. Computed tomography in adult obliterative bronchiolitis. Clin Radiol 1990; 41:116–119.
41. Eber CD, Stark P, Bertozzi P. Bronchiolitis obliterans on high-resolution CT: a pattern of mosaic oligemia. J Comput Assist Tomogr 1993; 17:853–856.
42. Skeens JL, Fuhrman CR, Yousem SA. Bronchiolitis obliterans in heart–lung transplantation patients: radiologic findings in 11 patients. AJR 1989; 153:253–256.
43. Lenz D, Bergin CJ, Berry GJ, Stoehr C, Theodore J. Diagnosis of bronchiolitis obliterans in heart–lung transplantation patients: importance of bronchial dilation on CT. AJR 1992; 159:463–467.
44. Morrish WF, Herman SJ, Weisbrod GL, Chamberlain DW. The Toronto Lung Transplant Group. Bronchiolitis obliterans after lung transplantation: findings at chest radiography and high-resolution CT. Radiology 1991; 179:487–490.
45. Aquino SL, Webb WR, Golden J. Bronchiolitis obliterans associated with rheumatoid arthritis: findings on HRCT and dynamic expiratory CT. J Comput Assist Tomogr 1994; 18:555–558.
46. Miravitlles M, Alvarez-Castells A, Vidal R, Vendrell M, Torrents C, de Gracia J. Scintigraphy, angiography and computed tomography in unilateral hyperlucent lung due to obliterative bronchiolitis. Respiration 1994; 61:324–329.
47. King TE Jr. Respiratory bronchiolitis-associated interstitial lung disease. Clin Chest Med 1993; 14:693–698.
48. Remy-Jardin M, Remy J, Gosselin B, Becette V, Edme JL. Lung parenchymal changes secondary to cigarette smoking: pathologic–CT correlations. Radiology 1993; 186:643–651.
49. Remy-Jardin M, Remy J, Boulenguez C, Sobaszek A, Edma JL, Furon D. Morphologic effects of cigarette smoking on airways and pulmonary parenchyma in healthy adult volunteers: CT evaluation and correlation with pulmonary function tests. Radiology 1993; 186:107–115.
50. Zerhouni EA, Herold CJ, Brown RH, Wetzel RC, Hirshman CA, Robotham JL, Mitzner W. High-resolution computed tomography—physiologic correlation. J Thorac Imaging 1993; 8:265–272.
51. Stern EJ, Webb WR. Dynamic imaging of lung morphology with ultrafast high-resolution computed tomography. J Thorac Imaging 1993; 8:273–281.
52. Brown RH, Herold CJ, Hirschman CA, Zerhouni EA, Mitzner W. In vivo measurements of airway reactivity using HRCT. Am Rev Respir Dis 1991; 144:208–212.
53. Herold CJ, Brown RH, Mitzner W, Links JM, Hirschman CA, Zerhouni EA. Assessment of pulmonary airway reactivity with HRCT. Radiology 1991; 181:369–374.
54. McNamara AE, Müller NL, Okazawa M, et al. Airway narrowing in excised canine lung measured by high-resolution computed tomography. J Appl Physiol 1992; 73:307–316.

55. Brown RH, Herold CJ, Hirschman CA, Zerhouni EA, Mitzner W. Individual airway constrictor response heterogeneity to histamine assessed by high-resolution CT. J Appl Physiol 1993; 74:2615–2620.
56. Stern EJ, Webb WR. Dynamic imaging of lung morphology with ultrafast high-resolution computed tomography. J Thorac Imaging 1993; 84:273–282.
57. Newman KB Lynch DA, Newman LS, Ellegood D, Newell JD Jr. Quantitative computed tomography detects air trapping due to asthma. Chest 1994; 106:105–109.
58. Goldin JG, Aberle DR, Matthias PM, Dauphinee B, McNitt-Gray MF, Johnson TD, Kleerup EB, Tashkin DP. Airway hyperreactivity (AHR) using helical CT following methacholine bronchoprovocation in asthmatics [abstr]. Am J Respir Crit Care Med 1995; 151:A673.

11

Emphysema

CAROLE J. DENNIE
Ottawa Civic Hospital
Ottawa, Ontario, Canada

CRAIG L. COBLENTZ
McMaster University Medical Centre
Hamilton, Ontario, Canada

I. Introduction

Emphysema is a common lung disease; according to postmortem studies, up to 66% of the population is affected (1,2). Unfortunately, the premortem diagnosis of mild to moderate disease is not often made because of the low sensitivity of standard chest radiographs (3–13) and pulmonary function tests (1,14). However, with the advent of conventional computed tomography (CT) and high-resolution CT (HRCT), we can diagnose emphysema and characterize it into specific subtypes at an earlier stage owing to the ability of these techniques to accurately identify changes in pulmonary morphology.

With renewed interest in surgery for emphysema, these radiographic techniques have been used to predict which patients may benefit from surgery to decrease dyspnea secondary to bullous disease and diffuse parenchymal involvement. Although nuclear medicine imaging is useful in the functional assessment of patients with emphysema, this chapter concentrates on the structural evaluators of this disease, such as conventional radiography and CT, as emphysema is defined in terms of structure, rather than symptoms or physiological parameters.

II. Pathology and Pathogenesis

Emphysema is defined pathologically as a pulmonary disease characterized by abnormal permanent enlargement of the airspaces distal to the terminal bronchiole. These changes are accompanied by destruction of the alveolar walls, without significant associated fibrosis (15,16). The most commonly used classification of the various structural subtypes of emphysema, formulated by Thurlbeck (15), characterizes emphysema according to the region of the acinus that is most severely affected: (1) centrilobular, (2) panlobular, (3) paraseptal, and (4) paracicatricial (Fig. 1).

Centrilobular emphysema is the most common type of emphysema and is related to cigarette smoking. It is believed that smoking increases the migration of alveolar macrophages into the distal terminal bronchioles. These macrophages then release chemotactic factors that attract circulating neutrophils and induce them to release proteolytic enzymes, specifically elastases, which result in alveolar wall destruction. Antielastase activity in the blood, such as α_1-antiprotease, is inhibited both by chemicals in cigarette smoke and oxidation by-products released by neutrophils.

The destruction of alveoli in centrilobular emphysema is distal to the respiratory bronchiole, primarily in the upper lung zones. This distribution of disease occurs as a result of less blood flow, with decreased delivery of plasma antiproteases to the upper lung zone, as well as a higher negative pleural pressure compared with the lower lobes (4,17).

Panlobular emphysema results in destruction of alveoli throughout the entire secondary lobule. This disease affects patients with α_1-antitrypsin deficiency, a rare autosomal recessive disease in which there is a deficiency of antiprotease in the plasma. As a consequence, circulating proteolytic enzymes are unopposed and destroy lung. The pulmonary destruction is diffuse, but is more severe in the lower lung zones owing to greater perfusion at the lung bases (18). Panlobular emphysema is also seen in elderly nonsmokers (17). Patients with panacinar emphysema who smoke may also develop centrilobular emphysema.

Paraseptal emphysema leads to destruction of alveoli in the immediate subpleural region, sparing lung elsewhere. This results in subpleural bullae, found most commonly in the anterior and posterior aspects of the upper lobes and the posterior aspects of the lower lobes. Paraseptal emphysema may be related to the development of spontaneous pneumothorax (4,17,19) and the vanishing lung syndrome (20–22). This latter syndrome occurs primarily in young men and is characterized by the presence of giant bullae in the upper lung zones. The underlying abnormality appears to be mainly paraseptal emphysema that coalesces into large bullae affecting one-third or more of a hemithorax.

The final subtype of emphysema, paracicatricial emphysema occurs around

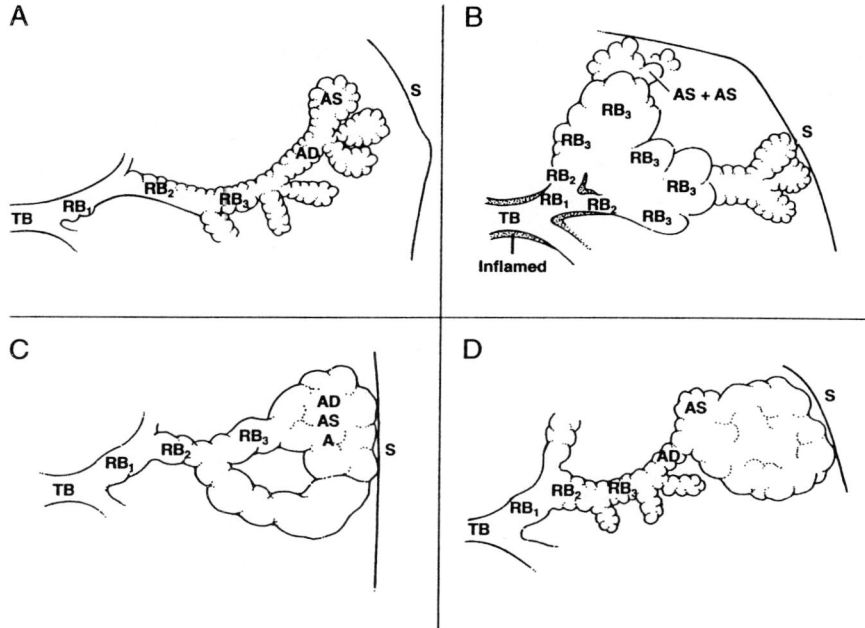

Figure 1 The secondary pulmonary lobule in normal individuals and in emphysema: (A) Normal secondary pulmonary lobule; (B) centrilobular emphysema; (C) panlobular emphysema; (D) paraseptal emphysema. TB, terminal bronchiole; RB, first-, second-, and third-order respiratory bronchioles; AD, alveolar duct; AS, alveolar sac; S, septum.

areas of fibrosis, usually as a result of granulomatous disease, prior pneumonia, or infarction (17). There is no consistent relation of the emphysematous destruction to any portion of the secondary lobule or acinus. It is of no clinical significance and, in fact, does not really meet the criteria of emphysema as set out by the National Heart, Lung, and Blood Institute (16).

The destructive changes secondary to emphysema may also result in the coalescence of airspaces forming air sacs larger than 1 cm in diameter in the distended state, referred to as *bullae*. Reid has further subclassified these bullae into three types (23). Type 1 bullae, which may be found in paraseptal emphysema, are located subpleurally in the lung apices or in the inferior aspect of the middle lobe or lingula. Type 2 bullae are also subpleural, most commonly arising along the anterior aspect of the upper and middle lobes and over the diaphragmatic surface of the lower lobes; however, this subgroup is associated with generalized emphysema. Type 3 bullae resemble type 2 bullae, but develop deep within the

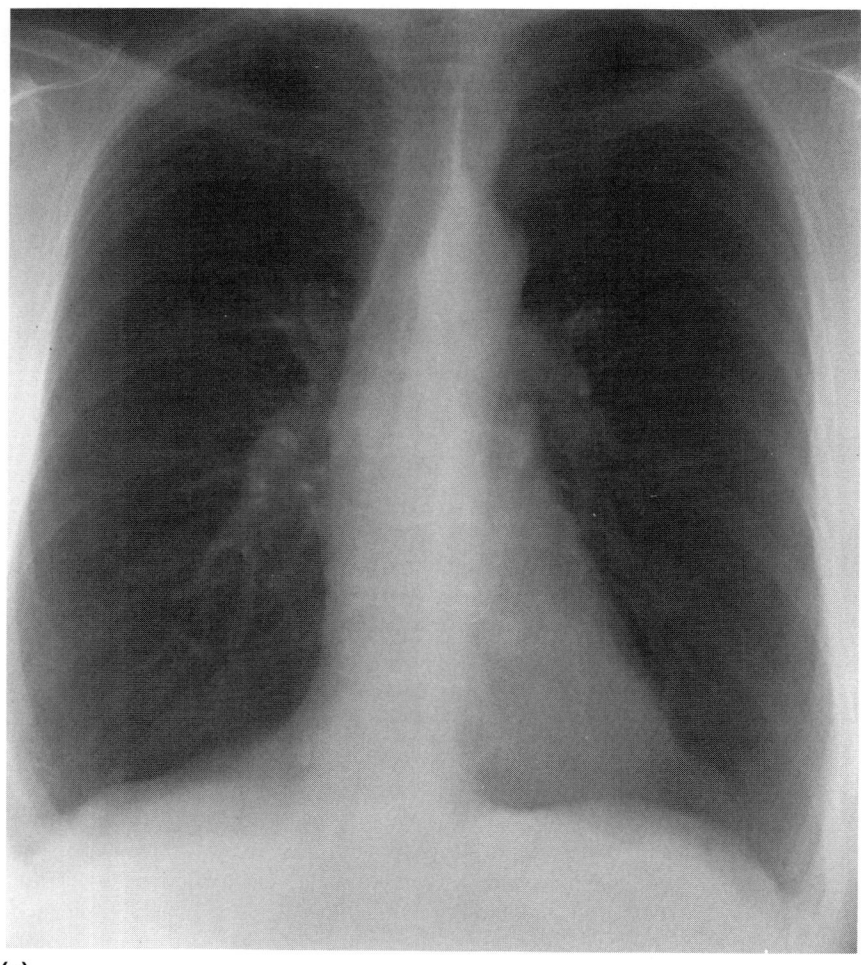

(a)

Figure 2 Radiographic appearance of centrilobular emphysema: (a) PA chest radiograph; note flattened hemidiaphragms and irregular areas of radiolucency; predominantly in the upper lung zones. (b) Lateral chest radiograph. The retrosternal airspace is increased and the diaphragm is flattened. The apex of the dome of the diaphragm is less than 2.6 cm from a line drawn from the costophrenic junction to the sternophrenic junction.

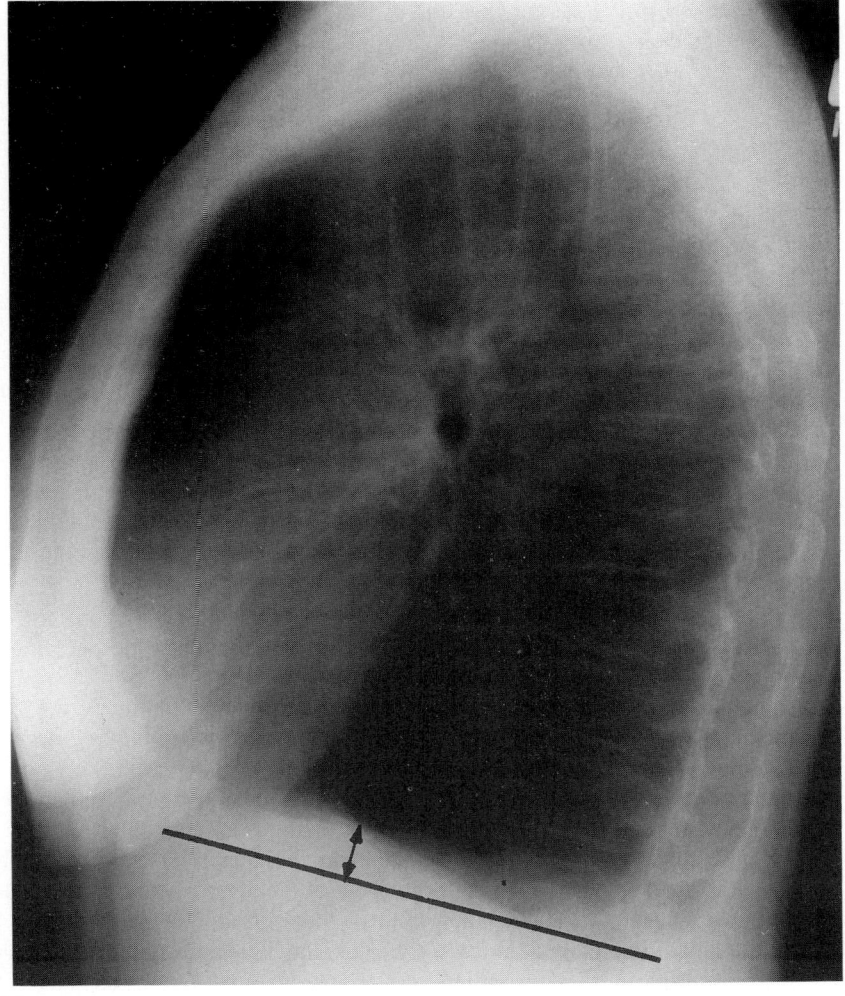

(b)

lung parenchyma and affect upper and lower lobes equally. They are also associated with generalized emphysema. It is important to differentiate between true bullae and blebs on the lung surface. *Blebs* are intrapleural collections of air that do not communicate with the airway and, therefore, do not collapse when the lung is deflated. Because blebs are commonly found in lungs in the absence of emphysema, they should not be considered characteristic of this disorder.

III. Pathological–Radiologic Correlation

To compare the pathological and radiologic grading of emphysema, most investigators have used the whole-lung paper-mounted technique, initially described by Gough and Wentworth (24), to delineate the pathological grade of the emphysematous disease. In this procedure, either whole lungs or a lobe resected at thoracotomy, are distended through a bronchus with formaldehyde. After fixation, the lung is sliced and the amount of emphysema is expressed as a percentage of involved lung. The gross parenchymal changes can also be addressed subjectively and by comparison with standards established by Thurlbeck and co-workers (25) or by using a "point-counting" system (25). The severity of emphysema can be classified as: trace (1–5%), mild (5–25%), moderate (25–50%), severe (>50%). This grading of emphysema can then be correlated with the degree of emphysema determined at chest radiography or CT.

IV. Radiology

A. Plain Radiography

In 1936, Kerley was the first to describe some of the classic radiographic features of emphysema that we still use today (26). In 1953, Simon and Galbraith further elucidated and summarized these conventional radiologic changes (27):

1. Depression or flattening of the diaphragm, with blunting of the costophrenic angles. Note that the level of the diaphragm is not as important for diagnostic purposes as its contour.
2. Irregular radiolucency of the lungs as a result of an inhomogeneous distribution of lung destruction.
3. On the lateral radiograph, the retrosternal airspace, as indicated by the distance between the posterior aspect of the sternum to the most anterior aspect of the ascending aorta, is larger than 2.5 cm.
4. Flattening or even concavity of the diaphragm on the lateral view, resulting in a 90° or larger sternodiaphragmatic angle (28; Fig. 2).

Unfortunately, as shown repeatedly, mild to moderate emphysema is very difficult to perceive on chest radiographs. The reason for this is as follows: chest radiographs are images of millions of superimposed alveoli (tiny air-filled holes) and bronchovascular structures. Emphysema destroys these alveoli. Because it is much more difficult for the human eye to appreciate when something is missing, compared with when something has been added to a complex image, the detection of early loss of alveoli with enlargement of these air-filled holes in emphysema is almost impossible.

The overall sensitivity of the chest radiograph in detecting emphysema has been variously quoted as 25–80%, (3,5,8,9,12,25). This wide range of sensitivities may partly relate to variations in the radiologic criteria used and to the use of pulmonary function testing (PFT) as a basis for making the clinical diagnosis in some studies. The use of PFTs for the detection of early emphysema is inherently flawed, as it has been estimated that 30% of the lung must be destroyed before symptoms of pulmonary function abnormalities become evident (29).

Although not sensitive, the specificity of plain chest radiography is quite high, resulting in few false-positive diagnoses (0–5%; 30). As disease severity increases, so does the accuracy of the chest radiograph; over 90% of patients with severe disease can be correctly diagnosed by a plain chest radiograph. The most specific criteria in predicting the presence of emphysema on chest radiographs are based mainly on the physiological changes that occur as result of airflow obstruction. The most useful include (30):

1. *Hyperinflation*, as depicted by flattening of the diaphragm on the lateral view (defined as a vertical distance of less than 2.6 cm from a line drawn from the costophrenic junction to the sternophrenic junction to the top of the diaphragmatic arc; 31; see Fig. 2).
2. The presence of *bullae*.
3. *Abnormal vascular branching* or *vascular deficiency*.

There are other signs of hyperinflation, such as an increase in lung length and width, vertical position of the heart, increased intercostal distance, increased anteroposterior diameter of the thorax, or an increased depth of the retrosternal airspace, but these do not improve the ability to recognize emphysema on plain chest radiographs (10,17).

Several different authors have devised complex equations, using regression analyses, to estimate changes in total lung capacity as compared with age- and weight-matched controls. Although these equations are valid, they have not been widely used because of their complexity. In addition, as their use for the prediction of total lung capacity requires prior knowledge of the lung disease in question, these equations are not useful for diagnostic purposes (32,33).

To overcome the problem of time taken to manually calculate lung volume from plain chest radiographs, we developed an automatic technique. The patient's chest images are obtained with a computed radiography system that makes use of a photostimulable phosphor plate, rather than film (Fuji AC1, Fuji Photo Film Co., Ltd, Tokyo Japan). The raw digital information is then read to a SUN SPARCstation (SUN Microsystems, California). With a mouse, the radiologist identifies five anatomical landmarks on the posteroanterior (PA) and lateral views (Fig. 3). These are used as starting points for an algorithm that searches for lung, heart, and diaphragm boundaries. From these the computer automatically calculates lung volumes using the multiple ellipsoid method of Barnhard et al. (34). Manually, the method takes 30 min, but less than 1 min with the computer. We found good

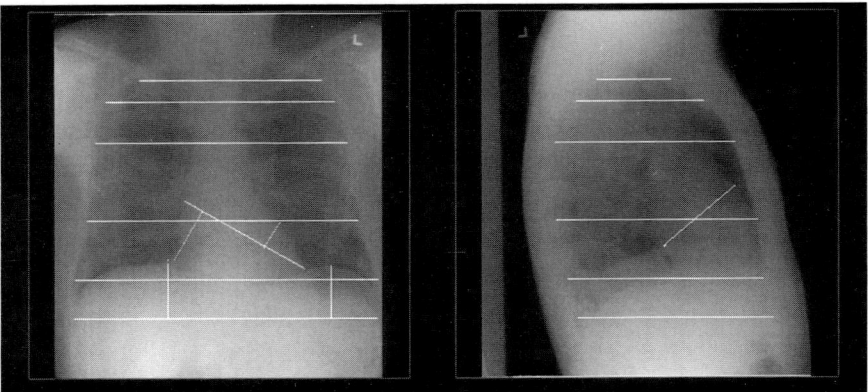

Figure 3 Automatic calculation of lung volume from computed chest radiographs. After the radiologist identifies five anatomical landmarks with a mouse pointing device on a computer workstation, the computer automatically creates multiple ellipsoids from which a variety of intrathoracic volumes are calculated. Patient height equals 175 cm; weight, 75 kg; total thoracic volume, 9339 ml; diaphragm volume, 1692 ml; heart volume, 867 ml; total lung volume, 6775 ml; total lung capacity, 5847 ml.

correlation between manual lung volumes and automatic lung volumes ($r = 0.9807$; mean relative error = 4.1%).

Not just lung volume can be estimated from a plain chest radiograph. Several authors have investigated whether an enlarged descending pulmonary artery diameter on plain chest radiographs is a useful indicator of pulmonary hypertension. The maximum transverse diameter in full inspiration for the interlobar artery, measured from its lateral aspect to the outer wall of the bronchus intermedius, is 16 mm in men and 15 mm in women (35). As Bush et al. indicate (36), the reported accuracy of whether enlargement indicates pulmonary hypertension is very variable. When they examined this, they were able to distinguish only 12 of 23 pulmonary hypertensive subjects undergoing cardiac catheterization when measuring the descending pulmonary artery diameter, even when taking radiographic magnification into account. To improve the detection of increases in pulmonary artery pressure, they scaled the pulmonary artery diameters for size of the subjects. They arbitrarily squared the diameter to exaggerate differences between patients and controls and divided this product by the lung volume, in an attempt to correct for body size. The new index distinguished 19 of 23 patients with pulmonary hypertension, and 1 false-positive diagnosis. It is unclear in emphysema patients whether a lung volume calculated from the chest radiograph will be as useful as the predicted lung volume. Further work is needed.

B. Computed Tomography

The CT findings of emphysema were first described in 1982 (37). Since then, several authors have demonstrated CT's superiority in the diagnosis of emphysema, as compared with conventional plain films. The advantage CT has over plain chest radiographs is its superior contrast resolution and ability to image in the axial plane, eliminating problems related to the superimposition of overlying structures. By using primarily densitometric measurements of pulmonary parenchyma, CT provides an accurate quantitative assessment of the severity of emphysema, even in very early stages of the disease, when the chest radiograph may be grossly normal (38). The reported correlations for CT scores with pathological grading are 0.59–0.91 (39–46). With technological improvements, scanning time and slice thickness have decreased, thereby improving the accuracy of CT. For example, with HRCT, very fine cuts are obtained through the lungs, and the images are reconstructed using a high-frequency algorithm, thereby further increasing resolution and enabling detection of emphysema at an earlier stage (46). Recent CT studies quote the overall sensitivity at about 90% and its accuracy at 80% (30).

Measurement of lung density in Hounsfield units (HU) allows identification of pulmonary emphysema. Normal lung tissue density measures between -400 and -900 HU on CT. In emphysema, focal areas of abnormally low density, measuring less than -900 HU, are seen. These areas of low density have no surrounding wall. The percentage of lung occupied by these low-density areas is proportional to the severity of emphysema.

Two different methods of quantifying the amount of emphysema can be used: visual inspection and density mask. The visual inspection method is a subjective technique in which the radiologist assesses each CT image individually and then estimates the percentage of the lungs affected by emphysema. The density mask method, a more objective technique introduced by Müller in 1988 (44), involves the use of a computer program, available on many CT scanners, designed to highlight areas of lung with densities lower than -900 HU. The computer then calculates the percentage of lung involvement for each CT slice, from which the total amount of emphysema can be calculated.

Although this correlates well with the pathological grade of emphysema, there are three drawbacks to CT scoring: (1) The scanner must be well-calibrated. (2) Unfortunately, although CT is very sensitive and specific in the diagnosis of emphysema, it is still unable to detect the very earliest changes when the low-density areas measure less than 5 mm in diameter (45); therefore, it consistently underestimates the extent and severity of disease. Occasionally, there are also false-positive scans (47,48). (3) The method is very time-consuming; each CT slice has to be analyzed individually, using a track ball to outline lung. As a result, the density mask technique can take up to 2 h per patient and, therefore, has been used only as an investigational tool. To decrease the time required to analyze a patient's entire lung, we developed two strategies.

In the first we created and validated a computer program that automatically determines lung volume and percentage of emphysema (%Emph) from CT images (49–52), using the same principles of pixel analysis used by the GE 9800 Density Mask Program (GE Medical Systems, Milwaukee, WI). Data from routine lung scans performed on a GE 9800 scanner are transferred digitally to a SUN SPARCstation for analysis. As distinct tissue types can be characterized with CT scans by their Hounsfield attenuation numbers, we selected a threshold of -400 HU to distinguish between lung tissue and the adjacent tissue of the heart, diaphragm, and ribs (53). We set the threshold between normal and emphysematous tissue at -900 HU, based on previous studies and results of a pilot study comparing pathology with CT emphysema score results in three pneumonectomy specimens scanned in vivo (54,55).

The boundaries of the lungs are extracted using a subrange filter, with a threshold of -400 HU. This creates a unit width-connected edge around each lung. These highlighted edges can be altered manually if required.

The center of each lung is found by counting all pixels within the CT range of normal lungs (-400 to -900 HU). The lungs are defined by expanding regions from these center points until the highlighted edges are reached. These two regions represent the total lung area of a given CT slice. The total lung volume is found by using the number of lung pixels $\times$ pixel-size^2 $\times$ slice-thickness. Within the extracted lung regions, emphysematous tissue area is calculated by counting all pixels less than -900 HU. The emphysema score is reported as the percentage of emphysema, calculated by dividing the total emphysema volume by the total lung volume multiplied by 100. The method is fully automated (Fig. 4). This program allows quick, accurate, and reproducible quantification of emphysema. The whole process can be accomplished in 1–2 min per patient versus 1–2 hr with the manual density mask method.

In the second strategy, we simply analyzed fewer slices. To validate this approach, we analyzed lung CT scans from 89 patients (56). The scan data were transferred digitally to our SUN SPARCstation for determination of %Emph for each slice. By weighted averaging all of a patient's slices together, we derived a total %Emph score. This was compared with the %Emph score derived from one, three, four, or five evenly spaced slices through the lungs. The mean difference between the %Emph and the one, three, four, and five slice model was 0.06% (SD 2.80), 0.01% (SD 1.11), 0.02% (SD 1.13), and 0.01% (SD 1.05), respectively. From this we concluded estimates of %Emph can be accurately calculated from a single midlung slice. However, the correlation is improved by using a three-slice model. Accuracy is not improved by increasing the number of slices. By using only three scans, one obtains a reasonably accurate quantification of emphysema,

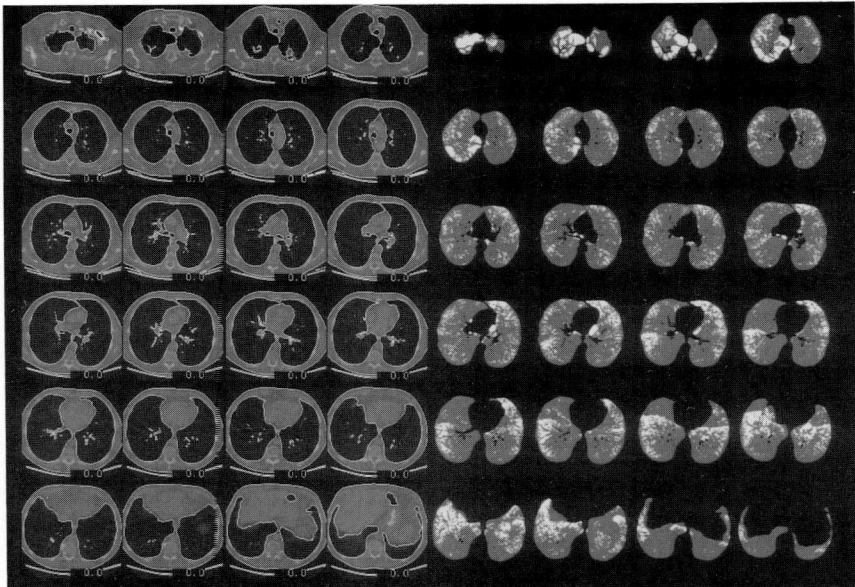

Figure 4 Automatic calculation of lung volume and percentage emphysema from computed tomography: The left side of the figure shows the patient's complete lung scan from which the lungs are automatically extracted, shown on the right side of the figure, by a computer workstation. Pixels with a value less than −900 HU, indicating emphysema, are identified (highlighted in white on the extracted lung images) and expressed as a percentage of the total lung volume. Lung volume; 4040 ml (20.3% emphysema).

with a minimum radiation dose to the patient and minimum amount of time required for analysis.

In addition to quantifying the amount of emphysema, CT can be used to characterize its type into its specific subgroups. The characteristic CT features of centrilobular emphysema are unmarginated focal areas of low attenuation, up to 1 cm in diameter, which first develop in the center of the secondary pulmonary lobule, on a homogeneous background of lung parenchyma (40). These changes have a propensity for the upper lung zones (Fig. 5). In panlobular emphysema, there are large and extensive areas of low density, characteristically in a lower lobe distribution (54). In contrast with centrilobular emphysema, the periphery of the secondary pulmonary lobule is not preserved, and pulmonary vascularity is decreased. As a result, panlobular emphysema is more difficult to detect on CT

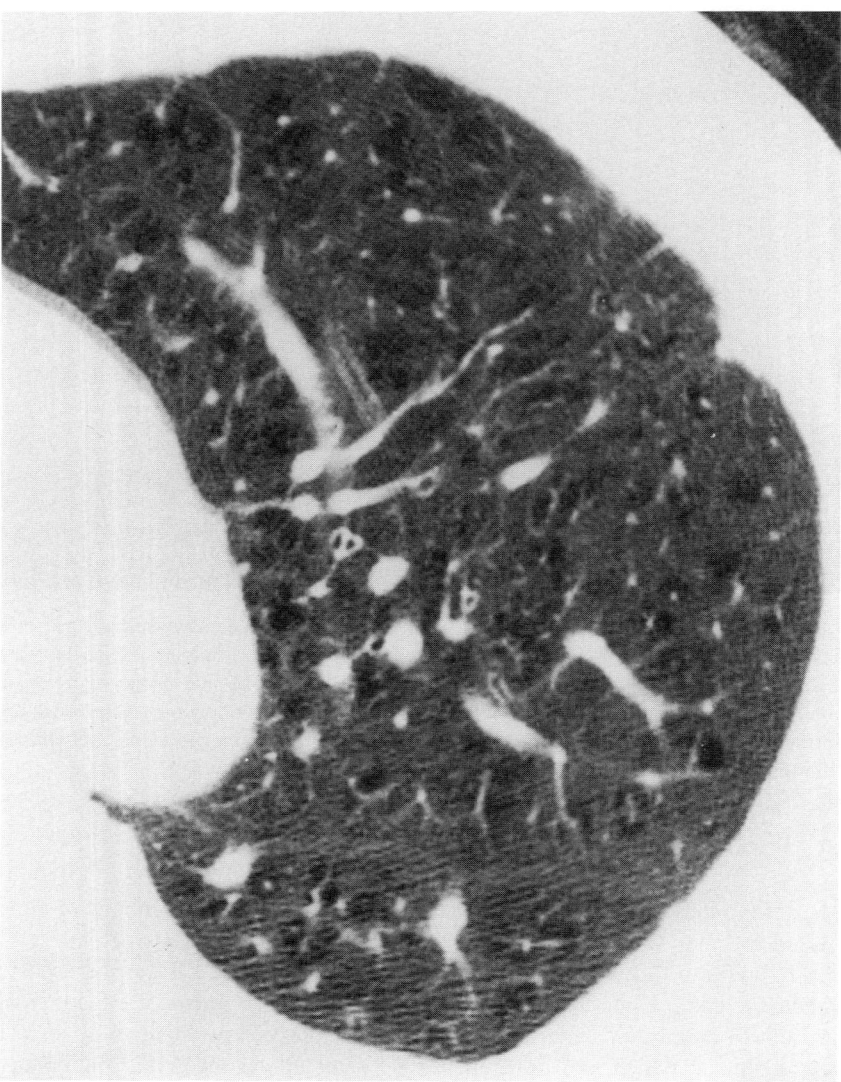

Figure 5 The HRCT appearance of centrilobular emphysema: 1.5-mm cut through the left upper lung zone demonstrates unmarginated foci of low density, measuring less than 1 cm in diameter in the center of secondary pulmonary lobules (arrow).

than other types, as there is no significant density difference between normal and abnormal lung (Fig. 6).

Paraseptal emphysema can be identified by the appearance of multiple subpleural airspaces, ranging from a few millimeters to 1 cm in diameter; Fig. 7), whereas paracicatricial emphysema appears as multiple, small airspaces surrounding a central scar (Fig. 8).

In dyspneic patients with abnormal diffusing capacity or evidence of decreased airflow (decreased FEV_1, FEF_{25-75}; 28,51,52), CT may identify emphysema as a cause of dyspnea, even when the chest radiograph is normal. Klein et al. (38) demonstrated this in a review of 47 cases with centrilobular emphysema in which 16 had normal chest radiographs. In addition, they found the CT changes correlated with impaired gas transfer (as measured by single-breath carbon monoxide-diffusing capacity) whereas the FEV_1 was normal in 10 of these patients. Unfortunately, despite CT's sensitivity and specificity in the diagnosis of emphysema, as discussed earlier, it is still unable to detect the earliest changes when the low-density areas measure less than 5 mm in diameter (45).

C. Preoperative Imaging

Some patients with moderate emphysema and large bullae may experience dyspnea secondary to compression of adjacent normal lung parenchyma. These patients' dyspnea may dramatically improve with resection of these large bullae. Predictors for which patients will improve following bullectomy include the presence of large, isolated bullae occupying more than one-third of the hemithorax, rapid progression of dyspnea, relatively normal remaining lung, and a restrictive defect on pulmonary function testing related to the compression of adjacent lung.

Linear tomography and angiography were used in the past to demonstrate compression of vascular structures by these large bullae. However, CT is now the modality of choice for preoperative imaging, as not only does it demonstrate the bullae, it also identifies whether emphysema is present.

Some patients with severe emphysema may not have large bullae to explain their dyspnea. These patients may benefit from lung volume reduction surgery, a procedure first introduced by Kress et al. in 1968 (57), that currently is undergoing a resurgence. In general this procedure is reserved for patients with debilitating diffuse emphysema whose only option would be single- or double-lung transplantation. Briefly, after patients undergo extensive medical rehabilitation, bilateral partial pulmonary resections are performed through a median sternotomy, in an effort to decrease the total lung capacity. The mechanism by which the surgery improves the patient's symptoms is not entirely clear, but probably partly relates to the restoration of optimal chest wall mechanics required for lung inflation. Patients with severe emphysema lose the mechanical advantage of the diaphragm,

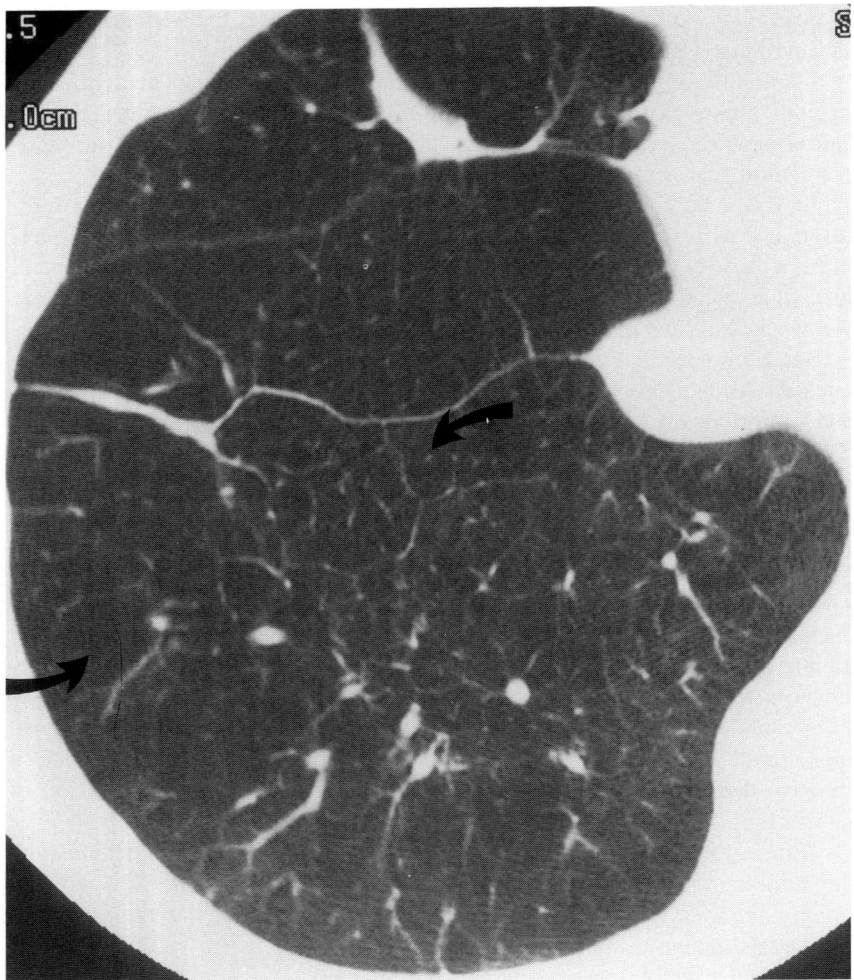

Figure 6 Panlobular emphysema: HRCT image of the right lower lung zone demonstrates large foci of hypodensity that involves entire secondary pulmonary lobules, as well as decreased vascularity (arrows).

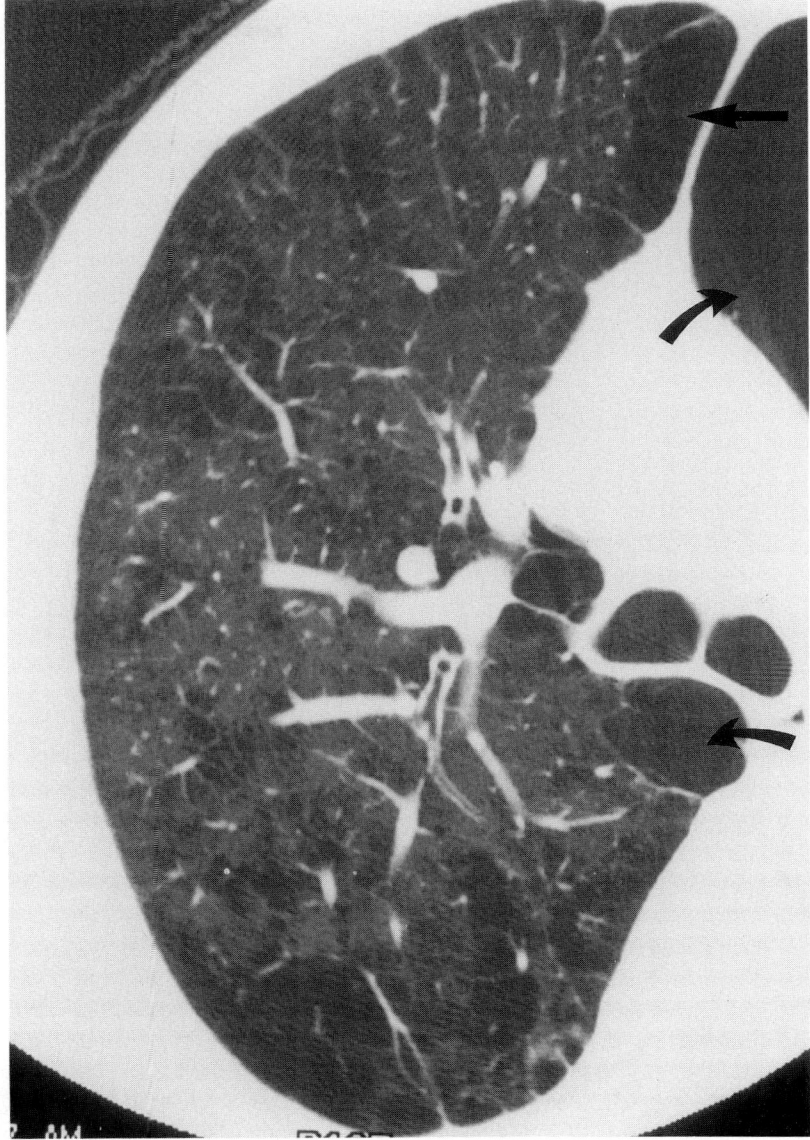

Figure 7 Paraseptal emphysema: HRCT image of the right upper lung zone shows subpleural areas of low density, measuring less than 1 cm in diameter (arrow). Some of these have coalesced to form subpleural bullae (curved arrows). There is mild centrilobular emphysema elsewhere in the lung.

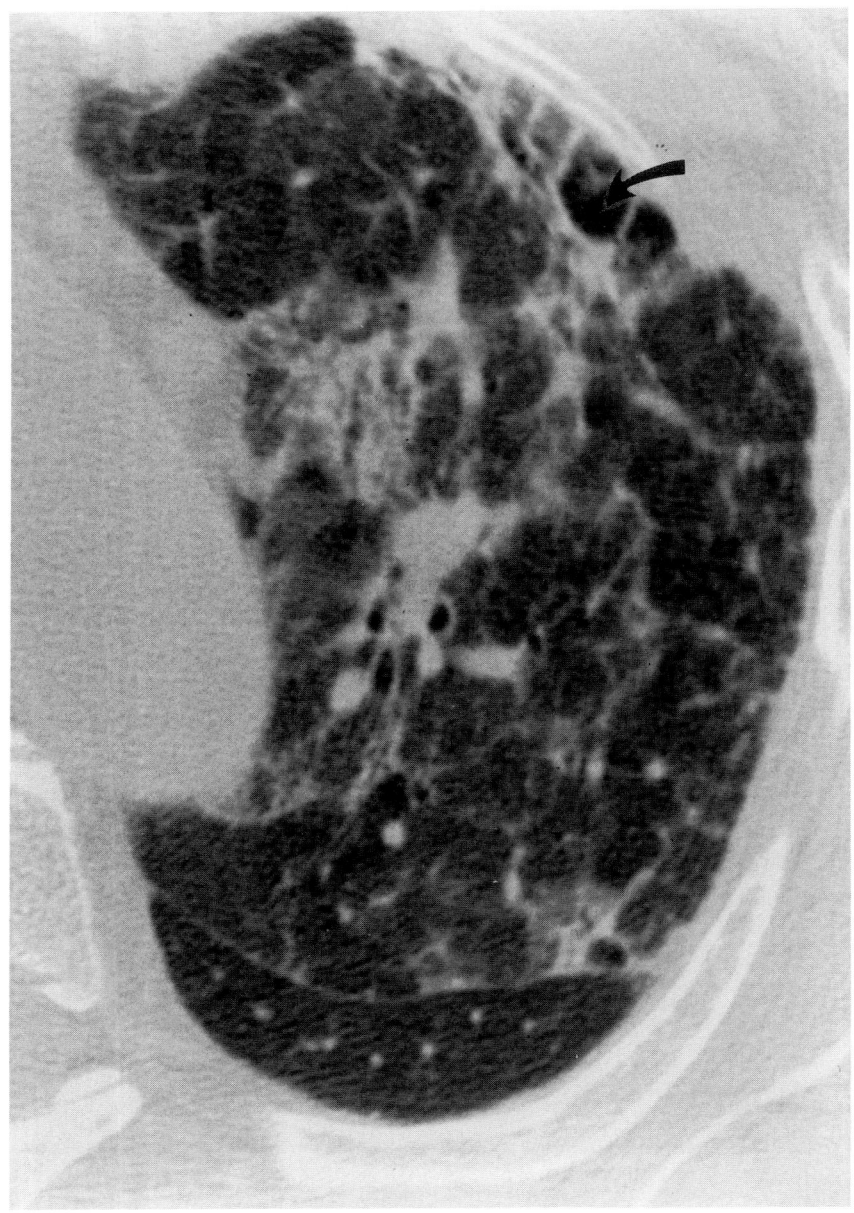

Figure 8 Paracicatricial emphysema: HRCT image of the left upper lung zone in a patient with stage 4 sarcoid. There are focal areas of low density adjacent to areas of scarring (arrow).

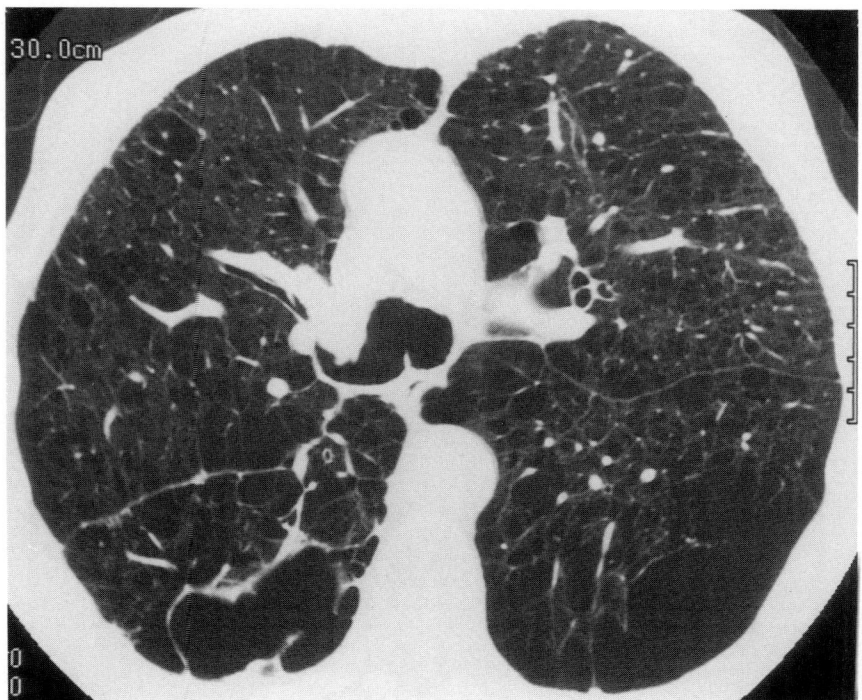

Figure 9 Heterogeneous emphysema: HRCT image at the level of the carina demonstrates severe diffuse emphysema, with bullae formation at the periphery of the posterior aspects of the lungs.

owing to thoracic compensatory hyperinflation. Advocates of the procedure believe that, by surgically reducing lung volumes, the diaphragm and chest wall assume a more normal configuration, improving respiratory mechanics. Unlike those who undergo a conventional bullectomy, patients are left with significant residual disease.

Preoperatively, the position of the diaphragm is almost identical on inspiratory and expiratory chest radiographs. Postoperatively, it assumes a more normal position and curve. The improvement in chest wall and diaphragmatic motion in patients with severe emphysema undergoing lung reduction surgery have been exquisitely demonstrated by both dynamic thoracic magnetic resonance imaging (MRI; 58) and CT (58,59).

The role of CT in the preoperative management of patients undergoing lung reduction surgery require clarification. Some surgeons use it to differentiate homogeneous versus heterogeneous emphysema. Surgical candidates with hetero-

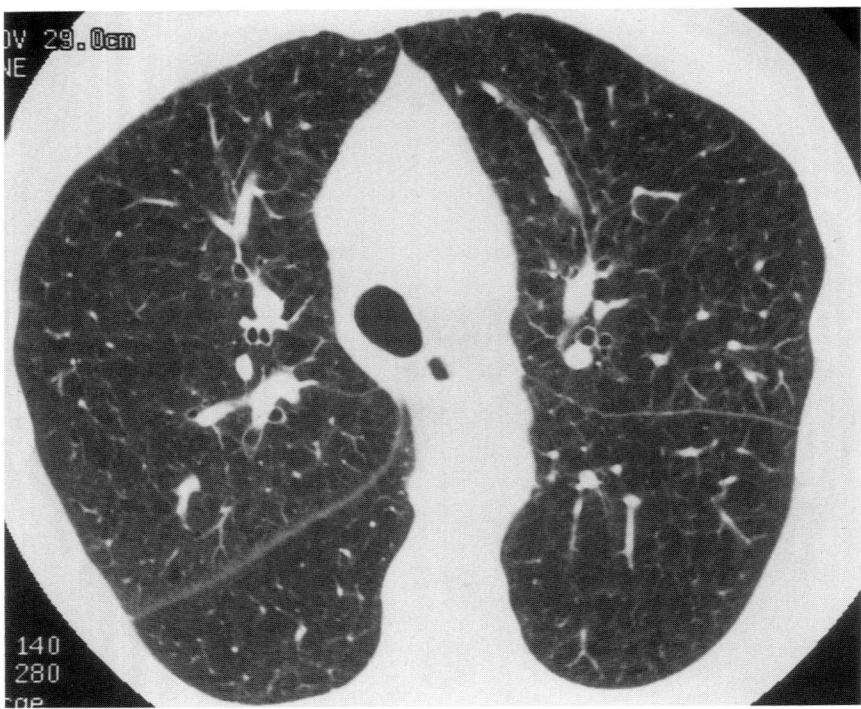

Figure 10 Homogeneous emphysema: HRCT image at the level of the aortic arch demonstrates severe emphysema, without bullae.

geneous disease have emphysema in the entire lung, but this is more severe at the lung's periphery, with formation of subpleural bullae (Fig. 9). Patients with widespread, but homogeneous, emphysema generally have no bullae (Fig. 10).

D. Imaging Sequence in the Patient with Suspected Emphysema

The chest radiograph is the initial imaging test of choice in the patient with suspected emphysema. If the radiograph is diagnostic of emphysema, no further imaging is usually necessary. If the type or severity of emphysema must be determined, CT may be performed. Specific roles for CT include: (1) monitoring the efficacy of treatment with α_1-protease inhibitor (Prolastin) for α_1-antitrypsin deficiency (60); (2) identifying emphysema in dyspneic patients in whom the chest radiograph is normal and the pulmonary function tests are either normal or there is an abnormal diffusing capacity; (3) demonstrating compression of adjacent lung parenchyma and rule out emphysema in patients whose chest radiograph demonstrates what is thought to be a single, large bulla, and pulmonary function tests show a restrictive defect; (4) identifying candidates for lung volume reduction surgery and differentiating homogeneous versus heterogeneous disease; (5) assessment of diaphragmatic and chest wall motion pre- and post-lung volume reduction surgery or bullectomy.

V. Conclusion

The radiologic diagnosis of emphysema is based on perceived changes in anatomical structure that results from parenchymal destruction. Importantly, many patients, clinically, have chronic obstructive pulmonary disease (COPD), as demonstrated by some pattern of airflow obstruction on pulmonary function testing, in the absence of the aforementioned criteria for the radiologic diagnosis of emphysema. We believe it is incorrect to equate the morphological term emphysema with the clinical term COPD. Because one can have emphysema with or without clinical COPD, the clinical term COPD should not be used in image interpretation. Imaging yields useful information about morphological emphysematous destruction, but not necessarily about physiological COPD.

References

1. Thurlbeck WM. Overview of the pathology of pulmonary emphysema in the human. Clin Chest Med 1983; 4:337–350.
2. Sobonya RE, Burrows B. The epidemiology of emphysema. Clin Chest Med 1983; 4:351–358.
3. Nicklaus TM, Stowell DW, Christiansen WR, Renzetti AD. The accuracy of the roentgenologic diagnosis of chronic pulmonary emphysema. Am Rev Respir Dis 1966; 93:889–899.
4. Fraser RG, Paré JAP, Paré PD, Fraser RS, Généreux GP. Diseases of the airways. In: Diagnoses of diseases of the chest. 3d ed. Philadelphia: WB Saunders, 1990:1969–2275.
5. Katsura S, Martin CJ. The roentgenologic diagnosis of anatomic emphysema. Am Rev Respir Dis 1967; 96:700.
6. Simon G. Principles of chest x-ray diagnosis. 3d ed. London: Butterworths, 1971:153.
7. Pugatch RD. The radiology of emphysema. Clin Chest Med 1983; 4:433–442.
8. Thurlbeck WM, Simon G. Radiographic appearance of the chest in emphysema. AJR 1978; 130:429–440.
9. Reid L, Millard FJC. Correlation between radiological diagnosis and structural changes in emphysema. Clin Radiol 1964; 15:306–311.
10. Simon G. Radiology and emphysema. Clin Radiol 1964; 15:293–306.
11. Laws JW, Heard BE. Emphysema and the chest film: a retrospective radiological and pathological study. Br J Radiol 1962; 35:750–761.

12. Sutinen S, Christoforidis AJ, Klugh GA, Pratt PC. Roentgenologic criteria for the recognition of nonsymptomatic pulmonary emphysema. Am Rev Respir Dis 1965; 91:69–76.
13. Heitzman ER, Markarian B, Solomon J. Chronic obstructive pulmonary disease. Radiol Clin North Am 1973; 11:49–75.
14. Zamel N, Hogg J, Gelb A. Mechanisms of maximal expiratory limitation in clinically unsuspected emphysema and obstruction of the peripheral airways. Am Rev Respir Dis 1976; 113:337–345.
15. Thurlbeck WM. Chronic airflow obstruction in lung disease. Philadelphia: WB Saunders, 1976.
16. National Heart, Lung, and Blood Institute, Division of Lung Diseases workshop report. The definition of emphysema. Am Rev Respir Dis 1985; 132:182–185.
17. Pratt PC. Emphysema and chronic airways disease. In: Dail DH, Hamar SP, eds. Pulmonary pathology. New York: Springer-Verlag, 1988; 651–669.
18. Cohen AB, ed. Symposium on proteases and antiproteases in the lung. Am Rev Respir Dis 1983; 127(suppl 2):S1–S58.
19. Lesur O, Delorme N, Fromaget JM, Bernadac P, Polu JM. Computed tomography in the etiologic assessment of idiopathic spontaneous pneumothorax. Chest 1990; 98:341–347.
20. Roberts L, Putman CE, Chen JT, Goodman LR, Ravin CE. Vanishing lung syndrome: upper lobe bullous pneumopathy. Rev Interamericana Radiol 1987; 12:249–255.
21. Burke RM. Vanishing lungs: a case report of bullous emphysema. Radiology 1937; 28:367–371.
22. Stern EJ, Webb WR, Weinaker A, Müller NL. Idiopathic giant bullous emphysema (vanishing lung syndrome): imaging findings in nine patients. AJR 1994; 162:279–282.
23. Reid L. The pathology of emphysema. London: Lloyd-Duke, 1967.
24. Gough J, Wentworth JE. The use of thin sections of entire organs in morbid anatomic studies. J R Microsc Soc 1949; 69:231–235.
25. Thurlbeck WM, Dunnill MS, Hartung W, et al. A comparison of three methods of measuring emphysema. Hum Pathol 1970; 1:215–226.
26. Kerley P. Discussion on emphysema. Proc R Soc Med 1936; 29:1307.
27. Simon G, Galbraith HJB. Radiology of chronic bronchitis. Lancet 1953; 2:850.
28. Pratt PC. Role of conventional chest radiography in the diagnosis and exclusion of emphysema. Am J Med 1987; 82:998–1006.
29. Predd PC, Kilburn KH. A modern concept of the emphysemas based on correlations of structure and function. Hum Pathol 1970; 1:443–463.
30. Sanders C. The radiographic diagnosis of emphysema. Radiol Clin North Am 1991; 29:1019–1029.
31. Reigh SB, Weinshelbaum A, Yee J. Correlation of radiographic measurements and pulmonary function tests in chronic obstructive pulmonary disease. AJR 1985; 144:695–699.
32. Thompson KR, Eyssen GE, Fraser RG. Discrimination of normal and overinflated lungs and prediction of total lung capacity based on chest film measurements. Radiology 1976; 119:721–723.

33. Teklu B, Gray WM, Mills RJ, Moran F. A critical appraisal of a rapid radiographic method of determining total lung capacity. Scott Med J 1986; 31:99–102.
34. Barnhard HJ, Pierce JA, Joyce JW, Bates JM. Roentgenographic determination of total lung capacity. A new method evaluated in health, emphysema, and congestive heart failure. Am J Med 1960; 28:51–60.
35. Chang CH. The normal roentgenographic measurement of the right descending pulmonary artery in 1085 cases. AJR 1962; 87:929–935.
36. Bush A, Gray H, Denison DM. Diagnosis of pulmonary hypertension from radiographic estimates of pulmonary arterial size. Thorax 1988; 43:127–131.
37. Codington R, Mera SL, Goddard PR, et al. Pathological evaluation of computed tomography images of lungs. J Clin Pathol 1982; 35:436–440.
38. Klein JS, Gamsu G, Webb WR, et al. HRCT diagnosis of emphysema in symptomatic patients with normal chest radiographs and isolated low diffusing capacity. Radiology 1992; 182:817–821.
39. Hayhurst MD, Flenley DC, McLean A, et al. Diagnosis of emphysema by computed tomography. Lancet 1984; 2:320–322.
40. Foster WL, Pratt PC, Roggli V, et al. Centrilobular emphysema: CT–pathologic correlation. Radiology 1986; 159:27–32.
41. Bergin C, Müller N, Nichols DM, et al. The diagnosis of emphysema: a computed tomographic–pathologic correlation. Am Rev Respir Dis 1986; 133:541–546.
42. Gould GA, Macnee W, McLean A, et al. CT measurements of lung density in life can quantitate distal airspace enlargement. Am Rev Respir Dis 1988; 137:380–392.
43. Hruban RH, Meziane MA, Zerhouni EA, et al. High-resolution computed tomography of inflation fixed lungs: pathologic–radiologic correlation of centrilobular emphysema. Am Rev Respir Dis 1987; 136:935–940.
44. Müller NL, Staples CA, Miller RR, et al. "Density mask"; an objective method to quantitate emphysema using computed tomography. Chest 1988; 94:782–787.
45. Miller FF, Müller NL, Vedal S, et al. Limitations of computed tomography in the assessment of emphysema. Am Rev Respir Dis 1989; 139:980–983.
46. Kuwano K, Masuba K, Ikeda T, et al. The diagnosis of mild emphysema: correlation of CT and pathological scores. Am Rev Respir Dis 1990; 141:169–178.
47. Adams H, Bernard MS, McConnochie K. An appraisal of CT pulmonary density mapping in normal subjects. Clin Radiol 1991; 43:238–242.
48. Knudson RJ, Standen JR, Kaltenborn WT, et al. Expiratory computed tomography for assessment of suspected pulmonary emphysema. Chest 1991; 99:1357–1366.
49. Archer DC, Coblentz CL, deKemp RA, et al. Automated in vivo quantification of emphysema. Radiology 1993; 188:835–838.
50. Spouge D, Mayo JR, Wellington C, Müller NL. Panacinar emphysema: CT and pathologic findings. J Comput Assist Tomogr 1993; 17:710–713.
51. Sakai F, Gamsu G, Im JG, et al. Pulmonary function abnormalities in patients with CT-determined emphysema. J Comput Assist Tomogr 1987; 11:963–967.
52. Sanders C, Nath PH, Bailey WC. Detection of emphysema with computed tomography: correlation with pulmonary function tests and chest radiography. Invest Radiol 1988; 23:262–266.

53. Hedlund LW, Anderson RF, Goulding PL, et al. Two methods for isolating the lung area of a CT scan for density information. Radiology 1982; 144:353–357.
54. Hayhurst MD, Flenley DC, McLean A. Diagnosis of pulmonary emphysema by computerised tomography. Lancet 1984; 2:320–322.
55. Müller NL, Staples CA, Miller RR, Abboud RT. "Density mask": an objective method to quantitate emphysema using computed tomography. Chest 1988; 94:782–787.
56. Archer DC, Coblentz CL, Norman G, Nahmias C. CT quantification of emphysema: how many sections is enough? [abstr]. Radiology 1992; 185(P):242.
57. Kress MB, Goco RV, Brantigan OC. The role of surgery in the management of generalized pulmonary emphysema without blebs and bullae. Dis Chest 1968; 53:427–435.
58. Slone RM, Gierada DS, Cooper JD, et al. Imaging evaluation of patients who undergo reduction pneumoplasty for treatment of severe debilitating emphysema [abstr]. Radiology 1994; 193(P):182–183.
59. Bae KT, Slone RM, Gierada DS. CT assessment of emphysema in candidates for volume-reduction surgery [abstr]. Radiology 1994; 193(P):233.
60. Hansell DM. HRCT in emphysema associated with alpha$_1$-antitrypsin deficiency. Clin Radiol 1992; 45:260–266.

12

Radiologic Assessment After Lung Transplantation

STEPHEN J. HERMAN

University of Toronto
and The Toronto Hospital
Toronto, Ontario, Canada

I. Introduction

Between 1963 and 1980, the 38 attempts at lung transplantation all failed, usually because of infectious complications associated with airway ischemia and dehiscence. In 1983, the first successful transplant was performed at the Toronto General Hospital, using improved methods of immunosuppression and omentopexy. Since that time, lung transplantation has been further developed to the point that it is now a well-accepted procedure for many patients with end-stage pulmonary parenchymal or pulmonary vascular disease that otherwise would prove fatal. It is currently being performed at many centers worldwide. Recently, of 131 patients undergoing single or bilateral transplant, with at least 5 months follow-up, there was a 92% hospital survival; there were 13 late deaths with 107 (81%) remaining alive, with a median follow-up period of 19 months (1).

Generally speaking, single-lung transplantation is performed for end-stage fibrotic lung diseases, primary pulmonary hypertension, Eisenmenger's syndrome, and in some instances, for obstructive disease. Double-lung transplantation is used in patients with septic conditions, such as cystic fibrosis, because a single transplanted lung would be vulnerable to spread of infection from the remaining lung, and in some centers, for obstructive diseases. Heart–lung transplantation is indicated in patients with irreversible disease of the heart and both lungs.

Patients undergoing single- and double-lung transplantation are subject to various unique problems, which include the reimplantation response, rejection phenomena, consequences of airway ischemia (including dehiscence and stricture formation), and cyclosporine-associated lymphoproliferative disorders. In addition, one must be aware of the presence of the intrathoracic omentum, infectious complications, and the consequences of transbronchial biopsies.

II. Reimplantation Response

Autotransplantation of the lung is itself associated with certain problems that form the *reimplantation response*. This response has been summarized as "the morphologic, roentgenographic and functional changes that occur in a lung transplant in the early postoperative period as a result of surgical trauma, ischemia, denervation, lymphatic interruption and other injurious processes (exclusive of rejection) that are unavoidable aspects of the transplant operation" (2). In practice, the reimplantation response is a diagnosis of exclusion and, radiographically, includes all changes beginning immediately after surgery that are not due to left ventricular failure, rejection, fluid overload, infection, or atelectasis.

In a recent review of the reimplantation response in 51 patients (24 single-lung, 27 double-lung transplants), the most common finding was airspace disease in the mid- and lower lungs (3; Fig. 1). Reticular interstitial disease in the same distribution was also commonly seen. The process was seen in all patients, almost always beginning on day 1 posttransplantation and always present by day 3. It frequently progressed over the first few days, but peaked by day 4 in all patients, so that any new process beginning after this time must be considered some other disease. The patients' films were reviewed for their first 21 days posttransplantation and, in most instances, the response persisted as mild reticular interstitial disease over this entire time period. In almost half of the double-lung recipients, the disease was asymmetric. In a previous paper in which patients were followed indefinitely, the reimplantation response was noted to gradually change from airspace to reticular interstitial disease over the first few weeks and then gradually clear (4). The time to complete clearing varied greatly from 11 days to 6 months.

Similarly, another group found that the process was present in 97% (144/148) of transplanted lungs, almost always beginning on day 1 and always present by day 3 (5). The process was most severe in the perihilar regions and lung bases and most often reached maximal severity on day 1 (46%) or day 3 (40%). There was poor correlation of the severity of the response with lung ischemia times.

It appears that the reimplantation response is milder in patents undergoing heart–lung transplantation. In one report, all ten patients developed an interstitial pattern that peaked, on average, on day 11; seven developed bilateral airspace disease, which persisted for an average of 7 days and then resolved (6). Another group reports the occasional presence of a "hilar butterfly pattern of pulmonary edema" following a few transplantations (7). One of four patients, in another study, developed mild transient interstitial disease (8). More recently, in a group of 20 patients, all developed at least mild disease on the first postoperative day, which became less evident by day 7, but gradually increased during the second week (9). It is not known why this response appears to be milder in patients undergoing heart–lung transplantation compared with those receiving lungs alone; presumably, it is related to differences in organ procurement and preservation.

There was poor correlation between the severity of the response, as measured by chest radiography, compared with physiological methods, including the $A-aPO_2$ gradient and FIO_2/PO_2 (manuscript in preparation). In addition, in a study involving dogs, it was noted that the chest radiograph is only fair in assessing the severity of the reimplantation response, compared with physiological methods (10).

In summary, the reimplantation response is a form of noncardiogenic pulmonary edema that occurs in most transplanted lungs within 24 hr of transplantation. Clinically, it appears as perihilar or basal airspace or interstitial disease that peaks in severity by day 4. Therefore, any pulmonary process beginning on or after this time should be considered to be due to some other cause, such as rejection or infection, and investigated accordingly.

III. Acute Rejection

Acute pulmonary rejection has been observed as early as 3 days posttransplantation and as late as several years following the procedure (11). By clinical criteria, it occurs at least once in nearly all recipients following the transplant. There are several manifestations of acute rejection, including clinical symptoms and signs, and laboratory changes in blood gas analysis, white blood cell counts, and pulmonary function testing, as well as in imaging. Patients may develop malaise, dyspnea, cough, tachypnea, fever, and on physical examination, may have rales and rhonchi (11). Laboratory investigations may reveal an elevated white blood cell count and a widened $A-aPO_2$ gradient on blood gas analysis. These, however, are nonspecific and may be caused by other processes. A similar comment can be made for pulmonary function testing, which may show an obstructive pattern (i.e., fall in FEV_1 and vital capacity) and a decreased Dco, with both acute rejection and infection (12). Bronchoscopy with bronchoalveolar lavage (BAL) is an excellent method for detection of opportunistic infections, but its ability to differentiate

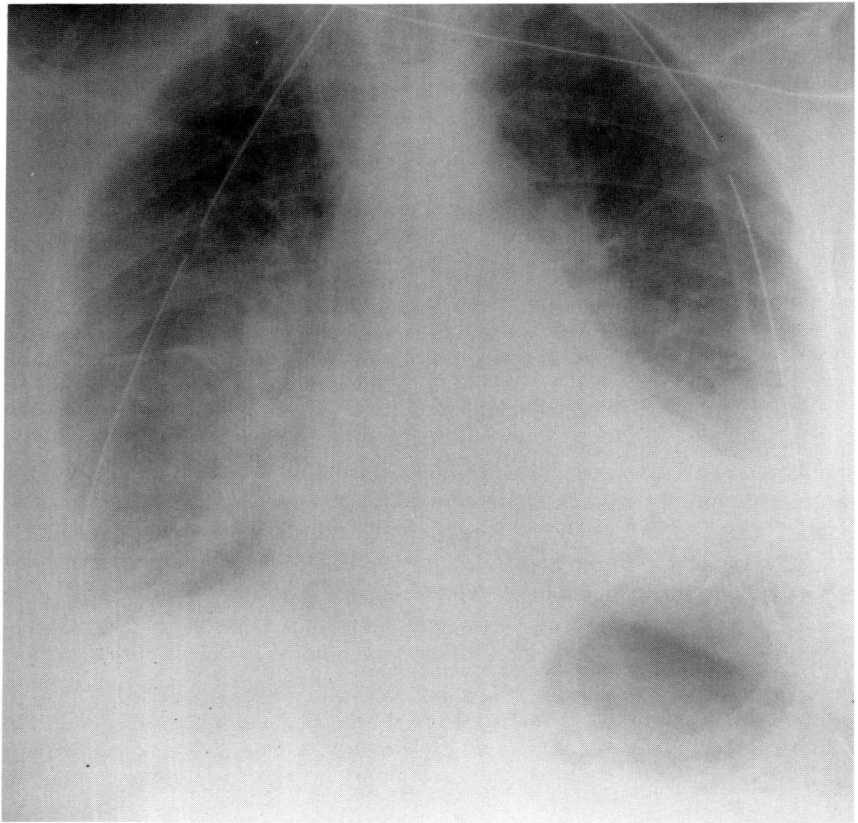

(a)

Figure 1 Reimplantation response: (a) Upright AP chest radiograph obtained 2 days post-bilateral lung transplantation. There is airspace disease in the perihilar regions and bases bilaterally. (b) Upright AP film obtained 8 days posttransplantation. There has been significant clearing, with mild residual reticular interstitial disease persisting.

between rejection and infection is controversial (11,13). However, in a recent study, the percentage of BAL lymphocytosis was higher in patients with grade 2 or 3 rejection than those with grades 1 or 0, suggesting a more definite role for this procedure in the future (14). There is now a consensus that the diagnostic gold standard is histopathology.

Tissue can be obtained for pathological examination by transbronchial biopsy (TBB) or by open-lung biopsy. The former is obviously less invasive and

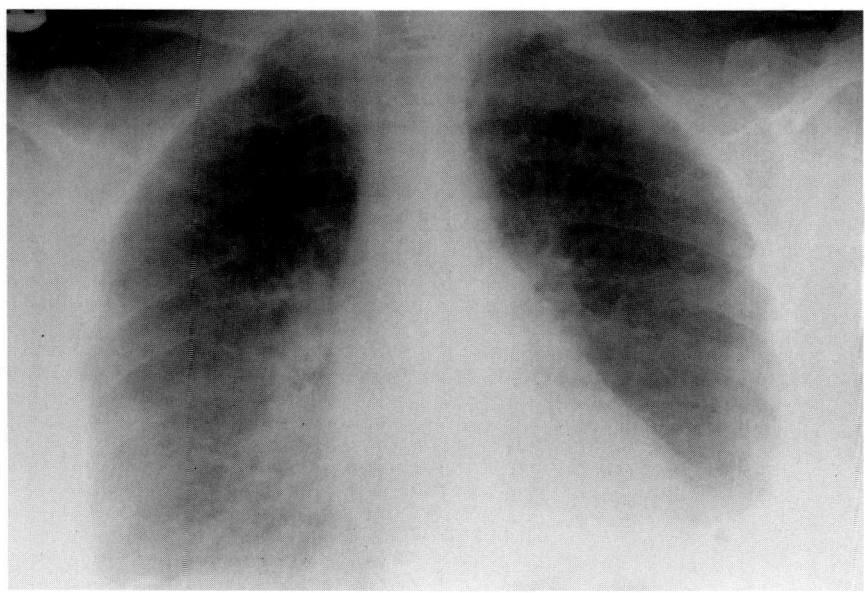

(b)

has emerged as the procedure of choice for making the diagnosis (11). With adequate sampling, a TBB sensitivity and specificity for acute rejection of 84 and 100%, respectively, can be obtained (15). However, this procedure is not without problems. Because of the small tissue samples obtained, interpretation is often difficult and there may be only nonspecific changes, again making acute rejection difficult to distinguish from infection. This problem may occur even with multiple biopsies (15).

Pathologically, acute rejection manifests initially as a perivascular lymphocytic infiltrate. With progression, this infiltrate becomes more widespread with extension into alveolar septae, resulting in an interstitial pneumonitis. With further progression, this diffuse perivascular, interstitial, and peribronchiolar infiltrate becomes associated with acute alveolar injury, reflected by airspace filling by neutrophils, red blood cells, and fibrin. This progression has been described as grades 1–4 acute rejection (least severe to most severe) in the classification of lung rejection proposed by the Lung Rejection Study Group (16).

Although occurring after the fact, response to administration of intravenous corticosteroids is also helpful in confirming the diagnosis; usually there is a dramatic response within 24 hr of steroid delivery.

In early studies, based on a clinical diagnosis, the most common radiographic abnormality was mid- or lower lung airspace disease (17,18; Fig. 2). Reticular interstitial disease in the same distribution was also seen (Fig. 3). In almost half of the instances of acute rejection, no radiographic changes were seen. In those patients in whom there were radiographic abnormalities, there was clearing within 48 hr of IV steroid therapy in almost all instances.

In a recent study, 21 of 42 lungs with pathologically proved acute rejection demonstrated mid- or lower lung reticular interstitial or airspace disease, or some combination of such (sensitivity = 0.50). This pattern was seen in 18 of 58 lungs

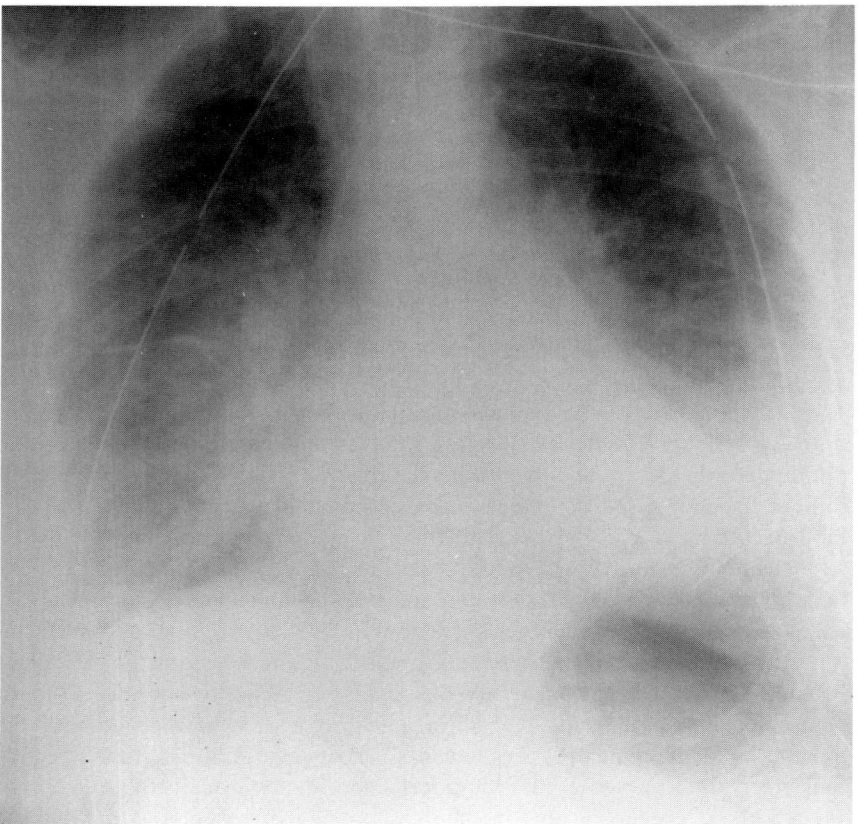

Figure 2 Acute rejection: Transbronchial biopsy revealed changes of acute rejection in this patient who had undergone bilateral lung transplantation 5 days earlier. This AP radiograph reveals right perihilar and basal airspace disease.

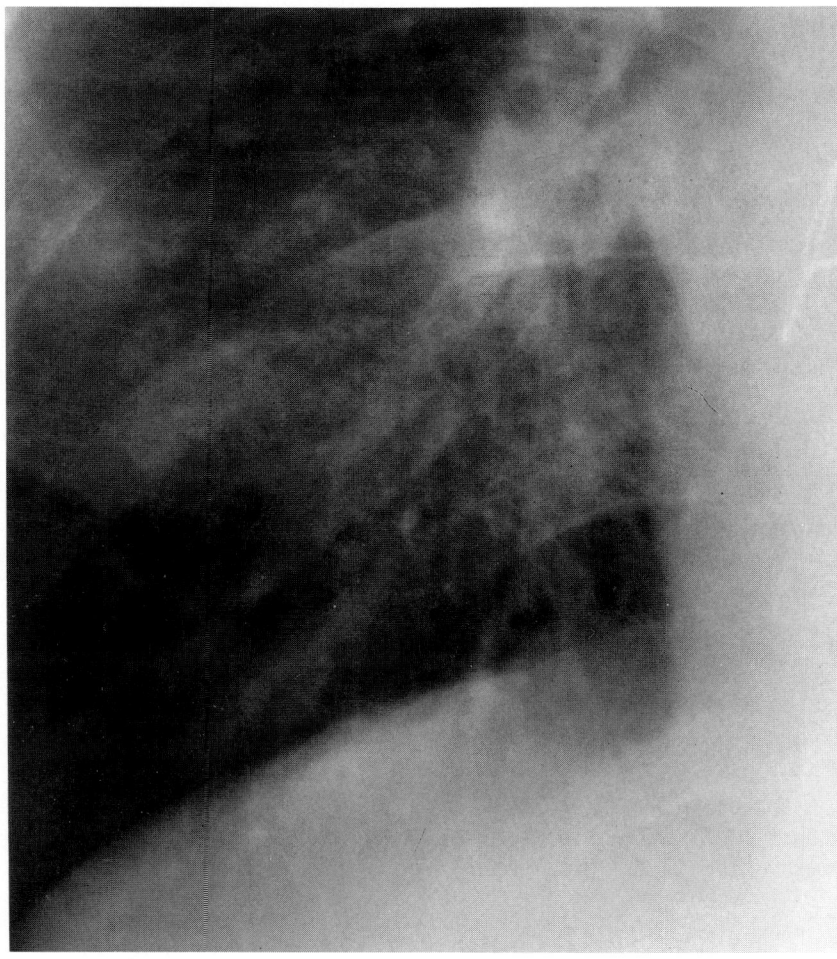

Figure 3 Acute rejection: Bilateral lung transplant recipient in whom transbronchial biopsy revealed acute rejection. Close-up view of right lower lung demonstrates mild reticular interstitial disease.

without acute rejection (specificity = 0.69 [40/58]). There was no difference in the appearance of the lungs between acute rejection grades 1 and 2. Normal lungs were noted in 20 instances (48%) of acute rejection (19).

Similarly, a low specificity was found in a study of children in which CT was unable to distinguish between acute rejection, chronic rejection, and infection (20).

However, in a study in adults who had undergone single-lung, double-lung, or heart–lung transplantation, high-resolution (HR)CT revealed ground-glass opacities in 65% of pathologic proved acute rejection episodes (21). These opacities were more widespread when more severe grades of rejection were present, although the numbers were small. In 20% of episodes, the HRCT was normal. Ground-glass opacities were also noted during cytomegalovirus pneumonia, but the specificity of this finding was still high (85%).

In one patient, who died from severe acute rejection, HRCT revealed relatively mild changes, consisting of interlobular septal thickening, patchy airspace disease, and increased attenuation in the walls of some airways (22). In a piglet experimental model, acute rejection was manifested on CT by worsening peripheral airspace disease in untreated animals, or as a densitometrically measured diffuse interstitial infiltration, with or without perihilar or peripheral airspace disease or bronchial wall thickening (23).

In the past, our clinicians have used aerosolized ^{99m}Tc-pentetate (DTPA) to assess the integrity of the alveolar capillary membrane (24), but this test was not found to add clinically useful information, and it is no longer performed in these patients. However, one group has found that this test, although relatively insensitive (0.69), was useful in conjunction with pulmonary function testing (25). In a small number of patients undergoing single-lung transplantation for primary pulmonary hypertension, rejection was manifested by a marked decrease in ventilation, with a mild decrease in perfusion on V/Q scanning (26). In a group of patients with single-lung transplantation for pulmonary fibrosis, acute rejection was associated with a shift of flow to the native lung at the time of acute rejection, which was reversible with the administration of steroids (27). Single-photon emission (SPE)CT lung perfusion imaging was very sensitive in the detection of acute rejection (pathologically proved), but nonspecific, with a sensitivity of 96% and specificity of 54% (28). A recent experimental study, using rats, found that nuclear scanning with ^{111}In-labeled lymphocytes was quite accurate in the detection of pathologically proved rejection (29). In a study using lymphoscintigraphy with radiocolloids in dogs, the presence of acute rejection was associated with disappearance of lymphatic drainage from the transplanted lung to the mediastinum (30).

By using a Doppler flow meter in the ascending aorta and left pulmonary artery in dogs, a decrease in pulmonary flow and an increase in pulmonary vascular resistance were found to be useful early indicators of acute rejection in animals that had undergone single-lung transplantation (31).

In summary, the chest radiograph is relatively insensitive and quite nonspecific in the diagnosis of pulmonary rejection. When they are present, changes usually consist of perihilar and basal reticular interstitial disease or consolidation. With double-lung transplants, the disease is not necessarily symmetric. Although nonspecific, the chest radiograph (CXR) can be the first suggestion that rejection is occurring and may help confirm a suspicion of rejection by the rapid response to intravenous steroid administration. Use of HRCT appears to improve both the sensitivity and specificity of the diagnosis.

IV. Bronchiolitis Obliterans

Bronchiolitis obliterans (BO), which is probably due to chronic rejection, develops in approximately 50% of long-term survivors of heart–lung transplantation (32,33). The incidence of this condition in lung transplant recipients is uncertain, but is also felt to approach 50% of long-term survivors (34). Recently, a clinical-staging scheme was proposed in an attempt to better define BO in lung transplant recipients (35). This system is based on progressive airway obstruction on pulmonary function testing, and it has been useful in the assessment of this group of patients (34). Clinically BO may cause progressive dyspnea, as well as a mixed pattern of restrictive and obstructive disease on pulmonary function testing (33). Although transbronchial biopsy may demonstrate the presence of BO, this method lacks sensitivity, because the disease can be quite patchy in distribution, and only a small number of airways may be sampled by this technique. Therefore, open-lung biopsy may be necessary.

In a small series of four patients who had pathologically proved BO following lung transplantation, a slight to moderate decrease in peripheral vascular markings and decrease in lung volumes, along with areas of subsegmental atelectasis and linear irregular opacities were noted by chest radiography (36). On HRCT, all four patients exhibited mild peripheral bronchiectasis, and three had decreased peripheral vascular markings (Fig. 4). In another study, 57 HRCT scans were reviewed from 100 single- or double-lung recipients (37). Bronchiectasis was noted on 28 of these scans. Of these 28, 12 had pathologically proved BO, whereas only 1 of the 29 patients whose HRCT did not show bronchiectasis had BO. This relation was statistically significant in the single-lung recipients (70% incidence of BO if bronchiectasis was seen, 5% incidence if not). In a more recent study, there was a close correlation between the number of dilated bronchi and pulmonary function testing, although the HRCT findings appeared later (38).

In a study of 40 transplant recipients, HRCT revealed bronchiectasis in 12 of

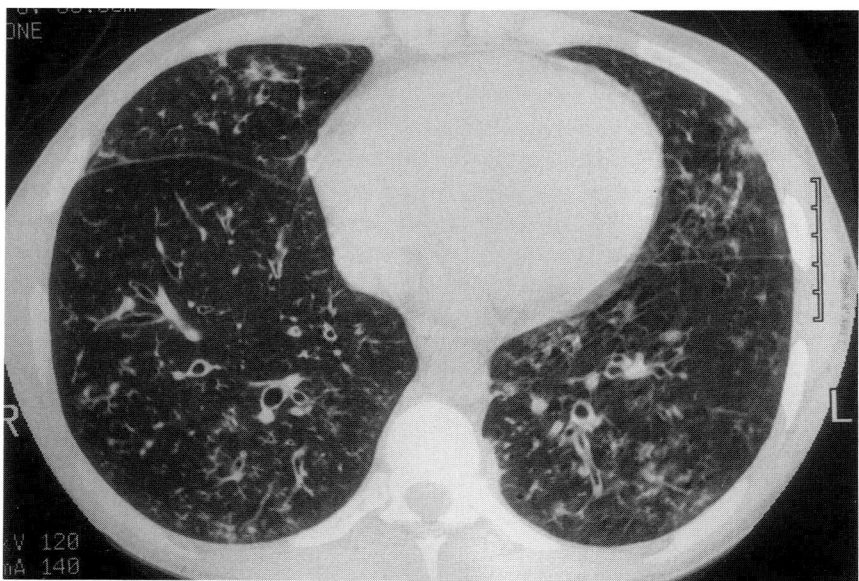

Figure 4 Bronchiolitis obliterans: Bilateral lung transplant recipient with bronchiolitis obliterans proved at open-lung biopsy. This HRCT image reveals diffuse bronchial dilation and wall thickening, areas of hyperlucency in the right lower lobe, and small linear and nodular opacities in a patchy distribution.

the 14 with the bronchiolitis obliterans syndrome (86%), but in only 6 of 20 (23%) without it (39). Bronchiectasis appeared within 1 month of the syndrome in 8 (67%) of 12 patients.

Two patients with BO following heart–lung transplantation had CXR changes consisting of decreased peripheral bronchovascular markings and hyperinflation (40). In another study of 11 heart–lung recipients with BO (10 proved pathologically, 1 clinically), the CXR revealed linear–nodular, nodular, confluent nodular, or diffuse alveolar opacities (41). In addition, central bronchiectasis was seen in 9 of the patients, but not in 5 randomly selected asymptomatic recipients. In a study of seven heart–lung recipients with clinical BO, there was good correlation between the percentage of dilated lower lobe bronchi and pulmonary function evidence of airway obstruction (42). No lower lobe bronchial dilation was seen in patients without clinical BO. In a case report of an asymptomatic heart–lung recipient, with pathologically proved BO, the chest radiograph and standard CT scan were normal, a perfusion scan was near normal, but an aerosol ventilation scan was abnormal (43). In addition, HRCT was abnormal.

In a study of inflation-fixed lungs from heart–lung recipients, two specimens exhibited chronic rejection pathologically (extensive severe BO, bronchiectasis, and peribronchial fibrosis; 44). On HRCT, the bronchiectasis was striking, but in the actual regions of pathological BO, the lungs were unremarkable.

Therefore, it appears that BO may be associated with HRCT evidence of bronchiectasis and peripheral areas of lucency, presumably related to distal airway obstruction, local hypoxia, and reflex vasoconstriction. The accuracy of HRCT is detecting BO and grading its severity is not yet clear because of problems with transbronchial biopsy as a gold standard and because there has not yet been a large prospective study. Also, the relation between bronchial dilation on HRCT and the presence of airways disease has been called into question (45).

Some patients develop bronchiolitis obliterans organizing pneumonia (BOOP), which differs considerably from the BO discussed in the foregoing (46). There is relatively rapid development of hypoxemia and restrictive abnormalities on pulmonary function testing in patients with BOOP. Pathologically, endobronchial granulation tissue plugs and endogenous lipoid pneumonia are seen. The chest radiograph reveals areas of consolidation. Patients respond to high-dose steroid administration with clearing of the radiographic and pulmonary function abnormalities. The exact etiology of BOOP in the posttransplantation population is unknown.

V. Airway Complications

Lung transplantation is unique, compared with other solid-organ transplants, in that a systemic arterial supply is not established at the time of transplantation. Ischemic-related airway necrosis and dehiscence was the cause of death in most of the early lung transplant failures. Recently, the avoidance of steroids and the use of the omental wrap in the early postoperative period have dramatically reduced both the number and severity of airway problems following lung transplantation. In fact, it now appears that the omentum itself may no longer be necessary, although most surgeons wrap the anastomosis with some form of vascularized tissue, such as pericardium or intercostal muscle. Similarly, low doses of steroids do not appear to seriously impair bronchial healing. In double-lung recipients, these problems have been further reduced now that bilateral single-lung transplants are performed, rather than en bloc transplantation of both lungs with a tracheal anastomosis. All of the 13 double-lung recipients in our early study had a tracheal anastomosis. Tracheal anastomotic blood supply is more tenuous than main bronchial supply because the donor airways are supplied by retrograde pulmonary-to-bronchial arterial flow through collateral pathways (47). Heart–lung recipients have less severe tracheal ischemia because of an adequate coronary–bronchial arterial anastomotic network (7).

Recent transplants have demonstrated a much lower incidence of airway problems than in those performed earlier. For example, in 38 patients undergoing bilateral lung transplantation, five complications were noted in 13 early patients (total of 26 anastomoses), whereas only two complications occurred in 25 later recipients (50 anastomoses) (48).

Although airway anastomotic problems have been significantly reduced, ischemic problems still occasionally occur. This is especially true in patients whose transplanted lung has been affected by rejection or infection, as these processes may reduce the retrograde pulmonary–bronchial arterial flow to the donor bronchus.

The two main airway problems that occur are dehiscence and stricture formation, and both are best assessed by bronchoscopy. Recently, however, spiral CT has provided excellent visualization of the bronchial tree, and this technique should become useful in assessing these airway problems. For example, CT (thin-section with reconstructions) has been excellent in detecting both the presence of extraluminal gas and the bronchial wall defect itself (49).

Airway dehiscence is manifested radiographically by the presence of extraluminal gas (Fig. 5). Although this can be detected by chest radiography, CT is much better. For example, mediastinal gas was noted on the chest radiograph in five of the six instances in which dehiscence occurred; however, in one double-lung recipient, this was not apparent until 7 weeks after the diagnosis was made at bronchoscopy. Presumably, this delay was due to the presence of only a small amount of extraluminal gas, the location of the gas being directly over an airway, or was due to suboptimal radiographic technique. Five of the six patients had a CT scan performed at the time of the dehiscence; in all, extraluminal gas was easily visualized.

In a study of 23 patients, in whom bronchoscopy demonstrated dehiscence in 17 (bilateral in four with 21 areas of dehiscence), CT allowed the identification of the bronchial defect in addition to extraluminal gas in all 17 (49). There were 18 airways noted by bronchoscopy to be intact and, in these, CT demonstrated a defect in 1 (which may have been missed by bronchoscopy) and extraluminal gas in 4. In these instances, the amount of extraluminal gas was always small, the gas was not always in direct contiguity with the anastomosis, and it was seen during the first 7–12 days posttransplantation. Pneumothorax was not helpful in predicting the presence of dehiscence; it was seen in 43% of 21 episodes of dehiscence, but also in 33% of intact anastomoses.

Also, CT was much better than plain radiography at visualizing airway strictures. Of the total of seven strictures (17,18), only three were visible on the radiographs, but all were evident at CT. Similarly, Silastic stents, which are used to treat significant strictures, were always seen by CT, but were only occasionally visible on chest radiography. One must be careful that the plane of the image being assessed is through the middle of the bronchus. An image through the superior or

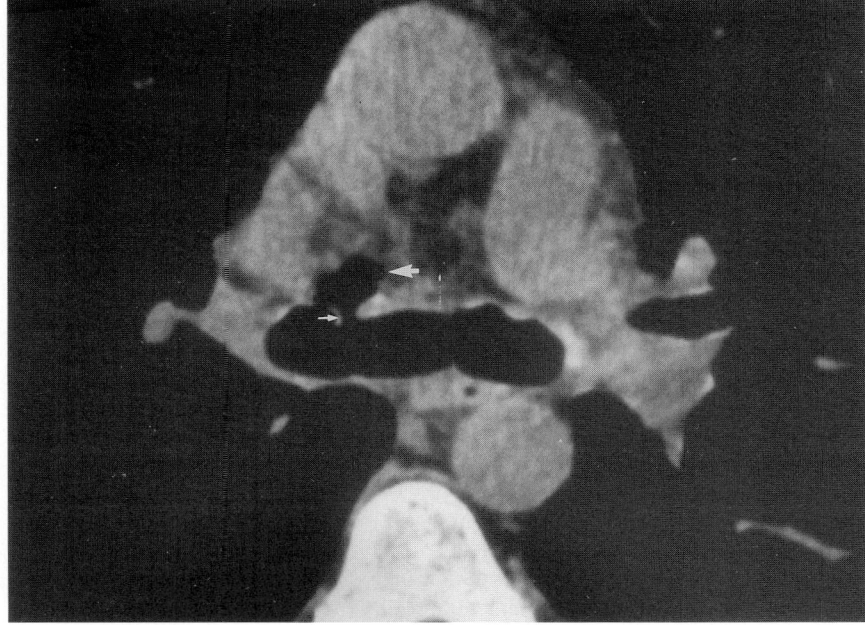

Figure 5 This CT scan reveals a small gas collection (large arrow) in the mediastinum anterior to the right main stem bronchus. The bronchial defect (small arrow) and tract leading to this collection are visible.

inferior aspect of one of the main bronchi may falsely make the lumen appear narrow. Also, because the donor or recipient airway is frequently "telescoped" into the other, mild airway irregularity and narrowing are expected.

VI. Infections

Infections may occur in 50–100% of patients following lung transplantation (50,51). Compared with other transplanted organs, the lungs are particularly susceptible to infection because of their direct communication with the atmosphere. The transplanted lung is affected more often than the native lung, probably because of impaired mucociliary function and cough reflexes (52). Because of the systemic immunosuppression, approximately 40% of infections in these patients are extrapulmonary.

Bacterial infections are most common, but are not as lethal as viral and fungal infections. Most bacterial pneumonias are due to gram-negative organisms, especially *Enterobacter* and *Pseudomonas* species,whereas bronchitis, which is also very common, is usually caused by *P. aeruginosa* and *Staphylococcus aureus*. *Pseudomonas cepacia* is frequently involved in patients with cystic fibrosis. Bacterial empyemas may be relatively asymptomatic. In one study, primary or secondary pulmonary hypertension and the presence of airway complications, were significant risk factors for bacterial pneumonia (51).

Cytomegalovirus (CMV) is the most significant viral infection and can take one of three forms. Primary infection, the most serious, occurs in 50–100% of seronegative recipients who receive a graft from a seropositive donor. Seropositive recipients may develop reinfection if the donor had been infected by a different CMV strain, or may reactivate their disease following immunosuppression. Cytomegaloviral infection most commonly develops between 1 and 4 months posttransplantation and may vary from asymptomatic disease to fulminant pneumonia, possibly with extrathoracic involvement (e.g., retinitis, hepatitis, gastritis, diffuse dissemination). This infection also appears to induce imunosuppression over and above that caused by immunosuppressive drugs, with inversion of the normal $CD4^+/CD8^+$ ratio. Other viral pathogens include herpes simplex (less common now that acyclovir prophylaxis is routine), varicella–zoster (most common manifestation is mucocutaneous involvement), and Epstein-Barr (which has an important role in the development of lymphoproliferative disorders).

Both *Aspergillus*, which may infect either the transplanted or the native lung, and *Candida* tend to occur more commonly in lungs that have been previously traumatized (e.g., by other infections, acute rejection, or other posttransplant complications). Fungi endemic to specific regions must always be considered in recipients from these regions as well as in those whose transplanted lung is from a donor who had resided in such a region. Because of the routine use of prophylaxis, *Pneumocystis carinii* pneumonia is uncommon.

The radiographic manifestations of these pneumonias are nonspecific for both the etiology of the pneumonia and even the diagnosis of pneumonia itself, since similar findings are seen with the reimplantation response, rejection, and fluid overload. However, the chest radiograph is still an important diagnostic tool, as it may be the first evidence that a pulmonary problem is present. Also, it (and CT) may be used in directing bronchoscopy or needle biopsy to the optimal location from which to obtain a suitable specimen.

VII. Lymphoproliferative Disorders

Lymphoproliferative disorders, now a well-known posttransplantation complication, occur in about 2% of transplant recipients (53). The disorder associated with cyclosporine therapy usually begins within the first 8 months posttransplantation and, generally, involves multiple organs with, for unknown reasons, sparing of the central nervous system (54). The disease ranges in severity from a benign slow-growing polyclonal proliferation, to an aggressive monoclonal tumor that is rapidly fatal. Most of the tumors are B cell type and are associated with Epstein-Barr virus (EBV) infection. This virus is known to induce a B-cell proliferation that is normally controlled by cytotoxic T cells. It is believed that cyclosporine inhibits this normal T-cell response, thereby allowing the uncontrolled growth of the infected B cells. The tumor may respond to a decrease in the cyclosporine dose, with or without administration of acyclovir. If this fails, and the tumor is not localized and resectable, the patient will probably die within 6 months (45).

In a review of the radiographic manifestations of 35 patients with intrathoracic manifestations of this process, the following findings were noted: pulmonary nodules (in 16 patients), airspace disease (in 3), hilar and mediastinal adenopathy (in 17), pleural fluid (in 4), pericardial thickening or fluid (in 2), and thymic enlargement (in 2) (55; Fig. 6).

VIII. Pulmonary and Cardiac Changes

The degree to which the mediastinum shifts following single-lung transplantation is quite variable. With fibrotic diseases, it tends to shift toward the remaining

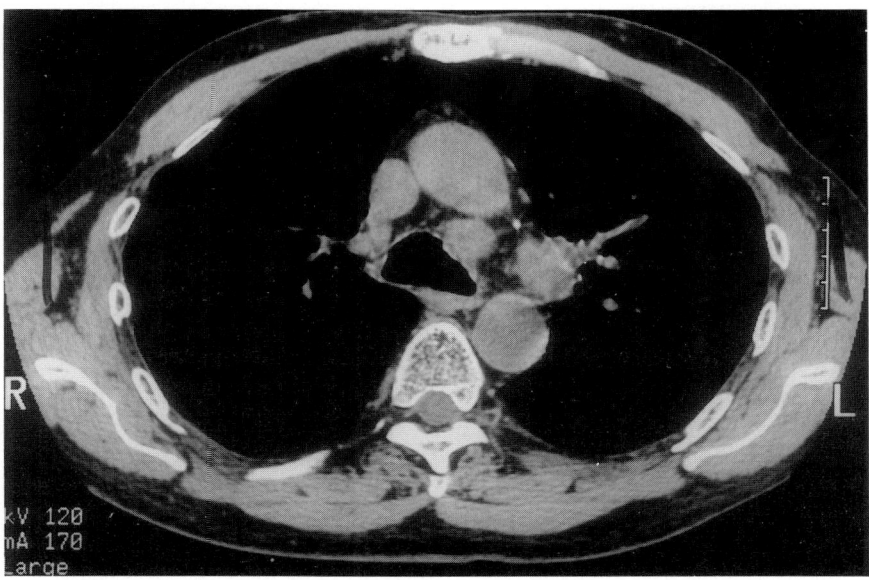

Figure 6 Lymphoproliferative disorder: High-resolution CT scan from a bilateral lung transplant recipient reveals a left tracheobronchial angle node. Biopsy revealed a polyclonal lymphoproliferation, and the patient responded to a lower doses of cyclosporine.

native lung owing to its reduced compliance compared with the transplanted lung. It was initially felt that single-lung transplantation would not be appropriate for patients with obstructive disease because the native lung, owing to its reduced compliance, would receive relatively more ventilation. This would lead to shift of the mediastinum toward the transplanted lung, further reducing its ventilation and causing V/Q mismatching (Fig. 7). In practice, however, this has not usually been a problem.

In an early group of 14 double-lung recipients, lung and cardiac sizes on both the preoperative posteroanterior radiograph and on the first postoperative and

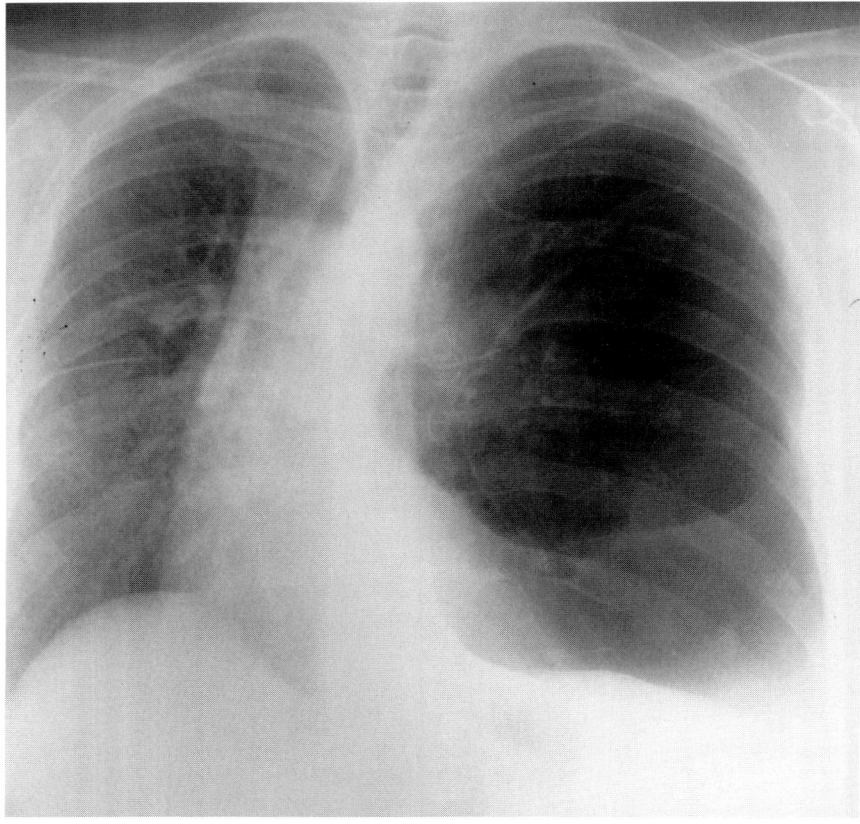

Figure 7 Mediastinal shift: This patient is post-right lung transplant for severe emphysema. There is significant shift of the mediastinum to the right owing to hyperinflation of the native left lung.

latest available posteroanterior radiographs were assessed. Lung size was evaluated by noting the height of the right hemidiaphragm in the midclavicular line relative to the posterior ribs, and cardiac size was measured by determination of the cardiothoracic ratio.

The average height of the right hemidiaphragm preoperatively was at rib 10.9 (range = 10–11). Its height on the early and late postoperative films did not differ; the mean level was rib 9.9 (range = 9.0–10.5). Similarly, this decreased lung size was noted on pulmonary function testing (56). The chest wall structures, therefore, appear to rapidly adapt to the new normal-sized lungs.

On the preoperative film, the average cardiothoracic ratio was 0.38 (10.8/28.2), the range being 0.32–0.51. As with the hemidiaphragm height, the cardiothoracic ratio did not differ on the early and late radiographs. The mean ratio was 0.51 (14.1/27.4) with a range of 0.45–0.59. Because the thoracic diameter changed very little (from 28.2 to 27.4) this increase in the cardiothoracic ratio was, therefore, due to an increase in the cardiac diameter itself (increasing from 10.8 to 14.1). This appeared to be partially due to the more transverse orientation of the heart secondary to the elevation of the diaphragm. More importantly, however, there was an increase in the size of the heart itself, possibly because of an increase in the venous return to the thorax following resection of the hyperinflated lungs.

Recently, MRI has been useful in assessing the arterial flow to transplanted single lungs (57). The ratio of flow to the transplanted lung, compared with the native lung, was 2.8 ± 0.83:1. The flow profile was noted to differ between the two lungs as well, in that there was forward flow during all of systole and most of diastole in the transplanted lung, but reversal of flow during most in diastole in the native lung. These differences were thought to be due to the greater vascular resistance in the native lung. Magnetic resonance imaging may become a valuable tool in assessing the vascular physiology of the transplanted lung (58). Nuclear studies have also been used to assess both perfusion and ventilation to the transplanted lung. In one study, patients with primary pulmonary hypertension undergoing single-lung transplantation had 93% of pulmonary flow going to the transplanted lung, with only 40% of ventilation to the native lung (59). In patients with COPD, α_1-antitrypsin deficiency, and idiopathic pulmonary fibrosis, about 68% of perfusion and 64% of ventilation went to the new lung.

IX. Omentum

When used during the transplant procedure, the intrathoracic omentum is frequently visible on the chest radiograph. In single-lung recipients, it appears as a perihilar density. In double-lung recipients it is most often seen as a lower right paratracheal mass or, occasionally, as a convexity over the left upper cardiac margin or in the left paraspinal region (18). Other findings include a cardiophrenic angle mass, pseudocardiomegaly, pseudoparenchymal infiltrate, and increased hilar opacity (60). Therefore, the omentum may be the cause of a "mass" on the chest radiograph, and it is important that it not be confused with a true pathological process, such as lymphoma. In situations for which one is uncertain, CT is extremely helpful. Because of its easily recognizable fat density, the course of the omentum is always accurately depicted, from its entry point into the thorax to the airway anastomosis (61).

X. Posttransbronchial Biopsy Changes

Focal nodular opacities have been reported in lung transplant recipients following transbronchial biopsy (62). New pulmonary nodules, felt to represent discrete areas of parenchymal hemorrhage, were noted on 35% of postbiopsy radiographs; such nodules were seen in only 8% of a control group. The nodules occasionally cavitated and persisted for 1–2 weeks. Changes seen on CT scans following transbronchial biopsy include areas of ground-glass density, consolidation, and nodules, which may or may not cavitate (63; Figs 8 and 9).

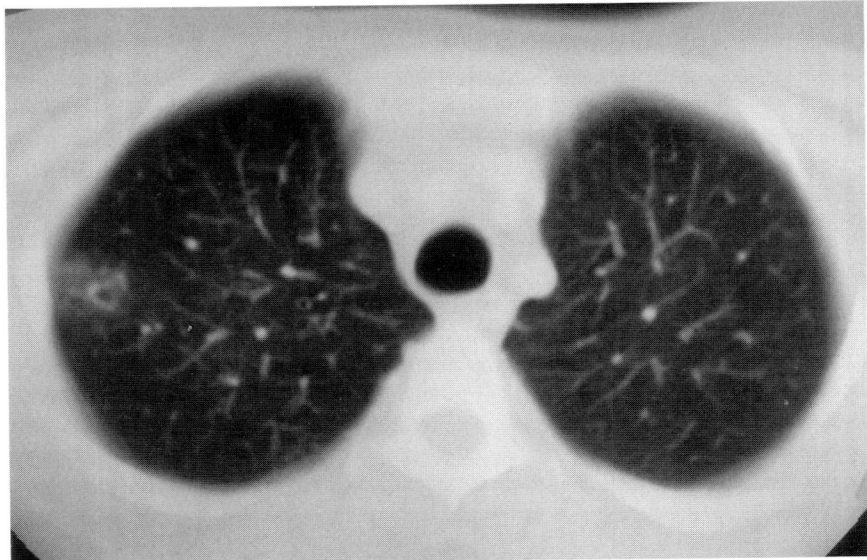

Figure 8 Changes postbronchoscopy: This CT scan reveals a small cavity in the right upper lobe, presumed to be due to a transbronchial biopsy obtained earlier the same day.

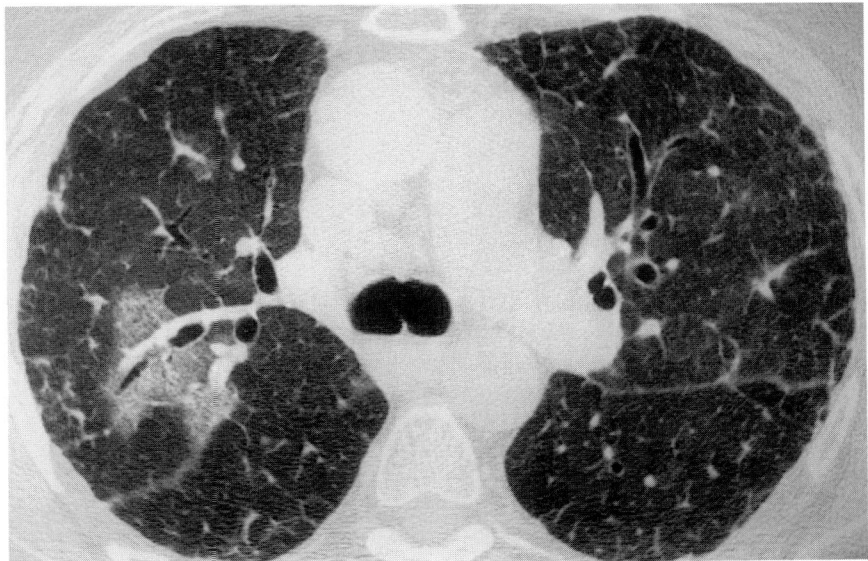

Figure 9 This HRCT reveals an area of ground-glass opacity in the right upper lobe, presumed to represent hemorrhage secondary to a transbronchial biopsy obtained a few hours earlier.

XI. Summary

Imaging studies played a major role in patients undergoing lung transplantation. These patients may develop unique problems, such as the reimplantation response, acute rejection, bronchiolitis obliterans, ischemia-induced airway complications, and immunosuppression-associated lymphoma; the radiologic manifestations for these conditions have been discussed. In addition, one must always keep in mind that these patients are also subject to the all of the usual problems associated with thoracic surgery, including atelectasis, infection, pneumothorax, and pleural effusion, conditions for which radiologic assessment is crucial.

References

1. Cooper JD, Patterson GA, Trulock EP, et al. Results of single and bilateral lung transplantation in 131 consecutive recipients. J Thorac Cardiovasc Surg 1994; 107:460–471.

2. Montefusco CM, Veith FJ. Lung transplantation. Surg Clin North Am 1986; 66: 503–515.
3. Herman SJ, Kundu S, Winton TL, Weisbrod GL, Rappaport DC. Radiographic manifestations of the reimplantation response following lung transplantation. Radiology 1993; 189(P):211.
4. Herman SJ. Radiologic assessment after lung transplantation. Clin Chest Med 1990; 11:333–346.
5. Anderson DC, Glazer HS, Semenkovich JW, et al. Lung transplant edema: chest radiography after lung transplantation—the first 10 days. Radiology 1995; 195: 275–281.
6. Chiles C, Guthaner DF, Jamieson SW, et al. Heart–lung transplantation: the postoperative chest radiograph. Radiology 1985; 154:299–304.
7. Griffith BP, Hardesty RL, Trento A, et al. Heart–lung transplantation: lessons learned and future hopes. Ann Thorac Surg 1987; 43:6–16.
8. Holland SA, Hutton LC, McKenzie FN. Radiologic findings in heart–lung transplantation: a preliminary experience. J Can Assoc Radiol 1989; 40:94–97.
9. Harjula ALJ, Baldwin JC, Silverman NE, et al. Implantation response following clinical heart–lung transplantation. J Cardiovasc Surg 1990; 31:1–6.
10. Keshavjee SH, Herman SJ, Yamazaki F, et al. Radiologic correlation of the early physiologic function of the transplanted lung. Invest Radiol 1990; 25:511–516.
11. Trulock EP. Management of lung transplant rejection. Chest 1993; 103:1566–1576.
12. Otulana BA, Higenbottam T, Scott J, Clelland C, Igboaka G, Wallwork J. Lung function associated with histologically diagnosed acute lung rejection and pulmonary infection in heart–lung transplant patients. Am Rev Respir Dis 1990; 142:329–332.
13. Higgenbottam T, Stewart S, Penketh R, Wallwork J. Transbronchial lung biopsy for the diagnosis of rejection in heart–lung transplant recipients. Transplantation 1988; 46:532–539.
14. DeHoyos A, Chamberlain D, Schvartzman R, et al. Prospective assessment of a standardized pathologic grading system for acute rejection in lung transplantation. Chest 1993; 103:1813–1818.
15. Kirby TJ, Mehta A, Rice TW, Gephardt GN. Diagnosis and management of acute and chronic lung rejection. Semin Thorac Cardiovasc Surg 1992; 4:126–131.
16. Yousem SA, Berry GJ, Brunt EM, et al. A working formulation for the standardization of nomenclature in the diagnosis of heart and lung rejection: lung rejection study group. J Heart Lung Transplant 1990; 9:593–601.
17. Herman SJ, Rappaport DC, Weisbrod GL, et al. Single–lung transplantation: imaging features. Radiology 1989; 170:89–93.
18. Herman SJ, Weisbrod GL, Weisbrod L, et al. Chest radiographic findings following bilateral lung transplantation. AJR 1989; 153:1181–1185.
19. Herman SJ, Lahrs A, Rappaport DC, Weisbrod GL, Winton T. Accuracy of chest radiograph in diagnosis of acute rejection after lung transplantation. Radiology 1994; 193(P):146.
20. Medina LS, Siegel MJ, Glazer HS, et al. Diagnosis of pulmonary complications associated with lung transplantation in children: value of CT vs histopathologic studies. AJR 1994; 162:969–974.

21. Loubeyre P, Revel D, Delignette A, Loire R, Mornex JF. High-resolution computed tomographic findings associated with histologically diagnosed acute lung rejection in heart–lung transplant recipients. Chest 1995; 107:132–138.
22. Hruban RH, Ren H, Kuhlman JE, et al. Inflation-fixed lungs: pathologic–radiologic (CT) correlation of lung transplantation. J Comput Assist Tomogr 1990; 14:329–335.
23. Hammainen P, Kivisaari L, Aarnio P, et al. Sequential CT in monitoring experimental lung transplant. J Comput Assist Tomogr 1992; 16:138–147.
24. Krasnow AZ, Isitman AT, Collier D, et al. Diagnostic applications of radioaerosols in nuclear medicine. In: Freeman LM, ed. Nuclear medicine annual 1993. New York: Raven Press, 1993:123–193.
25. Herve PA, Silbert D, Mensch J, et al. Increased long clearance of ^{99m}TcDTPA in allograft lung rejection. Am Rev Respir Dis 1991; 144:1333–1336.
26. Levine SM, Jenkinson SG, Bryan CL, et al. Ventilation–perfusion inequalities during graft rejection in patients undergoing single lung transplantation for primary pulmonary hypertension. Chest 1992; 101:401–405.
27. Grossman RF, Frost A, Zamel N, et al. Results of single-lung transplantation for bilateral pulmonary fibrosis. N Engl J Med 1990; 322:727–733.
28. Colt HG, Cammilleri S, Khelifa F, et al. Comparison of SPECT lung perfusion with transbronchial lung biopsy after lung transplantation. Am J Respir Crit Care Med 1994; 150:515–520.
29. Arai H, Yuda T, Goodgold HM, deMello DE, Hendershott L, Pennington DG. Detection of lung rejection with indium-111-labelled lymphocytes in heterotopic rat heart–lung transplantation. Circulation 1991; 84(suppl 3):355–363.
30. Ruggiero R, Thomas GA, Farris RH, Myles JL, Baciewicz FA Jr. Detection of canine allograft lung rejection by pulmonary lymphoscintigraphy. J Thorac Cardiovasc Surg 1994; 108:253–258.
31. Yamashita C, Yamamoto H, Tobe S, et al. Early diagnosis of acute rejection by pulmonary hemodynamics after single-lung transplantation. Ann Thorac Surg 1994; 57:1559–1563.
32. Burke CM, Theodore J, Baldwin JC, et al. Twenty-eight cases of human heart–lung transplantation. Lancet 1986; 1:517–519.
33. Burke CM, Theodore J, Dawkins KO, et al. Post transplant obliterative bronchiolitis and other late lung sequelae in human heart–lung transplantation. Chest 1984; 86:824–829.
34. Idolor L, Chaparro C, Rajagopalan, Kesten S, Mauer J. Bronchiolitis obliterans syndrome: usefulness of a clinical staging system to categorize post-transplant airways obstruction [abstr]. American Thoracic Society Conference. Boston, MA, May 21–25, 1994.
35. Cooper JD, Billingham M, Egan T, et al. A working formulation for the standardization of nomenclature and for clinical staging of chronic dysfunction in lung allografts. J Heart Lung Transplant 1993; 12:713–716.
36. Morrish WF, Herman SJ, Weisbrod GL, Chamberlain DW, Toronto Lung Transplant Group. Bronchiolitis obliterans after lung transplantation: findings at chest radiography and high-resolution CT. Radiology 1991; 179:487–490.
37. Granton J, DeHoyos A, Chamberlain D, et al. Bronchiectasis is related to the presence

of obliterative bronchiolitis in lung transplant recipients. Am Rev Respir Dis 1992; 145:A700.
38. Laurent F, Dromer C, Gayraud L, Latrabe V, Couraud L, Drouillard J. High-resolution CT findings of bronchiolitis obliterans in lung transplantation patients. Radiology 1993; 189(P):182.
39. Loubeyre P, Revel D, Delignette A, et al. Bronchiectasis detected with thin-section CT as a predictor of chronic lung allograft rejection. Radiology 1995; 194:213–216.
40. Holland SA, Hutton LC, McKenzie FN. Radiologic findings in heart–lung transplantation: a preliminary experience. J Can Assoc Radiol 1989; 40:94–97.
41. Skeens JL, Fuhrman CR, Yousem SA. Bronchiolitis obliterans in heart–lung transplantation patients: radiologic findings in 11 patients. AJR 1989; 153:253–256.
42. Lentz D, Bergin CJ, Berry GJ, Stoehr C, Theodore J. Diagnosis of bronchiolitis obliterans in heart–lung transplantation patients: importance of bronchial dilation on CT. AJR 1992; 159:463–467.
43. Halvorsen RA Jr., DuCret RP, Kuni CC, Olivari MT, Tylen U, Hertz MI. Obliterative bronchiolitis following lung transplantation—diagnostic utility of aerosol ventilation, lung scanning and high resolution CT. Clin Nucl Med 1991; 16:256–258.
44. Herve PA, Silbert D, Mensch J, et al. Increased lung clearance of ^{99m}Tc-DTPA in allograft lung rejection. Am Rev Respir Dis 1991; 144:1333–1336.
45. Lynch DA, Newell JD, Tschomper BA, Cink TM, Newman LS, Bethel R. Uncomplicated asthma in adults: comparison of CT appearance of the lungs in asthmatic and healthy subject. Radiology 1993; 188:829–833.
46. DeHoyos A, Maurer JR. Complications following lung transplantation. Semin Thorac Cardiovasc Surg 1992; 4:132–146.
47. Ladowski JS, Hardesty RL, Griffith BP. Pulmonary artery blood supply to the supracrainal trachea. Heart Transplant 1984; 4:40–42.
48. Ramirez J, Patterson GA. Airway complications after lung transplantation. Semin Thorac Cardiovasc Surg 1992; 4:147–153.
49. Semenkovich JW, Glazer HS, Anderson DC, et al. Bronchial dehiscence in lung transplantation: CT evaluation. Radiology 1995; 194:205–208.
50. Maurer JR, Tullis E, Grossman RF, et al. Infectious complications following isolated lung transplantation. Chest 1992; 101:1056–1059.
51. Horvath J, Dummer S, Loyd J, et al. Infection in the transplanted and native lung after single lung transplantation. Chest 1993; 104:681–685.
52. Dolovish J, Rossman C, Chambers C, et al. Mucociliary function in patients following single lung or lung/heart transplantation [abstr]. Am Rev Respir Dis 1987; 92:135–136.
53. Penn I. Cancers complicating organ transplantation [editorial]. N Engl J Med 1990; 323:1767–1768.
54. Harris KM, Schwartz ML, Slasky BS, et al. Posttransplantation cyclosporin-induced lymphoproliferative disorders: clinical and radiologic manifestations. Radiology 1987; 162:697–700.
55. Dodd GD III, Ledesma-Medina J, Baron RL, Fuhrman CR. Posttransplant lymphoproliferative disorder: intrathoracic manifestations. Radiology 1992; 184:65–69.

56. Toronto Lung Transplant Group. Double lung transplant for advanced chronic obstruction lung disease. Am Rev Respir Dis 1989; 139:303–307.
57. Mohiaddin RH, Paz R, Theodoropoulos S, Firmin DN, Longmore DB, Yacoub MH. Magnetic resonance characterization of pulmonary arterial blood flow after single lung transplantation. J Thorac Cardiovasc Surg 1991; 101:1016–1023.
58. Silverman JM, Julien PJ, Herfkens RH, Pelc NJ. Quantitative differential pulmonary perfusion: MR imaging versus radionuclide scanning. Radiology 1992; 185(P):217.
59. Medina LS, Royal HD, Trulock EP, Ettinger NA. Postoperative evaluation of single-lung transplant patients with quantitative ventilation–perfusion imaging. Radiology 1992; 185(P):283.
60. Glazer HS, Anderson DJ, Cooper JD, Molina PJ, Sagel SS. Omental flap in lung transplantation Radiology 1992; 185:395–400.
61. Bhalla M, Wain JC, Shepard JO, McLoud TC. Surgical flaps in the chest: anatomic considerations, applications, and radiologic appearance. Radiology 1994; 192: 825–830.
62. Root JD, Molina PL, Anderson DJ, Sagel SS. Pulmonary nodular opacities after transbronchial biopsy in patients with lung transplants. Radiology 1992; 184: 435–436.
63. Kazerooni EA, Cascade PN, Gross BH. Transplanted lungs: nodules following transbronchial biopsy. Radiology 1995; 194:209–212.

13

Imaging of the Pleura

PAUL BURROWES and JOHN H. M. MacGREGOR

University of Calgary
Foothills Hospital
Calgary, Alberta, Canada

I. Introduction

A. Recognition of Pleural Disease

The recognition of pleural disease leads to the consideration of a variety of processes and the involvement of physicians from many specialties. Diagnostic imaging has a key role in the detection, diagnosis, and treatment of pleural abnormalities. The increased number of imaging modalities and their rapid refinement present a challenge to both the radiologist and the referring physician to select those that are most appropriate.

This chapter will attempt to highlight the strengths and weaknesses of available imaging techniques and provide some guidance for their use.

B. Pleural Anatomy and Physiology

The visceral and parietal pleura both comprise a single layer of mesothelial cells, basement membrane, layers of collagen, and elastic tissue (1). The visceral pleura envelops the lung and extends into the interlobar fissures, whereas the parietal pleura covers the costal, mediastinal, and diaphragmatic surfaces of the thorax. Both layers of pleura become continuous at the hilum, through which the pulmonary and bronchial vessels, bronchi, and associated nerves and lymphatics pass. Microvilli, the function of which has been speculated to increase the absorptive surface of the pleura and possibly to decrease friction between the lung and chest wall, cover the surface of the pleural mesothelial cells (2).

Lymphatic drainage of the pleura occurs through small openings (stomata) between mesothelial cells of the parietal pleura that directly communicate with lymphatic lacunae (1). The lymphatics of the visceral pleura, in contrast, do not directly communicate with the pleural space (2).

Although some controversy still exists, the major blood supply of the visceral pleura appears to be by superficial branches of bronchial arteries, with drainage by the pulmonary veins into the left atrium (1). The blood supply to the parietal pleura is systemic from branches of the arteries to the adjacent chest wall. For example, the costal pleura is supplied by branches of the intercostal and internal mammary arteries, and the mediastinal pleura by branches of the bronchial, upper diaphragmatic, internal mammary, and mediastinal arteries (2). Drainage of the parietal pleura is by the azygos, hemiazygos, and internal mammary veins to the right atrium (2).

C. Pleural Fluid Formation and Absorption

Under normal conditions, it is estimated that 1.0–5.0 ml of pleural fluid is present in the pleural space, the formation of which is governed by the Starling equation (3). The parietal pleura, being supplied by systemic vessels, has a hydrostatic pressure of approximately 30.0 cm H_2O. This, coupled with the normally negative intrapleural pressure (-5.0 cm H_2O), forces fluid from the capillary bed of the parietal pleura (1). The visceral pleura is thought to contribute little to normal pleural fluid formation, owing to lower filtration pressure and the greater distance from the mesothelium of the pleural microvessels (1).

There are six basic mechanisms for increased pleural fluid (1,3): increased hydrostatic pressure; decreased oncotic pressure; decreased pressure in the pleural space; increased permeability of the microvascular circulation, which may be secondary to inflammatory or neoplastic causes; impaired lymphatic drainage from the pleural space; and movement of fluid from the peritoneal space through diaphragmatic defects or diaphragmatic lymphatics.

It is clinically helpful to differentiate between exudative and transudative causes of pleural fluid. *Transudates* are due to an increase in hydrostatic pressure, decrease in osmotic pressure, or movement of fluid from the peritoneal cavity into the pleural space (1). Common causes are cardiac failure, cirrhosis, and the nephrotic syndrome. *Exudates*, on the other hand, occur when inflammatory, infectious, or neoplastic processes result in increased capillary permeability or lymphatic obstruction (3).

Transudates are differentiated from exudates by biochemical analysis. Exudates must meet at least one of the following criteria: (1) pleural fluid/serum total protein ratio higher than 0.5; (2) pleural fluid/serum lactate dehydrogenase (LDH) ratio higher than 0.6; and (3) pleural fluid LDH value higher than two-thirds the upper limit of normal for the serum (1). Fluid with a specific gravity higher than 1.016, or a protein concentration over 3 g/100 ml is also generally considered an exudate (4). Measurement of pH may also be helpful. Light and associates (5,6) have suggested that chest tube drainage may be indicated when a parapneumonic effusion demonstrates a pH lower than 7.0.

II. Imaging of Pleural Fluid

A. Plain Radiography

The most sensitive view of the chest for detection of pleural fluid is the lateral decubitus, on which it is estimated that as little as 5 ml of pleural fluid may be detected. At least 75 ml is needed to blunt the posterior costophrenic angles in an upright film, and 175 ml to blunt the lateral costophrenic angles (7,8). Distribution of fluid in the free pleural space is governed by gravity and elastic recoil of the lungs. In an upright patient, fluid first accumulates in a subpulmonic position between the lung and diaphragm, with increasing amounts spilling into the costophrenic angles, first posteriorly, where the pleural reflection is deepest (9,10). The subpulmonic distribution of pleural fluid may be difficult to recognize and may be mistaken for an elevated hemidiaphragm. On a frontal film, the apex of the diaphragm may be shifted laterally, but this is seen in only 50% of patients and is better appreciated on expiration films (4). Another clue is lack of visualization of vessels through the pseudodiaphragmatic contour, owing to fluid being interposed between the lung and the diaphragm. In the left hemithorax, separation of the lung base from the gastric air bubble by more than 2.0 cm is suggestive of a subpulmonic pleural effusion (11). This sign, however, is not entirely reliable and is most dependable when compared with previous films. When fluid is suspected of being localized to a subpulmonic distribution, it may be confirmed with decubitus films. In comparison with subpulmonic fluid, fluid occurring in the costophrenic angles is usually much easier to recognize by causing blunting of the normal acute angles.

In the supine patient, pleural fluid may be obscured owing to layering posteriorly. However, if of sufficient quantity, a diffuse haziness of the hemithorax may result, as well as a pleural cap of fluid at the apex of the lung. The latter occurs because the apex is the most dependent portion of the thorax in the supine position. Costophrenic angle blunting may also occur (12,13).

Loculation and encapsulation of pleural fluid may result from adhesions secondary to pyothorax or hemothorax, and they may occur anywhere in the

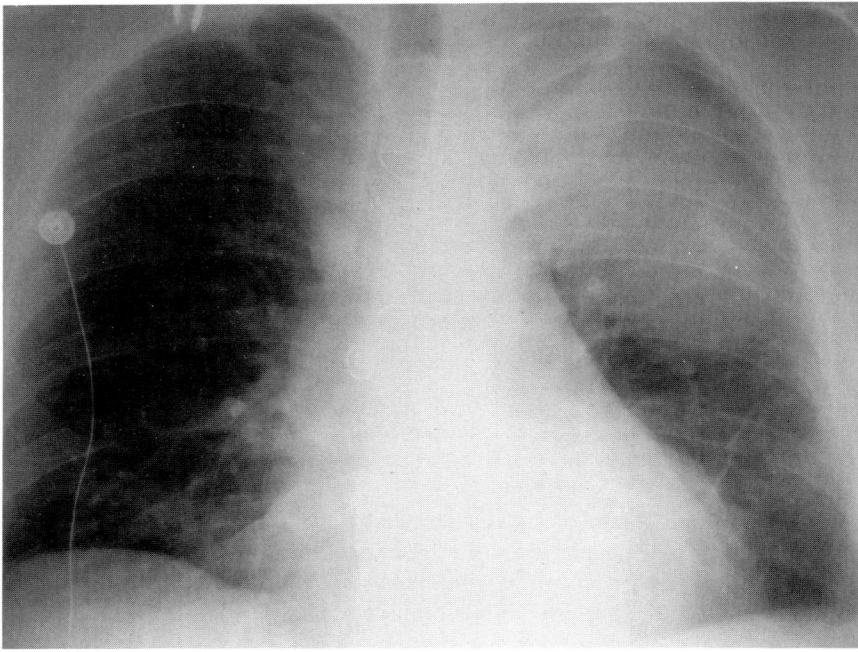

(a)

Figure 1 Pleural pseudotumor: (a) Frontal CXR shows a homogeneous opacity projecting in the left upper chest. Some of its margins are sharp and others are poorly defined, suggesting this is a pleural abnormality. (b) Lateral CXR places the "mass" in the expected position of the major fissure. Note how the inferior margin tapers into a normal-appearing fissure, confirming the mass is pleural fluid loculated in the major fissure.

pleural space. It may be difficult at times to differentiate these from parenchymal masses on plain radiographs, requiring further evaluation with computed tomography (CT) scans. Fluid may loculate also in the fissures, forming so-called pseudotumors. These may be suggested by identifying fluid elsewhere in the pleural space, recognizing its anatomical orientation along an interlobar fissure, usually the minor fissure (4), and often its rapid change in appearance over time. The localized fluid collection outlined by leaves of the pleura is often elliptical and well defined if the interface is in profile with the x-ray beam (Fig. 1).

The "incomplete pulmonary interlobar fissure sign" (14) occurs when fluid enters an incomplete major fissure from its superior and lateral aspects and, in so doing, creates an arcuate interface. This interface results from fluid meeting in the

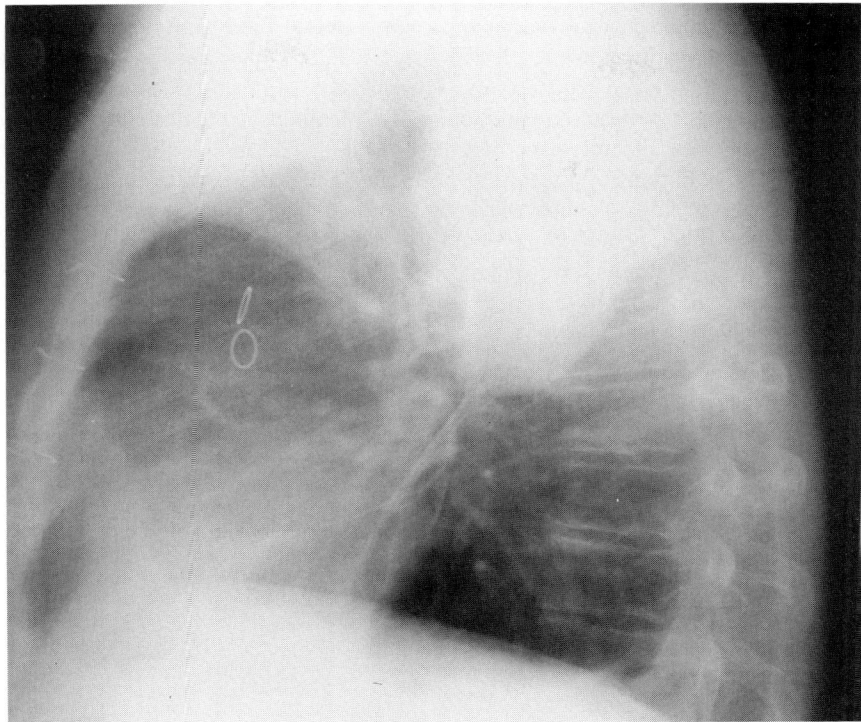

(b)

depths of the fissure. Heitzman and Raash (4) have shown significant degrees of incompleteness in the lower portions of the interlobar fissures (18% on the right and 32% on the left).

B. Computed Tomography

Computed tomography is a sensitive detector of pleural effusion and is particularly helpful in differentiating pleural from parenchymal disease. Free pleural fluid in the supine patient accumulates first in the most-dependent part of the chest posteriorly. If loculated, it is usually seen as a well-defined lentiform opacity, compressing adjacent lung. Some recent work (15) has indicated that, on CT, exudates may be differentiated from transudates by identifying parietal pleural thickening on contrast-enhanced scans.

It may be difficult to differentiate ascites from pleural fluid on CT examination. Four signs have proved to be helpful (16–18). The first is the diaphragm sign: Fluid seen central to the diaphragmatic contour represents ascites, and fluid seen outside the diaphragmatic contour represents pleural fluid. The displaced crura sign results when fluid in the pleural space displaces the crura away from the spine. This is not seen with ascites. The interface sign describes the apparent interface between pleural fluid and the liver. If the interface is ill-defined, fluid is most likely in the pleural space and, if well-defined, it is most likely related to ascites. The bare area sign results from ascites being prevented from extending behind the right lobe of the liver owing to reflections of the coronary ligaments (Fig. 2). Fluid seen behind the liver at this level, therefore, must be in the pleural space. On CT sections above or below the bare area, intraperitoneal fluid may extend posterior to the liver and be mistaken for pleural fluid.

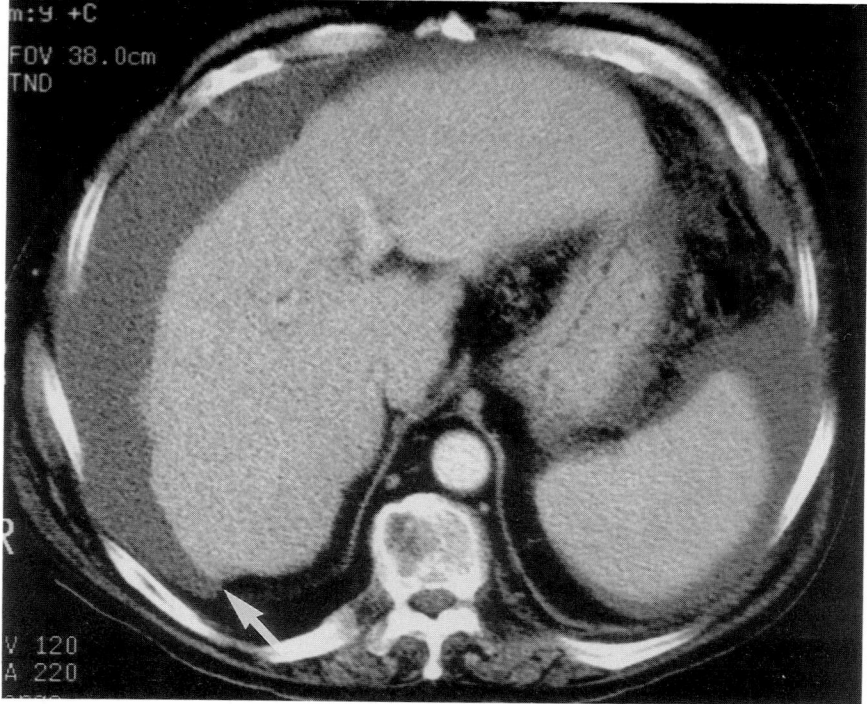

Figure 2 Pleural fluid versus ascites on CT: Fluid does not extend posterior to the liver, and its posterior extent is determined by the position of the coronary ligament (solid arrow) confirming its intra-abdominal position (ascites). The interface between the ascites and liver is also much better defined than with pleural fluid, as there is no interposed diaphragm.

Computed tomography may also be very useful for localizing and guiding drainage of loculated fluid. Use of CT-guided percutaneous catheter drainage ensures proper and successful catheter placement in a high percentage of patients (19).

C. Ultrasound

Ultrasound is a very valuable imaging modality for both the detection of fluid and localization of fluid before performing thoracentesis. It is of particular help in the diagnosis of small pleural effusions in severely ill patients when lateral decubitus films are unobtainable. Yang et al. (20) have recently used ultrasound to help differentiate transudates from exudates. In their study, anechoic effusions were either transudates or exudates, but heterogeneously echogenic pleural effusions, with or without septations, were always exudates (Fig. 3). Findings of thickened pleura and adjacent parenchymal lesions were also indicative of exudates.

Ultrasound is commonly used for guidance of pleural fluid drainage. It also has been used successfully for guidance of empyema drainage, pleural sclerotherapy, and pleural biopsy (20,21).

D. Magnetic Resonance Imaging

Currently, magnetic resonance imaging (MRI) has a limited role in the diagnosis of pleural effusion. Preliminary reports suggest that MRI may better differentiate transudates and exudates (22). Subacute or chronic hemorrhage can also be recognized by very high signal intensity on T1- and T2-weighted images. Chylous effusions also may be diagnosed by signal intensities similar to that of subcutaneous fat (23).

III. Empyema

As opposed to a simple parapneumonic effusion, empyema is diagnosed when pleural fluid is grossly purulent, when the white blood cell count of the fluid exceeds 5×10^9/L, or if organisms are identified by Gram stain or culture (24,25). In the presence of pneumonia, a pH lower than 7.0 is also considered diagnostic of empyema. Although most empyemas occur as a result of bacterial pneumonia or lung abscess, other predisposing causes include thoracic surgery, trauma, and mediastinitis. Currently, anaerobic bacteria are the most common organisms involved in empyema; this high incidence is explained by the usual indolent course of these infections, resulting in delayed presentation (24). Other bacterial causes include pneumococci, staphylococci, gram-negative enteric organisms, and tuberculosis (24).

The primary radiographic sign of empyema is pleural fluid. Therefore, it is clinically important to specifically look for its presence when evaluating a patient

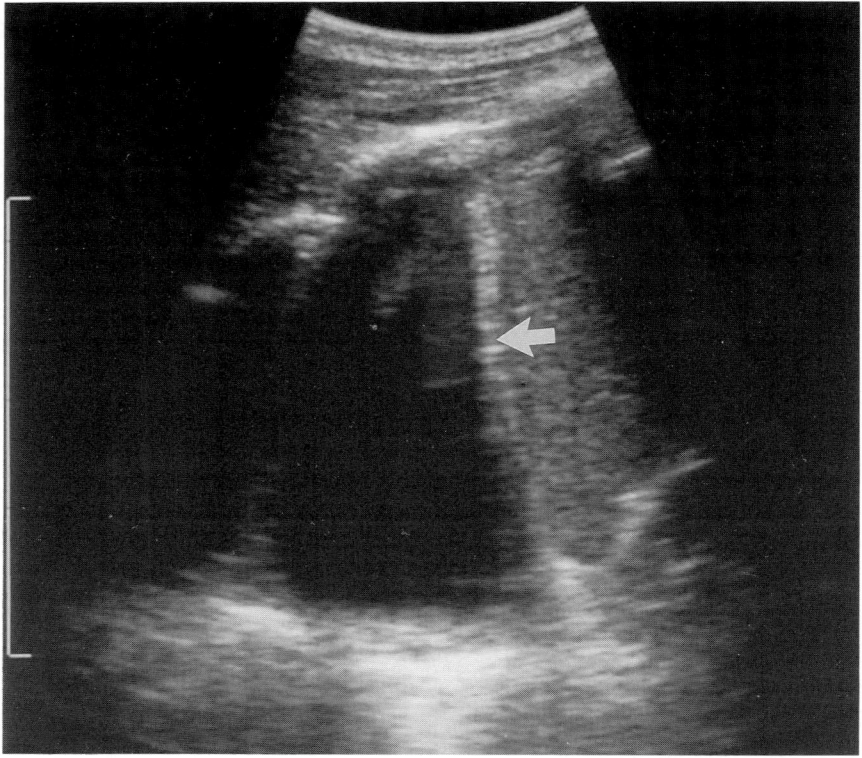

(a)

Figure 3 Chest ultrasound: (a) Image through the right lower chest demonstrates the diaphragm, which is seen as an echogenic band (arrow). Pleural fluid above (to the readers left) is anechoic and is displayed as black. The liver is seen to the readers right below the diaphragm. (b) Cephalad to image a multiple echogenic band (arrows) extend through the pleural effusion, indicating the effusion is not a simple transudate.

with pneumonia. Pleural fluid, however, may be difficult to differentiate from adjacent parenchymal consolidation or peripheral lung abscess and, at times, differentiation may be impossible. When seen, it is generally unilateral and, if bilateral, is asymmetrically increased on the infected side (25). Decubitus views may prove very helpful in detecting pleural fluid in the presence of parenchymal consolidation.

When loculated, empyema may be distinguished from a peripheral lung abscess by its lentiform shape, in contrast with the spherical shape of most lung abscesses. Also, pleural collections typically form an obtuse angle with the chest

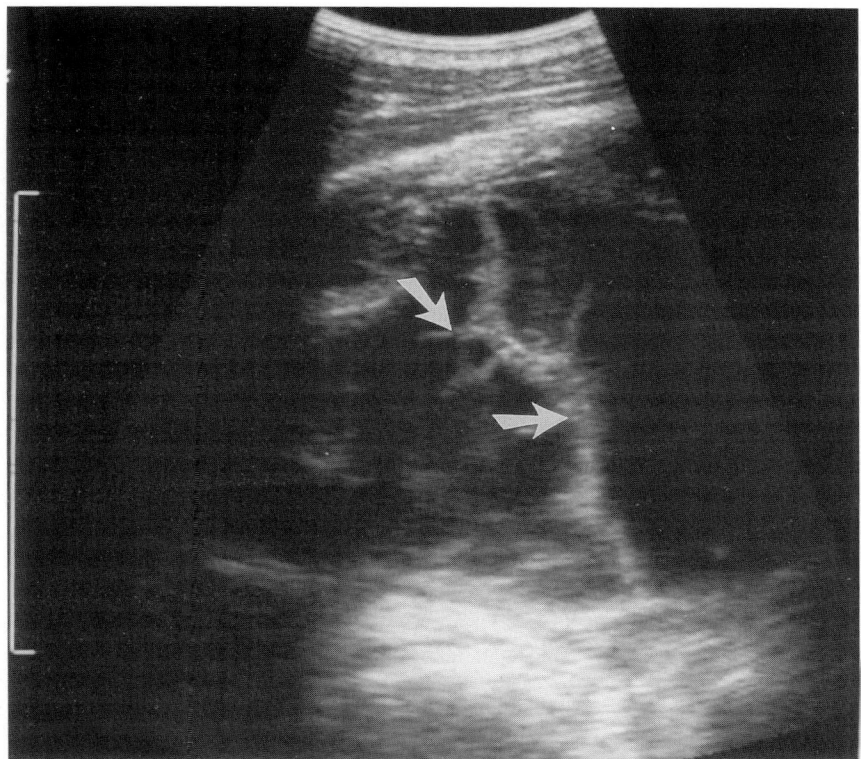

(b)

wall, as opposed to lung abscesses. If a bronchopleural fistula is present, differentiation of empyema, with an air–fluid level, from a peripheral lung abscess, with an air–fluid level, may be particularly difficult. Generally, a fluid level with empyema is disparate in length on frontal and lateral chest radiographs, whereas it is often of equal length in an abscess (26).

Computed tomography is currently the best-imaging modality for differentiating empyema from lung abscess. This differentiation is of therapeutic importance in that the treatment of lung abscesses does not generally include chest tube drainage. As with plain radiography, the recognition of the characteristic shapes of empyema and abscesses is helpful. The "split pleura sign" definitively localized an abnormality to the pleural space (27). This sign consists of identification on enhanced CT scans of a fluid collection interposed between enhancing visceral and parietal layers of pleura (Fig. 4). Another characteristic CT feature is displacement of adjacent bronchi and vessels away from an empyema, as opposed to the

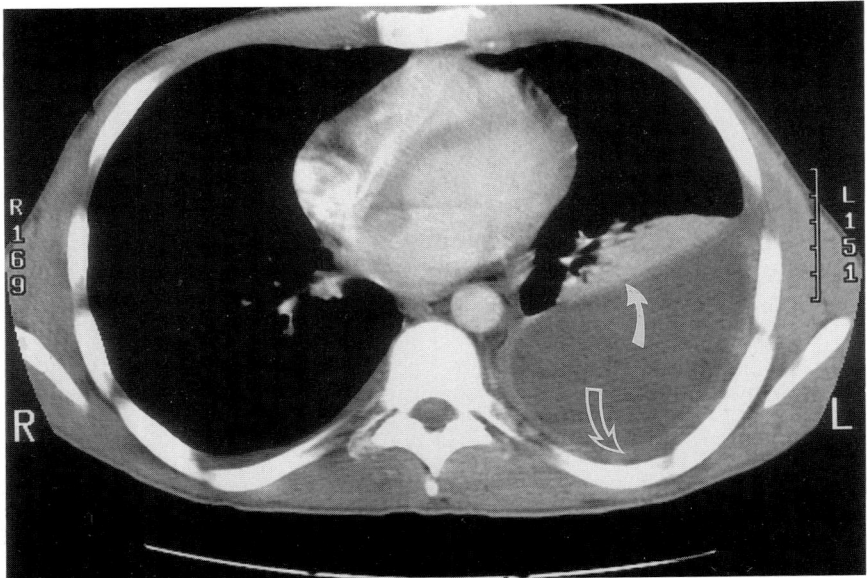

Figure 4 Empyema: CT demonstrates a fluid collection that is outside the lung bounded by the visceral (solid arrow) and the parietal pleura (open arrow). The pleura is thickened and enhances, which is suggestive of an empyema.

abrupt termination of bronchi and vessels at the margin of a lung abscess. Empyema also generally forms a well-defined border with the lung, whereas the boundary between a lung abscess and adjacent parenchyma is generally indistinct. Moreover, empyemas may have a smooth inner surface, compared with the thick, irregular wall of an abscess (28).

Computed tomography is of considerable value in guiding and ensuring accurate placement of pleural drainage tubes when empyema is loculated and, particularly, when multiple loculated collections exist (29,30). A pleural rind has generally been considered an indication for decortication. Recently, however, Neff et al. (31), in a series of ten patients, demonstrated resolution of pleural thickening in the presence of proven empyema treated with catheter drainage.

IV. Focal Pleural Diseases

A. Definition

A focal opacity is recognized as pleural by several radiographic signs. The opacity is peripheral on at least one projection, with sharply defined margins on part of its border, with other borders blending imperceptibly with surrounding structures. The opacity forms obtuse margins at its interface with the chest wall. Changes in adjacent ribs should always be looked for, as abnormality of the underlying rib is the only reliable means of separating pleural from extrapleural masses. As with other radiographic signs, the separation of pleural from parenchymal is not always possible, especially when the opacity is large.

Computed tomography is a powerful tool in recognizing pleural abnormalities. The interpretive rules are similar to those used for CXR. On CT, masses can more accurately be localized to the pleural space by analysis of angles of interface with the lung, the extent of contact with the chest wall, and detection of underlying rib changes, but it may be impossible, even with CT, to categorize every mass accurately.

B. Plaques

Pleural plaques are sharply demarcated, dense collections of collagenous tissue, usually located on the parietal pleural surface (32). The plaques are most frequently found along the posterior lateral margins of the seventh to tenth ribs and on the diaphragm's surface (33). The costophrenic angles and anterior pleural surfaces are usually spared. The distribution is usually bilateral and asymmetric, but is unilateral in 25% of patients. The plaques may calcify, and this can be recognized on CXR in about 25% of patients (34).

Plaque formation is the hallmark of asbestos exposure. The presence of plaques is related to the intensity of exposure, and the latency period is between 15 and 20 years (35). It should be remembered that, rarely, plaques will be secondary to causes other than asbestos exposure.

The recognition of plaques is important for several reasons. It is virtually pathognomonic of asbestos exposure and should prompt a careful work history. The detection of plaques in a patient with interstitial lung disease suggests the parenchyma process is asbestosis. An unnecessary workup for metastatic disease can be prevented if the plaques are not mistaken for multiple pulmonary nodules.

The CXR is the main technique for the detection of plaques, but its accuracy depends on factors, such as the strictness of the criteria used, the study population, and the experience of the observers. Sensitivities in the range of 30–80% and specificity in the range of 60–80% have been reported (36,37). The specificity is hampered by the difficulty in separating normal companion shadows caused by fat and muscles from those of plaques.

Conventional CT is useful and can separate plaques (Fig. 5) from subpleural fat, but high-resolution HRCT is superior to both conventional CT and CXR in the assessment of pleural plaques (38). On HRCT there is a normal 1- to 2-mm–thick stripe of soft tissue in the intercostal spaces. This intercostal stripe is mainly due to the innermost intercostal muscle. This muscle does not pass internal to the

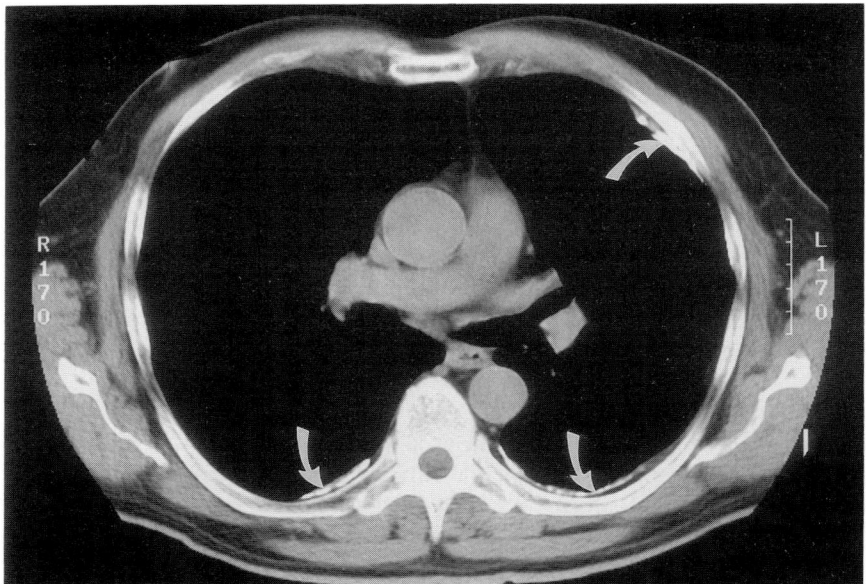

Figure 5 Pleural plaque: CT demonstrates multiple, bilateral, focal areas of pleural thickening. The plaques are calcified (arrows) in this patient with documented asbestos exposure. On CT it is always abnormal to see thickening along the inside margin of the ribs, and this suggests the presence of plaques, even if there is no calcification present.

rib and, in the normal person, the stripe is not seen over the internal aspect of the rib. Soft tissue that is internal to the rib is always abnormal (39).

The cost of HRCT limits its usefulness as a screening tool, but it plays a valuable role in excluding the CXR false-positive diagnose, caused by fat and intercostal muscles.

C. Neoplasm

Fibroma

These pleural neoplasms are uncommon and are not related to asbestos exposure. Pathological examination shows no epithelial differentiation, as seen in mesothelioma and, therefore, the term localized fibrous tumor is preferred (40). Sixty percent are benign and 40% are malignant. A strong association with hypertrophic pulmonary osteoarthropy is well known, but a recent series found clubbing in only 4% of cases (41).

Fibromas can be large and, in 40% of patients, are mobile owing to their attachment to the pleura by a pedicle. Acute angles, noted on CT, likely relate to the presence of a pedicle. Differentiation can be difficult, especially with larger masses. A variable enhancement pattern is seen, with many tumors giving a heterogeneous appearance (42).

Lipoma

The presentation is usually that of an asymptomatic mass found on CXR. The CT appearance is of a well-defined mass of fat attenuation, with obtuse margins (43). If the mass is heterogeneous, it suggests a liposarcoma.

Bronchogenic Carcinoma

Several studies have confirmed the poor predictive value of CT signs of pleural and chest wall involvement by primary lung cancer (44,45). The use of MRI scans offers theoretical advantages in the assessment of pleural and chest wall involvement. To date, its main use has been in the assessment of superior sulcus tumors.

Involvement of the visceral pleura indicates a T2 lesion, and parietal pleural involvement indicates a T3 lesion. Pleural involvement does not contraindicate resection, but the presence of a malignant pleural effusion makes the tumor T4, which is unresectable (46).

D. Positron Emission Tomography

Positron emission tomography (PET) is a new-imaging modality that, unlike other modalities, provides physiological information. It utilizes a glucose analogue, most commonly 2-[^{18}F]fluoro-2-deoxy-d-glucose (FDG) to demonstrate increased glucose metabolism in malignant cells (47). Unlike glucose, FDG becomes metabolically trapped within cells; this property, along with the increased uptake, forms the basis for imaging malignant tumors (47,48). Initial studies in the chest were used to evaluate pulmonary nodules (49), but the technique has great potential benefit in differentiating recurrent carcinoma from posttherapeutic fibrosis. Patz et al. (50) have recently demonstrated increased FDG activity in the pleura of patients with a diagnosis of recurrent malignancy (Fig. 6).

The great potential benefits of PET imaging are currently limited by accessibility and cost.

V. Diffuse Pleural Diseases

The definition of diffuse pleural thickening is arbitrary and controversial. The International Labor Office (ILO) classification of pneumoconiosis was designed as an epidemiological tool and not for diagnosis. It divides the asbestos-related

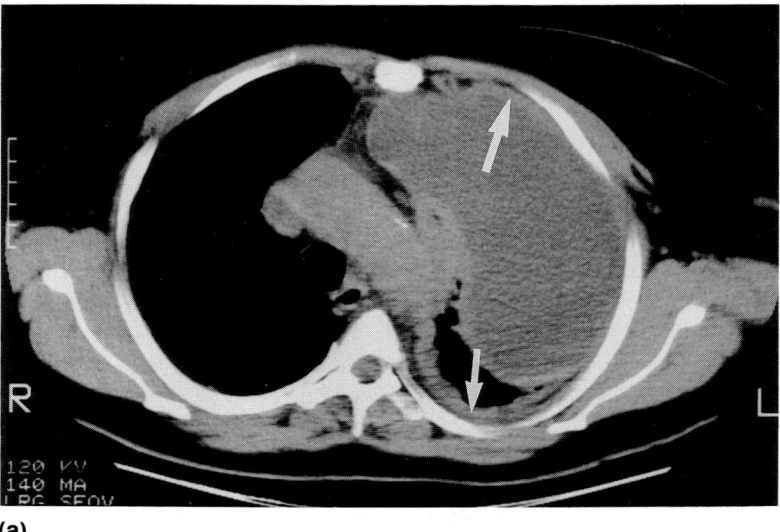

(a)

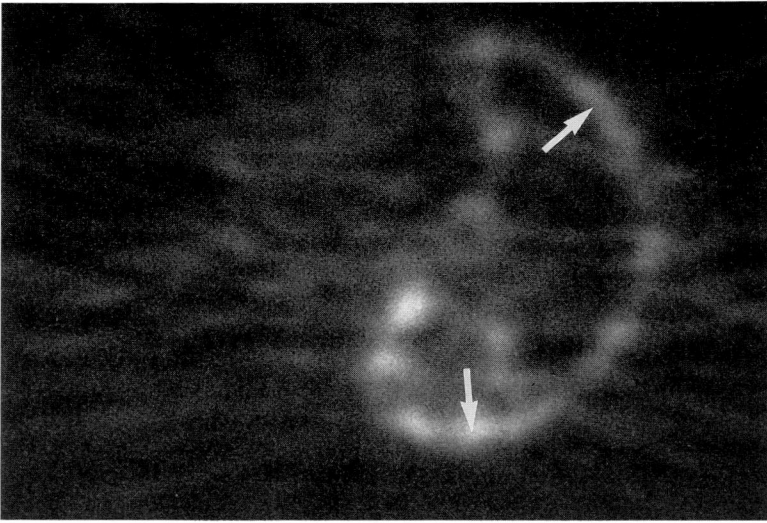

(b)

Figure 6 (a) A CT scan through the upper chest demonstrates pleural thickening (arrows) associated with pleural fluid. (b) A PET scan at the same level shows increased uptake in the pleura (arrows), strongly suggestive of malignant pleural disease.

pleural disease into circumscribed plaques and diffuse thickening, but criteria to distinguish these two forms of pleural disease are not specified.

McLoud and co-workers (51) have defined *diffuse pleural thickening* radiographically as smooth uninterrupted pleural opacity extending over at least one-fourth of the chest wall, with or without obliteration of the costophrenic angles.

Lynch et al. (52) have defined the CT criteria as thickening greater than 3 mm that extends more than 8 cm craniocaudally and 5 cm laterally.

The most common causes of diffuse pleural thickening are diffuse pleural fibrosis, mediastinal and pleural lipomatosis, metastatic carcinoma, and mesothelioma.

A. Diffuse Pleural Fibrosis

Fibrothorax is the fibrous obliteration of the pleural space usually secondary to empyema (including tuberculosis), pleural hemorrhage, and benign asbestos-related pleurisy. The diffuse changes of asbestos can be secondary to an exudative effusion or to confluent plaques.

Assessment of the underlying parenchyma for evidence of postinflammatory changes can suggest a cause for the pleural findings. The presence of heavy calcification in pleura is common in tubercular fibrothorax and hemothorax. Bilateral changes are suggestive of asbestos-related changes.

Bilateral disease is important to recognize because of the restrictive influence on pulmonary function (53,54). A CT scan can aid assessment by clearly displaying the extent of pleural change, differentiating it from subpleural fat, and assessing the underlying lung for fibrosis.

B. Mesothelioma

Malignant mesothelioma is strongly associated with asbestos exposure, with a latency period of 35 years (55). Only 20% of patients with mesothelioma will not have an exposure history.

The histology of the tumor can make its diagnosis difficult. It may be epithelial, mesenchymal (sarcomatous), or mixed (56). The epithelial and mixed tumors resemble adenocarcinoma, and the sarcomatous lesions can be mistaken for a postinflammatory fibrothorax.

The classic radiology findings are unilateral, nodular thickening of the pleural, with a pleural effusion. The mediastinum is midline or shifted to the ipsilateral side.

Computed tomography is superior in the assessment of suspected mesothelioma (57). The CT findings include pleural thickening, thickening of the interlobular fissures, pleural effusion, loss of volume of the hemithorax, invasion of the chest wall (Fig. 7), and lymphadenopathy. Despite its superiority to CXR,

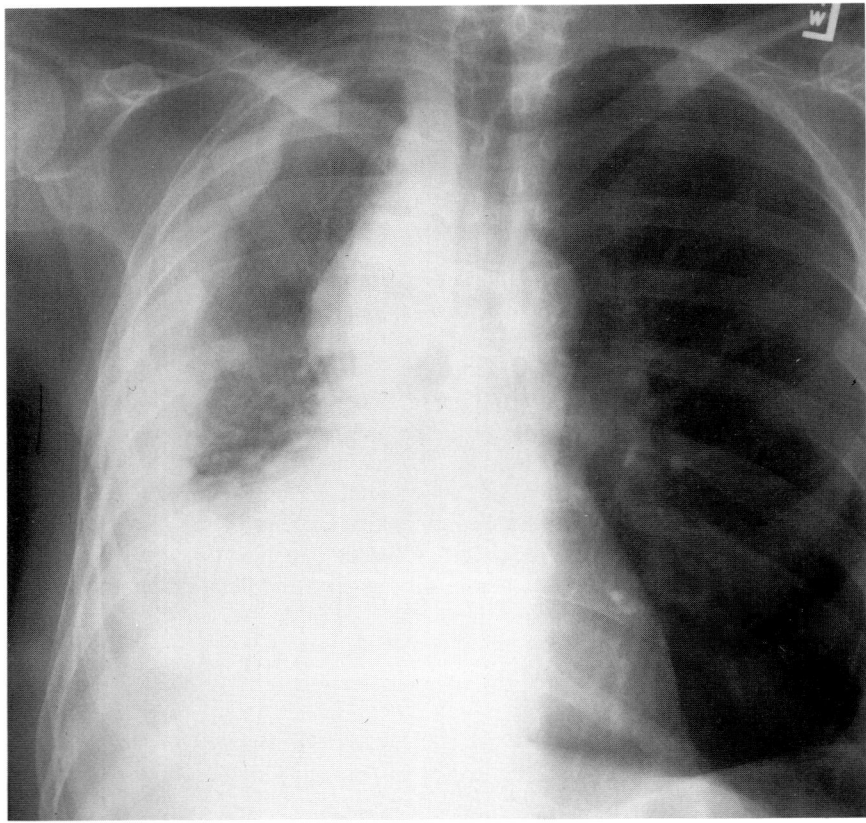

(a)

Figure 7 Mesothelioma: (a) Frontal CXR demonstrates pleural thickening on the right side that is lobulated and circumferential. (b) A CT section at the level of the aortic arch confirms the extensive distribution of the lobulated pleural thickening, which is of soft-tissue attenuation. The CT scan also demonstrates extension through the chest wall posteriorly (arrow).

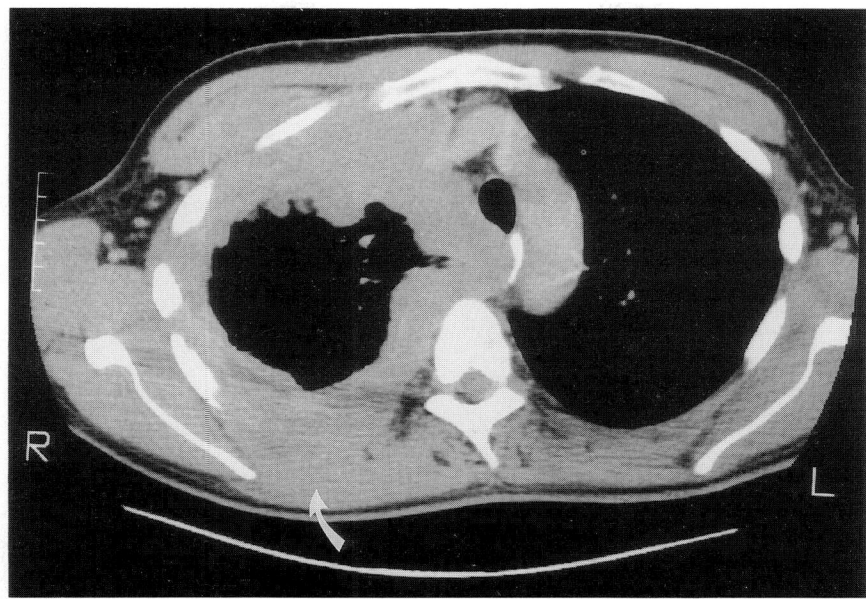
(b)

surgical series have shown that CT underestimates the extent of disease (58). Its preoperative value is in identifying patients with unequivocal evidence of unresectable disease, such as chest wall or mediastinal extension, involvement of the contralateral lung, or gross lymphadenopathy (59).

C. Pleural Metastases

Metastatic disease is a common cause of pleural disease, especially in the older-aged group (60). Adenocarcinoma, lymphoma, and malignant thymoma are neoplasms that tend to spread to the pleura. Pleural effusion is often the only sign of metastases, but focal masses and extensive pleural thickening, similar to mesothelioma are frequently seen.

D. Lymphoma

Hodgkin's lymphoma and non-Hodgkin's lymphomas usually produce small effusions if there is pleural involvement (61). However, direct involvement can produce changes similar to mesothelioma and metastases. This is usually seen in association with extensive lymphadenopathy or in recurrence of a known lymphoma.

VI. Role of Imaging in Diffuse Pleural Thickening

The differentiation of malignant from benign disease is often difficult on the basis of clinical findings and pleural biopsy. Even thoracotomy can fail to establish the diagnosis. Ryan et al. (62) reported a series in which 25% of 51 patients had a delay of diagnosis following thoracotomy, ranging between 12 days and 5 years.

Computed tomography can play a role in distinguishing malignant from benign pleural disease. Leung and co-workers (63) identified circumferential pleural thickening, nodular pleural thickening, parietal pleural thickening of more than 1 cm, and mediastinal pleural involvement as features helpful in separating thickening caused by mesothelioma and metastatic pleural disease from benign disease.

This correlates well with the pathological finding that malignant pleural disease tends to involve the entire pleural surface. Reactive pleurisy usually does not involve the mediastinal pleura.

The ability of CT to demonstrate the distribution of disease is an aid to the surgeon contemplating video-assisted thoracoscopy (VAT). Preoperative planning is important in VAT to ensure that abnormal areas are assessed, and CT's ability to depict anatomical relations can be a valuable asset.

References

1. Sahn SA. The pleura. Am Rev Respir Dis 1988; 138:184–234.
2. Pistolesi M, Miniati M, Giuntini C. Pleural liquid and solute exchange. Am Rev Respir Dis 1989; 140:825–847.
3. Müller NL. Imaging of the pleura. Radiology 1993; 186:297–309.
4. Heitzman ER, Raash BN. Diseases of the pleura. In: Groskin SA, ed. The lung, radiologic–pathologic correlation. 3rd ed., St. Louis: Mosby Year Book, 1993: 575–614.
5. Light RN, Girard WM, Jenkinson SG, George RB. Parapneumonic effusions. Am J Med 1980; 69:985–986.
6. Light RN, Pleural diseases. Philadelphia: Lea & Febiger, 1990:39–73.
7. Collins JD, Burwell D, Furmanski S, Lorber P, Steckel RJ. Minimal detectable pleural effusions. Radiology 1972; 105:51–53.
8. Moskowitz H, Platt RT, Schachar R, Mellins H. Roentgen visualization of minute pleural effusion. Radiology 1973; 109:33–35.
9. Hessen I. The localization of fluid in the free pleura. Acta Radiol 1951; 86:1–68.
10. Bryk D. Infrapulmonary effusion: effect of expiration on the pseudodiaphragmatic contour. Radiology 1976; 120:33–36.
11. Hessen I. Roentgen examination of pleural fluid. A study of the localization of free effusions. The potentialities of diagnosing minimal quantities of fluid and its existence under physiologic conditions. Acta Radiol [Suppl] 1951; 86.

12. Ruskin JA, Gurney JW, Thorsen MK, Goodman LR. Detection of pleural effusions on supine chest radiographs. AJR 1987; 148:681–683.
13. Woodring JH. Recognition of pleural effusion on supine radiographs: how much fluid is required? AJR 1984; 142:59–64.
14. Dandy WE. Incomplete pulmonary interlobar fissure sign. Radiology 1978; 128:21–25.
15. Aquino SL, Webb WR, Gushiken BJ. Pleural exudate and transudates: diagnosis with contrast-enhanced CT. Radiology 1994; 192:803–808.
16. Halvorsen RA, Fedyshin PJ, Korobkin M, Foster WL, Thompson WM. Ascites or pleural effusion? CT differentiation: four useful criteria. Radiographics 1986; 6:135–149.
17. Teplick JG, Teplick SK, Goodman L, Haskin ME. The interface sign: a computed tomographic sign for distinguishing pleural and intra-abdominal fluid. Radiology 1982; 144:359–362.
18. Griffin DJ, Gross BH, McCracken S, Glazer GM. Observations on CT differentiation of pleural and peritoneal fluid. J Comput Assist Tomogr 1984; 8:24–28.
19. Merriam MA, Cronan JJ, Dorfman GS, Lambiase RE, Haas RA. Radiographically guided percutaneous catheter drainage of pleural fluid collections. AJR 1988; 151:1113–1116.
20. Yang PC, Luh KT, Chang DB, Wu HD, Yu CJ, Kuo SH. Value of sonography in determining the nature of pleural effusion: analysis of 320 cases. AJR 1992; 159:29–33.
21. O'Moore PV, Mueller PR, Simeone JF, Saini S, Butch RJ, Hahn PF, Steiner E, Stark DD, Ferrucci JT. Sonographic guidance in diagnostic and therapeutic interventions in the pleural space. AJR 1987; 149:1–5.
22. Davis SD. MR imaging of pleural effusion. J Comput Assist Tomogr 1990; 14:192–198.
23. McLoud TC, Flower CDR. Imaging the pleura: sonography, CT, and MR imaging. AJR 1991; 156:1145–1153.
24. Strange C, Sahn SA. Management of parapneumonic pleural effusions and empyema. Infect Dis Clin North Am 1991; 5:539–557.
25. Hanna JW, Reed JC, Choplin RH. Pleural infections: a clinical–radiologic review. J Thorac Imaging 1991; 6:68–79.
26. Friedman PJ, Hellekant CAG. Radiologic recognition of bronchopleural fistula. Radiology 1977; 124:289–295.
27. Stark DD, Federle MP, Goodman PG, Podrasky AE, Webb WR. Differentiating lung abscess from empyema—radiography and computed tomography. AJR 1983; 141:163–167.
28. Baber CE, Hedlund LW, Oddson TA, Putman CE. Differentiating empyemas and peripheral pulmonary abscesses: the value of computed tomography. Radiology 1980; 135:755–758.
29. Silverman SG, Mueller PR, Saini S, Hahn PF, Simeone JF, Forman BH, Steiner E, Ferrucci JT. Thoracic empyema: management with image-guided catheter drainage. Radiology 1988; 169:5–9.
30. Westcott JL. Percutaneous catheter drainage of pleural effusion and empyema. AJR 1985; 144:1189–1193.

31. Neff CC, vanSonnenberg E, Lawson DW, Patton AS. CT follow-up of empyemas: pleural peels resolve after percutaneous catheter drainage. Radiology 1990; 176: 195–197.
32. Schwartz DA. New developments in asbestos-related pleural disease. Chest 1991; 99:191–198.
33. Rockoff SD, Kagan E, Schwartz A, Kriebel D, Hix W, Rohatgi P. Visceral pleural thickening in asbestos exposure: the occurrence and implications of thickened interlobar fissures. J Thorac Imaging 1987; 2:58–66.
34. Gefter WB, Conant EF. Issues and controversies in the plain-film diagnosis of asbestos-related disorders in the chest. J Thorac Imaging 1988; 3:11–28.
35. Schwartz DA, Fuortes LJ, Galvin JR, et al. Asbestos-induced pleural fibrosis and impaired lung function. Am Rev Respir Dis 1990; 141:321–325.
36. Wain SL, Roggli VL, Foster WL. Parietal pleural plaques, asbestos bodies, and neoplasia: a clinical, pathologic, and roentgenographic correlation of 25 consecutive cases. Chest 1984; 86:707–713.
37. Hourihane DO, Lessof L, Richardson PC. Hyaline and calcified pleural plaques as an index of exposure to asbestos: a study of radiological and pathological features of 100 cases with a consideration of epidemiology. Br Med J 1966; 1:1069–1074.
38. Aberle DR, Gamsu G, Ray CS. High-resolution CT of benign asbestos-related diseases: clinical and radiographic correlation. AJR 1988; 151:883–891.
39. Im JG, Webb WR, Rosen A, Gamsu G. Costal pleura: appearance at high-resolution CT. Radiology 1989; 171:125–131.
40. Fraser RG, Paré JAP, Paré PD, Fraser RS, Genereux GP. Diagnosis of diseases of the chest. 3rd ed. Philadelphia: WB Saunders, 1991: 2712–2793.
41. England DM, Hochholzer L, McCarthy MJ. Localized benign and malignant fibrous tumors of the pleura: a clinicopathologic review of 223 cases. Am J Surg Pathol 1989; 13:640–658.
42. Mendelson DS, Meary E, Buy JN, Pigeau I, Kirschner PA. Localized fibrous pleural mesothelioma: CT findings. Clin Imaging 1991; 15:105–108.
43. Buxton RC, Tan CS, Khine NM, Cuasay NS, Shor MJ, Spigos DG. Atypical transmural thoracic lipoma: CT diagnosis. J Comput Assist Tomogr 1988; 12:196–198.
44. Glazer HS, Duncan-Meyer J, Aronberg DJ, Moran JF, Levitt RG, Sagell SS. Pleural and chest wall invasion in bronchogenic carcinoma: CT evaluation. Radiology 1985; 157:191–194.
45. Scott IR, Müller NL, Miller RR, Evans KG, Nelems B. Resectable stage II lung cancer: CT, surgical, and pathologic correlation. Radiology 1988; 166:75–79.
46. Mountain C. A new international staging system for lung cancer. Chest 1986; 89: 225–233.
47. Hawkins RA, Hoh CK, Glaspy F, et al. PET–FDG imaging in cancer. Appl Radiol 1992; May:51–57.
48. Nolop KB, Rhodes G, Brudin LH, et al. Glucose utilization in vivo by human pulmonary neoplasm. Cancer 1987; 60:2682–2689.
49. Gupta NC, Frank AR, Dewan NA, et al. Solitary pulmonary nodules: detection of malignancy with PET with 2[F-18]-fluoro-2-deoxy-d-glucose. Radiology 1992; 184:441–444.

50. Patz DF, Lowe VJ, Hoffman JM, Paine SS, Harris LK, Goodman PC. Persistent or recurrent bronchogenic carcinoma: detection with PET and 2 [F-18]-fluoro-2-deoxy-*d*-glucose. Radiology 1994; 191:379–382.
51. McLoud TC, Woods BO, Carrington CB, Epler GR, Gaensler EA. Diffuse pleural thickening in an asbestos-exposed population: prevalence and causes. AJR 1985; 144:9–18.
52. Lynch DA, Gamsu G, Aberle DR. Conventional and high resolution computed tomography in the diagnosis of asbestos-related diseases. Radiographics 1989; 9:523–551.
53. Jones RN, McLoud T, Rockoff SD. The radiographic pleural abnormalities in asbestos exposure: relationship to physiologic abnormalities. J Thorac Imaging 1988; 3:56–66.
54. Hillerdal G, Malmberg P, Hemmingsson A. Asbestos-related lesions of the pleura: parietal plaques compared to diffuse thickening studied with chest roentgenography, computed tomography, lung function, and gas exchange. Am J Ind Med 1990; 18:627–639.
55. Antman KH, Corson JM. Benign and malignant pleural mesothelioma. Clin Chest Med 1985; 6:127–140.
56. Mossman BT, Gee JBL. Asbestos-related diseases. N Engl J Med 1989; 320:1721–1730.
57. Kawashima A, Libshitz HI. Malignant pleural mesothelioma: CT manifestations in 50 cases. AJR 1990; 15:965–969.
58. Rusch VW, Godwin JD, Shuman WP. The role of computed tomography scanning in the initial assessment and the follow-up of malignant pleural mesothelioma. J Thorac Cardiovasc Surg 1988; 96:171–177.
59. Adams H, Butchar EG. Computed tomographic assessment of patients following radical surgery for malignant mesothelioma. Clin Radiol 1992; 45:120–124.
60. Mathay RA, Coppage L, Shaw C, Filderman AE. Malignancies metastatic to the pleura. Invest Radiol 1990; 25:601–619.
61. Sahn SA. Malignant pleural effusion. In: Fishman AP, ed. Pulmonary diseases and disorders. 2nd ed. New York: McGraw-Hill, 1988:2159–2169.
62. Ryan CJ, Rodgers RF, Unni KK, Hepper NGG. The outcome of patients with pleural effusion of indeterminate cause at thoracotomy. Mayo Clin Proc 1981; 56:145–149.
63. Leung AN, Müller NL, Miller RR. CT in differential diagnosis of diffuse pleural disease. AJR 1990; 154:87–492.

14

Thoracic Interventional Procedures

JEFFREY S. KLEIN
University of Vermont School of Medicine
Burlington, Vermont

I. Transthoracic Needle Biopsy

A. Introduction

The advent of imaging intensifiers and cross-sectional imaging with computed tomography (CT) and ultrasound has permitted the accurate detection and characterization of pulmonary, mediastinal, hilar, and pleural lesions. These imaging techniques, along with the design of small-gauge needles providing cytological and histological tissue specimens and the availability of cytopathological and immunocytochemical analysis of biopsy specimens, have supported the growth of imaging-guided transthoracic needle biopsy (TNB) for the diagnosis of localized thoracic disease.

B. Indications for Transthoracic Needle Biopsy

A TNB may be performed for any undiagnosed intrathoracic lesion (Table 1), providing the patient is cooperative and there is safe access to the lesion.

Table 1 Indications for Transthoracic Needle Biopsy

Solitary pulmonary nodule or mass
Mediastinal mass
Pleural mass or diffuse pleural thickening
Enlarged hilar lymph nodes/mass[a]
Diffuse pulmonary disease[a]

[a]Usually following negative bronchoscopic biopsy.

C. Contraindications to Transthoracic Needle Biopsy

The contraindications to TNB are all relative (Table 2), and most can be addressed before the procedure.

D. Preoperative Evaluation

Consent

Because most patients undergo TNB as outpatients, the referring physician provides a brief explanation of TNB after radiologic consultation and before scheduling the procedure. When obtaining informed consent from the patient for TNB, the radiologist details the procedure, gives an estimate of the benefits and risks, and discusses alternative methods of diagnosis.

Review of Imaging Studies

The radiologist should review the medical and surgical history and any pertinent chest radiographs, CT scans, or magnetic resonance imaging (MRI) scans before the procedure. The size, location, and appearance of the lesion will determine the

Table 2 Contraindications to Transthoracic Needle Biopsy

Coagulopathy
PT value >1.5 control
Platelet count <50,000/cm^3
Inability to cooperate (i.e., lie prone, suspend respiration)
Pulmonary hypertension
Single lung
Suspected arteriovenous malformation or aneurysm
Suspected echinococcal cyst
Severe obstructive lung disease
Inability to manage complications

imaging modality and the technique used for biopsy. Pulmonary nodules easily seen on both frontal and lateral radiographs are best sampled fluoroscopically, whereas lesions visualized on only a single view or those within or adjacent to the mediastinum or hilum usually require CT guidance. Ultrasound is most useful for biopsy of anterior mediastinal masses, pleural-based parenchymal masses, and pleural masses.

Preoperative Testing

A complete blood count and coagulation profile (prothrombin time [PT] and partial thromboplastin time [PTT]) are obtained within 1 week of the procedure, and any abnormalities are corrected before the biopsy. Measurement of blood urea nitrogen (BUN) and creatinine is performed immediately before biopsy if scans with intravenous contrast are required. Pulmonary function testing is not routinely obtained before TNB, although there is evidence that functional obstructive lung disease predicts a higher rate of TNB-related pneumothorax.

Patient Instructions

Patients undergoing TNB may eat a light breakfast on the morning of the procedure. Routine medications should be taken. Anticoagulants and antiplatelet agents (aspirin and other nonsteroidal anti-inflammatory agents) should be suspended for a minimum of 7 days before the procedure. Any patient with an intractable cough should receive oral antitussives containing codeine phosphate or dextromethorphan hydrobromide 1 hr before TNB.

Pathology Consultation

The case is discussed in advance with the pathologist who will handle the specimen, as this enables him or her to make a more accurate interpretation of the biopsy specimen. It is particularly important to indicate any previous biopsy or resection for malignancy, because comparison of the specimens allows a more specific diagnosis of metastatic disease. If lymphoma is a diagnostic consideration, tissue specimens are optimally placed into B5 fixative so that cell markers and immunocytochemistry can be performed. If an infectious granuloma is considered likely, special stains for acid-fast bacilli and fungus are obtained. If cytopathology is to be used at the time of biopsy, provisions are made for the cytopathologist to perform a fast stain and view the specimen on site.

E. Technical Considerations

Imaging Guidance

The choice in imaging guidance is individualized to the specific characteristics of the patient and lesion, the cost and availability of the various modalities, and the preference of the radiologist performing TNB. C-arm or biplane fluoroscopy is widely available and relatively inexpensive, and provides real-time capabilities during tissue sampling (1,2). Pulmonary or pleural-based lesions, easily visualized on orthogonal views, are best approached under fluoroscopic guidance. Computed tomography is most useful for small lesions seen on only a single radiographic view. It provides direct visualization of bullae, blood vessels, and bronchi, thereby allowing safe access to central pulmonary, mediastinal, and hilar masses (3,4; Fig. 1). An additional convenience of CT is that patients referred for

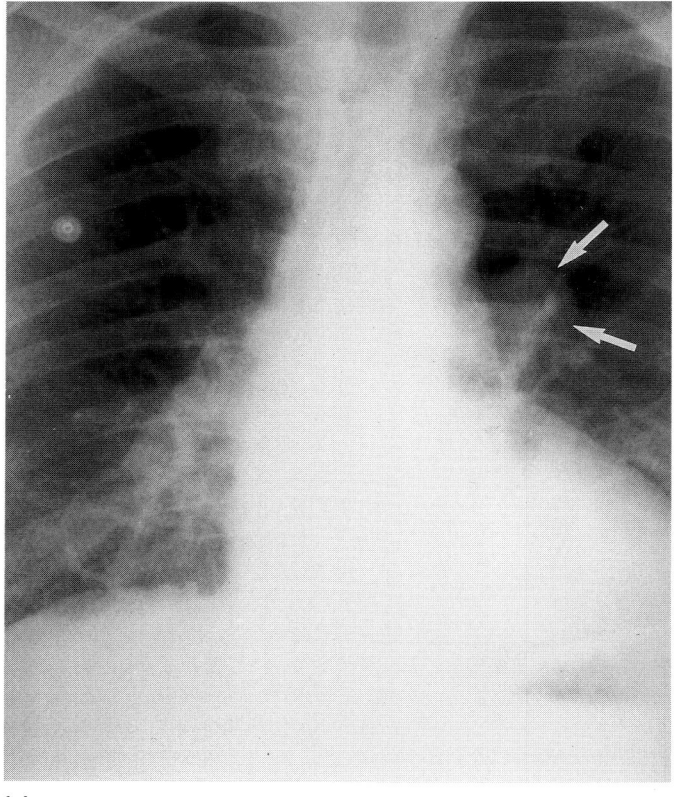

(a)

Figure 1 (a) Coned-down frontal radiograph shows a left hilar mass (arrows), which was not visible on the lateral film. (b) CT-guided biopsy, by a posterior approach with the patient prone, shows the biopsy needle at the edges of the lesion. Histological diagnosis was adenocarcinoma.

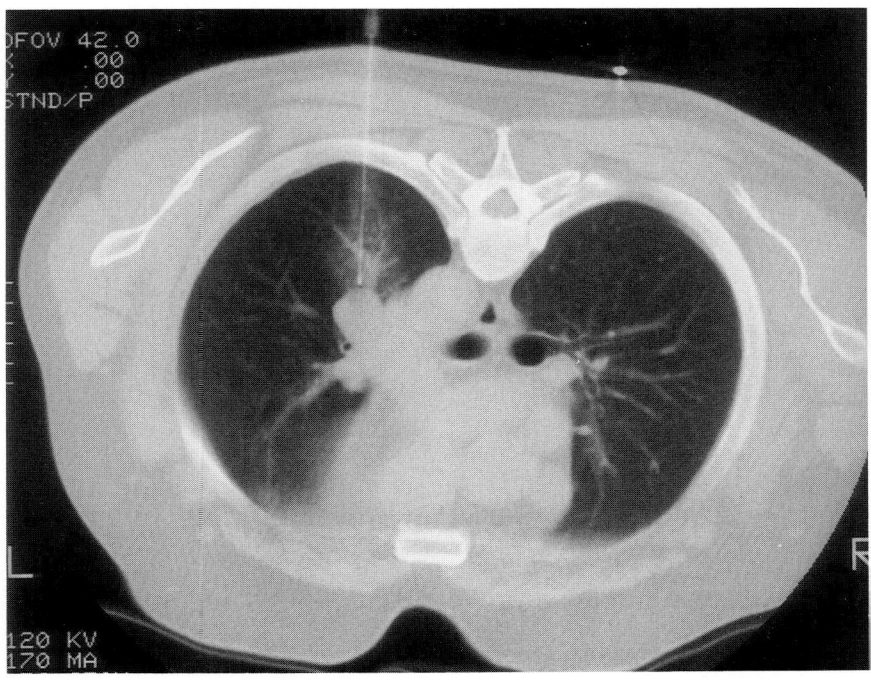
(b)

evaluation of a solitary pulmonary nodule can undergo CT-guided TNB immediately following indeterminate CT nodule densitometry. Ultrasound lacks ionizing radiation and provides real-time capabilities during tissue sampling. The usefulness of ultrasound is limited to lesions that provide an adequate acoustic window through the chest wall: anterior mediastinal masses that protrude laterally beyond the sternal margin or superiorly into the sternal notch, parenchymal masses with a broad area of contact against the pleural surface, and pleural masses (5). Ultrasound has proved useful in the biopsy of large peripheral lung masses by directing sampling toward viable tissue within the wall of the tumor and away from the necrotic center (6).

Needle Choices

A wide variety of biopsy needles is available for TNB. These needles are generally divided into fine-aspirating needles, used to obtain cytological specimens and material for stains and culture, and cutting needles, which routinely provide core specimens for histological examination. Most aspirating needles are 20- to 22-

gauge in diameter: these include the Chiba (Cook, Bloomington, IN), spinal, and Turner (Cook, Bloomington, IN) needles (7,8). When expert cytopathology is readily available, or when material for only stains or cultures is desired, aspiration biopsy will usually provide an adequate sample.

The most widely used cutting needles for TNB are disposable versions of the Tru-Cut needle that have been placed into a handle containing a spring-loaded mechanism that fires the inner side-notched stylet and outer cutting cannula in rapid succession at the press of a button (9). Recently, automated biopsy needles with an end hole cutting mechanism have been developed, but a reportedly high incidence of "zero" biopsies has precluded widespread use (10). The automated-cutting biopsy needles range from 14- to 20-gauge in diameter and include the ASAP gun (Meditech, Boston Scientific Co., Watertown, MA), Biopty gun (Bard, Covington, GA), and Temno needle (Bauer Medical, Clearwater, FL). These needles can routinely provide core biopsy specimens suitable for frozen section or paraffin-embedded histological examination, which may be particularly useful for the diagnosis of lymphoma and benign pulmonary lesions. Automated-cutting biopsy needles are generally reserved for large lesions, with a diameter exceeding the length of throw of the needle (usually 20–23 mm). They are routinely employed in the biopsy of pleural-based lung masses, mediastinal masses, and pleural tumors.

Biopsy Technique

The monitored patient is positioned on the biopsy table to allow the shortest vertical access to the lesion. If the patient is unable to lie comfortably in the optimal position, or if the lesion is inaccessible from a vertical approach, a nonvertical approach, with CT guidance, may be necessary. Intravenous analgesia and sedation are administered, as necessary, to reduce patient discomfort, but the patient should be able to follow commands to avoid inaccurate needle placement and to minimize complications.

To facilitate access to lesions near the anterior chest wall and lung apex, the CT gantry can be tilted in a craniocaudal or caudocranial direction to guide an oblique vertical approach (11). For anterior mediastinal masses that project beyond the lateral sternal margin, a parasternal approach, lateral to the internal mammary vessels and medial to the parietal pleura of the upper lobe, is best (12). A transsternal approach has been described for small anterior mediastinal masses that do not project far enough laterally to provide an extrapleural approach (13). Pleural fluid or air can provide an extrapleural access to mediastinal and medially situated lung masses, whereas a paravertebral approach, avoiding lung in the azygoesophageal recess, allows an extrapleural access to subcarinal masses (14; Fig. 2). An approach through consolidated or atelectatic lung that is distal to a central hilar or mediastinal mass should be used whenever possible, as an air leak

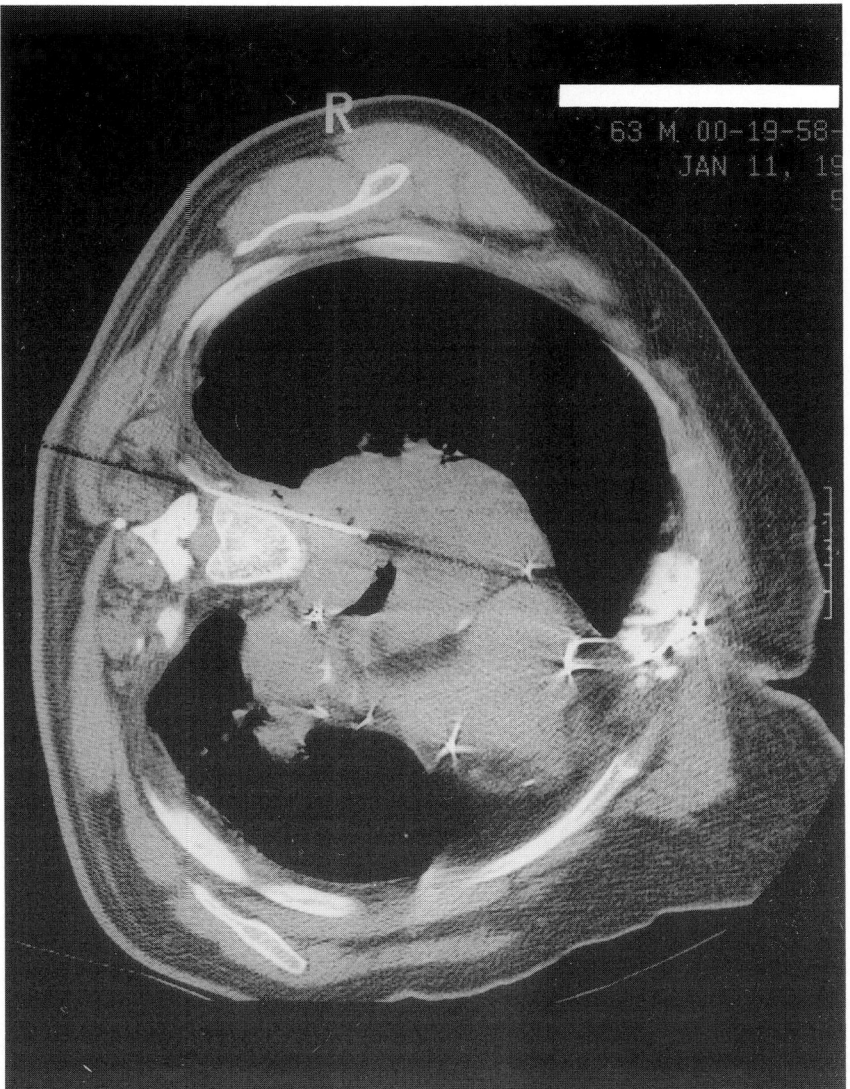

Figure 2 A CT-guided biopsy of a middle and posterior mediastinal mass through a paravertebral approach with the patient in the left lateral, decubitus position; 15 ml of lidocaine has been injected into the paravertebral space to provide a safe access to the lesion. Diagnosis was metastatic adenocarcinoma of lung.

(and resultant pneumothorax) will not develop following removal of the needle (15).

The chosen needle-entry site is marked with an indelible marker, and the skin is sterilely prepared and draped. Two percent lidocaine is used for local anesthesia to the level of the parietal pleura, and a small skin incision is made to ease the entry of the biopsy needle. A single-needle technique is effective for large pleural-based or mediastinal masses for which repeated passes are easily performed without transversing the visceral pleura. For small parenchymal lesions that are difficult to access, or when multiple samples are required, a coaxial technique should be used. This technique involves the initial placement of a needle over the superior margin of the rib and through the pleura to the edge of the lesion while the patient suspends respiration. Once the proper position of the guide needle is confirmed by lateral fluoroscopy, fine-collimation CT scan, or real-time ultrasound using a needle guide or biopsy transducer, a longer biopsy needle is placed through the lumen of the guide needle and into the lesion to provide a

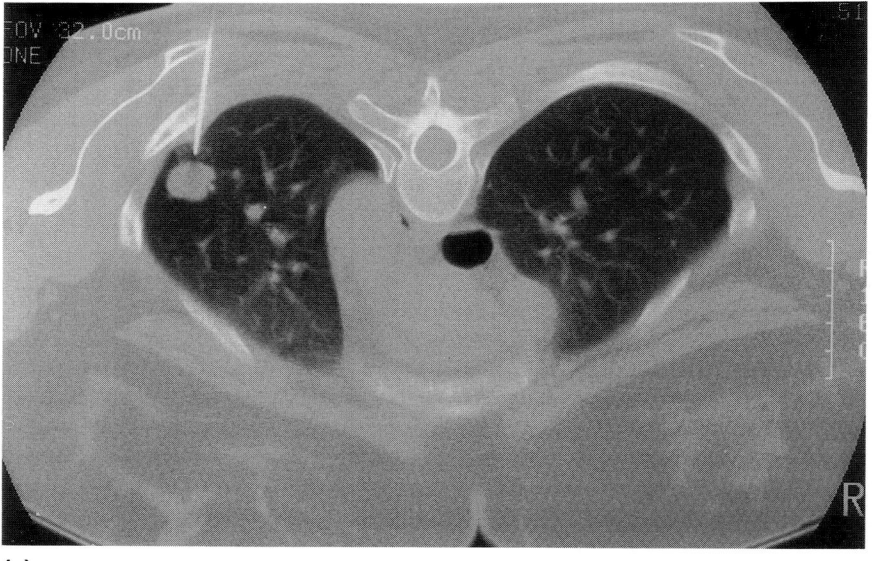

(a)

Figure 3 (a) A CT guided biopsy of a left upper lobe nodule with a 20-gauge, automated, core biopsy needle placed coaxially. The 19-gauge needle guide is seen at the edge of the nodule. (b) Photomicrograph (100×) of the core biopsy specimen shows central necrosis on the left, with lymphohistiocytic infiltrate and multinucleated giant cells (arrows) on the right, consistent with a granuloma.

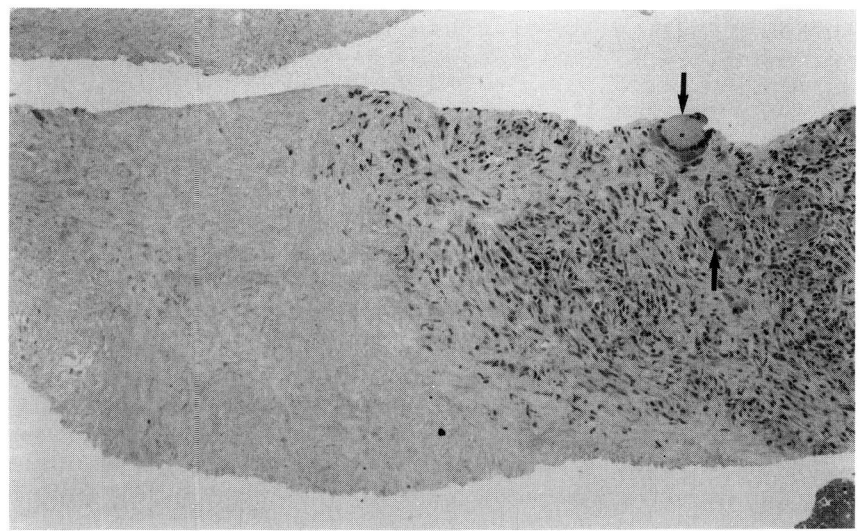

(b)

specimen. The coaxial technique allows repeated sampling of the lesion with either aspiration or cutting needles, thereby providing multiple cytological or histological specimens following a single pleural puncture. An aspirate for cytopathology or microbiological stains and cultures is obtained with a 20- or 22-gauge needle and attached syringe by piercing the lesion with a rapid repetitive up-and-down and rotary motion. Specimens for histological examination are reliably obtained with automated-cutting biopsy needles. Core tissue biopsy for histological examination is most useful in the diagnosis of lymphoma, malignant mesothelioma, and benign pulmonary lesions, such as granuloma and hamartoma (16,17; Fig. 3).

Specimen Handling

Aspirated specimens are expressed onto glass slides for immediate fixation in alcohol. An on-site cytopathologist then performs a fast stain with toluidine blue and examines the slide microscopically. A confident diagnosis of malignancy precludes further needle passes and indicates that the biopsy is complete. If additional material for repeat cytological examination or stains and cultures is necessary, a repeat aspiration is performed. If immediate cytopathological examination is unavailable, several aspirates are best obtained. When a core tissue biopsy is obtained with an automated-cutting needle, a saline-filled syringe and

25-gauge needle are used to produce a high-velocity saline stream and dislodge the tissue specimen from the slotted receptacle of the biopsy needle into the formalin (18). This technique avoids immersing the biopsy needle in formalin, thereby allowing repeated core biopsy with the same needle.

F. Postbiopsy Management

After the biopsy is completed, an assessment for pneumothorax is made by cross-table fluoroscopy, or by a single CT scan through the thorax. The biopsy needle is removed and the patient is immediately rolled from the biopsy table onto a gurney, with the biopsy site in a dependent position. A large or symptomatic pneumothorax is treated by immediate catheter drainage. If a small or asymptomatic pneumothorax is present, an expiratory upright anteroposterior (AP) radiograph is obtained to serve as a baseline for follow-up radiographs. Repeat radiographs are routinely obtained at 2 and 4 hr after biopsy. Patients with no pneumothorax, or those with a stable and asymptomatic pneumothorax, may be safely discharged home after 4 hr. Any patient found to have an enlarging or symptomatic pneumothorax proceeds to fluoroscopic drainage with an 8-French catheter. Once the air has been manually aspirated, the catheter is attached to a Heimlich valve or a three-chamber suction device, such as the Pleur-evac (Dek-natel, Fall River, MA).

G. Complications

A TNB-related pneumothorax occurs in 0–60% of cases (3,19), with most series reporting an incidence of 5–30% (20,21). Chest tube drainage is necessary in 0–15% of biopsies (22–24). Factors most often associated with an increased incidence of TNB-related pneumothorax include obstructive airway disease (25,26), intractable coughing, increased depth of the lesion (27), decreased size of lesion, the use of cutting needles or biopsy guns for core biopsy (28), multiple pleural punctures, increased duration of the procedure, cavitary lesions, and positive-pressure ventilation. The CT-guided procedures are associated with a relatively high pneumothorax rate, likely related to a long procedure time and the selection of small, deeply situated lesions.

There are several technical considerations during biopsy that may help reduce the incidence of TNB-related pneumothorax and the need for pneumothorax drainage. Subpleural bullae or cysts that lie along the anticipated needle path are most easily avoided by using CT guidance. A coaxial technique can provide a conduit for multiple aspiration or core biopsies following a single pleural puncture (29). The use of available extrapleural or transpleural routes avoids visceral pleural puncture and negates pneumothorax, and a needle pathway, coursing through airless lung toward a central mass, is associated with a 0% incidence of pneumothorax (15).

Two techniques have been described that attempt to diminish air leak from the puncture site following TNB, thereby reducing the incidence of pneumothorax and the need for chest tube insertion. The first involves the injection of an autologous blood clot through the guide needle of a coaxial system to help seal the pleural puncture site when the needle is withdrawn from the lung. Although recent retrospective and prospective studies suggest that the blood patch technique is of limited value in reducing air leak (30,31), several investigators have described the successful embolization of biopsy tracts using cyanoacrylate or collagen plugs (32,33). The second postprocedural technique involves immediate placement of the biopsy site in a dependent position following withdrawal of the biopsy needle (34–36). This maneuver theoretically diminishes alveolar volume adjacent to the puncture site and raises intrapleural pressure, thereby reducing air leak and the need for chest tube insertion for an enlarging pneumothorax (37). An additional advantage of dependent positioning is the prevention of transbronchial spread of any parenchymal hemorrhage complicating TNB.

The reported incidence of biopsy-induced hemorrhage ranges from 0–10%, and hemoptysis occurs in fewer than 5% of all patients (19–24; Fig. 4). The incidence of hemorrhage is higher for vascular lesions, including renal cell carcinoma, in patients with a bleeding diathesis, in those with pulmonary arterial or pulmonary venous hypertension, and when larger cutting needles are used to obtain histological specimens. Needle placement over the superior margin of the rib will prevent pleural or extrapleural bleeding from injury to the intercostal vessels (38). Similarly, biopsy of anterior mediastinal masses using a parasternal approach must avoid the internal mammary vessels, which are easily visualized by CT and lie approximately 1.25-cm lateral to the lateral sternal margin (39). Parenchymal hemorrhage is virtually always self-limiting, and is treated supportively by placing the biopsy side dependent to avoid aspiration of blood into normal lung.

Systemic air embolism is a rare complication of TNB. The mechanism is presumed to be air entry into a pulmonary vein, either directly through a needle open to the atmosphere or from a broncho- or alveolovenous fistula induced during needle placement (40). Maneuvers that increase airway pressure, including coughing and positive-pressure ventilation, increase the likelihood of air embolism. Systemic air embolism can lead to myocardial infarction, stroke, or death (41). Once the symptoms of air embolism are recognized, the patient should be placed in the left lateral decubitus position or Trendelenberg position to prevent any residual air within the left atrium from embolizing systemically. Blood pressure and ventilatory support must be provided, and 100% oxygen administered to promote the resorption of air bubbles. Immediate transfer to a hyperbaric unit may be necessary.

Seeding of biopsy tract and pleural space is a reported complication of TNB

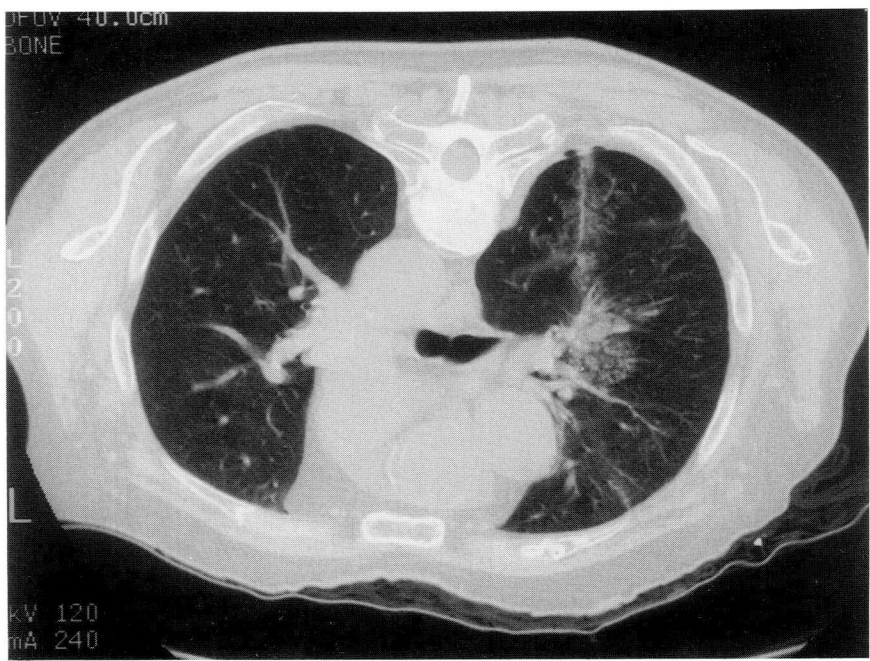

Figure 4 A CT scan after needle biopsy of a left upper lobe nodule by a posterior approach shows parenchymal hemorrhage in the parahilar portion of the upper lobe and superior segment of the lower lobe.

(42), although the results of several large series, using fine (< 20-gauge) needles, suggest that this is extremely rare and should not preclude the performance of TNB for diagnostic purposes.

H. Results

Several large series report overall yields for imaging-guided TNB of 85–97% (20–22, 43–45). The use of fine (20- to 22-gauge) aspiration needles and expert cytopathological technique has proved particularly useful in the diagnosis of intrathoracic malignancy, with sensitivities of 95–97% (20–22). The ability to accurately determine a specific cell type of bronchogenic carcinoma can be difficult in poorly differentiated tumors and is possible in approximately two-thirds of cases (46). However, the main factor determining treatment is the differentiation of small-cell and non–small-cell carcinoma, a distinction that is accurately made in the vast majority of cases. The diagnosis of intrathoracic lymphoma by TNB is somewhat more difficult, with yields of 60–75% by cytological examination (12,47). The diagnosis of lymphoma, and its distinction from thymoma, usually requires cutting biopsy for histological examination and immunohistochemical analysis of specimens.

Although the sensitivity of TNB for malignancy is high, the ability to obtain a specific benign diagnosis is lower, ranging from 16 to 68% (20–22, 44, 48, 49). The ability to provide a specific, benign diagnosis (e.g., granuloma, hamartoma, or abscess) and exclude malignancy can reduce the number of negative thoracotomies by as much as 55% (50). The key to increasing the yield for benign lesions is expert technique, with repeat sampling or biopsy if necessary, expert cytopathology, obtaining aspirates for microbiological stains and cultures, and the use of cutting needles to obtain histological specimens.

Transthoracic needle biopsy is useful in the diagnosis of focal pneumonitis and lung abscess in both normal and immunocompromised hosts, with reported yields of 73–94% (51,52). It not only provides diagnostic material in most patients with lung abscess, but the results of bacterial cultures can lead to an alteration in antibiotic therapy in approximately 50% of these patients (53).

II. Thoracic Drainage Procedures

A. Introduction

Imaging-guided percutaneous drainage of intrathoracic collections has developed as an extension of similar procedures in the abdomen and pelvis. The ability of CT and ultrasound to accurately detect and characterize parenchymal and pleural collections and advances in interventional techniques and catheter design have made percutaneous catheter drainage the treatment of choice for a variety of intrathoracic collections.

B. Pleural Drainage Procedures

Empyema–Complicated Parapneumonic Effusion

Infected pleural fluid collections may complicate pneumonia, chest trauma, or surgery; vertebral or chest wall infection; or develop from superinfection of a sterile pleural effusion (54). Approximately 40% of community-acquired pneumonias are associated with a parapneumonic pleural effusion (55), which most often resolves with therapy directed at the underlying infection. Those parapneumonic effusions that require drainage for definitive treatment are recognized by the presence of fluid with pH lower than 7.20, glucose values lower than 40 mg/dl, and lactate dehydrogenase (LDH) values higher than 200 IU ("complicated" parapneumonic effusion); or the identification of microorganisms of fluid Gram stain or culture, or the presence of frank pus (empyema) (55).

When physical examination suggests the presence of a parapneumonic effusion, decubitus chest radiographs should be obtained to assess for free-flowing or loculated collections. Computed tomography and ultrasound are used as adjuncts to the radiographs and accurately determine the extent of pleural disease and help guide diagnostic thoracentesis and drainage.

Infected pleural collections amenable to imaging-guided percutaneous catheter drainage include collections in patients with a short duration of symptoms, free-flowing or unilocular effusions, fluid that is easily aspirated by needle, and collections lacking a thick pleural peel on CT scan. Imaging guidance for free-flowing or peripherally loculated collections is best provided with ultrasound (56); CT is useful is characterizing complex pleural and parenchymal disease and provides direct visualization of the drainage tract.

A 10- or 12-French catheter provides adequate drainage of serous collections, whereas collections of thick, purulent or bloody material usually require

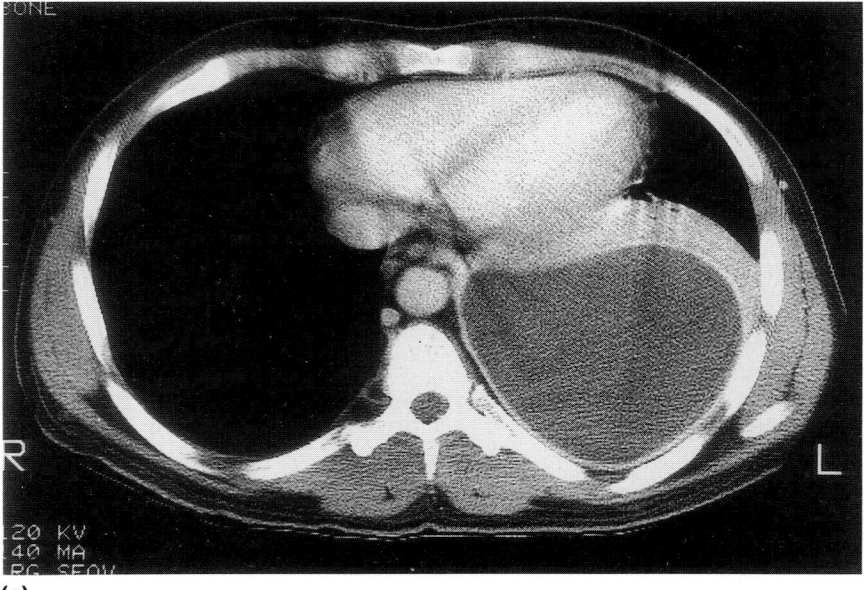

(a)

Figure 5 (a) Contrast-enhanced CT scan shows a large, loculated, left posterior pleural fluid collection with enhancing pleural surfaces, characteristic of an infected pleural collection. (b) Scan obtained following placement of a 12-French drainage catheter (arrows) with the patient in the right lateral decubitus position, and removal of 260 ml of purulent fluid shows complete evacuation of the collection (image rotated for comparison with panel a).

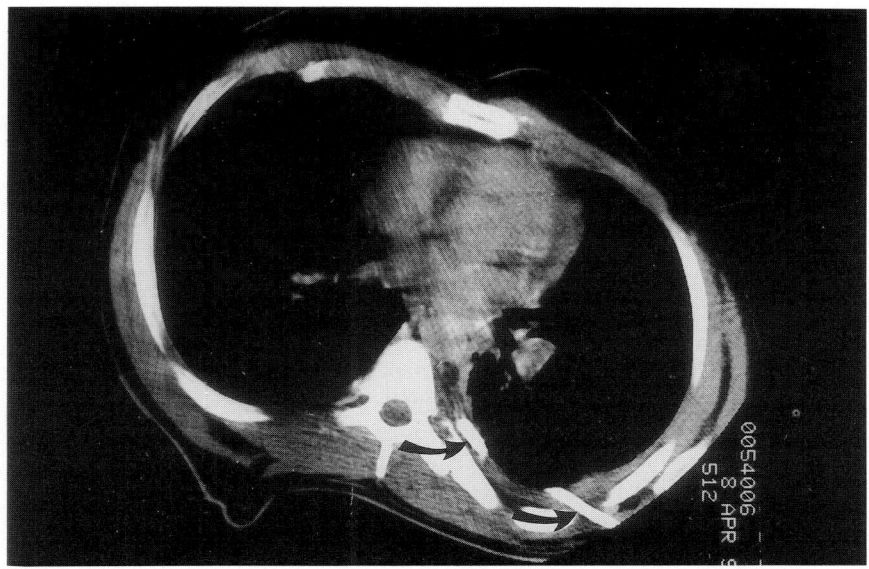
(b)

catheters of 12 to 28 French in diameter (57). Following placement of a diagnostic 18-gauge trocar needle into the thickest portion of the collection, fluid is aspirated and sent for Gram stain and culture. If purulent fluid is detected, or if there are microorganisms present, a drainage catheter is placed immediately. A floppy-tipped guidewire is placed through the needle and coiled in the collection and the tract is dilated in 2-French increments until the desired diameter is achieved. [ed.: Tract dilation is not necessary with hydrophilic catheter coating, allowing easier catheter insertion. (Glidex, Meditech, Boston Scientific Co., Watertown, MA).] The drainage catheter is then placed into the dependent portion of the collection and fluid is manually aspirated until resistance is encountered (Fig. 5). For large collections, a trocar technique may be used to place the catheter directly into the collection in tandem with the diagnostic needle. The patient is then reimaged to assess the adequacy of drainage, and additional catheters are placed as necessary. The catheter is attached to a Pleur-evac suction device (Deknatel, Inc., Fall River, MA).

The patency of the drainage catheter is maintained by twice-daily flushing of the catheter with saline. The response to drainage is assessed by monitoring fluid output, temperature, and peripheral white blood cell count. Chest radiographs or ultrasound examinations are obtained every other day to monitor progress. The catheter may be removed when output has diminished to less than 10 ml/day, there has been improvement in symptoms and signs of infection, and the collection has resolved radiographically. The average duration of catheter drainage is 5–10 days (58–60).

If pleural drainage is inadequate, despite proper catheter placement, a larger-diameter catheter may be necessary. New pleural locules will require additional catheters. In patients with collections containing multiple septations or loculations, fibrinolytic therapy with streptokinase or urokinase may be necessary to enhance drainage (61,62). The intrapleural administration of 80–100,000 units of urokinase, admixed in 100 ml saline and left dwelling in the pleural space for several hours, can aid in the management of loculated collections and can help avoid thoracoscopic or open-drainage procedures (63).

The success rate of imaging-guided catheter drainage of infected pleural collections is 72–88% (58–60), which compares favorably with the results from placement of large-bore surgical thoracostomy tubes (64,65). Although imaging-guided techniques are often successful at managing infected pleural fluid collections, patients that fail to respond rapidly to closed drainage should proceed to an open-drainage procedure for definitive treatment (66). Complications of imaging-guided pleural drainage are uncommon, but include bleeding from intercostal vessel injury, pneumothorax, and lung laceration.

Drainage and Sclerosis of Malignant Pleural Effusions

The term *malignant pleural effusion* refers to effusions associated with underlying malignancy that have either positive pleural fluid cytology or evidence of tumor infiltration on pleural biopsy. Most malignant pleural effusions are secondary to bronchogenic or breast carcinoma or lymphoma (67). Although some malignant effusions will respond to systemic therapy directed at the underlying malignancy, most will require tube drainage with sclerosis to prevent recurrence. Imaging-guided drainage with chemical pleurodesis, which can be accomplished with minimum patient discomfort, has become the initial treatment of choice for the management of malignant effusions. Alternative methods of treatment for malignant effusions include large-bore, closed thoracostomy tube placement, thoracoscopy with insufflation of talc poudrage, open pleural decortication, and pleuroperitoneal shunting (68,69).

As most malignant pleural effusions are large and free-flowing, ultrasound is used to guide catheter placement (70,71). With the patient sitting upright, an 8- or 10-French pigtail drainage catheter is placed through the posterior axillary line into the dependent portion of the collection, using a trocar technique. A quantity of fluid, not exceeding 1.5 L of fluid, is initially withdrawn to avoid the development of reexpansion pulmonary edema. Once affixed to the skin, the catheter is attached to a drainage system and -20 cmH_2O suction is applied to evacuate the pleural fluid.

Chemical pleurodesis with transcatheter sclerosing agents is usually possible within several days of catheter placement, when catheter output has diminished to less than 100 ml/24 hr, and the pleural effusion has resolved radiographically (72,73). The agents most often employed include doxycycline, minocycline, bleomycin, and talc (74–76). To perform pleurodesis, the sclerosing agent is admixed with lidocaine and administered at the bedside through the indwelling catheter. Once injected, the patient is rotated in an attempt to distribute the sclerosing agent throughout the pleural space. The catheter is then reattached to the drainage apparatus and suction applied to evacuate the sclerosing agent and appose the visceral and parietal pleural surfaces to achieve pleurodesis. The catheter is usually removed 24–48 hr later.

Successful catheter drainage and pleurodesis, defined as lack of reaccumulation of pleural fluid within 30 days, can be accomplished in 62–92% of patients (70,72,73,77). Complications of this technique are uncommon and include superinfection of pleural fluid, pneumothorax, intercostal artery laceration, and reexpansion pulmonary edema (70,77).

Pneumothorax

Pneumothorax may be traumatic or spontaneous in origin. Common causes of traumatic pneumothorax include blunt or penetrating chest trauma, central venous catheterization, and transbronchial and transthoracic needle biopsy. Asymptomatic patients with small or stable pneumothoraces are observed, whereas drainage is performed for large or symptomatic air collections.

Imaging-guided drainage is most often performed for pneumothorax complicating TNB, spontaneous pneumothorax, or loculated pleural air collections (78). Although simple catheter drainage will suffice for most patients with pneumothorax, patients with recurrent spontaneous pneumothorax or persistent bronchopleural fistula usually require additional therapeutic procedures, including chemical pleurodesis, thoracoscopy with talc poudrage, or bullectomy or stapling by thoracotomy (79–81).

Fluoroscopy is used to guide catheter placement for pneumothorax. Computed tomography may be used for pneumothorax complicating CT-guided procedures and to access loculated collections. There are several small-gauge (8- or 9-French) catheters available that are modified versions of catheters used for peripheral intravenous catheterization. With the patient in the supine position, an anterior approach through the second intercostal space in the midclavicular line is used. The catheter and inner hollow trocar, with attached syringe, are advanced through the chest wall in a cephalad direction over the third rib, with entry into the pleural space confirmed by the aspiration of air. The catheter–trocar combination is then advanced an additional centimeter to ensure intrapleural catheter position, and the catheter is advanced off the trocar and into the pleural apex (Fig. 6). The catheter is then affixed to the skin and the pneumothorax is manually aspirated

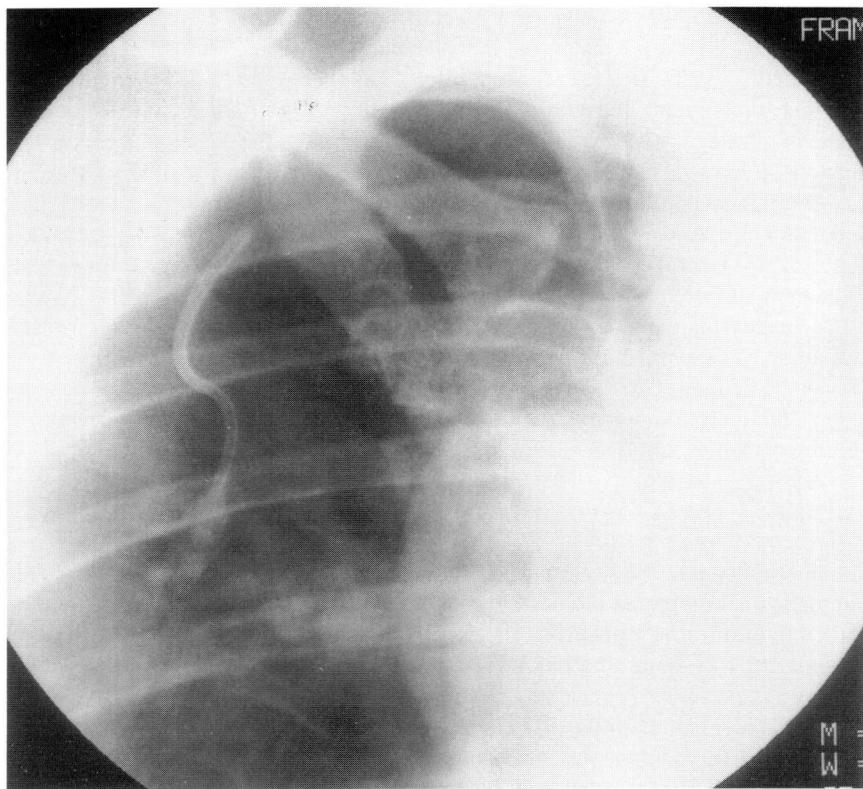

Figure 6 Spot film obtained following fluoroscopically guided drainage of a pneumothorax complicating CT-guided lung biopsy shows the drainage catheter curving over the right lung apex.

with a large syringe until resistance is encountered. The catheter is then attached with an adapter to an underwater seal device with suction (i.e., Pleur-evac) or to a flutter (Heimlich) valve.

The success of imaging-guided drainage of postbiopsy pneumothorax using small-bore catheters ranges from 87 to 93%, with a mean duration of pleural drainage of approximately 3 days (78,82,83). Failure of pneumothorax drainage may be secondary to catheter kinking or occlusion by blood or fibrin, inadvertent removal, or the presence of a large bronchopleural fistula (78,84). Wound infection, chest wall hematoma, and hemothorax may complicate catheter placement (85,86).

C. Parenchymal Drainage Procedures

Lung Abscess

Lung abscess is usually the result of aspiration of oropharyngeal bacteria in patients with altered levels of consciousness or defective swallowing mechanisms, but may result from endobronchial obstruction, superinfection of bullae or cysts, septic pulmonary embolus, or contiguous spread from a chest wall or vertebral osteomyelitis (87). The diagnosis is often first suggested on chest radiographs that show a round mass with central cavitation in a dependent portion of lung. Computed tomography scans are useful in patients with suspected lung abscess, as it provides superior characterization of the parenchymal process and allows differentiation of lung abscess from empyema with bronchopleural fistula.

The standard treatment of lung abscess is antibiotic therapy directed against the causative organisms, which are most often anaerobic bacteria. Conservative medical therapy is successful in 80–90% of patients (88). Those patients with persistent signs of sepsis, despite appropriate antibiotic therapy, failure of the abscess to resolve radiographically, or complicating features, including empyema, require more invasive methods of management. Although some patients will require resection for cure, closed drainage is a viable alternative mode of treatment in pleural-based abscesses and in patients who are poor operative candidates. Both surgical and imaging-guided thoracostomy tube drainage may be performed for treatment of lung abscess (89,90).

Catheter placement for lung abscess drainage is usually performed using CT or fluoroscopy, with sonography reserved for large, pleural-based abscesses (Fig. 7). The patient should be positioned with the abscess cavity down, to prevent soilage of the contralateral lung. A trocar-insertion technique at the point of contact between the abscess and pleural surface avoids traversing lung and is safely performed, because local pleural symphysis is invariably present. A relatively large-bore catheter (12-French or larger outer diameter) is necessary for adequate external drainage. Once the catheter is positioned dependently within the abscess cavity, the fluid is manually aspirated, and the drainage catheter is placed to underwater suction to evacuate residual pus and collapse the cavity.

The patient is assessed daily to assess response to therapy and to maintain catheter patency. When daily assessment by clinical parameters and chest radiographs indicate resolution of the abscess, the catheter is removed. A repeat CT scan is obtained when there is a lack of improvement, particularly if there is concern for a complicating bronchopleural fistula and empyema.

Successful imaging-guided percutaneous lung abscess drainage can be accomplished in nearly 100% of selected patients, with surgery avoided in 84% (90). The mean time to abscess resolution is approximately 10–15 days, although marked improvement in the clinical parameters of sepsis occurs within 48 hr of

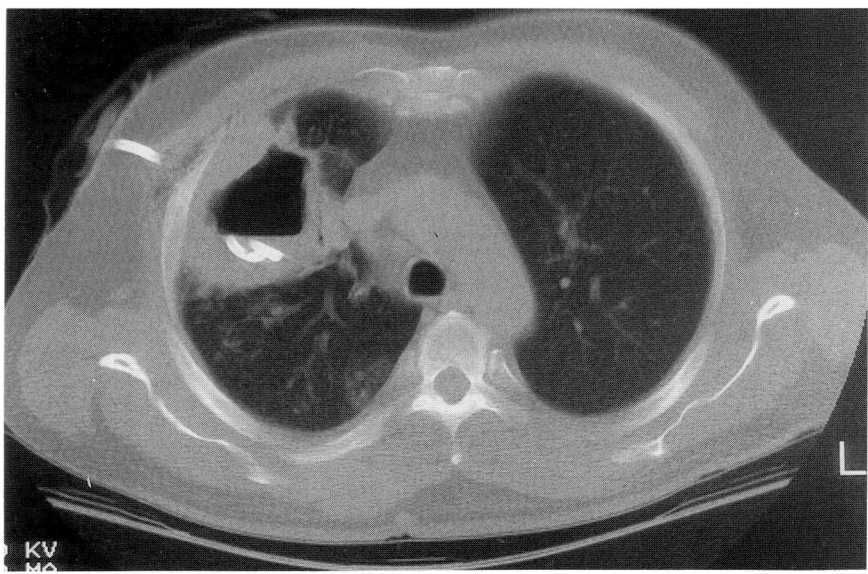

Figure 7 A 14-French pigtail drainage catheter has been placed into the dependent portion of a right upper lobe abscess, using CT guidance. Following aspiration of 40 ml of purulent fluid, a small amount of fluid remains in the cavity.

drainage (91). The complications of percutaneous abscess drainage are pneumothorax, bronchopleural fistula formation with empyema, and hemorrhage. The incidence of each of these complications is greater when normal lung is traversed by the drainage catheter.

References

1. Dahlgren SE, Nordenstrom B. Transthoracic needle biopsy. Chicago: Year Book Medical Publishing, 1966.
2. deGregorio Ariza MA, Alfonso Aguiran ER, Villavieja Atance JL, et al. Transthoracic aspiration biopsy of pulmonary mediastinal lesions. Eur J Radiol 1991; 12:98–103.
3. Fink I, Gamsu G, Harter L. CT-guided aspiration biopsy of the thorax. Comput Assist Tomogr 1982; 6:958–962.
4. Gardner D, vanSonnenberg E, D'Agostino HB, et al. CT-guided transthoracic needle biopsy. Cardiovasc Intervent Radiol 1991; 14:17–23.
5. Yang PC, Chang DB, Yu CJ, et al. Ultrasound-guided core biopsy of thoracic tumors. Am Rev Respir Dis 1992; 146:763–767.

6. Pan JF, Yang PC, Chang DB, et al. Needle aspiration biopsy of malignant lung masses with necrotic centers. Improved sensitivity with ultrasound guidance. Chest 1993; 103:1452–1456.
7. Gazelle GS, Haaga JR. Biopsy needle characteristics. Cardiovasc Intervent Radiol 1991; 14:13–16.
8. Yap J, Tan KP. A comparative study of the Chiba and Turner needles in percutaneous lung biopsy. Singapore Med 1988; 29:14–16.
9. Mladinich CR, Ackerman N, Berry CR, et al. Evaluation and comparison of automated biopsy devices: work in progress. Radiology 1992; 184:845–847.
10. Hopper KD, Adenroth CS, Sturtz KW, et al. CT percutaneous biopsy guns: comparison of end-cut and side-notch devices in cadaveric specimens. AJR 1995; 164: 195–199.
11. Stern EJ, Webb WR, Gamsu G. CT gantry tilt: utility in transthoracic fine-needle aspiration biopsy. Work in progress. Radiology 1993; 187:873–874.
12. Herman SJ, Holub RV, Weisbrod GL, Chamberlain DW. Anterior mediastinal masses utility of transthoracic needle biopsy. Radiology 1991; 180:167–170.
13. D'Agostino HB, Sanchez RB, Laoide RM, et al. Anterior mediastinal lesions: transsternal biopsy with CT guidance. Work in progress. Radiology 1993; 189:703–705.
14. Bressler EL, Kirkham JA, Mediastinal masses: alternative approaches to CT-guided needle biopsy. Radiology 1994; 191:391–396.
15. Haramati LB, Austin JHM. Complications after CT-guided needle biopsy through aerated versus nonaerated lung. Radiology 1991; 181:778.
16. Hamper UM, Khouri NF, Stitik FP, et al. Pulmonary hamartoma: diagnosis by transthoracic needle-aspiration biopsy. Radiology 1985; 155:15–18.
17. Goralnik CH, O'Connell DM, El Yousef SB, et al. CT-guided cutting-needle biopsies of selected chest lesions. AJR 1988; 151:903–907.
18. Wachsberg RH. The sticky biopsy specimen: a saline solution. AJR 1993; 161:1336–1337.
19. Tikkakoski T, Lohela P, Leppanen M, et al. Ultrasound-guided aspiration biopsy of anterior mediastinal masses. J Clin Ultrasound 1991; 19:209–214.
20. Stanley JH, Fish GD, Andriole JG, et al. Lung lesions: cytologic diagnosis by fine-needle biopsy. Radiology 1987; 162:389–391.
21. Westcott JL. Direct percutaneous needle aspiration of localized pulmonary lesions: results in 422 patients. Radiology 1980; 137:31–35.
22. Khouri NF, Stitik FP, Erozan YS, et al. Transthoracic needle aspiration biopsy of benign and malignant lung lesions. AJR 1985; 144:281–288.
23. Greene R, Szyfelbein WM, Isler RJ, et al. Supplementary tissue-core histology from fine-needle transthoracic aspiration biopsy. AJR 1985; 144:787–792.
24. Westcott JL. Percutaneous needle aspiration of hilar and mediastinal masses. Radiology 1981; 141:323–329.
25. Fish GD, Stanley JH, Miller KS, et al. Postbiopsy pneumothorax: estimating the risk by chest radiography and pulmonary function tests. AJR 1988; 150:71–74.
26. Miller KS, Fish GB, Stanley JH, et al. Prediction of pneumothorax rate in percutaneous needle aspiration in the lung. Chest 1988; 93:742–745.

27. Poe RH, Kallay MC, Wicks CM, et al. Predicting risk of pneumothorax in needle biopsy of the lung. Chest 1984; 85:232–235.
28. Parker SH, Hopper KD, Yakes WF, et al. Imaging-directed percutaneous biopsies with a biopsy gun. Radiology 1989; 171:663–669.
29. Moulton JS, Moore PT. Coaxial percutaneous biopsy technique with automated biopsy devices: value in improving accuracy and negative predictive value. Radiology 1993; 186:515–522.
30. Bourgouin PM, Shepard JO, McLoud TC, et al. Transthoracic needle aspiration biopsy: evaluation of the blood patch technique. Radiology 1988; 166:93–95.
31. Herman SJ, Weisbrod GL. Usefulness of the blood patch technique after transthoracic needle aspiration biopsy. Radiology 1990; 176:395–397.
32. Skupin A, Gomez F, Husain M, et al. Complications of transthoracic needle biopsy decreased with isobutyl 2-cyanoacrylate: a pilot study. Ann Thorac Surg 1987; 43:406–408.
33. Engeler CE, Hunter DW, Casteneda-Zuniga W, et al. Pneumothorax after lung biopsy: prevention with transpleural placement of compressed collagen foam plugs. Radiology 1992; 184:787–789.
34. Berger R, Smith D. Efficacy of the lateral decubitus position in preventing pneumothorax after needle biopsy of the lung. South Med J 1988; 81:1140–1143.
35. Moore EH, Shepard JO, McLoud TC, et al. Positional precautions in needle aspiration lung biopsy. Radiology 1990; 175:733–735.
36. Moore EH, LeBlanc J, Montesi SA, et al. Effects of patient positioning after needle aspiration lung biopsy. Radiology 1991; 181:385–387.
37. Zidulka A, Braidy TF, Rizzi MC, et al. Position may stop pneumothorax progression in dogs. Am Rev Respir Dis 1982; 126:51–53.
38. Milner LB, Ryan K, Gullo J. Fatal intrathoracic hemorrhage after percutaneous aspiration lung biopsy. AJR 1979; 132:280–281.
39. Glassberg RM, Sussman SK. Life-threatening hemorrhage due to percutaneous transthoracic intervention: importance of the internal mammary artery. AJR 1990; 154:47–49.
40. Aberle DR, Gamsu G, Golden JA. Fatal systemic arterial air embolism following lung needle aspiration. Radiology 1987; 165:351–353.
41. Tolly TL, Feldmeier JE, Czarnecki D. Air embolism complicating percutaneous lung biopsy. AJR 1988; 150:555–556.
42. Müller NL, Bergin CJ, Miller RR, et al. Seeding of malignant cells into the needle track after lung and pleural biopsy. J Can Assoc Radiol 1986; 37:192–194.
43. Nordenstrom B. Transthoracic needle biopsy. N Engl J Med 1967; 276:1081–1082.
44. Ikezoe J, Morimoto S, Kozuka T. Sonographically guided needle biopsy of thoracic lesions. Semin Intervent Radiol 1991; 8:15–22.
45. vanSonnenberg E, Casola G, Ho M, et al. Difficult thoracic lesions: CT-guided biopsy experience in 150 cases. Radiology 1988; 167:457–461.
46. Horrigan TP, Bergin KT. Correlation between needle biopsy of lung tumors and histopathologic analysis of resected specimens. Chest 1986; 90:638–640.
47. Wittich GR, Nowels KW, Korn RL, et al. Coaxial transthoracic fine-needle biopsy in patients with a history of malignant lymphoma. Radiology 1992; 183:175–178.

48. Calhoun P, Feldman PS, Armstrong P, et al. The clinical outcome of needle aspiration of the lung when lung cancer is not diagnosed. Ann Thorac Surg 1986; 41:592–596
49. Winning AJ, McIvor J, Seed WA, et al. Interpretation of negative results in fine needle aspiration of discrete pulmonary lesions. Thorax 1986; 41:875–879.
50. Linder J, Olsen GA, Johnston WW. Fine-needle aspiration biopsy of the mediastinum. Am J Med 1986; 81:1005–1008.
51. Castellino RA. Blank N. Etiologic diagnosis of focal pulmonary infection in immunocompromised patients by fluoroscopically guided percutaneous needle aspiration Radiology 1979; 132:563–567.
52. Yang PC, Luh KT, Lee YC, et al. Lung abscesses: ultrasound examination and US-guided transthoracic aspiration. Radiology 1991; 180:171–175.
53. Grinan NP, Lucena FM, Romero JV, et al. Yield of percutaneous needle lung aspiration in lung abscess. Chest 1990; 97:69–74.
54. Snider GL, Saleh SS. Empyema of the thorax in adults: review of 105 cases. Chest 1968; 54:12–17.
55. Light RW. Parapneumonic effusions and empyema. Clin Chest Med 1985; 6:55–62.
56. O'Moore PV, Mueller PR, Simeone JF, et al. Sonographic guidance in diagnostic and therapeutic interventions in the pleural space. AJR 1987; 149:1–5.
57. Klein JS, Schultz S, Heffner JE. Interventional radiology of the chest: image-guided percutaneous drainage of pleural effusions, lung abscess, and pneumothorax. AJR 1995; 164:581–588.
58. Silverman SG, Mueller PR, Saini S, et al. Thoracic empyema: management with image-guided catheter drainage. Radiology 1988; 169:5–9.
59. O'Moore PV, Mueller PR, Simeone JF, et al. Sonographic guidance in diagnostic and therapeutic interventions in the pleural space. AJR 1987; 149:1–5.
60. Merriam MA, Cronan JJ, Dorfman GS, Lambiase RE, Haas RA. Radiologically guided percutaneous catheter drainage of pleural fluid collections. AJR 1988; 151:1113–1116.
61. Robinson LA, Moulton AL, Fleming WH, Alonso A, Galbraith TA. Intrapleural fibrinolytic treatment of multiloculated thoracic empyemas. Ann Thorac Surg 1994; 57:803–814.
62. Lee KS, Im J-G, Kim YH, Hwang SH, Bae WK, Lee BH. Treatment of thoracic multiloculated empyemas with intracavitary urokinase: a prospective study. Radiology 1991; 179:771–775.
63. Moulton JS, Moore PT, Mencini RA. Treatment of loculated pleural effusions with transcatheter intracavitary urokinase. AJR 1989; 153:941–945.
64. Alfageme I, Munoz F, Pena N, Umbria S. Empyema of the thorax in adults. Chest 1993; 103:839–843.
65. Ali I, Unruh H. Management of empyema thoracis. Ann Thorac Surg 1990; 50: 355–359.
66. Lemmer JH, Botham MJ, Orringer MB. Modern management of adult thoracic empyema. J Thorac Cardiovasc Surg 1985; 90:849–855.
67. Anderson CB, Philpott GW, Ferguson TB. The treatment of malignant pleural effusions. Cancer 1974; 33:916–922.

68. Jensik R, Cagle JE Jr, Milloy F. Pleurectomy in the treatment of pleural effusion due to metastatic malignancy. J Thorac Cardiovasc Surg 1963; 46:322–326.
69. Reich H, Beattie EJ, Harvey JC. Pleuroperitoneal shunt for malignant pleural effusions: a one year experience. Semin Surg Oncol 1993; 9:160–162.
70. Morrison MC, Mueller PR, Lee MJ, et al. Sclerotherapy of malignant pleural effusions through sonographically placed small-bore catheters. AJR 1992; 158:41–43.
71. Goff BA, Mueller PR, Muntz HG, Rice LW. Small chest-tube drainage followed by bleomycin sclerosis for malignant pleural effusions. Obstet Gynecol 1993; 81:993–996.
72. Parker LA, Charnock GC, Delany DJ. Small bore catheter drainage and sclerotherapy for malignant pleural effusions. Cancer 1989; 64:1218–1221.
73. Seaton KG, Patz EF Jr, Goodman PC. Palliative treatment of malignant pleural effusions: value of small-bore catheter thoracostomy and doxycycline sclerotherapy. AJR 1995; 154:589–591.
74. Walker-Renard PB, Vaughn LM, Sahn SA. Chemical pleurodesis for malignant pleural effusions. Ann Intern Med 1994; 120:56–64.
75. Heffner JE, Standerfer RJ, Torstveit J, Unruh L. Clinical efficacy of doxycycline for pleurodesis. Chest 1994; 105:1743–1747.
76. Adler RH, Sayek I. Treatment of malignant pleural effusion: a method using tube thoracostomy and talc. Ann Thorac Surg 1976; 22:9–15.
77. Walsh FW, Alberts WM, Solomon DA, Goldman AL. Malignant pleural effusions: pleurodesis using a small-bore percutaneous catheter. South Med J 1989; 82:963–972.
78. Conces DJ Jr, Tarver RD, Gray WC, Pearcy EA. Treatment of pneumothoraces utilizing small caliber chest tubes. Chest 1988; 94:55–57.
79. Almind M, Lange P, Viskum K. Spontaneous pneumothorax: comparison of simple drainage, talc pleurodesis, and tetracycline pleurodesis. Thorax 1989; 44:627–630.
80. Daniel TM, Tribble CG, Rodgers BM. Thoracoscopy and talc poudrage for pneumothoraces and effusions. Ann Thorac Surg 1990; 50:186–189.
81. van de Brekel JA, Duurkens VA, Vanderschueren RG. Pneumothorax: results of thoracoscopy and pleurodesis with talc poudrage and thoracotomy. Chest 1993; 103:345–347.
82. Casola G, vanSonnenberg E, Keightley A, Ho M, Withers C, Lee AS. Pneumothorax: radiologic treatment with small catheters. Radiology 1988; 166:89–91.
83. Molina PL, Solomon SL, Glazer HS, Sagel SS, Anderson DJ. A one-piece unit for treatment of pneumothorax complicating needle biopsy: evaluation in 10 patients. AJR 1990; 155:31–33.
84. Minami H, Saka H, Senda K, et al. Small caliber catheter drainage for spontaneous pneumothorax. Am J Med Sci 1992; 304:345–347.
85. Mercier C, Page A, Verdant A, Cossette R, Dontigny L, Pelletier LC. Outpatient management of intercostal tube drainage in spontaneous pneumothorax. Ann Thorac Surg 1976; 22:163–165.
86. Samuelson SL, Goldberg EM, Ferguson MK. The thoracic vent: clinical experience with a new device for treating simple pneumothorax. Chest 1991; 100:880–882.
87. Moore AV Jr, Zuger JH, Kelley MJ. Lung abscess: an interventional radiology perspective. Semin Intervent Radiol 1991; 8:36–43.

88. Yellin A, Yellin EO, Lieberman Y. Percutaneous tube drainage: the treatment of choice for refractory lung abscess. Ann Thorac Surg 1985; 39:267–270.
89. Weissberg D. Percutaneous drainage of lung abscess. J Thorac Cardiovasc Surg 1984; 87:308–312.
90. vanSonnenberg E, D'Agostino HB, Casola G, Wittich GR, Varney RR, Harker C. Lung abscess: CT-guided drainage. Radiology 1991; 178:347–351.
91. Ha HK, Kang MW, Park JM, et al. Lung abscess. Percutaneous catheter therapy. Acta Radiol 1993; 34:362–365.

15

Digital Imaging of the Chest

ERIK J. KILGORE and ROBERT H. CHOPLIN
Bowman Gray School of Medicine–Wake Forest University
Winston-Salem, North Carolina

I. Introduction

During the past 20 years, computer-assisted techniques used in the acquisition and storage of radiographic images have resulted in a striking evolution, from an analog base toward a digital base. Computer-assisted radiography now accounts for up to 60% of radiographic images. Techniques that use computer assistance for the primary acquisition of images include computed tomography (CT), computed radiography, ultrasonography, nuclear medicine, magnetic resonance imaging (MRI), and digital subtraction angiography. The images produced with these techniques literally could not be obtained without sophisticated computer assistance.

Projection radiography is the term used to describe the nonsectional images produced by projecting an x-ray beam through a patient. The resulting images are the very common and familiar studies referred to as plain films, conventional films, conventional radiographs, or plain radiographs. Most plain radiographs are obtained by using the conventional analog technique of a screen–film combination and are displayed on the film. Digital projectional images may be acquired by film digitization, computed radiography, selenium detectors, and some prototype detectors that are under development. In this chapter, we review the advantages and limitations of having the data in electronic format, the characteristics of a projectional digital image, the acquisition methods, and methods of processing, displaying, transmitting, and storing the data.

II. Advantages and Limitations

Chest radiography accounts for up to 40% of the volume of most radiology practices in the United States (1). A considerable amount of work has been undertaken to understand the advantages and limitations of digital techniques applied to the chest radiograph in the past 10 years. Advantages of having the image in a digital format include simultaneous availability of the image to multiple users by computer, ability to manipulate the data to enhance the quality of the image or to select or deselect specific pieces of information, easy and relatively inexpensive storage in computers, and electronic transmission of the images to multiple sites inside or outside the institution of origin. The costs of film and film storage have slowly risen, whereas the costs of computers and computer storage have fallen over the past decade. These two phenomena have made storage of images in a digital format nearly competitive on an economic basis. Despite studies that describe decreased identification of abnormalities on video monitors, institutions have progressively adopted their use over the past 10 years. At least two hospitals in the United States and several more worldwide have eliminated all radiographic film and are now all digital radiology departments. The added benefits of having the images in the electronic format are thought to outweigh the decreased detectability of subtle processes.

The major disadvantage of the digital image is the high capital cost associated with computer networks and workstations. The equipment used to acquire the digital images is expensive, but this cost may be partially offset by the fact that fewer retakes are needed to obtain adequate images than when film is used as the image receptor. Digital radiographic equipment is more complex than film-based equipment, and radiologic technologists need additional training in its use. Support personnel must be available to assure that equipment can be repaired quickly in the event of failure. When radiographic installations that use an all-digital format perform the imaging, images may need to be recalled and printed to film weeks to months after their generation if those images are requested by an institution at which the images cannot be viewed in their original format.

III. Image Quality

A major concern of physicians who deal with digital images has been the quality of those images for diagnostic purposes. Although very high levels of digitization approach very closely the quality of an original film, the file sizes required are quite large. As a result, physicians have sought the minimum pixel sizes and contrast levels needed for adequate interpretation. Several studies have compared screen–film combinations with reprinted digitized films, computed radiography, and interpretation from video monitors. A limitation of all of these studies is that there is no established method of simultaneously assessing the broad range of tasks that must be accomplished in the realm of clinical radiology when interpreting a large volume of films, comparing several techniques, and assessing multiple interpreters (most commonly radiologists). Comparative studies, therefore, are carried out by assembling a set of images that are representative of diseases encountered, that represent a range of challenge to the techniques involved (some easy, some difficult), and that use multiple readers who interpret the images in random order. The clinical relevance of differences in detection of disease has been difficult to document. On the other hand, studies that evaluate the amount of time required between acquiring portable chest radiographs and transmitting the information to managing physicians in an intensive care unit (ICU) show shorter times for digital systems with electronic image transmission (2,3).

In general, studies show that interpretation at video monitors takes longer than interpretation from film, even when the interpreters are experienced in the use of the equipment. To some extent, this additional time is probably related to the ability to window and level, and to reprocess images by using multiple algorithms, features that simply are not available with film-based images. The extent to which such manipulations have been allowed has varied across studies. More importantly, interpretation of images from video monitors commonly, but not always, demonstrates decreased performance in comparison with interpretation of laser-printed films or conventional radiographs (4–7).

Studies comparing computed radiography and conventional radiography generally show no significant difference in detection of pneumothorax and pulmonary nodules, or in assessment of life-support hardware. Detection of larger low-contrast regions of increased density, as may be seen with some pneumonias and subtle interstitial lung disease, is slightly decreased. Despite these slight differences, observers frequently prefer computed radiographs because of their consistent density and contrast levels (8).

IV. Characteristics of a Digital Image

A digital image is made up of columns and rows of squares, each of which is assigned a specific color or shade of gray. The squares of a digital image are referred to as pixels, and they represent the smallest element of an image. The spatial resolution in a digital image is limited by pixel size (9). Spatial resolution is the ability to distinguish two independent points as separate entities. The higher the spatial resolution, the smaller and closer together the points can be. Spatial resolution of conventional film is measured in line pairs (lp) per millimeter (i.e., how many pairs of the fine lines of a test phantom can be detected by the system being used). Screen–film systems used for chest radiography have a resolution of approximately 5 lp/mm.

When an analog image is converted to a digital image, regions of the image are broken down into small squares, and a shade of gray or color is assigned to each square, according to the average that was in that region of the image (Fig. 1). The fewer the squares, the more block-like the picture appears (Fig. 2). Ultimately, as the number of squares decreases, the image becomes unrecognizable. As the number of squares increases, the image more closely resembles the original analog image. In a digital image, size is usually expressed in terms of the number of rows of pixels times the number of columns of pixels (e.g., 1280 × 1000). Unfortunately, because manufacturers frequently do not give information about the size of the pixel, it may be difficult to understand the true resolution of a system. Observer studies suggest that a maximum pixel size of 0.2 mm is neces-

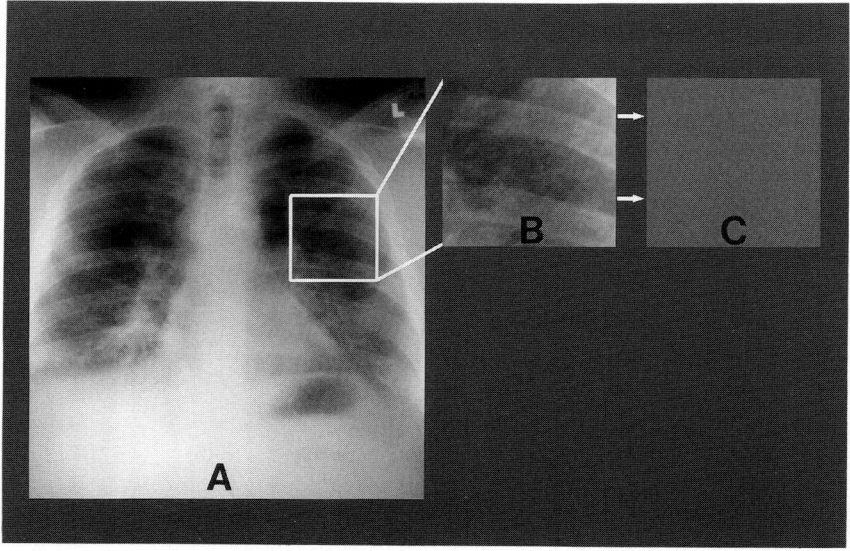

Figure 1 Image digitization: A standard analog chest radiograph (A) shows anatomical features that blend smoothly from one region of the image to another. Note the linear infiltrates in the lungs from lymphangitic spread of carcinoma. The square over the left lung is a stylized version of a pixel, which (B) was subsequently enlarged. In the first enlargement, the image has not yet been digitized. The ribs and pulmonary vessels are still visible within the square (arrow). (C) In the second enlarged square, the digitization process has occurred, and the pixel has been assigned the average density of all structures within the square.

sary to provide the minimum resolution necessary for proper interpretation of chest radiographs (10). With a 0.2-mm pixel size, an image matrix of approximately 2500 × 2000 pixels is required to cover the area of the thorax, as ois done with a 33.5 × 43-cm (14 × 17-in.) film (9). This corresponds to about 2.5 lp/mm. Importantly, this area measure only partially accounts for the file size that must be handled by the computer (see later discussion).

In conventional analog films, there is an infinite gray scale, with the shades of gray smoothly blending from lighter to darker and vice versa. In a digital image, the gray scale is divided into a stepwise pattern, with specific shades of gray assigned to each step. As the number of shades of gray increases, the gray-scale appearance of the image more closely approaches that of an analog image. When the number of shades of gray decreases, the image takes on a highly contrasting, harsh appearance. The importance of gray scale lies in the ability to reproduce subtle variations in attenuation in an accurate and acceptable way (9). Too small a gray scale can create artificial borders, an artifact known as *contouring*.

The number of shades of gray that can be assigned to a pixel depends on the number of bits chosen to be stored within each pixel. The higher the number of bits, the higher the number of shades of gray. The number of shades of gray = 2^N, where N = the number of bits. Observer studies have shown that a minimum of 256 shades of gray are needed; preferably, 1024 shades (10 bit) or 4096 shades (12 bit) are required for a superior display (9). The total size for a digital image, then, equals the number of rows of pixels times the number of columns of pixels times the bit depth. A 33.5 × 43-cm (14 × 17-in.) chest radiograph digitized to 2500 × 2000 × 12 bits is approximately 10 MB per image.

V. Image Acquisition

The most common means of producing digital images for projection radiography include film digitization, computed radiography, and wide-area image intensifiers. A selenium-based detector system that produces a digital image has recently been described, but is not widely used. Advanced multiple-beam equalization radiography (AMBER) is sometimes described as a digital imaging modality. This technique uses a computer to control the exposure of a screen–film detector and does not produce a digital image per se.

A. Conventional Chest Radiography

Because film digitization relies on a film as the starting point, a review of conventional radiography is appropriate. Conventional radiography is performed by passing an x-ray beam through the patient and acquiring the latent image by using a matched screen–film pair. When x-rays strike the screen, it becomes fluorescent and, in turn, exposes the film. The amount of light emitted at any point on the screen is proportional to the number and energy of the x-ray photons

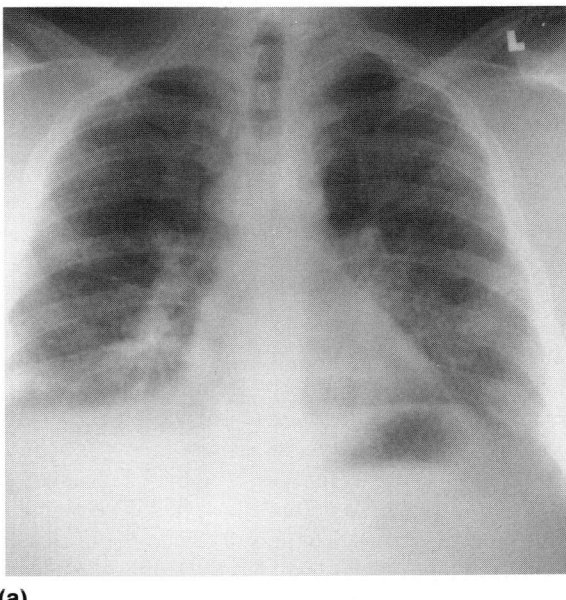

(a)

Figure 2 Image digitization: The chest radiograph in Figure 1 has been digitized to three different matrices: (a) 2048 pixels/in.; (b) 256 pixels/in., and (c) 64 pixels/in. The change between the 2048 image and the 256 image is noticeable by inspection of the L in the upper right corner of the image. The pixels become more apparent as the matrix size decreases. The linear infiltrates in the lungs are unrecognizable when the image matrix is small.

passing through the patient at that point. The greater the light emitted, the greater the film blackening.

Chest radiography is especially challenging because of the wide range of tissue attenuation that must be accommodated. The lungs and chest wall are relatively radiolucent, whereas the superimposed mediastinum and spine are significantly radiopaque. For proper exposure of both regions, a wide exposure range is needed. Each screen–film combination has its own exposure characteristics, and these may be plotted as the density (or amount of film blackening) achieved for a given amount of exposure (Fig. 3). Because the characteristic curves for conventional film are sigmoidal, the exposure density must be on the region of linear response to obtain interpretable films. Consequently, a limited range of densities can be recorded simultaneously. With the large difference in tissue attenuation in the chest, an exposure must be chosen that provides the best balance between visualization of the lungs and visualization of the mediastinum and spine.

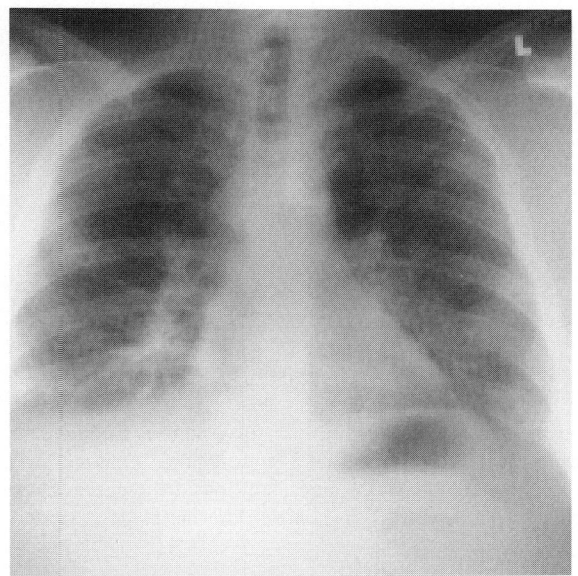

(b)

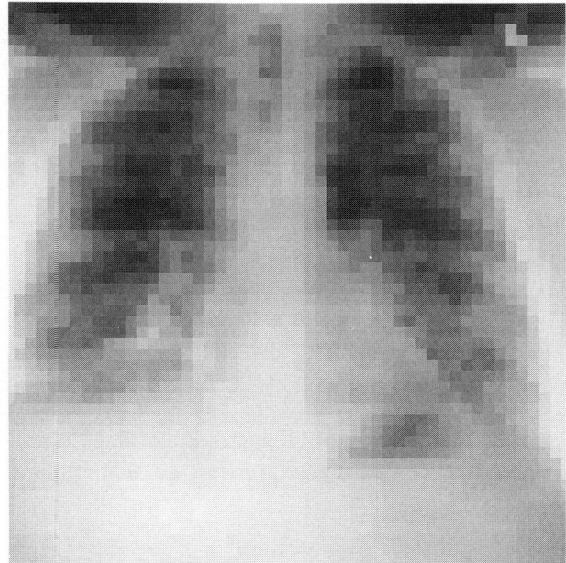

(c)

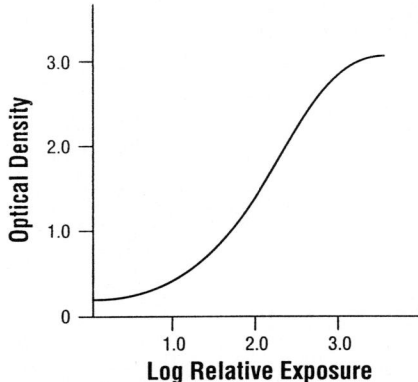

Figure 3 Exposure response for x-ray film: A curve plotting the log of film density versus the log of exposure for a film results in an S-shaped curve. Optimal images are obtained when exposure is in the middle of the linear portion of the curve. Differing films have curves of differing shapes, and the curves have differing slopes.

Typical chest radiography with a fixed radiographic unit employs a moderately high-kilovoltage peak technique (120–140 kVp), which allows better penetration of radiodense structures, such as the mediastinum. It also allows a decrease in exposure time in comparison with techniques that employ lower kilovoltage. Unfortunately, this high-kilovoltage technique results in a relatively high proportion of scatter radiation, which increases noises and decreases contrast. A grid made of a series of thin lead strips is used to decrease the effect of scatter radiation. These images are most frequently acquired with a phototimer to control the length of exposure and, therefore, the overall degree of film blackening.

Acquiring a high-quality film is more difficult with portable radiography. Patients are frequently unable to assist themselves, are uncooperative, or are difficult to position properly. Reliable, easily usable phototimers for portable radiography are not available, and exposures must be made manually. Because grids are somewhat difficult to align properly and are heavy, they frequently are not used. Finally, low-kilovoltage technique is frequently used because portable generators lack sufficient power output for high-kilovoltage techniques (8). This technique frequently results in long exposures, so that motion degrades the images.

B. Film Digitization

A low-cost method of obtaining digital images is through the use of film digitization. Conventional screen–film radiographs can be converted to digital images by using video cameras, linear diode array cameras, scanning microdensitometers, charge-coupled devices, and laser film scanners. Laser scanners provide the best spatial resolution and contrast (11).

Current laser scanners have resolutions of approximately 2500×2000 pixels, with 1024 shades of gray (9). Very high-resolution scanners, with resolutions of 4000×4000 pixels and 4096 shades of gray, have been developed and are just now becoming commercially available.

Once digitized, the image can be manipulated in much the same way as can other digital images. The primary disadvantage of film digitization is that it relies on conventional film for its source. The result of the digitization process is affected by the quality of the initial film. Moderate degrees of overexposure and underexposure may be corrected, but severe degrees cannot be completely repaired, as the information needed for a high-quality image is unavailable. By using a laser digitizer, MacMahon et al. (12) were able to recover 70–87% of improperly exposed images. Image-processing algorithms may be applied to improve contrast relations or to highlight various anatomical features. A higher percentage of images may be recovered as higher-resolution scanners and more sophisticated image-processing software becomes available. The overall cost of film digitization depends upon how the film is used. If the digitized images are routed to a computer network for display and no new films are created, the overall cost is reasonably low. If all of the digitized images are reprinted on film and subsequently stored, the cost of imaging is significantly higher. These cost calculations are quite complex and may differ from institution to institution, depending on the existing organizational structure.

C. Computed Radiography

Computed radiography, also known as storage phosphor radiography, is the most commonly used direct digital capture system. It was developed by the Fuji Photo Film Company (Japan) in the late 1970s (13). The storage phosphor plates are composed of a plastic base coated with a photostimulable phosphor, most commonly europium-activated barium fluorohalide. These reusable plates replace the x-ray screen in a conventional cassette (Fig. 4). When exposed to x-rays, the europium atoms are ionized and release electrons into the crystalline matrix. These electrons are trapped by the halogen ions in a semistable state, thereby creating a latent image on the plate.

After exposure, the cassette is placed in the image processor, and the image plate is automatically removed. The plate is scanned by a finely collimated helium–neon laser beam, which releases the captured electrons from the halogen ions. The electrons subsequently are reclaimed by the europium ions. During this process, energy is discharged as a blue-purple light, with a wavelength of 390–400 nm and a light emission life of 0.8 μsec that allows reading a larger surface

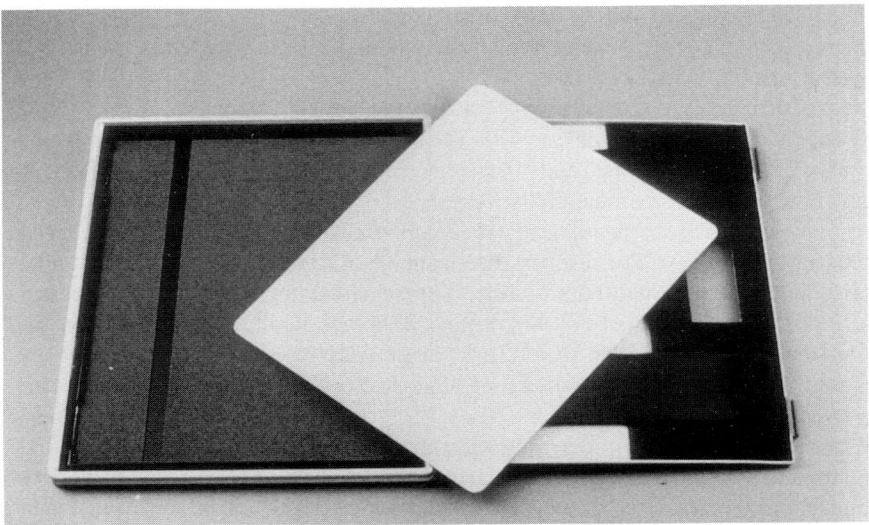

Figure 4 Computed radiography imaging plate: A plate used for computed radiography appears similar to a conventional x-ray-intensifying screen and fits within a conventional cassette. These cassettes may be used in fixed installations or in portable radiography systems.

area in a short time. The emitted light is detected by a photomultiplier tube and subsequently amplified and converted into an electrical signal. This signal is digitized, and computer processing permits automatic control of density, contrast, and presentation of detail, according to preset parameters that correspond to the imaged body part (e.g., chest or abdomen). Once the image is read out, the plates are erased by exposure to bright light.

One of the chief advantages of computed radiography is the linear relation of light emitted by the phosphor over a wide range of exposures to x-ray irradiation (1:10,000; Fig. 5). By comparison, the exposure range for conventional film is relatively narrow (1:100). The two-step–reading process for the phosphor plates provides the proper contrast and density according to the preset processing algorithm (14). This feature is of greatest importance in portable radiography, in which accurate exposure is difficult to achieve, and overexposure and underexposure are common. Uniformity of exposure in multiple films of the same patient can lead to a more accurate determination of radiographic change, without concern about variability attributable to technique (Fig. 6). Because of this wide exposure range,

Digital Imaging of the Chest

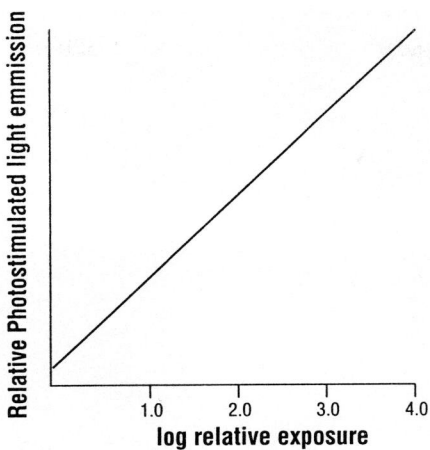

Figure 5 Exposure response for computed radiography: Curve plotting the output of photostimulated light versus the log of exposure for computed radiography (compare with Fig. 3). Note that the response is linear and that it extends over a wider dynamic range than does film.

repeat rates can be reduced from 4.5 to 1% (15). Most of the remaining repeat rate is the result of improper positioning.

It was initially hoped that computed radiography would result in decreased exposure of patients to x-rays. This hope has not been realized in practice, as the amount of exposure required to obtain satisfactory images is similar to that of conventional radiography. Underexposure of an image may be more difficult to recognize than with a conventional screen–film system, because the storage phosphor plates are sensitive to low levels of radiation, and computer processing provides for proper density settings when printing a film. Underexposure of an image can be suggested from evaluation of the sensitivity number that is printed on the film. This number is roughly inversely proportional to the quantity of radiation incident upon the imaging plate. As this number increases, the image becomes progressively more noisy and takes on a mottled appearance, known as quantum mottle (14). As this appearance worsens, portions of the film may be interpretable, but the increased granularity can make it impossible to detect subtle lesions or to evaluate the images properly for interstitial disease (Fig. 7).

Optimal processing of an imaging plate requires that the correct algorithm be entered by the technologist. If an algorithm for the wrong body part is selected (i.e., the abdomen algorithm is used for a chest radiograph), the resulting image may not have the correct contrast and exposure latitude. Such mistakes may result

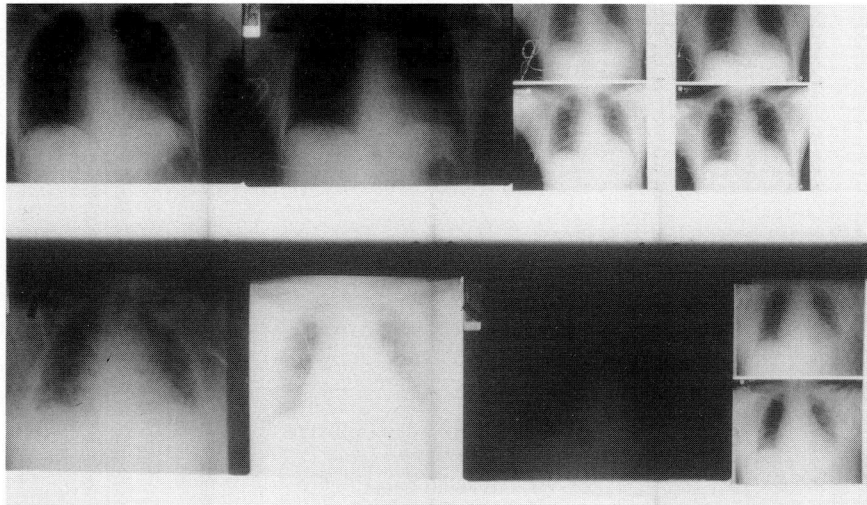

(a)

Figure 6 Uniform exposure from computed radiography: (a) Portable radiography with conventional film–screen examinations commonly produces nonuniform exposures. Two panels from an alternator loaded with five radiographs taken with conventional film as well as three computed radiography (smaller vertically oriented double images) images. Note the nonuniform exposures that are commonly seen with conventional screen–film technique. (b) Two panels from an alternator loaded with portable radiographs taken with computed radiography demonstrate much more uniform exposure.

in significant errors in interpretation if not recognized. In most instances, the image can be recovered by using the correct algorithm, and an appropriate interpretation can be rendered.

A comparison of the features and costs associated with conventional radiography, film digitization, and computed radiography is presented in Table 1.

D. Selenium-Detector Radiography

In contrast with the phosphorescent materials used in conventional and computed radiography, amorphous selenium can be used to convert X-ray energy directly into electrical signals (17). The detector is made by vacuum evaporation of selenium onto a 50-cm metallic drum. The thickness of the selenium layer is 500 μm. Arsenic (0.5%) is added to the substrate to enhance its thermal stability. A 1-μm organic polymer layer is then placed on top of the selenium to prevent its interaction with air.

Digital Imaging of the Chest

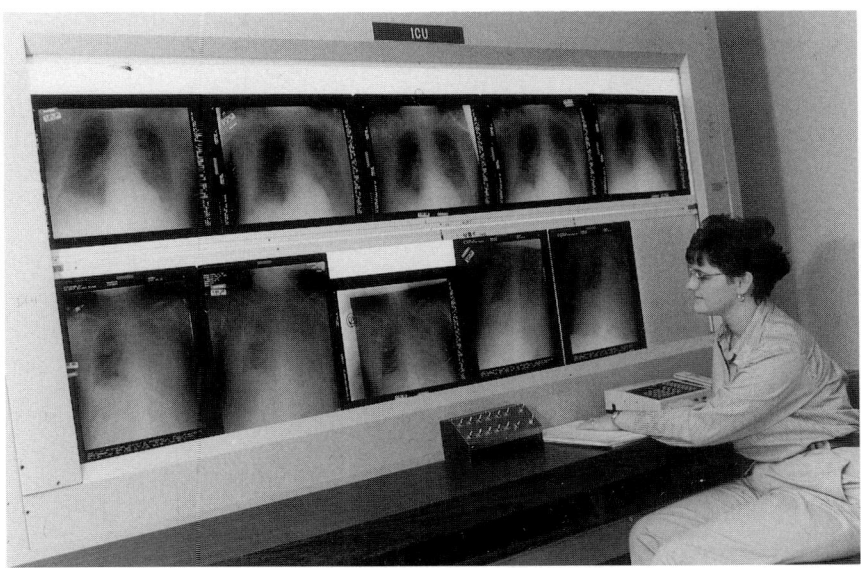

(b)

To generate an image, a positive charge is placed on the selenium layer of the plate by exposing it to a corona charging device. At the same time, a negative charge is applied to the metal substrate. When the plate is exposed to X-rays, the relative charge in the selenium layer decreases in proportion to the intensity of the X-ray exposure. Therefore, the residual charge on the imaging plate represents the x-ray image. The imaging plate may be read out by a series of microelectrometer probes, or it may be scanned with a laser coupled to an electrical probe. When the microelectrometer probes are used, the plate is scanned at a distance of 100 μm from its surface. The probes sense the surface charge on the plate through capacitive coupling. The signal from the probes is then amplified and digitized. Alternatively, photo-induced discharge within the selenium can be measured by scanning with a laser beam attached to a conduction probe. As the laser beam passes over the surface, the selenium absorbs the light (blue light is the most readily absorbed) and causes displacement of the stored charge (18). A probe, connected to a preamplifier, measures the displaced charge. After either technique, the plate can be recharged with the corona device, and it is then ready for reuse.

The drum design facilitates rapid readout and charging of the plate, but requires use as a fixed piece of equipment. The selenium system also has the advantage that it is virtually free of sources of intrinsic noise, unlike storage phosphor technology, in which luminescence and granularity contribute to the

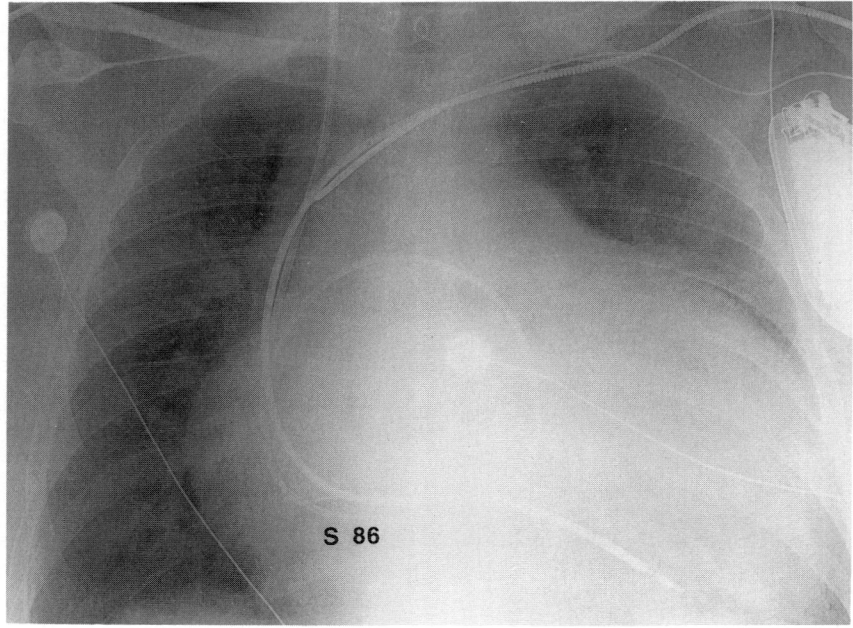

(a)

Figure 7 Quantum mottle: Underexposed computed radiography images have a grainy quality that is most noticeable in the uniformly dense regions of the radiograph: heart, chest wall, and upper abdomen. (a) Examination performed with higher-exposure factors has an S number of 86 and shows a smooth image. (b) Examination performed with lower-exposure factors has an S number of 515. Note the grainy appearance in the dense regions mentioned above.

system noise. Therefore, the detection efficiency exceeds that of storage phosphors and even screen–film systems (9).

E. Other Imaging Systems

Although the most promising technologies for imaging are storage phosphor radiography and selenium detectors, several other techniques are under development. Many modern radiographic image intensifiers have digital output, but are not large enough to encompass the entire chest on most patients. Large-area image intensifiers have been constructed, but are expensive and limited to use in fixed sites. Still under development is another system that employs a large, flat array of thin-film photodiode sensors and thin-film transistors in conjunction with a con-

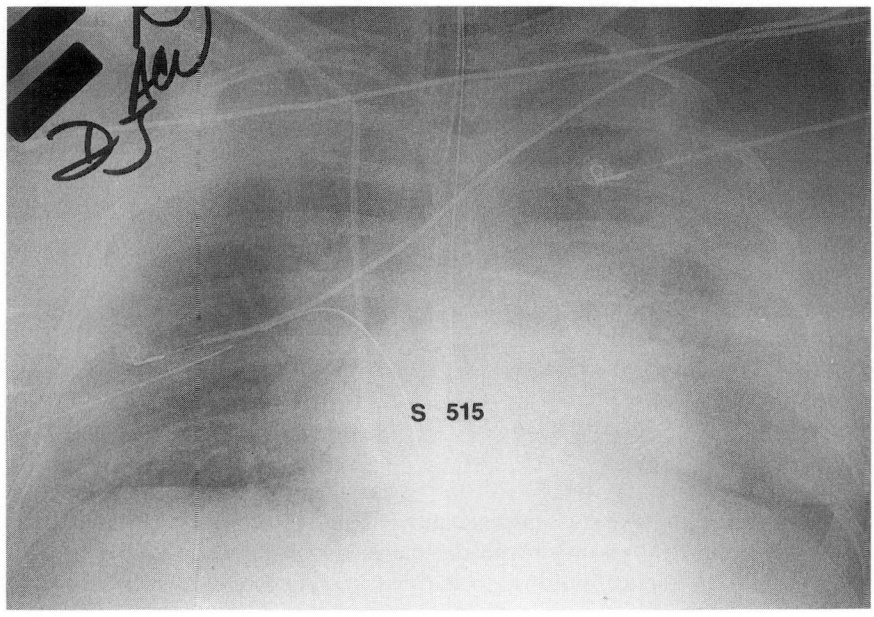

(b)

ventional x-ray screen (19). Most of the circuitry needed for signal acquisition and processing will fit into a container the size of a conventional cassette. Currently, the largest image format is about 23 × 23 cm (9 × 9 in.), and the resolution is insufficient for adequate evaluation of lung disease. Rapid gains are being made with this technology, however, and it is one of the most promising for the field of digital radiology.

F. Beam Equalization Radiography

The exposure difficulties resulting from the wide differences in attenuation of the radiographic beam by structures within the chest may also be addressed by modulation of the radiographic beam by means of the technique known as AMBER (20). Because this equipment scans the chest through a slit collimator, the x-ray beam is fan-shaped. A bank of 21 detectors placed between the patient and the film continuously monitors x-ray exposure. As the x-ray beam scans the thorax from bottom to top, feedback from the detectors controls the slit collimator to ensure uniform exposure of the film. The position of the modulators is adjusted 186-times during the 1-sec scanning time.

Table 1 Comparison of a Conventional Screen–Film System, Laser Digitizer, and Computed Radiography

Characteristic	Conventional screen–film	Laser digitizer	Computed radiography
Resolution	Excellent	Good	Fair
Low-frequency MTF[a]	Good	Fair	Good
Noise	Good	Good	Poor
Dynamic range	Poor	Good	Excellent
Image processing	Not applicable	Available	Available
Connection to PACS[b]	Not applicable	Available	Available
Initial cost	Low	Moderate	High
Running cost	Low	Low	High

[a]MTF, modulation transfer function.
[b]PACS, picture archiving and communication system.
Source: Modified from Ref. 16.

Use of AMBER improves the image quality in areas of low transmission, such as the mediastinum, without overexposing the lungs. Unfortunately, this method results in a higher radiation dose to the patient. Standard posteroanterior and lateral views of the chest result in an estimated radiation dose of 0.14 mSv, versus 0.086 mSv for conventional technique. Other disadvantages include relatively high cost and lower reliability because of the complexity of the equipment. Finally, artifactual distortion may occur at edges, for example, between the heart and lungs (21).

VI. Image Processing

A major advantage of digital radiography over conventional radiography is image processing. Perhaps the most useful image-processing technique is correction of density and contrast of suboptimally exposed radiographs. When the image is printed on film, the density and contrast are fixed. When digital images are viewed on workstations, windowing and leveling may be used, producing changes in brightness and contrast. Another algorithm, digital unsharp mask imaging (commonly referred to as edge enhancement), can partially compensate for the lower spatial resolution of digital radiographs (9). By masking some of the lower spatial frequencies, the high spatial frequencies found at the sharp borders within an image can be made more prominent. The result is enhancement of image details at higher spatial frequencies relative to lower frequencies, while maintaining the tone scale of the image. Algorithms have also been developed to remove some of the effects of scatter radiation and to improve contrast (22).

VII. Display

Currently, most digital radiographs are printed onto film and displayed on a viewbox in the traditional way. This method permits the most rapid presentation of the full-resolution image to the physician. It also facilitates direct comparison with any previous conventional radiographs. Alternatively, images may be displayed on specially designed computer workstations that use high-resolution video monitors (Fig. 8). No ideal workstation is currently available that can carry out all the tasks related to radiographic imaging in an acceptable time frame at a cost low enough for wide deployment. Workstations vary in their capabilities and cost, depending on their intended use. The most powerful workstations have considerable amounts of memory and high-resolution monitors. They can display multiple modalities, and they have software for presenting images in two-dimensional, three-dimensional, or cine versions. Most commonly, 2000-line (2K) monitors are used in these workstations. The cost of 2K monitors, approximately 20,000–30,000 dollars, limits the feasibility of their wide dissemination for interpretation of digital images in the near future. Monitors with even higher resolution may be necessary to evaluate very detailed images, such as mammograms. Lower-cost workstations can provide image review of patient data, but they have less sophisticated software and lower resolution monitors. Monitors with a minimum of 1000 lines have become rather inexpensive over the last few years and will probably be acceptable for review workstations.

Video monitors have lower levels of illumination than do viewboxes. The luminance of monitors ranges from 30 to 70 foot-lamberts, whereas the luminance of a conventional viewbox is as high as 500 foot-lamberts. A lower luminance level requires a darker room for interpretation of images and is thought to contribute to fatigue, when a large number of studies must be viewed. This concern is most important to radiologists, who spend large blocks of time viewing images, but presumably, causes less difficulty for physicians who intermittently view images throughout their day. Progress in monitor design continues to improve screen brightness.

Software is available to allow viewing of images on personal computers and is commonly used in teleradiology applications. The quality of the image is a function of the intrinsic resolution of the image and the monitor on which the image is displayed. Because the resolution of computed tomography and other sectional imaging studies is 512×512 or less, images may be displayed at full resolution. A digitized chest radiograph cannot be displayed as a single image at its highest resolution with these monitors, but the commonly available pan-and-zoom function makes it possible to view portions of the image at full resolution. Usually, these images are visually appealing and are satisfactory for much diagnostic imaging. Abnormalities most likely to be missed are fine nodularity or

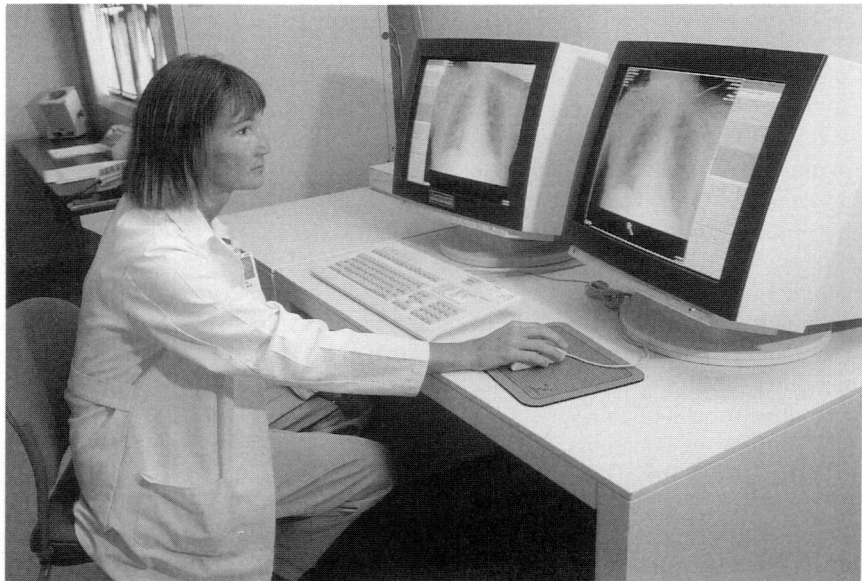

Figure 8 Digital imaging workstation: A two-screen workstation displays portable radiographic images. The workstation may be controlled by keyboard, function keys, or by a mouse.

linearity. These patterns, albeit important, are seen rather infrequently in most clinical practices. Most physicians with an interest in imaging technology believe that as electronic imaging becomes more commonplace, primary interpretation will be done at workstations with high-resolution monitors, and the images will be transmitted to review workstations or personal computers for review by clinical physicians.

VIII. Transmission and Storage

From the standpoint of computer engineering, an *image* is a data set, and the more pixels that are required to make up an image, the larger the data set that must be manipulated, transmitted, and stored. Because of the large-file sizes associated with radiologic imaging, the time needed to transmit an image file across computer networks is potentially quite large. A state-of-the-art network uses fiberoptic cable and appropriate transmission protocols to ensure transmission of the greatest amount of data per unit of time. For institutions with less sophisticated equipment and longer transmission times, electronic imaging may be accomplished through techniques such as transmission of data at off-peak hours. Unless these techniques are used, the time required for image transmission limits the usefulness of networks for image evaluation.

Storage technology has progressed rapidly in the last decade. Methods available for storage include magnetic disks (fixed or "floppy"), optical disks, magneto-optical disks, magnetic tape, and optical tape (23). Magnetic disks may be used independently, or they may be arranged in a variety of architectures to provide mass storage. For storage of very large amounts of data, jukeboxes are available that use any of the kinds of optical or magnetic devices for storage. A progressive decline in the price of storage media over the last decade has helped to bring electronic storage into a price range that makes it competitive with storage on film.

Data compression is a technique of extracting the essential information needed to reproduce an image from the full data set and deleting the unneeded data, thereby decreasing the size of the file to be stored. Data compression is classified as either reversible or irreversible. Reversible data compression allows the entire data set to be reconstructed by software. Data can be compressed up to two to four times (expressed as a compression ratio of 2:1 or 4:1). Irreversible data compression, which can achieve much higher levels of compression (10:1–60:1); it works by various methods, but most commonly by removing redundant data from the original data set. Although there is a significant increase in compression, data is lost from the original image, so that when uncompressed, the resulting image may be degraded. Degradation is most problematic when high-compression rates are used. A balance must be reached between compression and image quality. Recent studies indicate that data compression of up to 25% may satisfactorily retain the diagnostic accuracy of digital data (24).

References

1. Aberle DR, Hansell D, Huang HK. Current status of digital projectional radiography of the chest. J Thorac Imaging 1990; 5:10–20.
2. De Simone SD, Kundel HL, Arenson RL, et al. Effect of a digital imaging network on physician behavior in an intensive care unit. Radiology 1988; 169:41–44.
3. Humphrey LM, Fitzpatrick K, Atallah N, Ravin CE. Time comparison of intensive care units with and without digital viewing systems. J Digit Imaging 1993; 6:37–41.
4. Thaete FL, Fuhrman CR, Oliver JH, et al. Digital radiography and conventional imaging of the chest: a comparison of observer performance. AJR 1994; 162: 575–581.
5. Slatsky BS, Gur D, Good WF, et al. Receiver operating characteristic analysis of chest image interpretation with conventional, laser-printed, and high-resolution workstation images. Radiology 1990; 174:775–780.
6. Frank MS, Jost RG, Molina PL, et al. High-resolution computer display of portable,

digital, chest radiographs of adults: suitability for primary interpretation. AJR 1993; 160:473–477.
7. Ishigaki T, Endo T, Ikeda M, et al. Diagnostic efficacy of hard- and soft-copy images from computed radiography for detection of subtle pulmonary disease: comparison with conventional radiography. Radiology 1995; 197(P):528–529.
8. Niklason LT, Chan H-P, Cascade PN, Chang CL, Chee PW, Mathews JF. Portable chest imaging: comparison of storage phosphor digital, asymmetric screen–film, and conventional screen–film systems. Radiology 1993; 186:387–393.
9. MacMahon H, Vyborny C. Technical advances in chest radiography. AJR 1994; 163:1049–1059.
10. MacMahon H, Vyborny CJ, Metz CE, Doi K, Sabeti V, Solomon SL. Digital radiography of subtle pulmonary abnormalities: an ROC study of the effect of pixel size on observer performance. Radiology 1986; 158:21–26.
11. Glazer HS, Muka E, Sagel SS, Jost RG. New techniques in chest radiography. Radiol Clin North Am 1994; 32:711–729.
12. MacMahon H, Xu XW, Hoffmann KR, et al. Clinical experience with an advanced laser digitizer for cost-effective digital radiography. Radiographics 1993; 13:635–645.
13. Tateno Y, Iinuma T, Takano M, eds. Computed radiography. Tokyo: Springer-Verlag, 1987.
14. Cowen AR, Workman A, Price JS. Physical aspects of photostimulable phosphor computed radiography. Br J Radiol 1993; 66:332–345.
15. Sagel SS, Jost RG, Glazer HS, et al. Digital mobile radiography. J Thorac Imaging 1990; 5:36–48.
16. Yoshimura H, Xu XW, Doi K, et al. Development of a high quality film duplication system using a laser digitizer: comparison with computed radiography. Med Phys 1993; 20:51–58.
17. Neitzel U, Maack I, Günther-Kohfahl S. Image quality of a digital chest radiography system based on a selenium detector. Med Phys 1994; 21:509–516.
18. Rowlands JA, Hunter DM, Araj N. X-ray imaging using amorphous selenium: a photoinduced discharge readout method for digital mammography. Med Phys 1991; 18:421–431.
19. Antonuk LE, Yorkston J, Huang W, et al. A real-time, flat-panel, amorphous silicon, digital x-ray imager. Radiographics 1995; 15:993–1000.
20. Geleijns J, Broerse JJ, Julius HW, et al. AMBER and conventional chest radiography: comparison of radiation dose and image quality. Radiology 1992; 185:719–723.
21. Lehmann KJ, Busch HP, Drescher P, Loose R, Georgi M. New imaging methods in thoracic diagnosis. A study to evaluate digital storage screen radiography, the slit technique ("AMBER"), asymmetric ("Insight") and conventional film–screen. Akt Radiol 1993; 3(1):14–19.
22. Baker JA, Floyd CE Jr, Lo JY, Ravin CE. Observer evaluation of scatter subtraction for digital portable chest radiographs. Invest Radiol 1993; 28:667–670.
23. Hindel R. Digital image storage technology. Invest Radiol 1993; 28:454–458.
24. MacMahon H, Doi K, Sanada S, et al. Data compression: effect on diagnostic accuracy in digital chest radiography. Radiology 1991; 178:175–179.

# 16

Imaging of the Pulmonary Circulation

TONY P. SMITH and GLENN E. NEWMAN
Duke University Medical Center
Durham, North Carolina

I. Introduction

For a discussion of imaging of the pulmonary circulation, several methods of classification could be applied. Anatomically, one could divide the system into arteries and arterioles, capillaries, or veins and venules. It is also reasonable to divide the topic by imaging techniques: plain chest radiography, scintigraphy, angiography, computed tomography, or other. Finally, it could be divided into normal and disease processes. In reality, it is probably best to incorporate all of these divisions, as none are all-encompassing, and there are advantages to each.

The main focus here will be a discussion of the methods of imaging the pulmonary circulation while highlighting the applications of these techniques for more common disease entities. As this topic has been covered extensively in a previous volume of *Diagnostic Imaging in the Lung*, this review will concentrate mostly on newer techniques and updates of previously used imaging methods (1). Although imaging can be applied to many diseases of the pulmonary circulation (Table 1), the most common application of these techniques in the adult population is in the diagnosis of pulmonary embolus. Therefore, a large portion of this discussion will concentrate on pulmonary embolus, for it is prevalent, difficult to

Table 1 Applications for Pulmonary Imaging

Pulmonary hypertension
  Arterial–precapillary
    Hyperdynamic–hyperkinetic
      Hypoxia
      Vasoconstrictive drugs
      Increased pulmonary blood flow
    Vascular obstruction
      Thromboembolism
      Arteritis
      idiopathic
  Venous or postcapillary
    Left ventricular failure
    Mitral valve disease
    Pulmonary capillary or venous disease
Pulmonary arteriovenous malformations
Pulmonary artery aneurysms
Congenital heart or venous disease
  Pulmonary artery stenosis
  Anomalous pulmonary venous return

diagnose without imaging techniques, and allows comparison of the usefulness and future of many of the techniques described.

II. Chest Radiograph

The standard chest radiograph is relatively simple to obtain, is inexpensive, and is universally available. It has long been used as the first line for the diagnosis of pulmonary vascular disease because it gives an image, although somewhat limited, of the pulmonary vascular system, while also providing much information about the lungs, pleura, chest wall, and so on. It provides a roadmap of the pulmonary vascular systems and can reflect primary or secondary diseases of the circulatory system. The sequellae of pulmonary artery hypertension are demonstrated by enlarged central arteries, with distal, rapid tapering. Interstitial pulmonary edema can be indicative of pulmonary venous hypertension. Certainly pulmonary nodules may have features suggesting arteriovenous malformations (AVM; i.e., a nodule or nodules with vessels [arteries or veins] leading from them). Finally, the chest roentgenogram also provides an inexpensive, easily obtained, method of following changes or progression in disease.

There have actually been relatively few changes in the performance of chest roentgenograms. Probably the most important change has been the acquisition of images in a digital format (Fig. 1). Instead of the standard radiographic film, the radiation beam strikes a sensor panel after exiting the patient. The data is thus obtained in a digital format, much like computed tomography (CT) and can be postprocessed to highlight areas of concern and areas difficult to visualize. Digital radiography provides several advantages, especially as use for bedside radiographs, and may overcome some of the limitations of film–screen techniques for image display and for film archival (2). The initial concerns with digital images were for the spatial resolution of this format. Recent studies have shown that film interpretation is comparable between digital and film–screen systems when the interpretation is made from high-quality laser camera-produced images, rather than from the cathode ray tube (CRT; i.e., television screen) (3). However, these data have mostly been generated from visualization of lung opacities and nodules and not so much from subtle changes, such as mild interstitial edema or areas of decreased vascular perfusion, which is required to adequately evaluate the pulmonary circulation. Certainly, digital techniques hold promise, but currently await analysis of larger series, particularly involving subtle differences, to determine if they are comparable with film–screen techniques.

Nowhere is the chest radiograph more difficult to interpret than in the diagnosis of pulmonary embolus (Fig. 2). Chest radiography alone is inaccurate in the diagnosis of pulmonary embolus with a true-positive rate of 39% and a false-negative rate of 61%, when compared with pulmonary angiography (4). Because the lung has a limited response to injury, the radiographic findings are nonspecific and include pleural effusions, oligemia, atelectasis, interstitial or airspace opacities, elevation of the hemidiaphragm, or enlarged hila (Fig. 3). However, that is certainly not to say the chest radiograph is without value in the evaluation of the patient with suspected pulmonary embolus. Stein et al. (5) found, in a subset of patients in the collaborative trial of the Prospective Investigation of Pulmonary Embolism Diagnosis (PIOPED), that most patients (92%) with acute pulmonary embolus had abnormal chest radiographs. These authors also reviewed 123 patients, enrolled in the same trial, in whom there was no underlying cardiopulmonary disease. They found (6) that patients with prominent central arteries or cardiomegaly had higher pulmonary arterial mean pressures than did patients with atelectasis, pleural effusions, or a pulmonary parenchymal abnormality. The most important reasons to obtain chest films in patients suspected of having pulmonary embolus are to exclude diagnoses that clinically mimic this disorder and to aid in the interpretation of the ventilation–perfusion (V/Q) imaging of the lungs (7). Certainly, a recent chest roentgenogram clearly enhances the diagnostic accuracy of V/Q scanning, which does not decrease in diagnostic usefulness even in the presence of preexisting cardiac or pulmonary disease by chest radiograph (8,9).

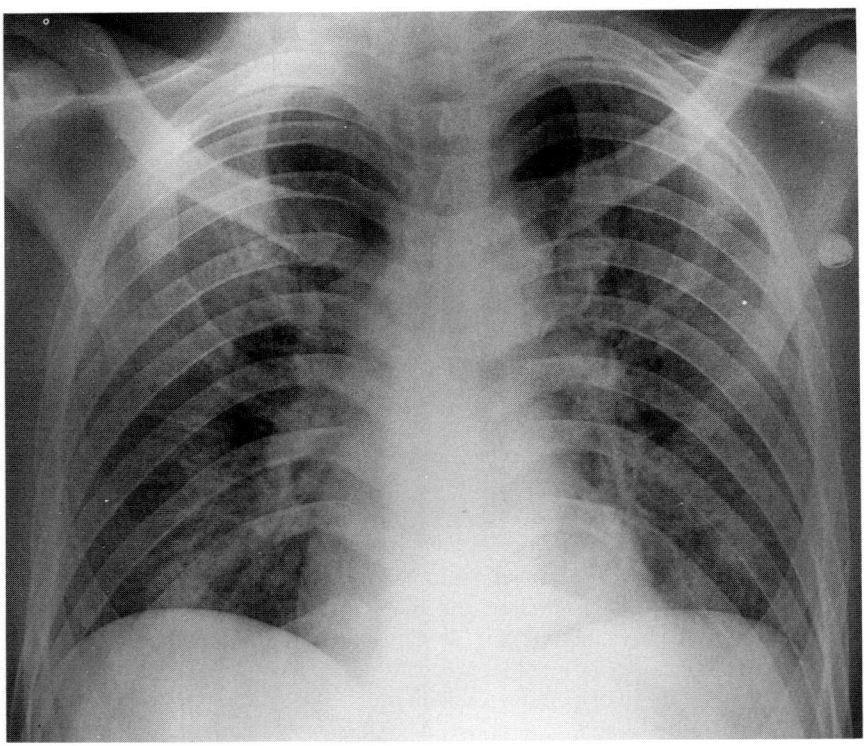

(a)

Figure 1 (a) Digital chest radiograph compared to (b) conventional radiograph obtained on the same day. Although the digital radiograph represents an excellent means of obtaining a portable image, the definition, particularly of the peripheral pulmonary vessel, is difficult particularly when compared with the quality of the conventional radiograph in panel b.

III. Nuclear Scintigraphy

A. Ventilation and Perfusion Imaging

Ventilation and perfusion (V/Q) imaging, for the most part, is limited to the diagnosis of pulmonary embolus. It can be used to determine the degree of perfusion to lung tissue in other disease conditions, but this application is quite limited.

Ventilation imaging can be performed with various agents composed of either a gas or an aerosol. Gases are an ideal medium, because they do not settle with gravity and are not aggravated by turbulence. However, they are limited by

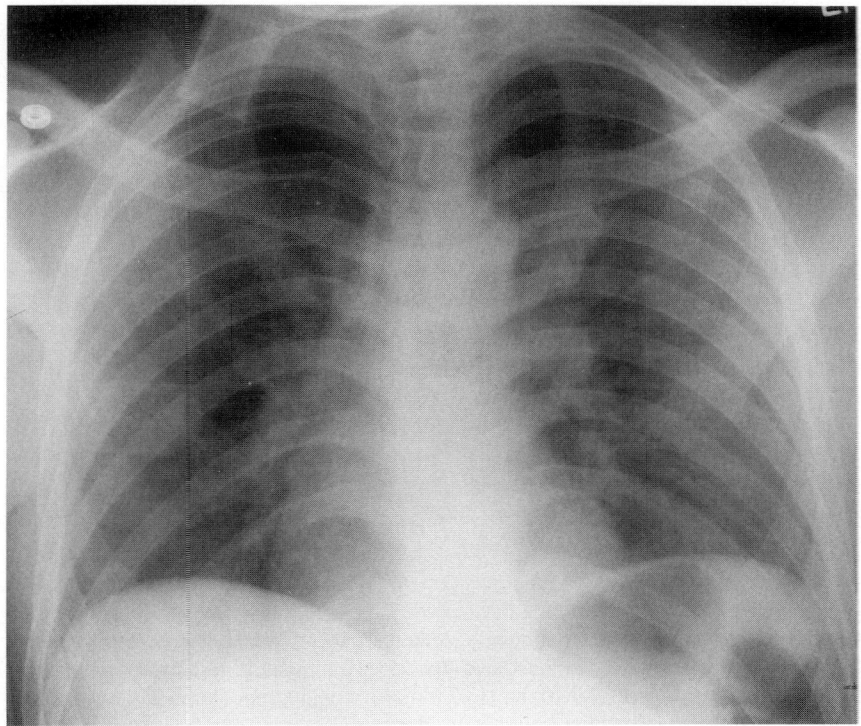

(b)

other properties, mostly related to technical preparations. The most commonly used gases are ^{133}Xe, ^{127}Xe, and ^{81m}Kr. Aerosols were tried almost 30 years ago, but the droplets were too large to act as an ideal agent (i.e., a gas). Recent advances have allowed the droplet size to be reduced to several microns, making them a much better agent. The most commonly used agent is technetium Tc 99m diethylenetriaminepentaacetic acid (pentetic acid; DTPA) aerosol. Technegas Tc 99m is the newest agent, although it is currently not available in the United States. This agent actually has fine carbon particles with adherent technetium, that are prepared to behave much like a gas.

Perfusion imaging is most often performed with ^{99m}Tc microaggregates of albumin (MAA). One usually injects on the order of 500,000 particles and approximately 0.1–0.2% of the pulmonary capillary bed is embolized. The timing of the perfusion scan relative to the ventilation scan is still somewhat debatable. Ideally, the ventilation portion could be reserved until after perfusion imaging, as

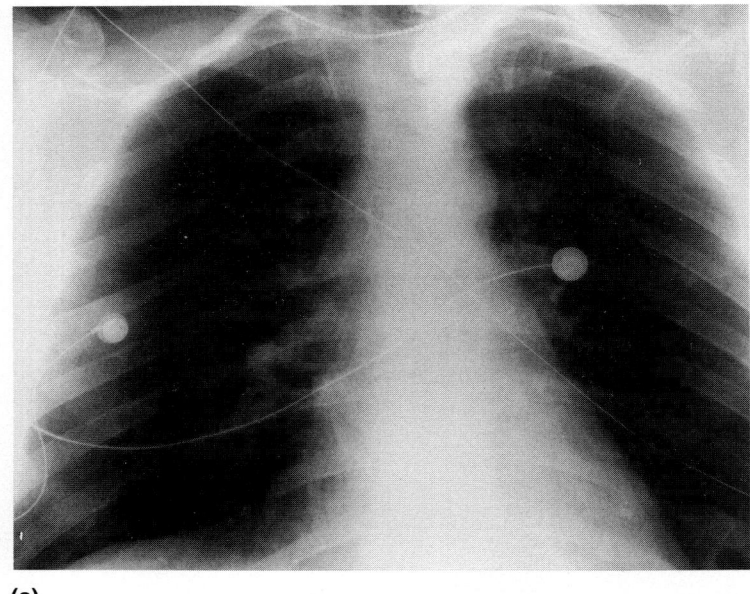

(a)

Figure 2 The findings of pulmonary embolus can be subtle on chest radiography. (a) Chest radiograph that demonstrates decreased pulmonary vascularity to the right upper lung, but this is quite subtle. (b) Pulmonary angiogram shows large pulmonary embolus (arrow) occluding the right upper lobe.

it may often be unnecessary. However, if the perfusion study is done first, only about 1 mCi of MAA may be used, because the radiotracer activity of the second agent (ventilation) must override the first during imaging. This has its own technical limitations. In general, most perform the perfusion imaging following the ventilation study.

Performing ventilation–perfusion imaging is a relatively simple issue when compared with image interpretation, which remains the center of an everchanging controversy. A number of diagnostic strategies have been used to classify the findings relative to the diagnosis of pulmonary embolus. Most often the terms are more related to the probability of pulmonary embolus, rather than to its diagnosis (Figs. 4 and 5; also see Fig. 9) The generally applied probability terms of normal, near normal, low probability, indeterminate–intermediate–moderate, and high probability have been used and are basically at the heart of much of the controversy. Several sets of probability criteria have found widespread use, including those set forth by Biello, McNeil, and PIOPED (10–13) The specifics of each set

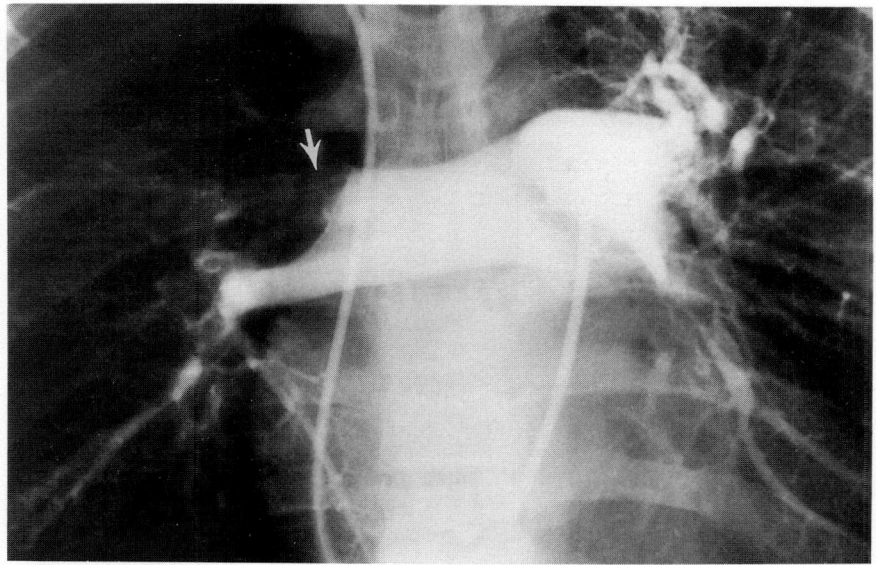

(b)

of criteria are unnecessary for this chapter. However, the main differences in each can be divided into the likelihood of predicting pulmonary emboli and the number of intermediate studies produced. Certainly, the ideal set would consist of the most favorable likelihood of correctly predicting pulmonary embolus, with very few studies being interpreted as intermediate. There is still no agreement among those interpreting the studies on the best available set or sets of such criteria. The PIOPED criteria and their recent modifications are the one used today in many centers (14). These criteria originated from the Prospective Investigation of Pulmonary Embolism Diagnosis (PIOPED) study, which was a multi-institutional study of large centers. One set of these modified criteria for the reading of pulmonary embolus on V/Q scanning and the one mostly used at Duke University Medical Center is provided in Table 2 (15).

With use of the modified PIOPED criteria, as outlined in Table 2, about 40% of patients with pulmonary embolism have high-probability V/Q scans, 40% have intermediate scans, and 20% have low-probability scans. Less than 1% of patients with normal scans will have pulmonary embolus. Obviously, patients with normal scans have effectively had pulmonary embolus excluded. However, looking at the same data in a different light, 87% of the patients with high-probability scans have pulmonary embolus, 30% of patients with intermediate scans, and 14% with low-

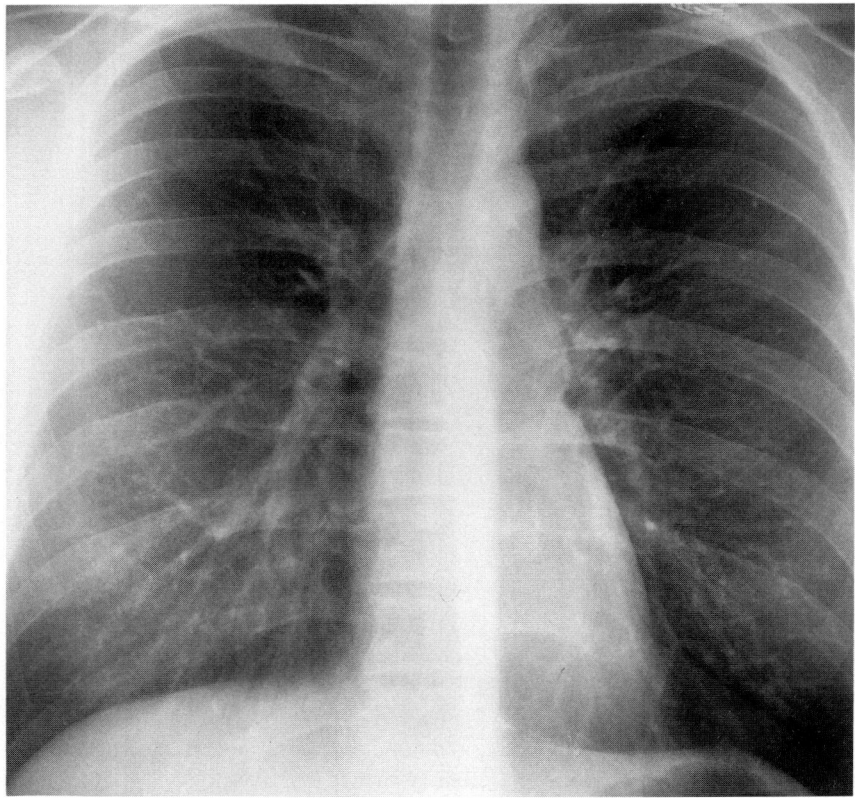

(a)

Figure 3 Chest radiograph in the same patient before and after pulmonary embolus. (a) The chest film is normal. The patient returned 15 months later with chest pain and shortness of breath. (b) The film demonstrates interval enlargement of both hila from pulmonary embolus, confirmed by angiography.

probability scans have pulmonary embolus. In addition, interobserver agreement for classifying scans as intermediate or low-probability is not as good as for high. Therefore, clinical suspicion must be combined with the V/Q results. When a high degree of clinical suspicion is combined with a high-probability scan, about 90% of the patients have pulmonary embolus. Conversely, when there is a low degree of clinical suspicion and a low-probability scan, only 4% of patients have pulmonary embolus. Unfortunately, all other situations fall somewhere in between (see Table 2). Although it may appear frustrating to assign only probabilities, rather

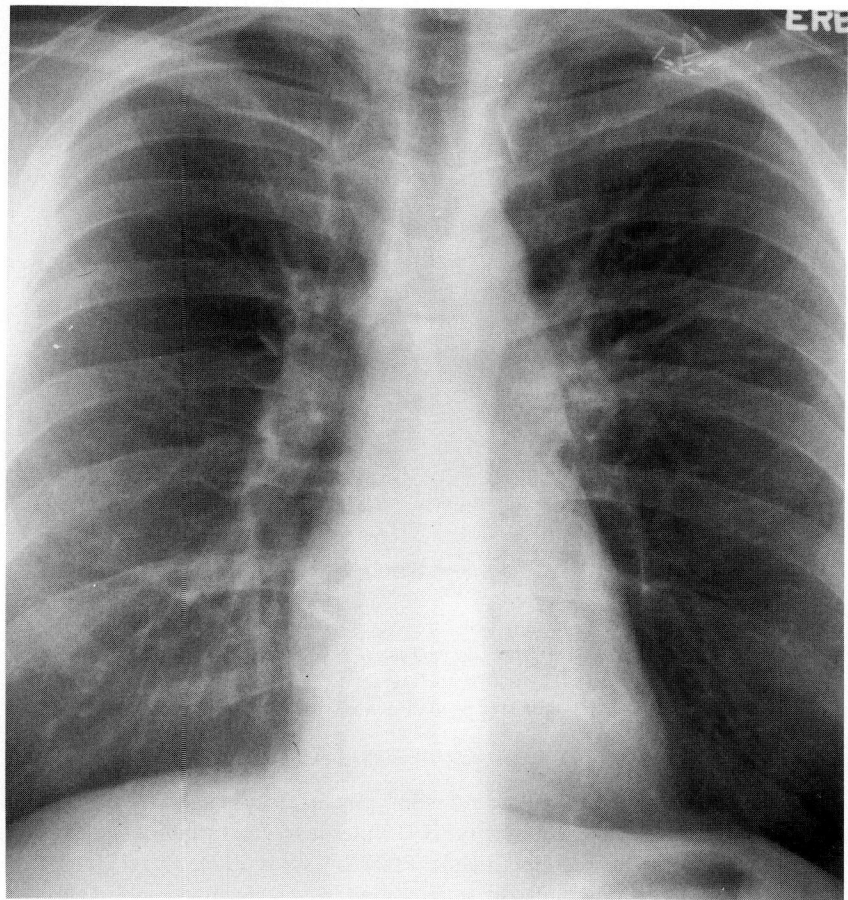

(b)

than a diagnosis, to the images, one must remember that V/Q scanning does not directly visualize thromboembolism, but visualizes only its secondary effects (16).

Given the results of V/Q imaging, it is often questionable about what the next step should be, whether it be treatment or further diagnosis (17). Certainly, the interpretation of the images and clinical data is important. Much of the weakness in V/Q imaging is also in reporting the results. So difficult is the disease clinically and so confusing are the diagnostic criteria (as seen in Table 2 and the previous paragraphs outlining those criteria) that interobserver variability is high

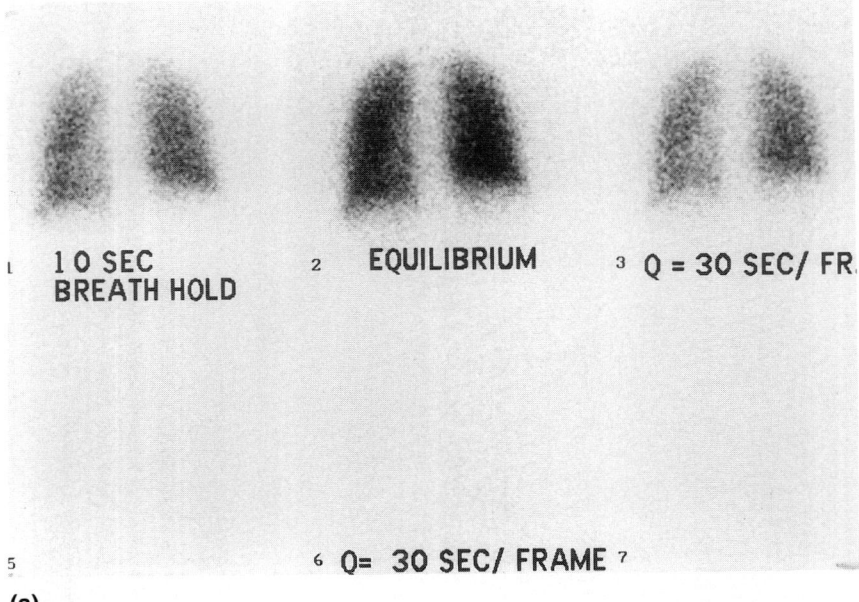

Figure 4 (a) Ventilation scan and (b) perfusion scan. (a) The ventilation images are essentially normal. (b) No segmental or subsegmental defects are noted in the perfusion images. This scan demonstrates a low probability for pulmonary embolus.

and great confusion exists among referring physicians over the meaning of the generated nuclear medicine report (18,19). Interobserver variability occurred in more than 20% of the readings in the PIOPED study (13). Even given these limitations, V/Q imaging is currently the noninvasive screening study of choice in the patient suspected of having pulmonary embolus following the chest roentgenogram. The probability of pulmonary embolus is then used for evidence of treatment, or as the guide for a study that directly visualizes the thromboembolus. Therefore, clinical judgment plays a major role, and there is a need for improved noninvasive testing to assess the pulmonary circulation for thromboembolic disease.

B. Other Scintigraphic Imaging

The most promising use for single-photon emission computed tomography (SPECT) in evaluating the pulmonary circulatory system is as a complementary-imaging tool for ventilation–perfusion imaging. This technique is not yet widely applied (20). It usually involves the injection of 6 mCi of ^{99m}Tc-MAA after the patient has been supine for at least 15 min to allow equalization of blood flow.

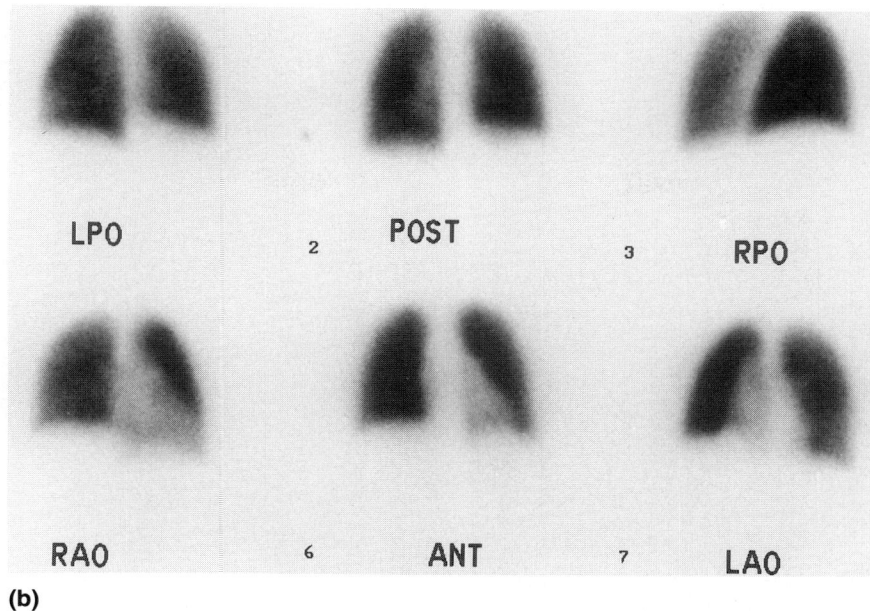
(b)

Acquisition of at least 64 angles with a 360° rotation is used to produce diagnostic images. The details of image postprocessing, including smoothing and filtering, will depend on available software, which is obviously in a constant state of change. With SPECT imaging, aerosol ventilation is often postponed for 18 hr to allow decrease in radiation within the lungs.

The overwhelming advantage of SPECT perfusion is the precise definition of the size and configuration of anatomical defects. SPECT imaging, with its inherent depiction of information in three dimensions, may add additional specificity to the diagnosis, when compared with planar imaging. The borders and configurations of the perfusion defects may be better defined with SPECT, and their confirmation to pulmonary blood flow distribution may be better assessed. Additional exciting work is being performed, including closely registered V/Q studies obtained from simultaneously acquired ^{81m}Kr ventilation studies and ^{99m}Tc perfusion studies, with V/Q ratio images obtained in three dimensions. However, SPECT images can be quite difficult to interpret (14,21,22). Much of the work described here is in the early stages of development and will require further evaluation before determining its ultimate use in the clinical arena.

Other than for the evaluation of pulmonary embolus, the distribution of perfusion and ventilation in the setting of chronic pulmonary disease may be assessed in three dimensions using SPECT imaging and, thus, may have some

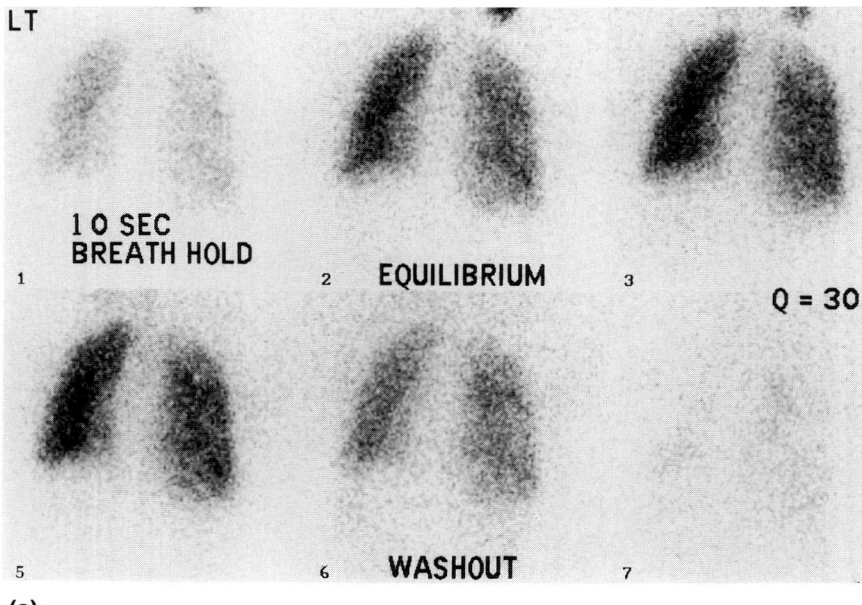

(a)

Figure 5 (a) Ventilation scan and (b) perfusion imaging. (a) The ventilation images demonstrate abnormal lung volume in the right apex. There is mildly diminished ventilation in the right midlung in a location that matches an opacification on chest radiograph. (b) The perfusion images demonstrate an inhomogeneous, mildly diminished defect in the right midlung. There is a subsegmental perfusion defect occupying most of the right apex. This V/Q scan pattern is consistent with an intermediate probability for pulmonary embolism.

quantitative value. In addition, tumor blood flow using ^{99m}Tc-hexamethyl-propyleneamineoxine (HMPAO) SPECT may offer valuable information concerning tumor blood flow (23).

Positron emission tomography (PET) has thus far seen little application for the pulmonary circulation. It has been used in experimental animal studies to evaluate regional pulmonary blood flow in noncardiogenic pulmonary edema (24). Certainly, given its promise in other areas of the chest, such as tumor evaluation, PET may have a future in evaluating the pulmonary circulation.

IV. Computed Tomography

Computed tomography (CT) has, since its inception, diagnosed pulmonary circulatory abnormalities. Many of these have been incidental, for direct imaging of the pulmonary circulation has had many limitations. Because of respiratory and

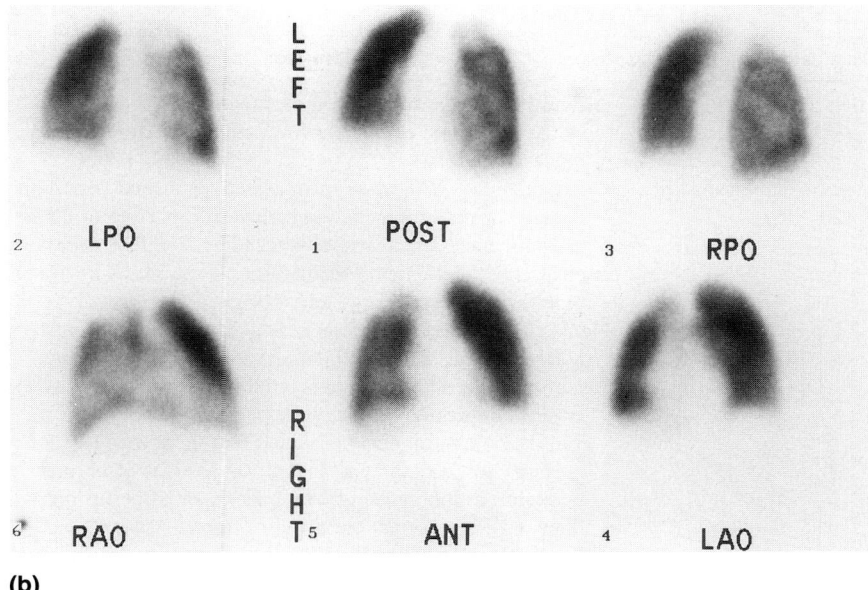

(b)

cardiac and vascular motion, the quality of imaging was significantly limited (25). In addition, as scan slices were thick and variable in location relative to one another based on different involuntary motion artifacts during multiple breath-holds, it was difficult to image structures in an axial plane. Basically, CT needed thinner sections and faster image acquisition, and it has undergone rapid changes in these areas. Visualization of very small structures has become possible with high-resolution (HR) CT. High-resolution CT has the ability to visualize vessels to approximately the 16th order and has shown identifiable changes in vessels with vascular loading and hypoxia in animal models (26). New ultrafast (electron beam) and volumetric (helical or spiral) scanners make possible the acquisition of images at a very rapid rate. Electron beam tomography uses an electron beam to strike onto target rings, producing radiation that passes through the patient to detectors. It eliminates the mechanics of typical slower rotating gantries. An entire chest can be scanned in 12 sec with state-of-the-art models. Although details of the technical changes for volumetric scanners are beyond the scope of this chapter, three main changes in the scanners are responsible for making this faster acquisition possible: the development of the slip-ring gantry, improved detector efficiency, and greater tube cooling (27). Interestingly, all of these can be incorporated into a conventional-appearing apparatus and, therefore, a helical scanner can be placed at virtually any radiology site currently using CT, and it outwardly

Table 2 Revised PIOPED Criteria

Scan category	Definition
High probability (≥80%)	At least two large mismatched segmental perfusion defects or the arithmetic equivalent in moderate or large and moderate defects[a]
Intermediate probability (20–79%)	One moderate to two large mismatched segmental perfusion defects, or the arithmetic equivalent in moderate or large and moderate defects;[a] one matched V–P defect, with a clear chest radiograph;[b] difficult to categorize as low or high, or not described as low or high
Low probability (≤19%)	Nonsegmental perfusion defects (e.g., cardiomegaly, enlarged aorta, enlarged hila, elevated diaphragm); any perfusion defect with a substantially larger abnormality at chest radiography; perfusion defects matched by ventilation abnormality[b] provided that there are (1) normal chest radiographs and (2) some areas of normal perfusion in the lungs; any number of small perfusion defects with a normal chest radiograph
Normal	No perfusion defects, perfusion outlines exactly the shape of the lungs seen on the chest radiograph (hilar and aortic impressions may be seen, and the chest radiograph or ventilation scan may be abnormal)

[a]Two large mismatched perfusion defects are borderline for high probability. Individual readers may correctly interpret individual scans with this pattern as showing high probability for PE. In general, it is recommended that more than this degree of mismatch be present for inclusion in the high-probability category.
[b]Very extensive matched defects can be categorized as indicative of low probability. Single V–P matches are borderline for low probablity, and thus should be categorized as intermediate in most circumstances by most readers, although individual readers may correctly interpret individual scans with this pattern as showing low probability.
Source: Ref. 15.

appears identical with conventional CT. Other advantages include smaller contrast doses and image reconstruction. Smaller volumes of contrast can be used to visualize the vascular structures of the thorax when compared with conventional scanners (28). However, there is as yet no definitive dose for contrast. The continuity of the truly volumetric data obtained in a helical manner allows three-dimensional reconstruction of the images, which may play an integral part in pulmonary vascular imaging in the future. In general, the downside of these scanners is really only economic, as conventional imaging can also be performed on them.

Most of the attention of CT imaging of the pulmonary circulation has been limited to pulmonary embolus and confirmation of pulmonary AVM (Figs. 6 and 7). A CT diagnosis of pulmonary embolus, using conventional scanners, was initially made incidentally (29,30). This is not really unexpected, for pulmonary embolism may not be clinically apparent. It generally required large emboli centrally (31). Volumetric and fast scanners, however, have prompted investigators to look at CT as a primary-imaging modality in the diagnosis of pulmonary embolus. Initial animal studies demonstrated thromboembolism within the pulmonary vascular system (32). Although smaller clinical studies and case reports using CT have flourished, Remy-Jardin et al. published (33) one of the first prospective studies of 42 patients in the diagnosis of pulmonary embolus, comparing the results of spiral CT with angiography. Twenty-three patients had normal CT and normal angiograms. In the remaining 19 patients, emboli were visualized from the second to the fourth division of pulmonary vessels. The sensitivity and specificity of CT were 100 and 96%, respectively. They concluded spiral CT was a safe procedure and could be used in patients felt to be at high risk for angiography; as a complement to angiography in patients with chronic pulmonary embolus, as it may help to analyze central vascular irregularities secondary to organized thrombus; and to monitor patients with documented central emboli to demonstrate recanalization of the vascular bed. As a follow-up to this, Teigen et al. (34), using electron beam CT, imaged the pulmonary vascular system in 86 patients and found comparable results, with sensitivities and specificities of 95 and 80%, respectively. However, these studies were in very controlled patient populations and, in general, not applicable to difficult clinical situations. Goodman et al. (35) looked at patients in whom clinical data and V/Q studies failed to answer the question of pulmonary embolus, and found helical CT was only 63% sensitive, with subsegmental emboli being the most difficult to diagnose. In effect, they were applying the technique in a clinical situation. They concluded that CT has a limited role in the evaluation of pulmonary embolism, with pulmonary angiography remaining the study of choice.

Certainly, the final results for helical and fast CT in the diagnosis of pulmonary embolus have yet to be determined. Although conflicting reports are in the literature, it is difficult to state its current role. The future appears bright, as continued modifications and improvements occur. Besides visualizing proximal thrombus, CT has also been able to analyze pulmonary arteries distal to occlusions (36). Although stenoses and vascular distortions are more difficult to visualize, as would be expected, parenchyma distal to stenoses or obstructions can be well evaluated (37). For example, areas of pulmonary infarction can be easily identified. Finally, CT allows visualization of other structures within the thorax, such as the mediastinum.

For pulmonary AVM, CT is a sensitive method to diagnosis the disease and has made angiography probably unnecessary, unless treatment is planned (38; Fig.

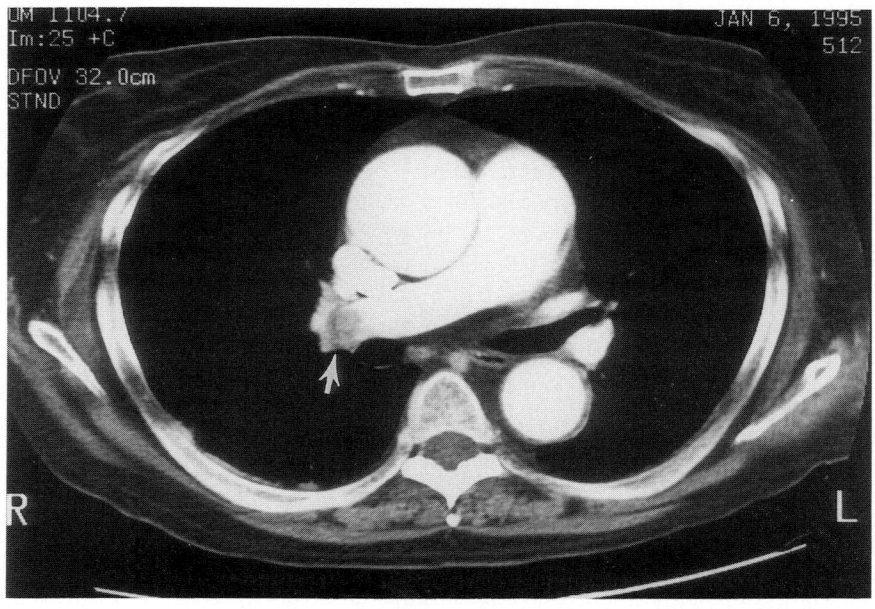

(a)

Figure 6 (a) CT scan shows a pulmonary embolus that involves the right pulmonary artery (arrow). (b) Pulmonary angiogram on the same patient demonstrates pulmonary embolus in the same location (arrows).

8). Computed tomography tends to be much more precise in providing anatomical detail than does magnetic resonance imaging (MRI), chest roentgenograms, or V/Q imaging (39,40). Knowledge of whether pulmonary AVMs are simple or complex (the latter occurs in 20% of cases), the number, and the location, all are important before treatment, which is usually embolotherapy (41). Remy et al. (42) also showed CT to be useful for recurrence, demonstrating an unembolized feeding vessel or flow existing through the embolic agent in up to 10% of patients. Finally, CT is probably the best-screening tool for patients in families at high risk for pulmonary AVM (43).

V. Magnetic Resonance Imaging

Magnetic resonance imaging (MRI) can be divided roughly into traditional imaging of tissues and imaging of flow, the latter being termed MR angiography. The basic scan consists of short-repetition time, short-echo time, as well as spin-echo

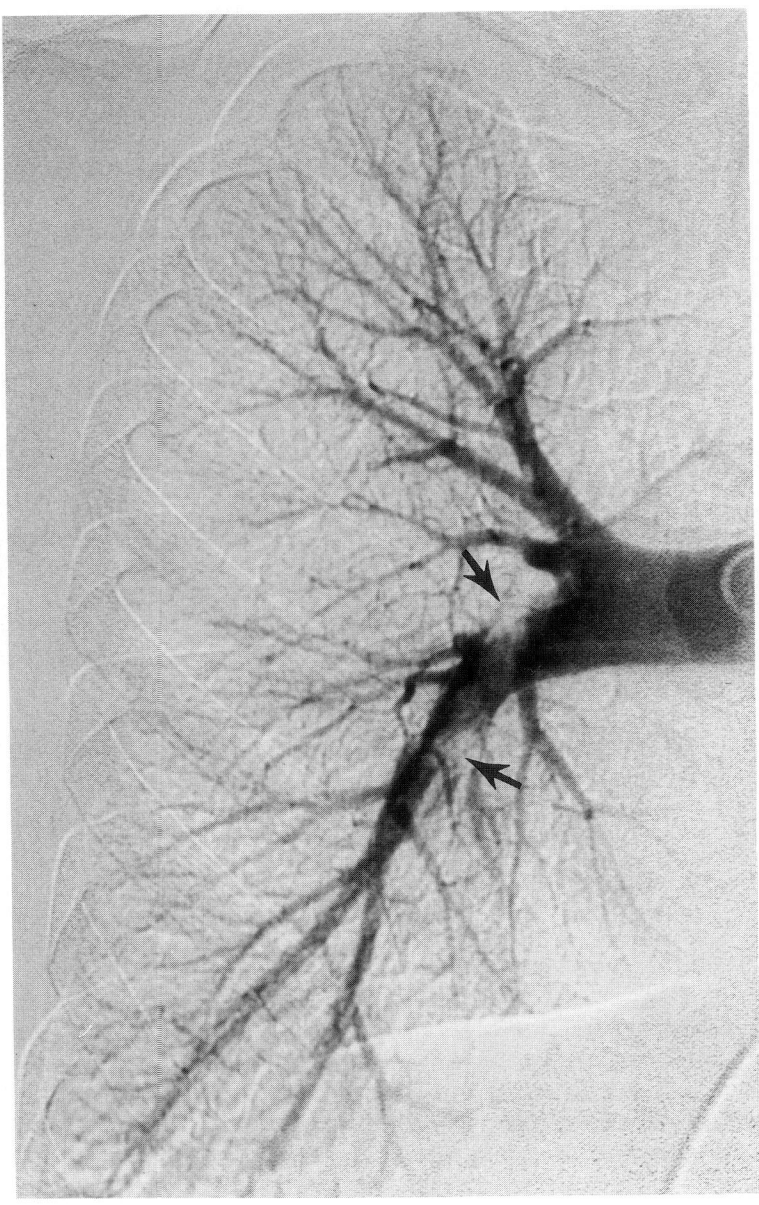
(b)

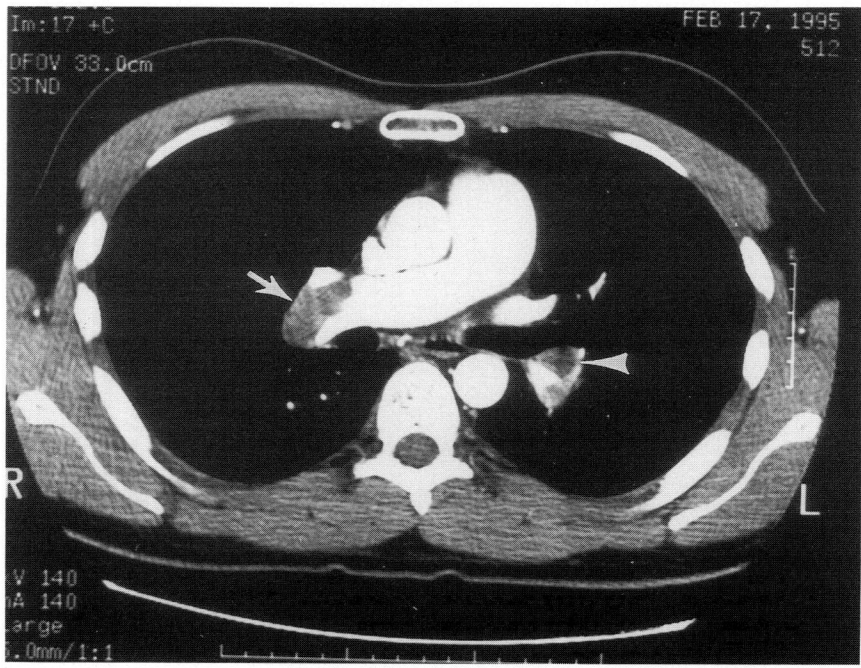

(a)

Figure 7 The CT scans demonstrate (a) bilateral pulmonary emboli centrally (arrow) as well as (a and b) peripherally (arrowheads).

sequences. For magnetic resonance angiography (MRA), some form of gradient echo technique is employed. In addition, electroencephalography (ECG) and respiratory gating are usually used. Overall, the exact sequences vary with the currently available hard- and software and are usually tailored for a specific application by a specific group.

Much like CT, MRI has the ability to visualize the pulmonary circulation as well as other structures in the mediastinum. It may also have an enhanced ability to visualize the central as well as the peripheral pulmonary arteries. Finally, a major potential advantage is to provide physiological information (44). An MRI scan is capable of identifying vascular involvement by extrinsic or intrinsic masses, as well as the identification of central thromboemboli. Its capability to show involvement of the central pulmonary arteries and veins by hilar, mediastinal, or lung masses can play a key role in lung tumor staging. Unfortunately, MRI is depen-

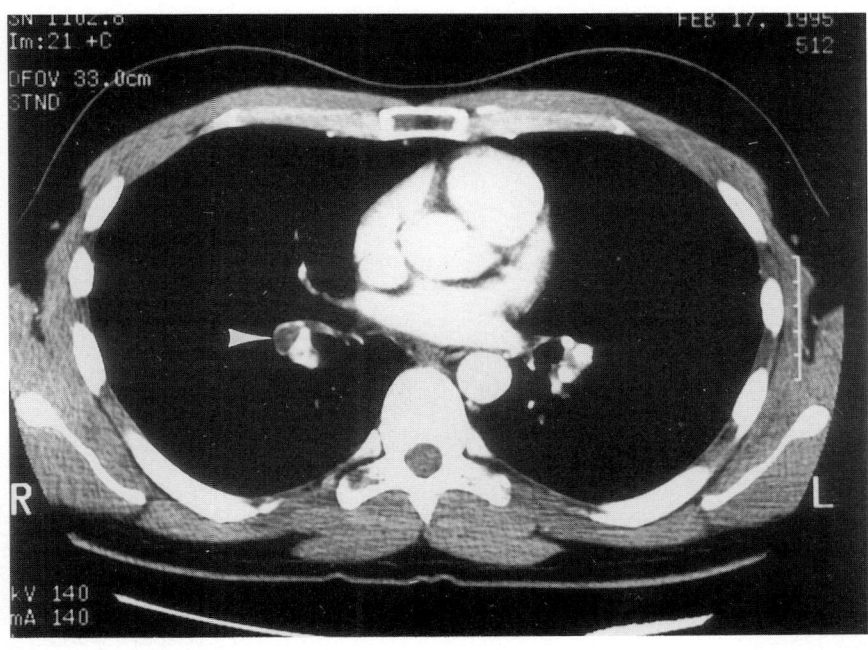
(b)

dent on the degree of flow, and slow flow can provide confusing artifacts, which also include adjacent air-containing bronchi.

Magnetic resonance imaging is an accurate, noninvasive modality to quantitate and characterize pulmonary blood flow. Recently, it has been as effective as V/Q imaging for assessment of relative and absolute differential pulmonary perfusion (45). This is most often used before lung transplantation.

Magnetic resonance angiography has obvious advantages. It does not require catheterization, as does standard angiography, and does not require iodinated contrast, as does CT. It has the potential to provide three-dimensional display of vessels from virtually any angle. It may also have the ability to quantitate blood flow. Velocity mapping with MRI has been applied to the pulmonary arteries in patients with pulmonary artery hypertension (46). This can also be applied to the venous system and is particularly promising in patients with mitral valve disease (47).

Magnetic resonance has found some use in the diagnosis of peripheral pulmonary AVM. These techniques most often consist of MRA, and can easily differentiate flowing blood in AVM from solid tumors. Early experience with MRA demonstrates that vessels to the sixth or seventh order can be identified (48);

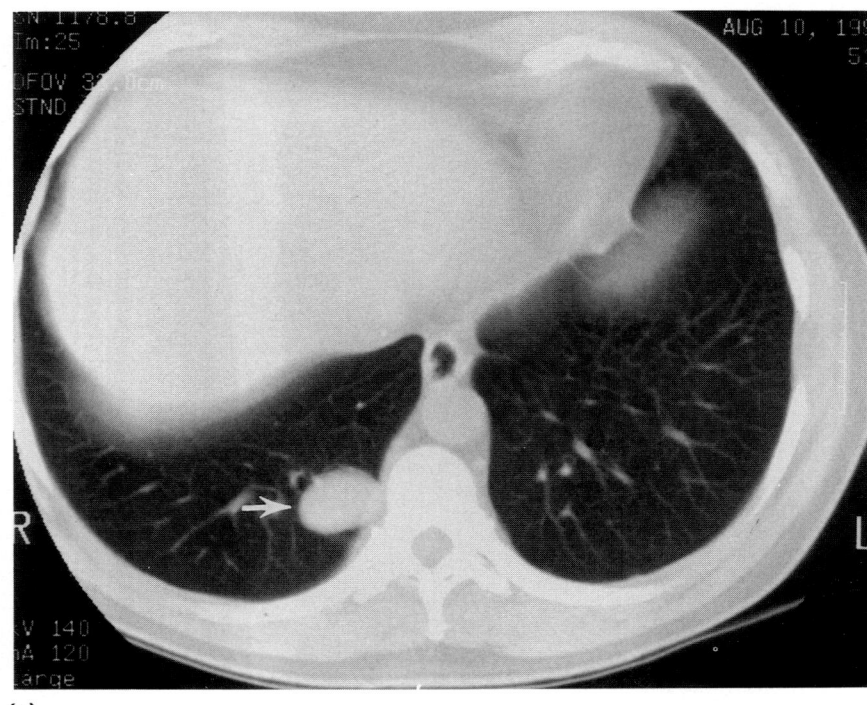

(a)

Figure 8 A CT scan (lower and higher images) demonstrates (a) a pulmonary nodule (arrows), (b) with vessels leading from it (arrowheads), consistent with pulmonary AVM. (c) Angiogram confirms the AVM (arrows). This was treated by embolization.

however, this is somewhat controversial. Although small AVM can be identified, there still exists problems, including breath-holding, in this group of patients.

In thromboembolic disease, MRI can visualize the vessel wall and mural clots, thereby giving a unique depiction of the degree of disease (Figs. 9 and 10). In a prospective study by Grist et al. (49), in which 20 studies were interpreted by blinded observers, the sensitivity of MRI for diagnosing pulmonary embolus was 100%, but the specificity was only 62%. Erdman et al. (50) compared V/Q imaging with that of MRI using angiography for correlation: MRI had a sensitivity of 90%, a specificity of 77%, with a positive predictive value of 86%, and a negative predictive value of 83%. In 21 patients with intermediate probability scans, MRI established a diagnosis of pulmonary embolism in 12 of 12 patients and absence of pulmonary embolism in 7 of 9 patients. The emboli were limited to large and medium size in a symptomatic population. Despite using the most

Imaging of Pulmonary Circulation

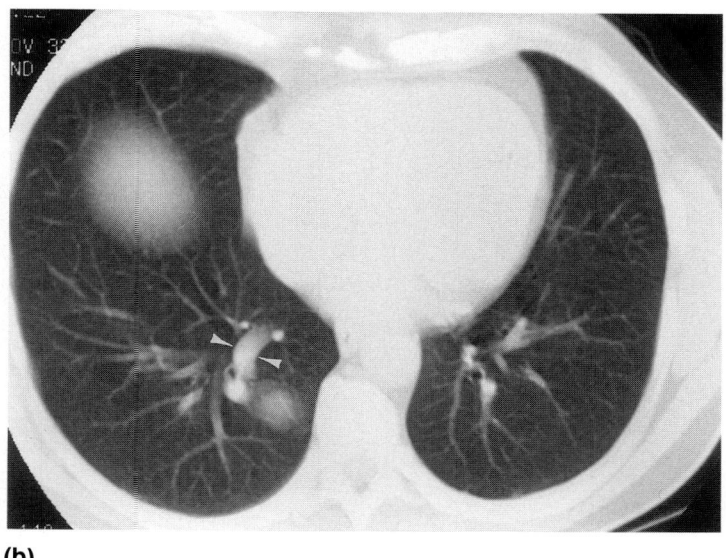

(b)

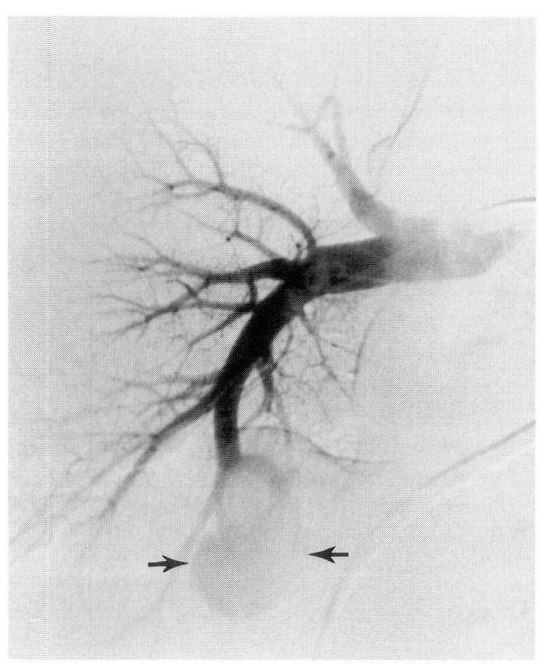

(c)

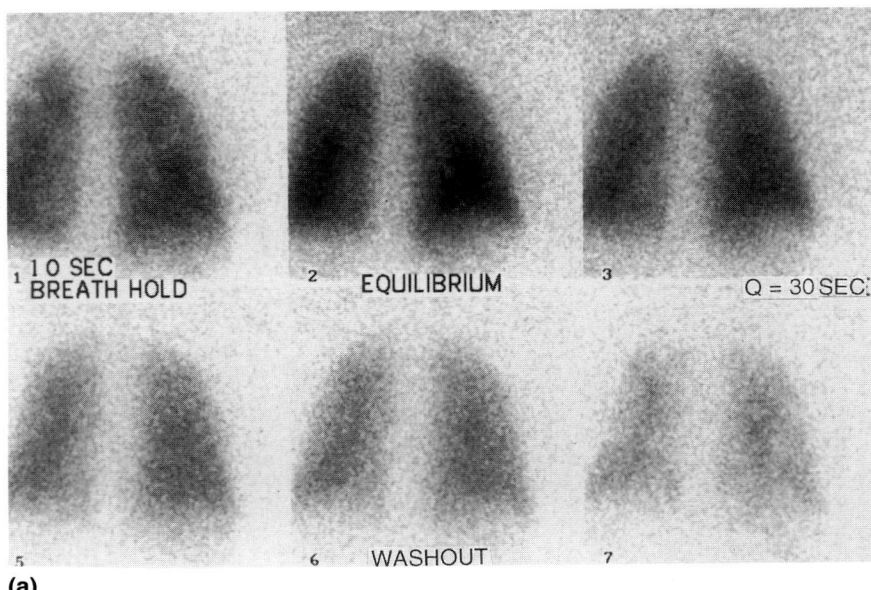

Figure 9 (a) Ventilation and (b) perfusion imaging: (a) The ventilation study shows evidence of obstructive lung disease that is most prominent at the left base in the right midzone. (b) The perfusion study shows multiple segmental perfusion defects throughout both lungs. The largest perfusion abnormality is the right lung base where the ventilation is most normal. In addition, there are other segmental mismatches. This study carries a high probability for pulmonary embolism. (c) MRI demonstrates decreased signal intensity representing flow void extending into left pulmonary artery (arrow) consistent with pulmonary embolus.

advanced techniques, emboli smaller than 4 mm could not be identified. To that end, Loubeyre et al. (51) found no value in the detection of peripheral emboli by MRI.

Much of the current work in MRI of pulmonary embolus centers around the pulse sequences and other technical factors. Schiebler et al. (52) demonstrated acute pulmonary emboli larger than 1 cm using MRA techniques, requiring only 15 sec and found these images comparable with those obtained with longer pulse sequences. Contrast agents also tend to increase the visualization of the pulmonary vessels (53). Techniques for pulmonary MRA are continually being developed for visualization of the pulmonary arteries and veins (54).

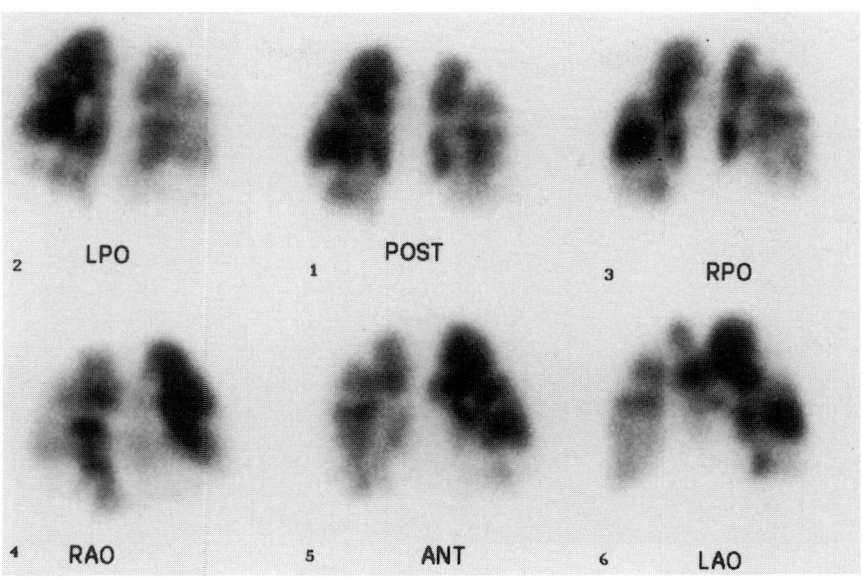

(b)

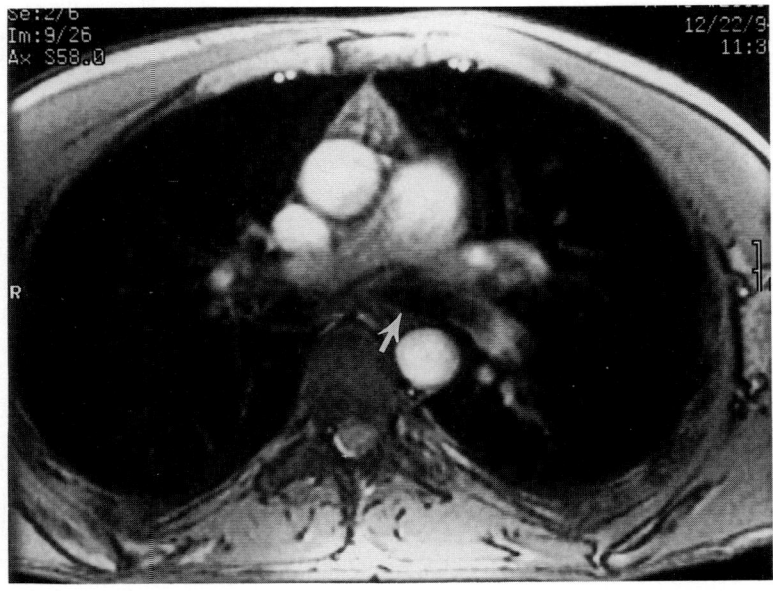

(c)

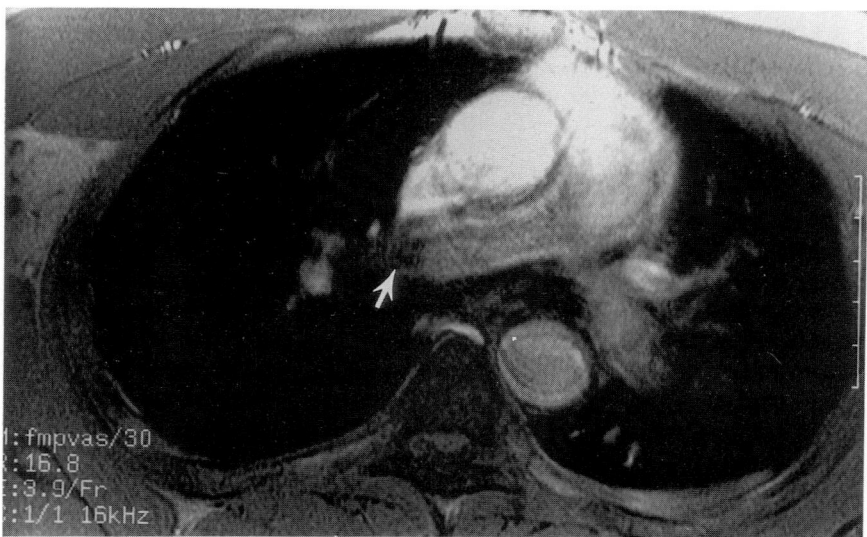

Figure 10 An MRI scan demonstrating decreased signal intensity, representing a difference in blood flow. The image demonstrates decreased signal in the right pulmonary artery from pulmonary embolus (arrow). Although one can see the signal abnormalities, which were confirmed with other imaging modalities, there are confusing artifacts within the images that can make them difficult to interpret.

VI. Sonography

The sonographic evaluation of the pulmonary circulation is mostly limited to the main and proximal right and left pulmonary arteries, as well as findings within the heart that reflect pulmonary arterial hypertension. Intraluminal thrombus is occasionally seen in the pulmonary arteries by sonography. Kasper et al. (55) reported a 13% frequency, with the right pulmonary artery being the most common site. These thrombi are typically quite mobile and serpiginous, suggesting their origin in the pelvic or lower limb venous system. In addition to transthoracic sonography, esophageal sonography has been used to diagnose central pulmonary emboli. In addition to actual imaging, much information concerning pulmonary flow can be assessed by obtaining flow velocities. Finally, newer techniques, such as intravascular ultrasound, have been used in the diagnosis of pulmonary emboli in the animal model (56). Unfortunately, use of this device is quite invasive and may be only an adjunct to angiography or, possibly, useful when one is trying to avoid contrast material.

VII. Pulmonary Angiography

The most common and most direct manner in which to visualize the pulmonary circulation is still pulmonary angiography (see Figs. 6b and 8c). It allows visualization of the arteries as well as the venous system and allows physiological pressure measurements. Pulmonary angiography in most centers has undergone few changes. It is usually performed from a femoral venous access, although the brachial or internal jugular veins are also possible sites. Peripheral intravenous digital subtraction techniques have been used, but are not routinely applied in most centers. There are many catheter styles, but most often some form of pigtail is used. Pulmonary artery pressures are routinely measured in most institutions before the injection of contrast material, particularly in patients suspected of having increased pulmonary artery pressures. Angiography is then performed, most often using nonionic low-osmolar agents, with the catheter initially in the main right or left pulmonary artery. The angiogram itself is tailored to the particular patient and the underlying disease process that is being evaluated.

Pulmonary angiography for AVM is usually performed before treatment, which is most often by endovascular means. Angiography is important to delineate the size and number of feeding arteries and draining veins for each AVM, as well as the number of AVM present. Since the process is often bilateral, both lungs must be injected.

Pulmonary angiography is most often performed to exclude the diagnosis of acute pulmonary embolus, or to define the extent of chronic pulmonary embolus. In most centers, noninvasive imaging, particularly V/Q imaging, has been performed before pulmonary angiography. Some have made the case for proceeding directly to pulmonary angiography, although this is not a widely held opinion (57).

When discussing any invasive procedure, particularly compared with the growing population of noninvasive procedures, one must determine the risks of the procedure and the benefits. To that end, the complications of pulmonary angiography and its diagnostic accuracy must be known. Complications of pulmonary angiography are well known. As with CT, an iodinated contrast medium needs to be administered; therefore, patients must not be allergic, or at least must be pretreated with some regimen before angiography if an allergy exists. This pretreatment varies among institutions. It is best if the patient has normal coagulation parameters. Patients are probably at an increased risk of complete heart block if an underlying left bundle-branch block exists. In these situations, it is best if one is prepared for either external or transvenous pacing should a problem arise. Finally, there is the fear of death from the procedure, related to acute cor pulmonale.

All of these potential complications have resulted in a reluctance to perform pulmonary angiography. This reluctance is demonstrated in a study by Cooper et al. (58), who surveyed 126 hospitals in the United Kingdom and found that 47,000

V/Q scans were performed over a 1-year interval compared with only 490 pulmonary angiograms, despite the availability of angiography in most centers. Much of the fear of pulmonary angiographic complications has arisen from Duke University. Mills et al. (59) published a report on a series of 1350 patients who underwent pulmonary angiography for pulmonary embolus. They had three deaths (0.2%) and an overall complication rate of 5%, including 20 endocardial–myocardial injuries, and cardiac perforation. The common thread to all three deaths was elevated pulmonary arterial pressures, and all deaths were from cor pulmonale. Unfortunately, additional data concerning the number of overall patients with pulmonary hypertension, including those in whom angiography was safely performed, were not included. Perlmutt et al. in 1987 (60) presented a follow-up to the previous series and found 388 (27%) with pulmonary hypertension (systolic > 40 mmHg) out of a total of 1434 patients who underwent pulmonary angiography. This series found two deaths, again in patients with elevated pressures. However, two major changes in the technique of pulmonary angiography have occurred at Duke. Since 1987, all patients have received nonionic low-osmolar contrast media. In addition, angiography is performed exclusively with pigtail-type catheters. Recently, a review of 1432 patients who underwent pulmonary angiography at Duke since the advent of nonionic media and the use of pigtail catheters was undertaken (61). There were no cardiac perforations and no deaths related to pulmonary angiography. Lack of cardiac perforation certainly relates to the use of pigtail catheters, rather than the endhole catheters popular in the previous series. However, there were no deaths in the prior series from cardiac perforation. Recently, Stein et al. (62) published the angiographic complication rates from the PIOPED series of 1111 patients. In all patients, ionic contrast media was used, and there were two deaths during angiography. The lack of deaths in the most recent series from Duke probably relates to the use of low-osmolar nonionic contrast media (61).

Despite this increased safety, pulmonary angiography remains an invasive procedure. Is it worth putting the patient to this risk, particularly with the growing number of less invasive procedures available? Pulmonary angiography has historically been the gold standard for the diagnosis of pulmonary arterial disease, most notably pulmonary embolus (63). However, as any angiographer will attest, these images can be anything but simple to interpret. For example, the angiographic criteria for pulmonary embolus can be divided into primary and secondary signs. Primary signs consist of an intraluminal-filling defect or the demonstration of an occluded pulmonary artery, with or without a trailing edge (tail) of clot (64). Secondary criteria are quite nonspecific and include diminished flow, abnormal parenchymal stain, and delayed venous return. If one limits the diagnosis to the primary findings in large central arteries, pulmonary angiography should be 100% specific, but have little sensitivity. However, this is not the case. Hull et al. (65) found 37% of pulmonary angiograms were either nondiagnostic or the procedure could not be performed. Quinn et al. (66) found that interobserver agreement was only 86% in a study of 60 patients with three blinded observers, and the greatest disagreement occurred in the subsegmental vessels. However, with the advent of new digital acquisition systems, and the perceived increased safety of pulmonary angiography with low-osmolar nonionic media, pulmonary angiography is still the gold standard, and it will be the basis against which other less invasive procedures will be compared in the near future.

VIII. Summary

Imaging of the pulmonary circulatory system continues to effectively apply standard techniques, and newer techniques are rapidly being developed. The essentials of imaging are demonstrated in the diagnosis of pulmonary embolus. Although invasive pulmonary angiography remains the standard for diagnosis, noninvasive imaging is taking a more active role, not only for screening, but also in the definitive diagnosis. Future trends will be for continued development of noninvasive imaging. This will not only enhance diagnoses of the same diseases, as currently imaged, but also expand into diagnostic arenas not yet appreciated by the currently available methods.

References

1. Carroll FE, Loyd JE. Diagnostic imaging in pulmonary vascular diseases. In: Putman CE, ed. Diagnostic imaging of the lung. New York: 1990:117–197.
2. Glazer HS, Muka E, Sagel SS, Jost RG. New techniques in chest radiography. Radiol Clin North Am 1994; 32:711–729.
3. Thaete FL, Fuhrman CR, Oliver JH, et al. Digital radiography and conventional imaging of the chest: a comparison of observer performance. AJR 1994; 162: 575–581.
4. Greenspan RH, Ravin CE, Polansky SM, McCloud TC. Accuracy of the chest radiograph in diagnosis of pulmonary embolism. Invest Radiol 1982; 17:539–543.
5. Stein PD, Alavi A, Gottschalk A, et al. Usefulness of noninvasive diagnostic tools for diagnosis of acute pulmonary embolism in patients with a normal chest radiograph. Am J Cardiol 1991; 67:1117–1120.
6. Stein PD, Athanasoulis C, Greenspan RH, et al. Relation of plain chest radiographic findings to pulmonary arterial pressure and arterial blood oxygen levels in patients with acute pulmonary embolism. Am J Cardiol 1992; 69:394–396.
7. Worsley DF, Alavi A, Aronchick JM. Chest radiographic findings in patients with acute pulmonary embolism: observations from the PIOPED study. Radiology 1993; 189:133–136.
8. Moses DC, Silver TM, Bookstein JJ. The complementary roles of chest radiography, lung scanning, and selective pulmonary angiography in the diagnosis of pulmonary embolism. Circulation 1974; 49:179–188.

9. Stein PD, Coleman RE, Gottschalk A, et al. Diagnostic utility of ventilation/perfusion lung scans in acute pulmonary embolism is not diminished by pre-existing cardiac or pulmonary disease. Chest 1991; 100:604–606.
10. Webber MM, Gomes AS, Roe D. Comparison of Biello, McNeil, and PIOPED criteria for the diagnosis of pulmonary emboli on lung scans. AJR 1990; 154:975–981.
11. McNeil BJ. Ventilation–perfusion studies and the diagnosis of pulmonary embolism: concise communication. J Nucl Med 1980; 21:319–323.
12. Biello DR. Radiological (scintigraphic) evaluation of patients with suspected pulmonary embolism. JAMA 1987; 257:3257–3259.
13. The PIOPED Investigators. Value of the ventilation/perfusion scan in acute pulmonary embolism. JAMA 1990; 263:2753–2759.
14. Gottschalk A, Sostman HD, Coleman RE, et al. Ventilation–perfusion scintigraphy in the PIOPED study. Part II. Evaluation of the scintigraphic criteria and interpretations. J Nucl Med 1993; 34:1119–1126.
15. Sostman HD, Coleman RE, DeLong DM, Newman GE, Paine S. Evaluation of revised criteria for ventilation–perfusion scintigraphy in patients with suspected pulmonary embolism. Radiology 1994; 193:103–107.
16. Gurney JW. No fooling around: direct visualization of pulmonary embolism. Radiology 1993; 188:618–619.
17. Ralph DD. Pulmonary embolism. Radiol Clin North Am 1994; 32:679–687.
18. Lensing AWA, van Beek EJR, Demers C. Ventilation–perfusion lung scanning and the diagnosis of pulmonary embolism: improvement of observer agreement by the use of a lung segment reference chart. Thromb Haemost 1992; 68:245–249.
19. Gray HW, McKillop JH, Bessent RG. Lung scan reporting language: what does it mean? Nucl Med Commun 1993; 14:1084–1087.
20. Elissa L, Kramer J. Clinical applications of SPECT in the chest. In: Elissa L, Kramer J. eds. Clinical SPECT imaging. New York: Raven Press, 1995:179–204.
21. Donaldson RM, Kahn O, Raphael MJ, et al. Emission tomography in embolic lung disease: angiographic correlations. Clin Radiol 1982; 33:389–393.
22. Palla A, Singer SJ, Tumeh SS, et al. Segmental pulmonary anatomy in man: a method of study with angiography and single photon emission computed tomography. J Nucl Med Allied Sci 1989; 33:247–251.
23. Rowell NP, McCready VR, Tait D, et al. Technetium-99m HMPAO and SPECT in the assessment of blood flow in human lung tumours. Br J Cancer 1989; 59:135–141.
24. Hamvas A, Kaplan JD, Markham J, Schuster DP. The effects of regional pulmonary blood flow on protein flux measurements with PET. J Nucl Med 1992; 33:1661–1668.
25. Ritchie CJ, Hsieh J, Gard MF, et al. Predictive respiratory gating: a new method to reduce motion artifacts on CT scans. Radiology 1994; 190:847–852.
26. Zerhouni EA, Herold CJ, Brown RH, et al. High-resolution computed tomography—physiologic correlation. J Thorac Imaging 1993; 8:265–272.
27. Zeman RK, Fox SH, Silverman PM, et al. Helical (spiral) CT of the abdomen. AJR 1993; 160:719–725.
28. Costello P, Dupuy DE, Ecker CP, et al. Spiral CT of the thorax with reduced volume of contrast material: a comparative study. Radiology 1992; 183:663–666.

29. Godwin JD, Webb WR, Gamsu G, Ovenfors CO. Computed tomography of pulmonary embolism. AJR 1980; 135:691–695.
30. Kalebo P, Wallin J. Computed tomography in massive pulmonary embolism. Acta Radiol 1989; 30:105–107.
31. Verschakelen JA, Vanwijck E, Bogaert J, Baert AL. Detection of unsuspected central pulmonary embolism with conventional contrast-enhanced CT. Radiology 1993; 188:847–850.
32. Geraghty JJ, Stanford W, Landas SK, Galvin JR. Ultrafast computed tomography in experimental pulmonary embolism. Invest Radiol 1992; 27:60–63.
33. Remy-Jardin M, Remy J, Wattinne L, Giraud F. Central pulmonary thromboembolism: diagnosis with spiral volumetric CT with the single-breath-hold technique—comparison with pulmonary angiography. Radiology 1992; 185:381–387.
34. Teigen CL, Maus TP, Sheedy PF, et al. Pulmonary embolism: diagnosis with electron-beam CT. Radiology 1993; 188:839–845.
35. Goodman LR, Curtin JJ, Mewissen MW, et al. Detection of pulmonary embolism in patients with unresolved clinical and scintigraphic diagnosis: helical CT versus angiography. AJR 1995; 164:1369–1374.
36. Kereiakes DJ, Herfkens RJ, Brundage BH, et al. Computerized tomography in chronic thromboembolic pulmonary hypertension. Am Heart J 1983; 106:1432–1436.
37. Tardivon AA, Musset D, Maitre S, et al. Role of CT in chronic pulmonary embolism: comparison with pulmonary angiography. J Comput Assist Tomogr 1993; 17:345–351.
38. Remy J, Remy-Jardin M, Giraud F, et al. Angioarchitecture of pulmonary arteriovenous malformations: clinical utility of three-dimensional helical CT. Radiology 1994; 191:657–664.
39. Moser RJ, III, Tenholder MF. Diagnostic imaging of pulmonary arteriovenous malformations. Chest 1986; 89:586–589.
40. Gutierrez FR, Glazer HS, Levitt RG, Moran JF. NMR imaging of pulmonary arteriovenous fistulae. J Comput Assist Tomogr 1984; 8:750–752.
41. White RI, Jr, Mitchell SE, Barth KH, et al. Angioarchitecture of pulmonary arteriovenous malformations: an important consideration before embolotherapy. AJR 1983; 140:681–686.
42. Remy-Jardin M, Wattinne L, Remy J. Transcatheter occlusion of pulmonary arterial circulation and collateral supply: failures, incidents, and complications. Radiology 1991; 180:699–705.
43. White RI, Jr, Pollak JS. Pulmonary arteriovenous malformations: diagnosis with three-dimensional helilcal CT—a breakthrough without contrast media. Radiology 1994; 191:613–614.
44. Gefter WB, Gupta KB, Holland GA. MR, CT enhance diagnosis of pulmonary emboli. Diagn Imaging 1993; 15:80–85.
45. Silverman JM, Julien PJ, Herfkens RJ, Pelc NJ. Quantitative differential pulmonary perfusion: MR imaging versus radionuclide lung scanning. Radiology 1993; 189:699–701.
46. Kondo C, Caputo GR, Masui T, et al. Pulmonary hypertension: pulmonary flow

quantification and flow profile analysis with velocity-encoded cine MR imaging. Radiology 1992; 183:751–758.
47. Galjee MA, Van Rossum AC, Hofman M, et al. Correlation of hemodynamic parameters and pulmonary venous flow in mitral regurgitation measured by magnetic resonance velocity mapping. In: Books of Abstracts: 11th Annual Meeting of the Society of Magnetic Resonance in Medicine. Berkeley CA: Society for Magnetic Resonance Medicine 1992; 2:2508.
48. Gefter WB, Hatabu H. Evaluation of pulmonary vascular anatomy and blood flow by magnetic resonance. J Thorac Imaging 1993; 8:122–136.
49. Grist TM, Sostman HD, MacFall JR, et al. Pulmonary angiography with MR imaging: preliminary clinical experience. Radiology 1993; 189:523–530.
50. Erdman WA, Peshock RM, Redman HC, et al. Pulmonary embolism: comparison of MR images with radionuclide and angiographic studies. Radiology 1994; 190:499–508.
51. Loubeyre P, Revel D, Douek P, et al. Dynamic contrast-enhanced MR angiography of pulmonary embolism: comparison with pulmonary angiography. AJR 1994; 162:1035–1039.
52. Schiebler ML, Holland GA, Hatabu H, et al. Suspected pulmonary embolism: prospective evaluation with pulmonary MR angiography. Radiology 1993; 189:125–131.
53. Frank H, Weissleder R, Bogdanov AA, Jr, Brady TJ. Detection of pulmonary emboli by using MR angiography with MPEG-PL-GdDTPA: an experimental study in rabbits. AJR 1994; 162:1041–1046.
54. Isoda H, Masui T, Hasegawa S, et al. Pulmonary MR angiography: a comparison of 2D and 3D time-of-flight. J Comput Assist Tomogr 1994; 18:402–407.
55. Kasper W, Meinertz T, Henkel B, et al. Echocardiographic findings in patients with proved pulmonary embolism. Am Heart J 1986; 112:1284–1290.
56. Tapson VF, Davidson CJ, Gurbel PA, et al. Rapid and accurate diagnosis of pulmonary emboli in a canine model using intravascular ultrasound imaging. Chest 1991; 100:1410–1413.
57. Windebank WJ. Controversies in nuclear medicine. Nucl Medi Commun 1990; 11:151–157.
58. Cooper TJ, Hayward MWJ, Hartog M. Survey on the use of pulmonary scintigraphy and angiography for suspected pulmonary thromboembolism in the UK. Clin Radiol 1991; 43:243–245.
59. Mills SR, Jackson DC, Older RA, et al. The incidence, etiologies, and avoidance of complications of pulmonary angiography in a large series. Radiology 1980; 136:295–299.
60. Perlmutt LM, Braun SD, Newman GE, et al. Pulmonary arteriography in the high-risk patient. Radiology 1987; 162:187–189.
61. Hudson ER, Smith TP, McDermott VG, et al. Pulmonary angiography using low osmolar nonionic contrast material: complications in 1432 patients. Radiology 1996; 198:61–65.
62. Stein PD, Athanasoulis C, Alavi A, et al. Complications and validity of pulmonary angiography in acute pulmonary embolism. Circulation 1992; 85:462–468.

63. Robin ED. Overdiagnosis and overtreatment of pulmonary embolism: the emperor may have no clothes. Ann Intern Med 1977; 87:775–781.
64. Newman GE. Pulmonary angiography in pulmonary embolic disease. J Thorac Imaging 1989; 4:28–39.
65. Hull RD, Hirsh J, Carter CJ, et al. Diagnostic value of ventilation–perfusion lung scanning in patients with suspected pulmonary embolism. Chest 1985; 88:819–828.
66. Quinn MF, Lundell CJ, Klotz TA. Reliability of selective pulmonary arteriography in the diagnosis of pulmonary embolism. AJR 1987; 149:469–471.

Part Two

CARDIAC IMAGING

17

Imaging the Coronary Circulation

LAWRENCE M. BOXT

Columbia University College of Physicians and Surgeons
and Columbia–Presbyterian Medical Center
New York, New York

I. Introduction

Myocardial infarction is the most frequent cause of mortality in the United States and Western Europe (1,2). More than 1.5 million acute myocardial infarctions were expected to occur in the United States in 1995, resulting in nearly 500,000 deaths (3); half of these deaths would occur suddenly, in patients in whom premorbid coronary artery disease was not suspected (4). These statistics suggest that our traditional criteria for clinical monitoring and intervention are insensitive to the biological mechanisms that result in acute coronary occlusion.

Our concept of "significant" coronary artery disease is based on the angiographic–hemodynamic correlate of flow-limiting arterial stenosis (5,6). That is, a significant coronary stenosis is one in which blood flow to a myocardial bed is critically decreased (Fig. 1). In conventional practice, one would expect that a lesion producing a 20%-diameter reduction would be of little hemodynamic significance, and that a lesion of more than 80% luminal narrowing would. This presumption is based on the observation that a 75% reduction in the luminal area of an artery is required to decrease coronary blood flow (long-segment stenoses of smaller diameter narrowing are felt to be equally flow-limiting). It is clear that this concept, however useful for the planning and

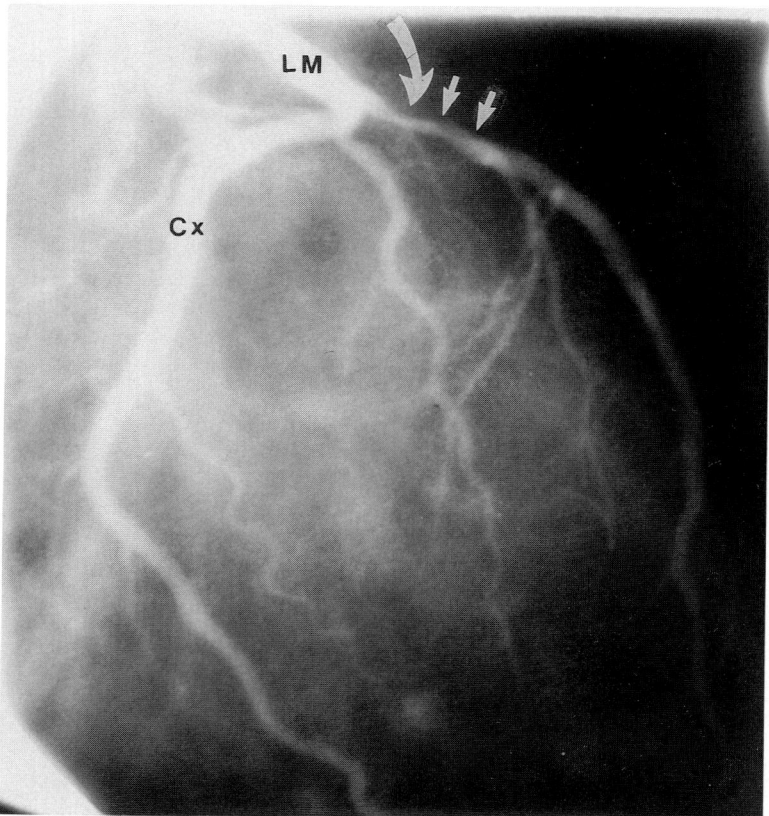

Figure 1 Left coronary arteriogram in RAO projection. The left main (LM) and circumflex (Cx) coronary arteries are normal. There is a long-segment narrowing of the proximal left anterior descending coronary artery (arrows), with most severe narrowing (curved arrow) in the proximal portion.

management of patients with myocardial ischemia, is limited. Numerous investigations have demonstrated discrepancies between angiographic findings and postmortem examination of the coronary arteries (7–9). Furthermore, in clinical series (10,11), retrospective review of preinfarction arteriography revealed irregularity in the region of sites of future coronary occlusions, even if the degree of coronary narrowing was minimal (12). That is, in patients studied angiographically before and after a sudden cardiac event, more than 90% of acute myocardial infarctions were the result of sudden occlusion of a coronary artery, and in more than 50% of acute myocardial infarctions, the coronary artery branch perfusing the infarcted territory was only mildly or moderately narrowed (13). Furthermore, in this same study, more than half the significant coronary stenoses that progressed to complete occlusion did not produce a myocardial infarction. Thus, conventional measurement of luminal narrowing seems not to aid in the identification of prognostically significant coronary arterial lesions.

Our understanding of the mechanics and vascular biology of the arterial wall and, in particular, for mechanisms of coronary atherosclerosis, have increased greatly in the past 30 years (14,15). We now believe that chronic endothelial injury is caused by local mechanical factors, such as abnormal wall shear stress (16) and mural tensile stress (17), which result from disturbed blood flow commonly found at bending points and areas near arterial branch points (15). For example, atherosclerotic plaques occur preferentially in the anterior descending coronary artery, just opposite its origin from the left main coronary artery (18), and in the right coronary artery in regions of relatively low-flow velocity (19).

Atherosclerotic disease follows a morphological progression (14) through five phases (20), each characterized by changes in lesion morphology and clinical findings. In phase 1, the earliest recognizable intimal lesions (type I) are characterized by the presence of "foam cells"—isolated macrophages containing oxidized lipid droplets. Acquisition of increasing lipid content characterizes the progression from type I to type II (flat fatty streak) and type III (raised fatty streaks) lesions. These three lesions are small and evolve slowly as a result of chronic endothelial injury and risk factors, increased vascular permeability to lipids and macrophages, and proliferation of smooth-muscle cells. If the process of lipid influx continues, and exceeds lipid efflux, then the lesion progresses into phase 2, a period of continuous slow lesion progression, leading to changes of types IV and Va lesions. The type IV lesion has a predominance of diffuse extracellular lipid that expands an extensive, but well-defined, region of the intima, the so-called lipid core. Formation of the lipid core precedes an increase in the collagen and smooth-muscle content of the lesion, resulting in the type Va lesion. These lesions have a high, mainly localized lipid content, and a very thin capsule. Both lesions progress slowly (over months to a few years) into more stenotic and fibrotic type Vb and Vc lesions.

However, more commonly, these lesions may suddenly rupture and acquire thrombus, changing shape, leading to the type VI complicated lesion. If the thrombus formed is mural, with or without development of clinical signs and symptoms of angina, this progression is referred to as phase 3; if the thrombus is occlusive, with clinical evidence of myocardial infarction, unstable angina, or ischemic sudden death, then the progression is phase 4. Organization of the thrombus by connective tissue contributes to a rapid evolution (phase 5), into types Vb (severely stenotic) or Vc (occlusive fibrotic) lesions.

Elucidation of this mechanism highlights the need to develop techniques for characterization of individual arterial plaque morphology, rather than simply measure the resultant percentage of luminal narrowing. Technical advances in the visualization of the coronary circulation must be directed toward early detection of prognostically significant coronary artery disease. In an era with great emphasis on decreasing the cost of individual examinations, as well as the cost of caring for patients with coronary heart disease, rapid, safe (i.e., non- or minimally invasive) diagnostic modalities appear more attractive than ever. However, to impinge significantly on this disease, patients at serious risk must be more accurately diagnosed. Therefore, not only must we develop noninvasive methods of coronary visualization, but also techniques that provide clues to the underlying disordered vascular biology of the arterial plaque.

In this chapter, I will review new, noninvasive means of detecting coronary arterial stenosis, namely magnetic resonance coronary arteriography, and transthoracic and transesophageal echocardiography. In addition, I will review the computed tomographic (CT) evaluation of coronary arterial calcification, a manifestation of disordered coronary arterial biology, and the use of intracoronary ultrasound to characterize individual arterial plaques. The purpose of this chapter is not to be a detailed review of these subjects, but rather, to point out for the interested reader the current state of these evolving technologies, emphasizing their limitations and potential utility.

II. Magnetic Resonance Coronary Arteriography

Magnetic resonance imaging (MRI) is very well suited for evaluation of the heart because it provides excellent soft-tissue contrast, without the need for administration of intravascular contrast agents; it provides a three-dimensional data set; and allows acquisition in any arbitrary anatomical section. However, all MRI scans are exquisitely sensitive to artifacts induced by motion and turbulent blood flow. Cardiac MRI is especially sensitive to cardiac and respiratory motion, and coronary MR arteriography (MRA) attempts to demonstrate vessels smaller than, or equal to, 5 mm in caliber running along the epicardial surface of the heart.

Conventional electrocardiographic (ECG)-gated spin-echo (Figs. 2 and 3) and gradient-reversal (Fig. 4) MRI has always provided occasional glimpses of portions of the epicardial coronary arterial tree. However, coronary arterial visualization by these methods is of limited temporal resolution, and they cannot be relied on for precise morphological diagnosis. Recent advances in fast MRI have nearly eliminated respiratory and cardiac motion artifacts, and this has offered the possibility of noninvasive visualization of the epicardial coronary arteries (Fig. 5).

Newly developed two-dimensional acquisition sequences, using electrocardiographically gated gradient-echos, depict laminar blood flow as bright signal, and turbulence or absent blood flow as signal voids. Use of fat-suppression

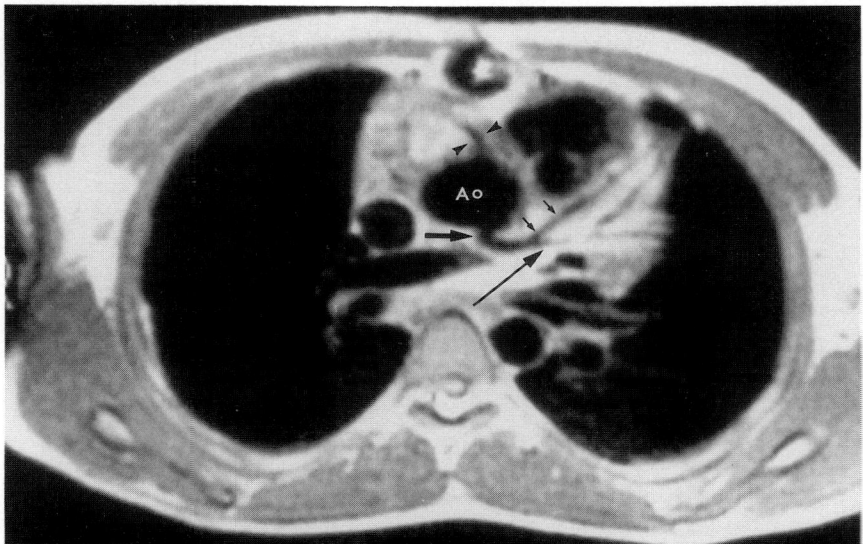

Figure 2 Axial spin-echo MR image obtained through the aortic root (Ao). The origin of the right coronary artery (arrowheads) is from the anterior aortic sinus of Valsalva. The left main (black arrow) and anterior descending (short arrows) coronary arteries as well as the origin of the left circumflex artery (long arrow) may be seen.

techniques increases the contrast of the epicardial coronary arteries by decreasing the relative signal produced by the epicardial fat surrounding the arteries (Fig. 6). In addition, rapid-acquisition sequence allow image acquisition during a single breath-hold, with and without use of k-space segmentation, to provide rapid visualization of the epicardial coronary tree (21–25). Examination of these preliminary series was often performed with the patient prone on a surface coil, sandwiched between the anterior chest wall and the examination table to decrease distance between the anterior surface of the heart and the source and receiver of RF stimulation. More conventional supine examination can be performed, and this may be preferred because of increased patient comfort.

In a preliminary evaluation of the use of fat-suppressed single–breath-hold MRA with k-space segmentation (21) in 25 subjects (including 19 healthy volunteers and 6 patients undergoing diagnostic coronary arteriography) the left main coronary artery (LMCA) was identified in 24 (96%) subjects. The left anterior descending coronary artery (LAD) and right coronary artery (RCA) were visualized in all 25 individuals. The left circumflex artery (LCx) was seen in 19 (76%). Diagonal branches of the LAD were identified in 20 (80%) subjects. In the 6

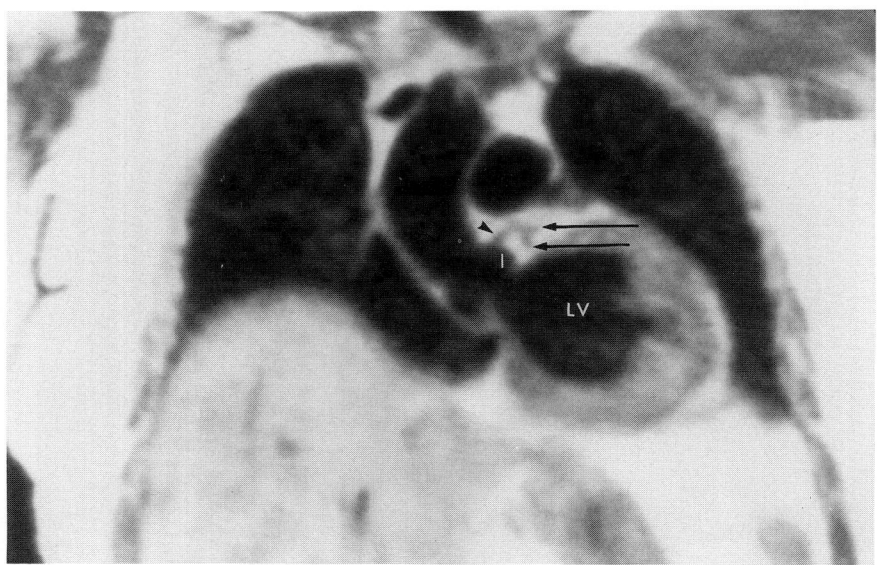

Figure 3 Coronal spin-echo MR image through the aortic root. The posterior left sinus of Valsalva (I) and origin of the left main coronary artery (arrowhead) is seen. Bifurcation of the left main into anterior descending (upper horizontal long arrow) and circumflex (lower horizontal arrow) arteries within the epicardial fat of the left ventricle (LV) is labeled.

patients in this series with angiographically proved coronary artery occlusion, all occlusions were identified by coronary MRA as total absence of signal distal to the area of occlusion. In a similar series (25), 39 adults referred for diagnostic coronary arteriography, underwent single–breath-hold gradient-echo coronary MRA, with incremented flip angle series and k-space segmentation, within 1 week of their conventional arteriograms. Conventional coronary arteriography demonstrated moderate to severe proximal coronary artery narrowing in 74% of patients. Overall sensitivity and specificity of the MRA examination for correctly identifying individual coronary vessels with hemodynamically significant ($\geq 50\%$) stenosis was 90 and 92%, respectively. Sensitivity and specificity of the technique for the LMCA were 100, 87, and 92% for the LAD, 71 and 90% for the LCx, and 100 and 78% for the RCA, respectively.

Subsequent studies with larger patient populations showed less optimistic results. Duerinckx and Urman (22) reported the use of a similar two-dimensional MRA coronary arterial technique in 20 patients undergoing both conventional and coronary MRA. These authors found 50% sensitivity for stenosis of the LMCA, 73% sensitivity for stenosis of the LAD, 0% for the LCx, and 62% sensitivity for significant stenosis of the RCA (overall sensitivity = 63%). Specificity in this

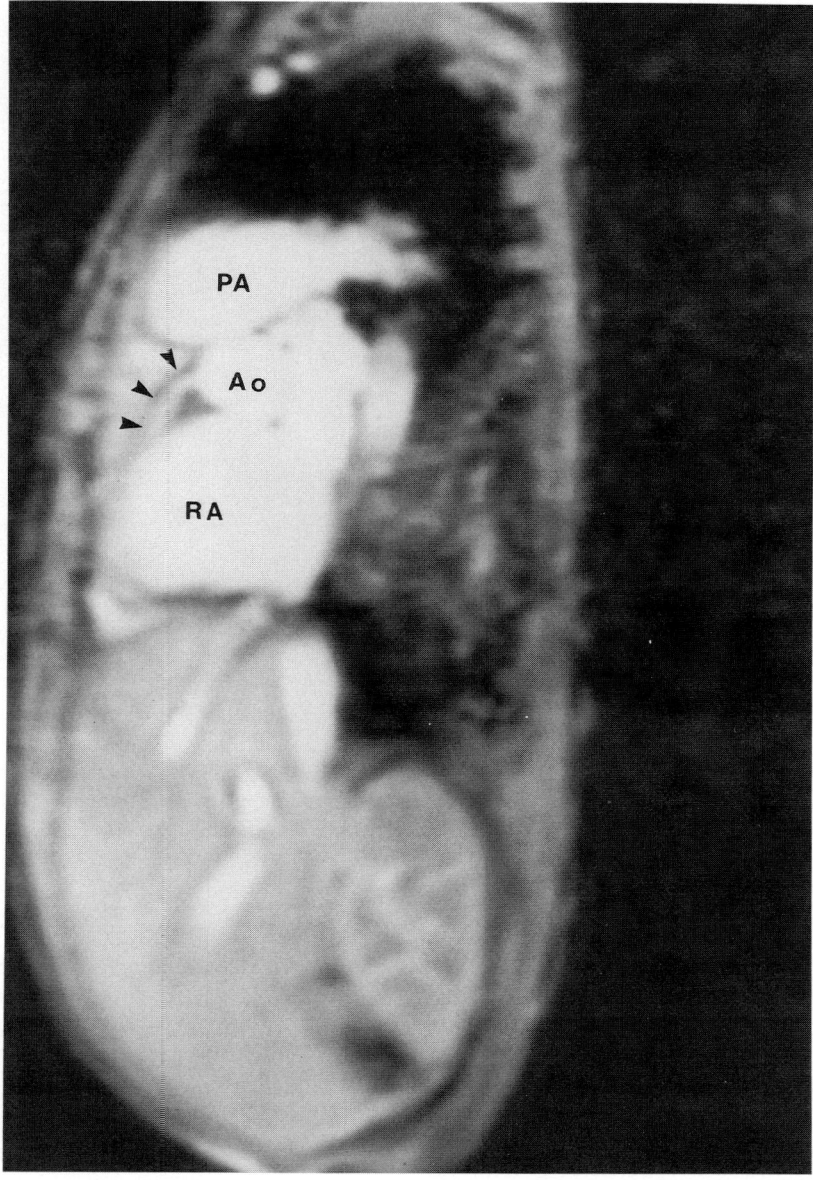

Figure 4 Short-axis gradient-reversal MR image through the aortic root (Ao). The dilated right atrium (RA) and main pulmonary artery are seen in this patient with pulmonary hypertension. The origin and proximal portion of the right coronary artery (arrowheads) is visualized.

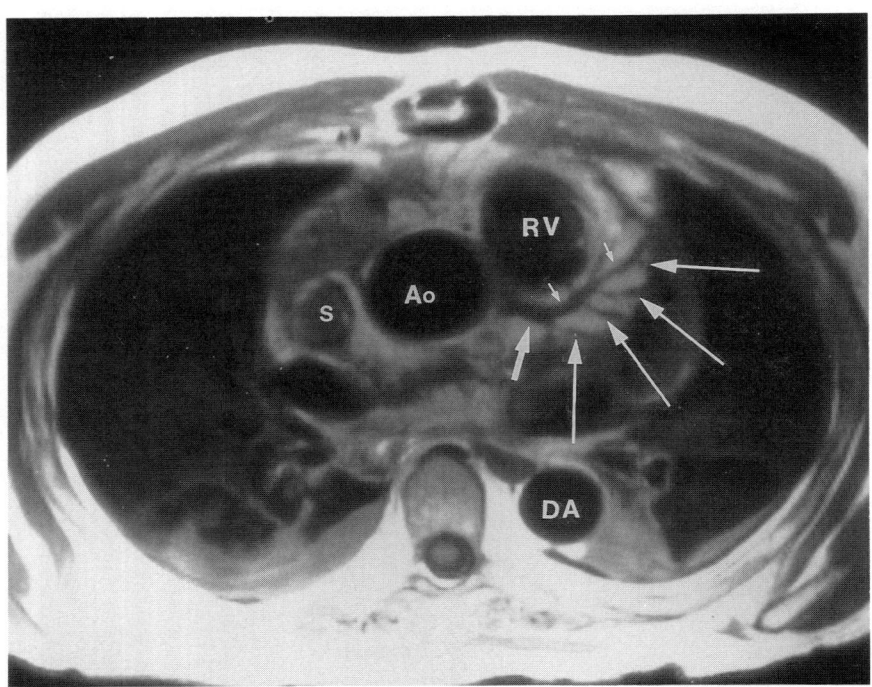

Figure 5 Axial fast spin-echo MR image at the level of the aortic root (Ao). The right ventricular outflow tract (RV), superior vena cava (S), right upper lobe pulmonary vein (curved arrow), and descending aorta (DA) are labeled. The left main (large arrow), anterior descending (small arrows), and diagonal branches of the anterior descending artery (long arrows) are identified. (Courtesy of Richard D. White, M.D., Cleveland, Ohio.)

series was 84% for the LMCA, 37% for the LAD, 82% for the LCx, and 56% for the RCA. Similarly, Pennell et al. (24) reviewed this technique of coronary MRA in a group of 21 healthy controls and 5 patients with angiographically proved coronary artery disease. Twenty-two (85%) of the 26 subjects were successfully imaged. The LMCA was identified in 95%, the LAD in 91%, the left circumflex in 76%, and the RCA in 95% of studies. All 5 coronary occlusions in their series were identified by coronary MRA. Although most missed vessels occurred early in their series, imaging the circumflex artery was problematic throughout their experience.

Preliminary experience with the use of an alternative technique for coronary MRA, three-dimensional, rapid, gradient-echo acquisition (23) provided similar findings. The proximal coronary tree was not identified in all subjects. The LMCA

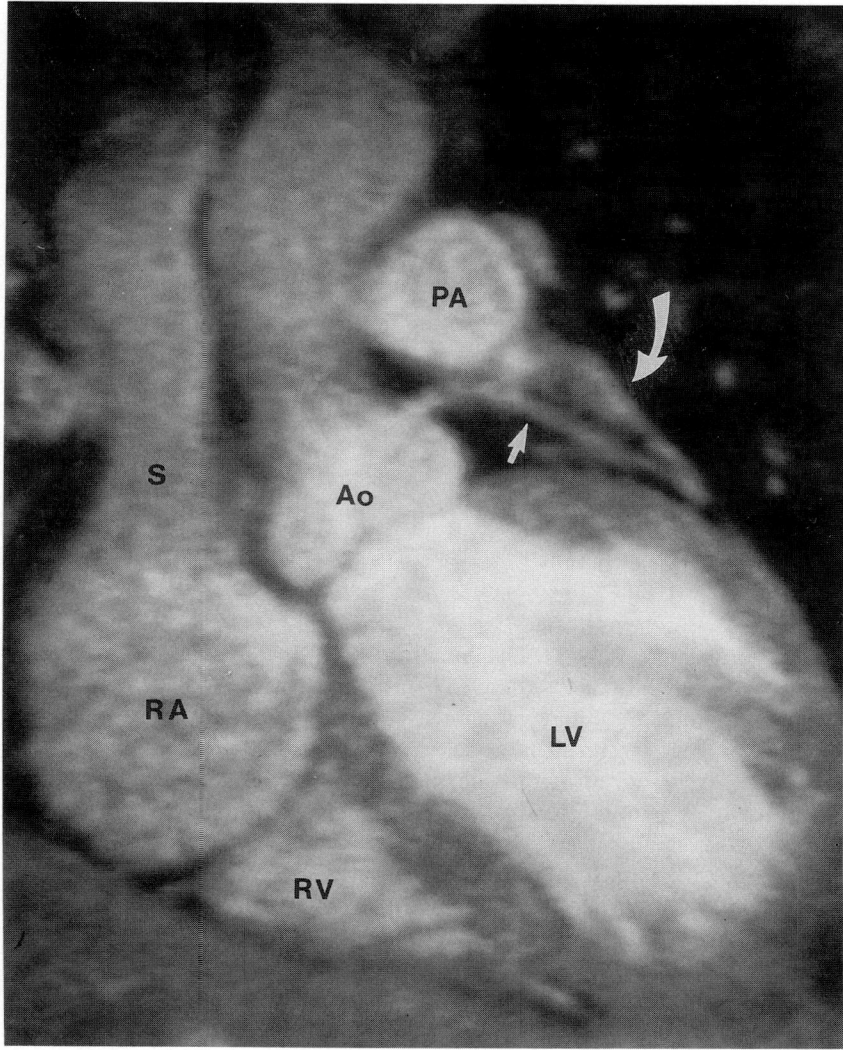

Figure 6 An RAO sagittal fat-suppressed breath-hold gradient reversal MR image through the aortic root (Ao). The left ventricular chamber (LV), superior vena cava (S), right atrium (RA), right ventricle (RV), and main pulmonary artery (PA) are identified. The left anterior descencing coronary artery (straight arrow) is seen coursing in the (fat-suppressed) epicardial fat between the left atrial appendage (curved arrow) and myocardium of the left ventricle. (Courtesy of Richard D. White, M.D., Cleveland, Ohio.)

was identified in four (57%) of seven healthy volunteers. In this same group of volunteers, the LAD was identified in four (57%) of seven, the LCx in two (29%), and the RCA in all seven (100%). Seven patients studied by conventional coronary arteriography and coronary MRA had 17 diseased arterial segments. Coronary MRA demonstrated altered signal intensity in 13 (76%) of these segments.

Coronary MRA cannot as yet provide complete and reliable noninvasive demonstration of the epicardial coronary arteries and their branches. Needless to say, advances in pulse sequence design, as well as hardware considerations (such as dedicated chest surface coils and higher RF gradients) will undoubtedly improve our ability to demonstrate the coronary arteries by these techniques. However, technological advances aside, the question of which vessels we are able to identify by MRA must be addressed. We must ask whether our ability to demonstrate the coronary arteries per se, improves our ability to diagnose coronary artery disease and identify patients at risk for future cardiac events. In other words, for coronary MRA to become a useful modality in the evaluation and management planning of patients with coronary heart disease, it must first be able to reliably demonstrate the entire epicardial coronary tree. (Can one imagine the growth in utilization of coronary arteriography if it allowed visualization of only the proximal epicardial arteries in only 80% of cases?) Then we must improve sensitivity and specificity for the detection of less severe ($< 50\%$) luminal narrowing; otherwise, its usefulness in detecting non–flow-limiting plaques, the major source of acute coronary occlusion and sudden cardiac events, will be limited. Furthermore, if coronary MRA is to become a noninvasive replacement for conventional catheter coronary arteriography, then the sensitivity and specificity for detection of significant vessel stenosis must increase. Claims of MRI eventually providing combined morphological and functional analysis of the heart do not offset its current limited spatial resolution and the difficulties in the sensitive and specific imaging of the circumflex coronary artery, the branches of the epicardial coronary arteries, and differentiation between coronary arteries and cardiac veins.

III. Echocardiography

Transthoracic echocardiographic imaging (TTE) has been used in the demonstration of coronary artery aneurysms in pediatric patients with Kawasaki's disease (26,27; Fig. 7) and the demonstration of congenital anomalies of the proximal coronary arteries in children with congenital heart disease (28; Fig. 8). Transthoracic examination of the coronary arteries is severely limited by technical difficulties inherent in examination of the chest. These include artifacts caused by the interposition of the chest wall between transducer and heart, decreased ultrasound beam penetration of the middle mediastinum where the coronary arteries reside, cardiac and respiratory motion, as well as problems caused by abnor-

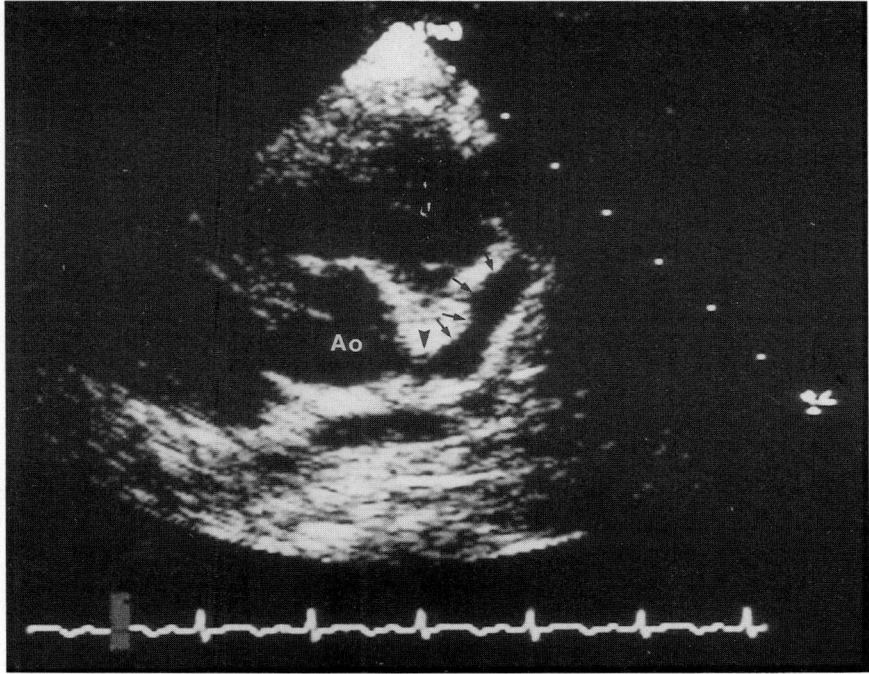

Figure 7 Parasternal short-axis transthoracic echocardiogram through the aortic root (Ao). There is aneurysmal dilation of a long segment of the anterior descending coronary artery (small arrows) extending from its origin from the left main coronary artery (arrowhead).

malities in chest wall configuration and the not infrequent presence of obstructive lung disease.

Clinical application of TTE in adults with atherosclerotic coronary artery disease, using a 2.25-MHz–phased, array ultrasound transducer, was attempted in a series of 73 patients, 21 of whom had more than 50%-lumen–diameter reduction (29). The LMCA was adequately visualized in 36 of 52 subjects (69%) with normal LMCAs and in 16 of the 21 with significant stenosis (76%). In 34 of the 36 subjects with normal LMCA, no intraluminal abnormalities were found. Of the 16 patients with significant stenosis, asymmetric, high-intensity–echo wall density or disruption of the arterial lumen was found in 12. Three of the 36 subjects with normal LMCAs had false-positive echocardiographic examinations, and 4 of the 16 patients with significant stenosis had false-negative examinations. These authors did not attempt visualization of the more distal coronary arteries or their branches.

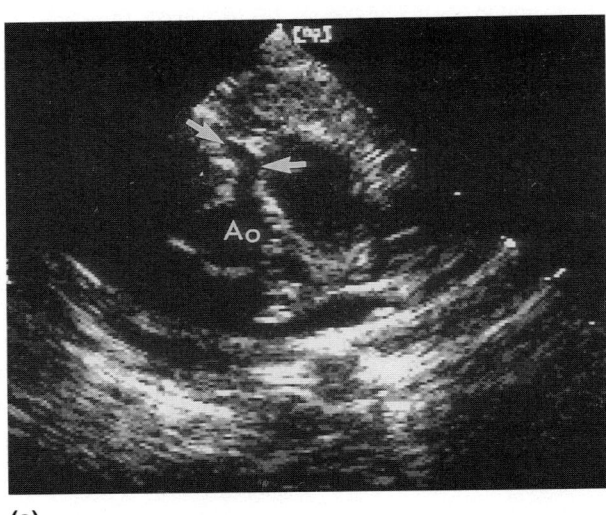

(a)

Figure 8 Parasternal short axis transthoracic echocardiogram: (a) The origin of the right coronary artery from the aortic root (Ao), and its normal course through the anterior atrioventricular ring (arrows) is shown. (b) Same patient: Image obtained with more lateral angulation of the transducer. The right ventricular outflow tract (R) is separated from the main pulmonary artery by the pulmonary valve (small arrows). The origin of the anomalous left main coronary artery from the posterior pulmonary sinus of Valsalva (arrowhead), and bifurcation of the anomalous artery into anterior descending (arrow 1) and circumflex (artery 2) branches, is labeled.

By using a 3.5- and 5.0-MHz–phased array transducer, more detailed examination of the epicardial coronary arteries was achieved (30). In a study group of 35 subjects, including 18 normal subjects and 17 patients with heart disease (9 with valvular, 5 patients with coronary, 2 patients with congenital, and 1 patient with cardiomyopathic heart disease), the LMCA was seen in 30 (86%), and its bifurcation was seen in 15 (43%). The LAD was seen in 30 (86%), the LCx in 11 (31%), and the RCA in 32 (91%). Diagonal and septal branches of the LAD were visualized in 11 (31%), and a marginal branch of the LCx in 1 (3%). In the 5 patients in their series with angiographically documented coronary artery disease, lesions were echocardiographically demonstrated in 4 (80%); 2 LAD, 1 LMCA, and 1 RCA. The proximal coronary arteries were obscured by heavy aortic valve calcification in the fifth patient.

Although TTE is an appealing method for noninvasive coronary artery diagnosis, it produced suboptimal examinations in a significant number of adult

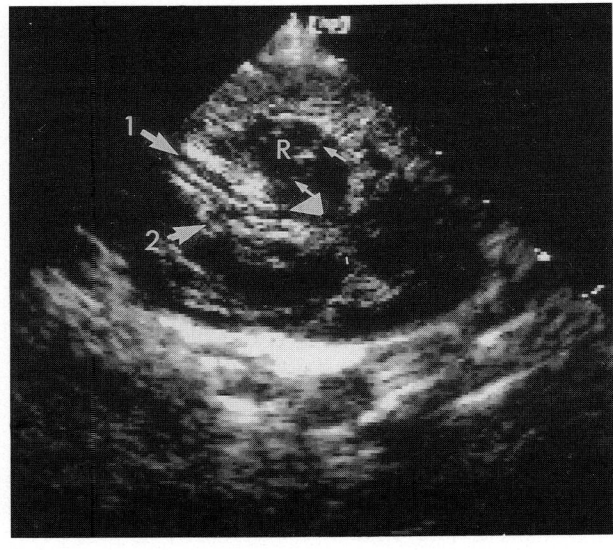
(b)

patients. Furthermore, limitations in TTE's ability to visualize side branches, as well as the entire length of the eparterial coronary tree, limit its diagnostic sensitivity and specificity. Imaging through the lungs prevents application of an adequately high-frequency transducer to resolve mural coronary arterial abnormalities, limiting arterial plaque detection and characterization, precluding any significant clinical usefulness, for the diagnosis of occlusive coronary artery disease.

Transesophageal echocardiography (TEE) brings the ultrasound transducer closer to the proximal coronary arteries, and avoids interposition of the chest wall between transducer and coronary arterial segments. This allows the utilization of higher-frequency transducers and, thereby, increased spatial resolution and more-detailed imagery. In a series of 111 consecutive patients in whom intraoperative TEE and coronary arteriography were performed (31), TEE provided complete visualization of the LMCA as far as its bifurcation in 103 of 111 patients (93%). The artery was not visualized in 7 patients, and was incompletely visualized in 1. The coronary artery was angiographically normal in 4 of these patients; distal stenosis was present in 4 and proximal stenosis in zero. The RCA was adequately visualized in 55 (49%) of the 111 patients. Significant coronary artery stenosis was correctly diagnosed by TEE in 47 (88%) of 53 lesions; 23 (96%) of 24 LMCA stenoses, 11 (78%) of 14 LAD lesions, and 6 (75%) of 8 LCx lesions. All proximal

RCA stenoses were identified by TEE. In these anesthetized patients, there were no complications caused by performance of the TEE examination.

In a series of 45 patients studied by nonintraoperative TEE and conventional coronary arteriography (32), the LMCA was visualized in all cases. All 6 patients with LMCA stenosis were identified by this technique. No patient with an angiographically normal LMCA had a false-positive TEE diagnosis. Visualization of the LAD was limited, however. Proximal, midportion, and distal segments of the LAD were visualized in 69, 31, and 16% of patients, respectively. In only 25 and 16% of patients were the first and second diagonal branches of the LAD identified. In this series, 10 patients had angiographically significant LAD stenosis; TEE correctly identified 8 (80%) of these lesions. The proximal, midportion, and distal LCx was visualized in 80, 51, and 20% of patients, respectively. The first marginal branch was identified in 18% of patients, and the second marginal branch in 11%. Eight (88%) of nine patients with angiographically significant LCx stenosis were correctly diagnosed by TEE. The proximal RCA was visualized in 84% of patients; the mid- and distal RCA was visualized in 16 and 11% of patients, respectively. No false-positive diagnosis of stenosis of the LAD, LCx, or RCA disease was made by TEE. Both groups of investigators (31,32) found use of pulsed color Doppler evaluation helpful in evaluation of the orifice of the LMCA, but of less value in evaluation of the more distal vessels. Improvement in coronary arterial visualization with TEE is encouraging, but limitation in visualization of the complete coronary tree, and need for esophageal intubation preclude its routine use.

IV. Coronary Artery Calcification and Very Rapid Computed Tomography

Although a close relation between the presence and extent of coronary arterial calcification and the presence and severity of coronary atherosclerosis (33–37) has been known for years, the only reasonably sensitive means for detection of coronary calcification had been cardiac fluoroscopy, a decidedly operator-dependent technique. Thus, investigation of coronary calcification as a detector of coronary atherosclerosis, and quantitating the degree and distribution of calcification as a function of clinical status and prognosis, have been severely limited.

Observation of coronary artery calcification on CT scans of the chest (38; Fig. 9) stimulated development of a scoring system for coronary calcification, to allow quantitative correlation between calcification and decrease in luminal stenosis (as evaluated by conventional coronary arteriography). However, conventional CT evaluation is limited by artifacts introduced by structure superimposition and motion during image acquisition. The introduction of electron beam (EB) CT now allows direct quantification of signal within voxel-sized regions of interest (Fig. 10).

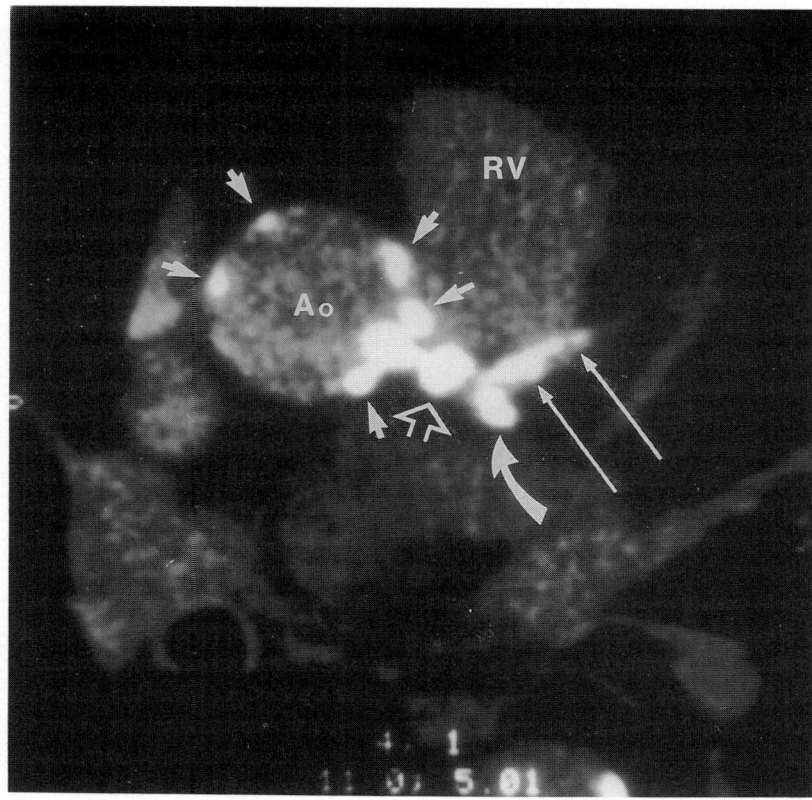

Figure 9 Conventional CT image of the heart through the aortic root (Ao) and right ventricular outflow tract (RV). Aortic calcification (short arrows) as well as calcification of the left main (open arrow), anterior descending (long arrows), and proximal circumflex (short arrows) coronary arteries is vividly demonstrated. (Courtesy of William Stanford, M.D., Iowa City, Iowa.)

The marked increase in temporal resolution of these new scanners eliminates motion artifacts caused by cardiac contraction and, to a lesser degree, those caused by respiratory motion (39,40). In fact, increasing coronary artery calcification score, as determined by EBCT (39–42) correlates well with significant coronary artery stenosis (e.g., > 70% luminal narrowing) as determined by conventional coronary arteriography.

The clinical utility of EBCT-derived calcification scores is controversial, however. Although such scores correlate with the presence of significantly stenosed coronary arteries, current understanding of the development and progres-

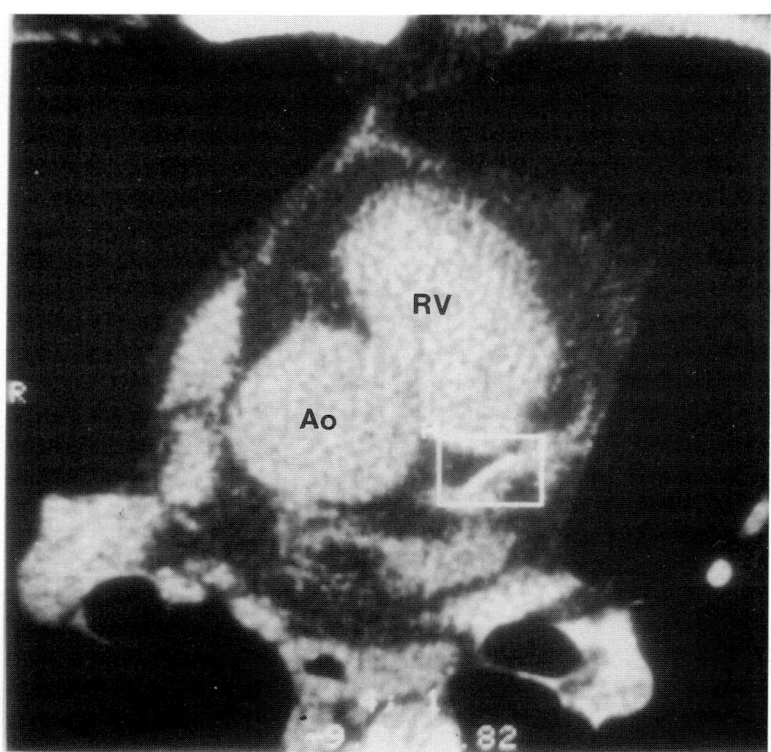

Figure 10 Electron beam computed tomographic image obtained through the aortic root (Ao) and right ventricular outflow tract (RV). The calcified proximal anterior descending coronary artery has been localized within the rectangular region of interest for quantitative analysis.

sion of coronary atherosclerosis (43) casts question on the clinical importance of lesions identified as containing advanced calcification. We know that a mature atherosclerotic plaque is usually covered by a smooth, fibromuscular capsule, which separates flowing blood from the plaque contents. On occasion, the plaque may rupture, exposing the plaque itself to the arterial lumen. Lumenal blood dissects into the plaque, forming a thrombus, which greatly increases the size of the plaque, and may extend into the vessel lumen to decrease its caliber as well. In some percentage of plaques, the intraplaque hematoma organizes and calcifies.

Coronary atherosclerotic lesions may be characterized by their angiographic appearance (44), a reflection of the status of their plaque capsule. A smooth coronary arterial wall is associated with an intact plaque capsule; a ruptured plaque capsule is associated with irregular margins. The variance between progression of a mild or moderate arterial stenosis to acute occlusion (10–12) and the presence of arterial wall calcification suggests that lesions identified by EBCT calcification scoring may not be culprit lesions in acute myocardial infarction. Thus, unless an association between coronary artery calcification and previous plaque rupture can be established, and whether, in fact, this association is associated with a future plaque rupture, then, cardiac prognosis may be more reliably predicted by the presence of an irregular plaque capsule than merely by the presence of mural calcification as quantitated by EBCT. The usefulness of EBCT is tantalizing, but its value is as yet unproved.

V. Intravascular Ultrasound

Catheter-based two-dimensional intracoronary ultrasound provides accurate dimensional information concerning the arterial lumen and wall structures (45–48). The use of very high-frequency transducers (20 MHz) mounted on the end of very small-caliber (5.5-F and 3.5-F) catheters allows advancement of the devices into the proximal coronary arterial tree. The spatial and contrast resolution of such systems allows the analysis of plaque morphology and the determination of morphological features of atherosclerotic coronary arteries that correlate with clinical syndromes.

Normal echographic intimal echoes are less than 150–300 mm and medial echoes are less than 200 mm in thickness (49,50). By using intravascular ultrasound, morphological plaque features can be classified (51). Soft plaques, presumably lesions with a high thrombus, lipid, or fibromuscular content, were identified as thickened intimal echoes with homogeneous echodensity, less than that seen for adventitia, and the absence of calcification (Fig. 11). Fibrous plaques were identified by the presence of thickened, dense intimal echoes with homogeneous echodensity greater than that seen in the adventitia, and the absence of calcification. Calcified plaques demonstrated bright echoes within the plaque and acoustic shadowing behind. Ultrasonographically mixed plaques, representing plaques with varying degree of thrombus, lipid, fibromuscular, as well as dense fibrous or calcific components, appeared to contain bright echoes and acoustic shadowing encompassing less than 90% of the vessel wall circumference. With this classification, the authors found no difference in the angiographic percentage of vessel area narrowing between patients with unstable versus stable angina. However, the authors did find that soft plaque was more common in patients with unstable angina (74%) than in patients with stable angina (41%; $p < 0.01$). Conversely, patients with stable angina pectoris had a higher incidence of calcific and mixed plaque morphology (59%) than did patients with unstable angina (25%; $p < 0.01$). Calcium deposition was found significantly more frequently in patients

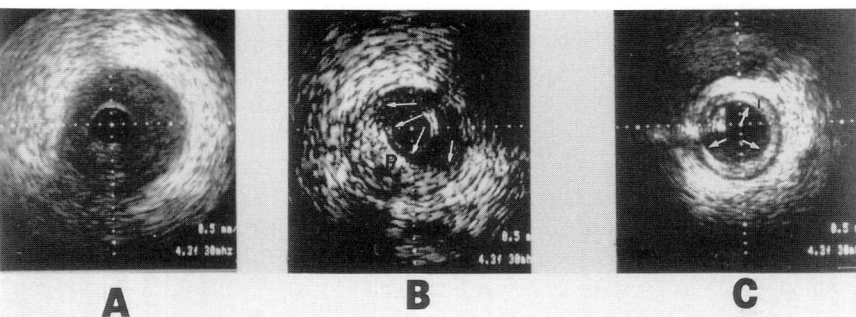

Figure 11 Intravascular ultrasonographic images obtained from adult patients with syndrome X. Marker dots are separated by 0.5 mm. (A) Normal segment from the midportion of the anterior descending coronary artery. The signal void of the catheter is located at the intersection of the marker dots. The normal arterial intimal layer cannot be differentiated from the arterial media (M). (B) Image obtained from the midright coronary artery in a patient with an atherosclerotic plaque (P). The large eccentric atheroma (outlined by arrows) occupies nearly 50% of the luminal area. (C) Segment of the anterior descending coronary artery in a patient with concentric thickening of the intima (arrows). The locus of increased signal in the left upper quadrant is the artifact produced by an intracoronary guide wire. (Courtesy of Dr. Marc Apfelbaum, New York, NY.)

with stable angina (10 of 22 patients; 45%) than in patients with unstable angina (7 of 43 patients, 16%; $p < 0.01$). Furthermore, correlation of ultrasonographic findings with angiographic morphology (52) revealed that patients with ultrasonographically soft plaque had clinically unstable angina in 32 of 41 cases (78%); angiographically, 17 of 21 patients (81%) with unstable angina had type II eccentric plaque. Thus soft plaque was found more often in patients with unstable angina than angiographic type II eccentric lesions.

Clearly, these findings indicate the great potential of ultrasonographic evaluation of patients with coronary artery disease. However, they also denote important limitations of its use. Although the problems of interposition of the chest wall and abnormal chest configuration found in transthoracic echocardiographic analysis of the coronary arteries are eliminated by use of the transesophageal approach, limited visualization of long segments of the coronary arteries, and most pointedly, that of the mid- and distal portions of the arteries, preclude use of this technique for routine evaluation of patients with atherosclerotic coronary artery disease. On the other hand, as a screening tool, for the evaluation of major coronary arterial anomalies in the preoperative evaluation of patients with congenital heart disease, TEE provides useful information in a safe manner. Direct analysis of the diseased arterial wall by intracoronary ultrasonography represents a tremendous advance in the evaluation of patients with subcritical or mild coronary arterial lumenal narrowing. However, the risks of conventional coronary arteriography in patients with chronic ischemia may not be significantly greater than those of intracoronary ultrasonography. Its full potential for investigating the natural history and biology of coronary atherosclerosis has not yet been fulfilled. With the development of higher resolution and smaller transducers, the use of this modality will undoubtedly grow and find greater applicability in the evaluation of patients with coronary heart disease.

References

1. Cooper ES. Prevention: the key to progress. Circulation 1993; 24:629–632 [AHA Medical/Scientific Statement].
2. WHO-MONICA Project. Myocardial infarction and coronary deaths in the World Health Organization Monica Project: registration procedures, event rates, and case–fatality rates in 38 populations from 21 countries in four continents. Circulation 1994; 90:583–612.
3. Heart and stroke facts. Dallas, TX: American Heart Association, 1992; 1–2.
4. Fuster V, Badimon L, Cohen M, et al. Insights into the pathogenesis of acute ischemic syndromes. Circulation 1988; 77:1213–1220.
5. Gould KL, Lipscomb K, Hamilton GW. Physiologic basis for assessing critical coronary stenosis: instantaneous flow response and regional distribution during coronary hyperemia as measures of coronary flow reserve. Am J Cardiol 1974; 33:87–94.
6. Gould KL, Lipscomb K. Effects of coronary stenoses on coronary flow reserve and resistance. Am J Cardiol 1974; 34:48–55.
7. Grondin CM, Dyrda I, Pasternac A, et al. Discrepancies between cineangiographic and postmortem findings in patients with coronary artery disease and recent myocardial revascularization. Circulation 1974; 49:703–708.
8. Isner JM, Kishel J, Kent KM, et al. Accuracy of angiographic determination of left main coronary arterial narrowing. Angiographic–histologic correlative analysis in 28 patients. Circulation 1981; 63:1056–1064.
9. White CW, Wright CB, Doty DB, et al. Does visual interpretation of the coronary arteriogram predict the physiologic importance of a coronary stenosis? N Engl J Med 1984; 310:273–279.
10. Haft JJ, Al-Zarka AM. Comparison of the natural history of irregular and smooth coronary lesions: insights into the pathogenesis, progression, and prognosis of coronary atherosclerosis. Am Heart J 1993; 129:551–561.
11. Ambrose JA. Coronary angiographic analysis and angiographic morphology, J Am Coll Cardiol 1989; 13:1492–1494.
12. Little WC. Angiographic assessment of the culprit coronary artery lesion before acute myocardial infarction. Am J Cardiol 1990; 66:44G–47G.
13. Ambrose JA, Tannenbaum MA, Alexopoulous D. Angiographic progression of coronary artery disease. J Am Coll Cardiol 1988; 12:56–62.
14. Fuster V. Lewis A. Conner Memorial Lecture. Mechanisms leading to myocardial

infarction: insights from studies of vascular biology. Circulation 1994; 90:2126–2146.
15. Glagov S, Zarins C, Giddens DP, Ku DN. Hemodynamics and atherosclerosis. Arch Pathol Lab Med 1988; 112:1018–1031.
16. Fry DL. Responses of arterial wall to certain factors. In: Porter R, Knight J, eds. Atherogenesis initiating factors. Amsterdam: Elsevier Scientific, 1973: 93–125.
17. Burton AC. Relation of structure to function of the tissues of the wall of blood vessels. Physiol Rev 1954; 34:619–642.
18. Svindland A. The localization of sudanophilic and fibrous plaques in the main left coronary arteries. Atherosclerosis 1983; 48:139–145.
19. Sabbah HN, Khaja F, Brymer JF, et al. Blood velocity in the right coronary artery: relation to the distribution of atherosclerotic lesions. Am J Cardiol 1984; 53:1008–1012.
20. Fuster V, Badimon L, Badimon JJ, Chesebro JH. The pathogenesis of coronary artery disease and the acute coronary syndromes. N Engl J Med 1992; 326:242–250.
21. Manning WJ, Li W, Boyle NG, Edelman RR. Fat-suppressed breath-hold magnetic resonance coronary arteriography. Circulation 1993; 87:94–104.
22. Duerinckx AJ, Urman MK. Two-dimensional coronary MR angiography: analysis of initial clinical results. Radiology 1994; 193:731–738.
23. Li D, Paschal C. B. Haacke EM, Adler LP. Coronary arteries: three-dimensional MR imaging with fat saturation and magnetization transfer contrast. Radiology 1993; 187:401–406.
24. Pennell DJ, Keegan J, Firmin DN, et al. Magnetic resonance imaging of coronary arteries: technique and preliminary results. Br Heart J 1993; 70:315–326.
25. Manning WJ, Li W, Edelman RR. A preliminary report comparing magnetic resonance coronary angiography with conventional angiography. N Engl J Med 1993; 328:828–832.
26. Yoshikawa J, Yanagihara K, Owaki T, et al. Cross-sectional echocardiographic diagnosis of coronary artery aneurysms in patients with the mucocutaneous lymph node syndrome. Circulation 1979; 59:133–139.
27. Hiraishi S, Yashiro K, Kusano S. Noninvasive visualization of coronary artery aneurysm in infants and children with mucocutaneous lymph node syndrome with two dimensional echocardiography. Am J Cardiol 1979; 43:1225–1233.
28. Pasquini L, Sanders SP, Parness IA, Colan SD. Diagnosis of coronary artery anatomy by two-dimensional echocardiography in patients with transposition of the great arteries. Circulation 1987; 75:557–564.
29. Chen CC, Morganroth J, Ogawa S, Mardelli TJ. Detecting left main coronary artery disease by apical, cross-sectional echocardiography. Circulation 1980; 62:288–293.
30. Douglas PS, Fiolkoski J, Berko B, Reichek N. Echocardiographic visualization of coronary artery anatomy in the adult. J Am Coll Cardiol 1988; 11:565–571.
31. Samdarshi TE, Nanda NC, Gatewood RP Jr, et al. Usefulness and limitations of transesophageal echocardiography in the assessment of proximal coronary artery stenosis. J Am Coll Cardiol 1992; 19:572–580.
32. Tardif J-C, Vannan MA, Taylor K, et al. Delineation of extended lengths of coronary arteries by multiplane transesophageal echocardiography. J Am Coll Cardiol 1994; 24:909–919.

33. Eggen DA, Strong JP, McGill HC. Coronary calcification: relationship to clinically significant coronary lesions and race, sex, and tomographic distribution. Circulation 1965; 32:948–955.
34. Bartel AG, Chen JT, Peter RH, et al. The significance of coronary calcification detected by fluoroscopy. Circulation 1974; 49:1247–1253.
35. Kelley MJ, Huang EK, Langou RA. Correlation of fluoroscopically detected coronary artery calcification with exercise stress testing in asymptomatic men. Radiology 1978; 129:1–6.
36. Warburton RK, Tampas JP, Soule AB, et al. Coronary artery calcification: its relationship to coronary artery stenosis and myocardial infarction. Radiology 1968; 91:109–115.
37. Hamby RI, Tabrah F, Wisoff HC. Coronary artery calcification: clinical implication and angiographic correlates. Am Heart J 1974; 87:565–570.
38. Moore EH, Greenberg RW, Merrick SH, et al. Coronary artery calcifications: significance of incidental detection on CT scans. Radiology 1989; 172:711–716.
39. Kaufmann RB, Sheedy PF, Maher JE, et al. Quantity of coronary artery calcium detected by electron beam computed tomography in asymptomatic subjects and angiographically studied patients. Mayo Clin Proc 1995; 70:223–232.
40. Mautner GC, Mautner SL, Froehlich J, et al. Coronary artery calcification: assessment with electron bean CT and histomorphometric correlation. Radiology 1994; 192:619–623.
41. Simons DB, Schwartz RS, Edwards WD, et al. Noninvasive definition of anatomic coronary artery disease by ultrafast computed tomographic scanning: a quantitative pathologic comparison study. J Am Coll Cardiol 1992; 20:1118–1126.
42. Kaufmann RB, Peyser PA, Sheedy PF, et al. Quantification of coronary artery calcium by electron beam computed tomography for determination of severity of coronary artery disease in younger patients. J Am Coll Cardiol 1995; 25:626–632.
43. van der Wal AC, Becker AE, van der Loos CM, Das PK. Site of intimal rupture or erosion of thrombosed coronary atherosclerotic plaques is characterized by an inflammatory process irrespective of the dominant plaque morphology. Circulation 1994; 89:36–44.
44. Levin DC, Fallon JT. Significance of the angiographic morphology of localized coronary stenoses: histopathologic correlations. Circulation 1982; 66:316–320.
45. Nishimura RA, Edwards WD, Warnes CA, et al. Intravascular ultrasound imaging. In vitro validation and pathologic correlation. J Am Coll Cardiol 1990; 16:145–154.
46. Gussenhoven EJ, Essed CE, Lancee CT, et al. Arterial wall characteristics determined by intravascular ultrasound imaging. J Am Coll Cardiol 1989; 14:947–952.
47. Mallery JA, Tobis JM, Griffith J, et al. Assessment of normal and atherosclerotic arterial wall thickness with an intravascular ultrasound imaging catheter. Am Heart J 1990; 119:1392–1400.
48. Bartorelli AL, Potkin BN, Almagor Y, et al. Plaque characterization of atherosclerotic coronary arteries by intravascular ultrasound. Echocardiography 1990; 7:389–395.
49. Fitzgerald PJ, Goar FG, Kao AK, et al. Intravascular ultrasound imaging of the coronary arteries: is three layers the norm? [abstr]. J Am Coll Cardiol 1991; 17(suppl A):217A.
50. Nissen SE, Gurley JC, Grines CL, et al. Intravascular ultrasound assessment of lumen

size and wall morphology in normal subjects and patients with coronary artery disease. Circulation 1991; 84:1087–1099.
51. Hodgson J McB, Reddy KG, Suneja R, et al. Intracoronary ultrasound imaging: correlation of plaque morphology with angiography, clinical syndrome and procedural results in patients undergoing coronary angioplasty. J Am Coll Cardiol 1993; 21:35–44.
52. Ambrose JA, Winters SL, Stern A, et al. Angiographic morphology and the pathogenesis of unstable angina pectoris. J Am Coll Cardiol 1985; 5:609–616.

18

Imaging of the Pericardium

J. JEFFREY CARR, JAMES G. WARNER, JR., and KERRY M. LINK
Bowman Gray School of Medicine–Wake Forest University
Winston-Salem, North Carolina

I. General Background

This chapter reviews the imaging of the anatomy and abnormalities of the pericardium, with emphasis on processes commonly seen in clinical practice. Rarer entities are described so that the reader may identify unique imaging characteristics. Particular attention is given to imaging with echocardiography, computed tomography (CT), magnetic resonance imaging (MRI), and chest radiography. A brief overview of relative anatomy and embryology is provided.

A. Anatomy and Embryology

The pericardium was recognized as the strong sac that surrounds the heart and the proximal great vessels early in medical history. Both Homer and Galen commented on the pericardium and its disease processes (1). The pericardium consists of two distinct layers: a visceral and parietal pericardium. Between these layers is the pericardial sac, which under normal circumstances contains a small amount of pericardial fluid. The embryology of the heart is beyond the scope of this chapter; however, a brief review will be helpful in understanding the anatomy of the pericardium. The following synopsis is from Moore's textbook on embryology, to which the interested reader is referred for the illustrations depicting the development of the cardiovascular system (2).

The primordial analogues of the heart and pericardium are present in embryos of 18–19 days. The pericardial coelom is directly adjacent to paired cardiogenic cords. The cardiogenic cords eventually form the paired endocardial heart tubes. These endocardial heart tubes then fuse to create the bulbus cordis, primitive ventricle, and primitive atria. The bending of the primitive heart forms the characteristic bulboventricular loop. During the formation of the bulboventricular loop, the primitive heart migrates in such a way that it becomes enveloped by the pericardial cavity (coelom). This invagination of the pericardial coelom creates a dorsal mesentery (or mesocardium) that attaches the heart to the body stock. The dorsal mesentery eventually leads to the pericardial reflections in the adult. The central portion of the dorsal mesentery undergoes degeneration, and the resulting hole is the transverse pericardial sinus seen in adults (2).

Histologically, the visceral pericardium or epicardium is composed of a single serousal layer of mesothelial cells. This monolayer of mesothelial cells is in direct contact with the epicardial fat and forms a continuous lining for the pericardial sac by reflecting back on itself at the root of the heart. This serousal layer continues as the inner component of the parietal, or fibrous, pericardium. The mesothelial cells of the pericardium are covered with microvilli and cilia. These cells have a large surface area for the production of pericardial fluid and other functions (3). The visceral pericardium extends over the proximal aspects of the ascending aorta and main pulmonary artery, as well as the pulmonary veins and superior and inferior vena cava (Fig. 1). Within the parietal or fibrous pericardium, in addition to the serousal layer, are multiple layers of wavy collagen fibers, intermixed with elastic fibers, which are responsible for its unique properties (4,5). The fibrous pericardium blends with the adventitia of the vessels, as well as extending and blending with the deep cervical fascia. The pericardium is connected to the body by attachments to the aorta, inferior vena cava, and pulmonary veins. In addition, it has strong attachments with the central tendon of the diaphragm. Anteriorly, the fibrous pericardium is attached to the sternum by means of superior and inferior sternopericardial ligaments.

The pericardium, similar to other tissues, has nerves, lymphatics, and blood vessels. The pericardium receives its blood supply from branches of the internal thoracic (mammary) arteries and small branches originating from the descending thoracic aorta. Lymph channels are present within the parietal pericardium and drain to corresponding mediastinal lymph nodes. The pericardial sac is predominantly innervated by means of the phrenic nerve, although the posterior aspect of the pericardial sac receives branches from the vagus nerve (4).

The pericardium plays an extensive role in cardiac function and physiology. Beyond the physical support functions of the pericardium, the serousal membrane reduces friction and provides a barrier to inflammation and neoplastic disease from the surroundings tissues. Beyond its role in limiting the acute distension of the heart, the pericardium plays a role in the left ventricular pressure-volume curve and in the diastolic coupling of the ventricles. The effects of the pericardium on cardiac physiology are beyond the scope of this chapter, and the interested reader is referred to other sources for a discussion of the subject (4–6).

Imaging of the pericardium has rapidly expanded with the development of cross-sectional and multiplanar imaging techniques. Before the development of CT and ultrasonography, the normal pericardium could not be imaged apart from the remaining cardiac structures that compose the cardiac silhouette on conventional radiography. With the development of echocardiography, CT, and MRI, the pericardium could be imaged noninvasively and separately from the myocardium. The thickness of the pericardium, when measured in normal volunteers with CT, is 2–2.3 mm ($\pm$ 0.6 mm) (7), and with MRI, 1.2–1.7 mm ($\pm$ 0.5 mm) (8). These measurements compare with specimen measurements of the pericardium of 0.4–1.0 mm (9). The parietal pericardium is thought to be responsible for most of the thickness visualized with both CT and MRI. Fluid within the pericardial sac is believed to account for some of the increased thickness on imaging studies when compared with pathological measurement. Imaging artifacts, particularly with MRI, also play a role in the pericardial thickness, determined by imaging studies. The pericardium varies in thickness, increasing near its attachment to the great vessels (Fig. 1) (8,10,11).

B. Normal Pericardial Fluid

The pericardial space contains a serous fluid, which is an ultrafiltrate of plasma. Normal pericardial fluid is present in volumes between 15 and 50 ml (4,9,10,12). Normal pericardial pressures are negative and vary with pleural pressures during the respiratory cycle. Acute increases in the pericardial contents (generally fluid) can lead to rapid elevation of the intrapericardial pressure and life-threatening cardiac tamponade, as is discussed in a subsequent section. Subacute and chronic changes in pericardial volume are better tolerated by the body. The pericardium can compensate in the long-term setting by structural changes in size of the pericardial sac, as well as changes that alter pericardial compliance (5).

II. Imaging Anatomy of the Pericardium

With the advent of CT and, subsequently, MRI of the chest, a thorough understanding of the pericardium and pericardial recesses became a necessity. Pericardial fluid in these recesses can be mistaken for an abnormality, generally mediastinal adenopathy. In addition, the intimate relation of the ascending aorta to the superior pericardial recess and the retroaortic segment of the transverse sinus is a potential pitfall, if unrealized, for the identification of abnormalities of the ascend-

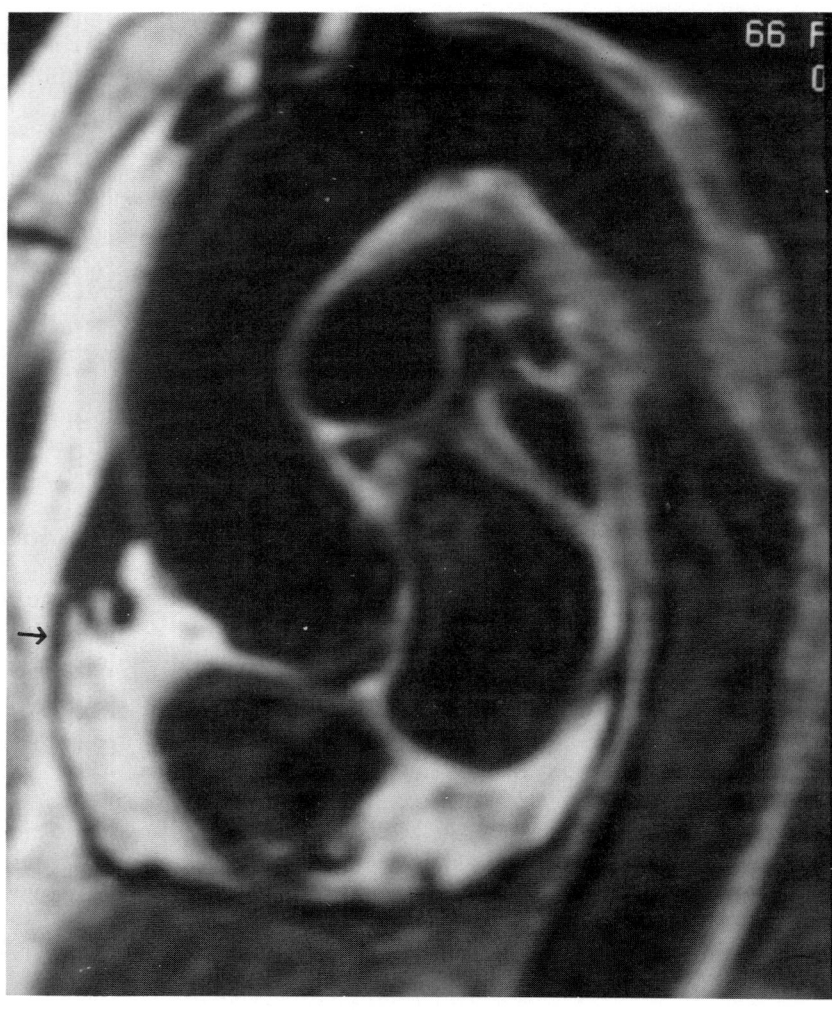

(a)

Figure 1 Reflection of pericardium over the great vessels: Two images from a sagittal oblique cardiac-gated, T1-weighted MRI study of the heart and aorta demonstrate the reflection of the pericardium (arrows) over (a) the ascending aorta and (b) main pulmonary artery. Note that the pericardium appears as a dark band between the high signal intensity of the epicardial and paracardial fat. Note also the continuation of the pericardium around the heart.

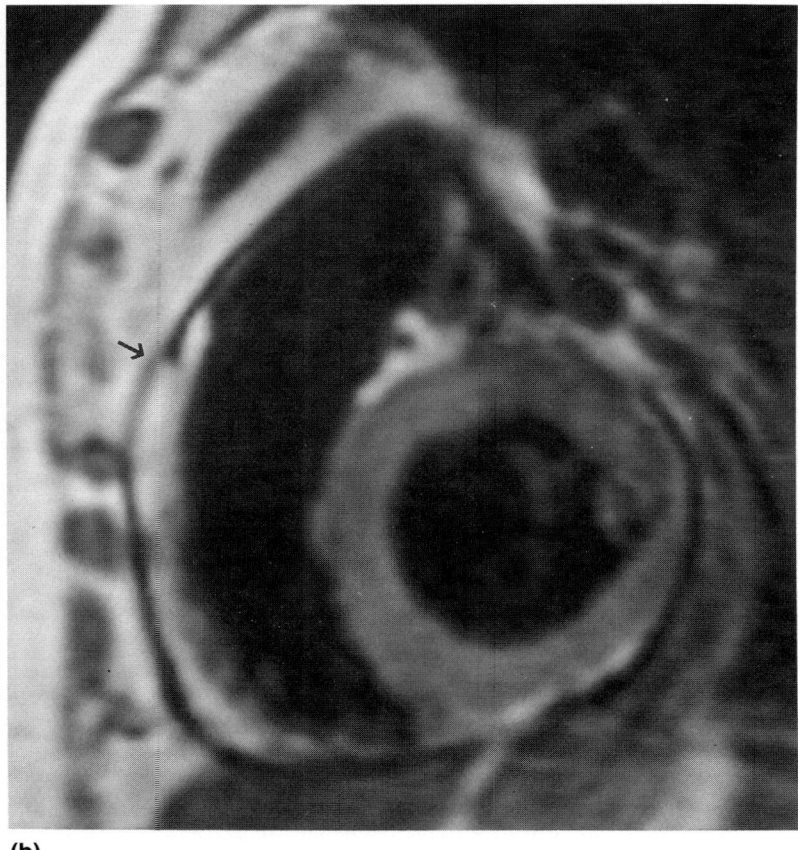

(b)

ing aorta. The superior pericardial recess and its continuation as the retroaortic segment of the transverse sinus can masquerade as a dissection flap or wall abnormality in the ascending aorta to those unaware of this anatomy (Fig. 2).

The superior pericardial recess is located primarily on the anterior (or ventral) aspect of the ascending aorta and main pulmonary artery. When fluid fills the superior pericardial recess, a characteristic extension of fluid between the ascending aorta and main pulmonary artery can be identified (Fig. 3). The superior pericardial recess continues around the right lateral portion of the ascending aorta before becoming contiguous with the retroaortic segment of the transverse sinus of the pericardium. The transverse sinus of the pericardium is located on the dorsal aspect of the main pulmonary artery and ascending aorta. The inferior and posterior relations are the atria and pulmonary veins. As mentioned in Section I.A,

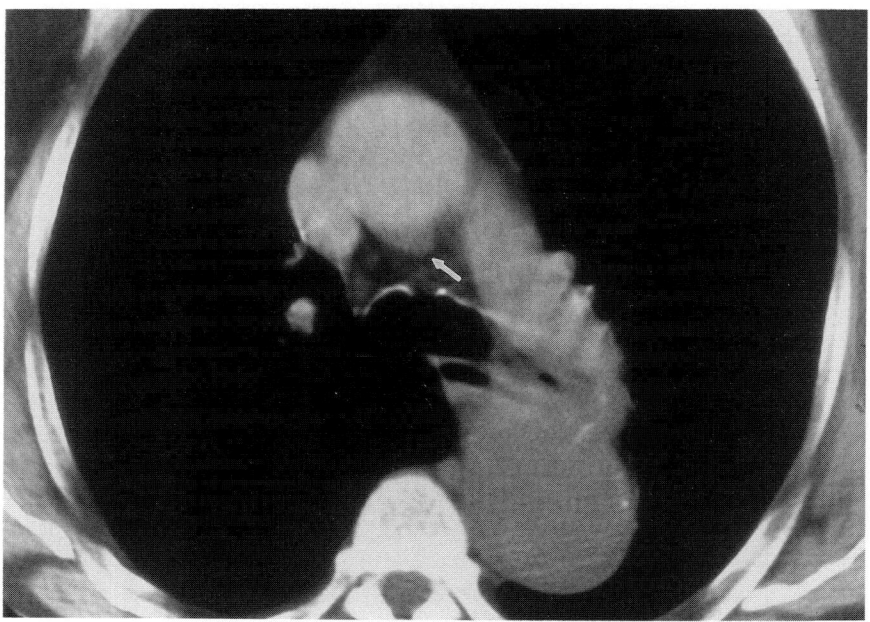

(a)

Figure 2 Retroaortic portion of the superior pericardial recess and transverse sinus of the pericardium: Corresponding (a) axial CT and (b) T1-weighted and (c) cine gradient-echo MRI scans demonstrate the characteristic appearance of pericardial fluid in this recess located dorsal to the ascending aorta (arrow). Correct identification will prevent confusion with aortic wall abnormalities and dissection flaps. Fluid in the transverse sinus and superior pericardial recess may appear pulsatile on flow-sensitive sequences, such as the cine gradient-echo sequence. Note the dissection flap in the descending aorta in this patient with a type III or Stanford B aortic dissection. (From Ref. 19.)

the transverse sinus is the result of atrophy of the central portion of the primitive dorsal mesentery of the heart. The transverse sinus communicates with the pericardial sac posteriorly at the level of the left superior pulmonary vein. The oblique sinus of the pericardium is located directly posterior to the left atrium. It is enclosed by the reflection of the pericardium over the inferior vena cava and pulmonary veins. The oblique sinus has a large opening to the pericardial sac, which is located between the left inferior pulmonary vein and the reflection between the right inferior pulmonary vein and the inferior vena cava. The oblique sinus is physiologically important as one of the major areas of reserved volume for the pericardial sac. Numerous other small recesses can be identified adjacent to the pericardial reflections around the pulmonary arteries and veins (13–19).

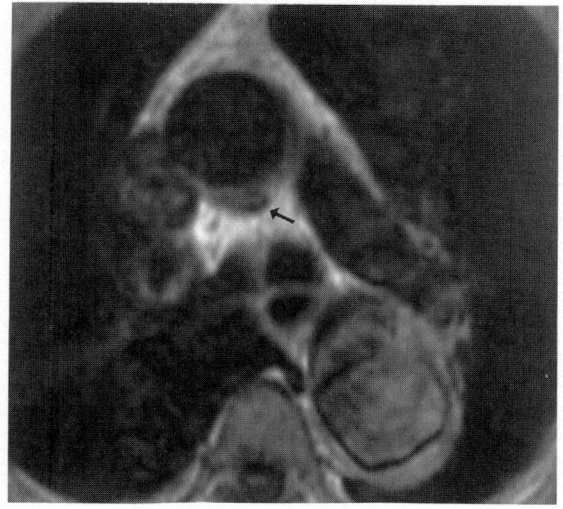

(b)

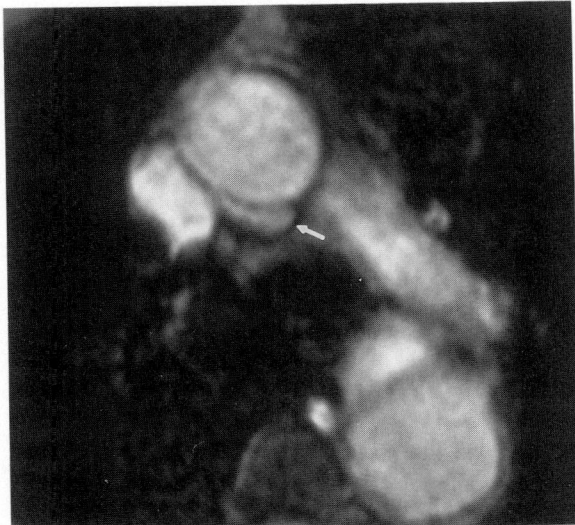

(c)

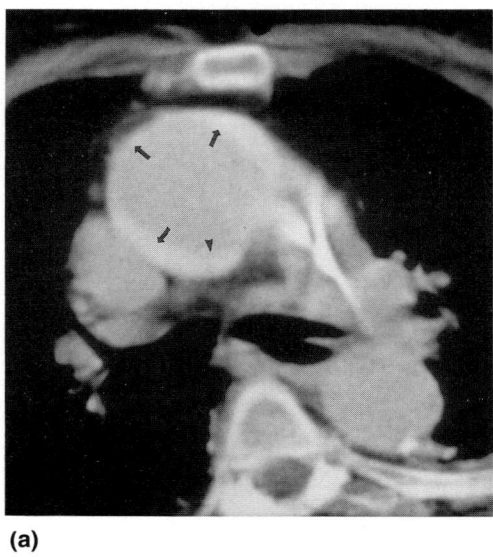

(a)

Figure 3 Contrast in the pericardial sac: This CT scan of the chest obtained immediately after catheter arthrectomy of a coronary artery demonstrates contrast in the pericardial sac resulting from coronary artery perforation. (a) The superior pericardial recess can be identified anterior to the ascending aorta and extending along the right lateral aspect of the aorta (arrows) before forming the retroaortic portion of the transverse sinus (arrowheads). (b) On a lower slice, contrast in the superior pericardial recess between the ascending aorta and main pulmonary artery (*) is noted. (c) More inferiorly, contrast fills the entire pericardial sac encircling the heart.

III. Pericardial Abnormalities and Their Imaging

A. Absence of the Pericardium

Absence of the pericardium includes a spectrum of pericardial defects. These defects include total absence of the pericardium, as well as partial and complete defects on the left or right side. Most frequently, absence of the pericardium occurs on the left side. Right-sided and anterior defects, although rare, have been reported (Fig. 4). Left-sided pericardial defects are more common than right-sided defects or total absence of the pericardium. According to Miller et al. (20), only 16 right-sided pericardial defects have been reported. In the Mayo Clinic series (21) of 15 patients with partial or complete absence of the pericardium, identified between 1951 and 1991, 7 had complete left-sided absence, 5 had partial left-sided absence, 1 had a partial defect on the right side, 1 had an anterior defect, and 1 had

Imaging of the Pericardium

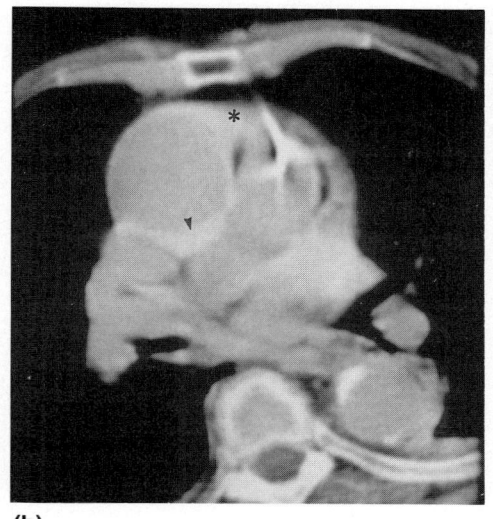

(b)

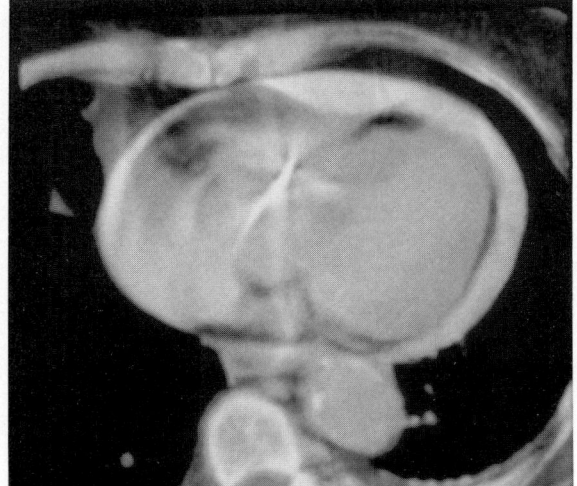

(c)

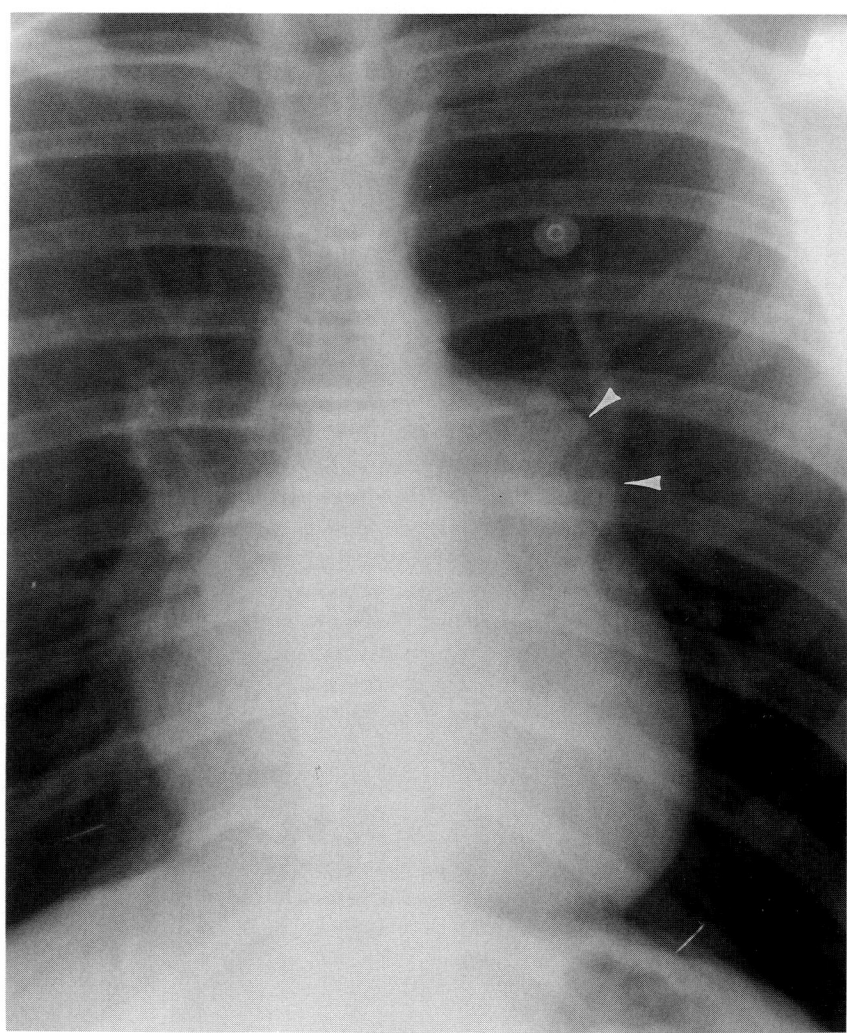

Figure 4 Partial absence of the pericardium: A contour abnormality (arrowheads) along the lateral heart border on this chest radiograph was surgically confirmed as a partial absence of the left pericardium, with herniation of the left atrial appendage. (Courtesy of Vincent D'Souza, M.D., Winston-Salem, NC.)

bilateral or complete absence of the pericardium. In 14 of these 15 patients, the pericardial defect was considered asymptomatic. Of this group of patients, 10 underwent surgical repair of congenital heart anomalies, 1 underwent coronary artery revascularization, 1 had aortic valve replacement, 1 underwent pericardiectomy, and in 1 the descending thoracic aorta was repaired (21). Left-sided defects have an associated defect in the parietal pleura that can permit herniation of cardiac structures into the pleural space and vice versa (22). The condition is thought to be secondary to premature atrophy of the left common cardinal vein (duct of Curvier), which supplies blood to the pleuropericardial membrane of the embryo. The persistence of the corresponding right common cardinal vein as the superior vena cava may explain the rarity of right-sided pericardial defects (20).

Although in most cases the absence of the pericardium is asymptomatic and an incidental finding, deaths have reportedly resulted from cardiac strangulation through a partial left-sided defect (23). The left atrial appendage, atrium, ventricle, or entire heart could potentially become entrapped through the pericardial defect. Sudden death from cardiac strangulation has not been reported with right-sided defects, although asymptomatic herniation of the right atrial appendage has been reported (20). The rather high association (30–50%) of absence of the pericardium with a variety of other congenital anomalies of the heart, lung, diaphragm, or chest wall has been noted (6,10,21,24,25).

The diagnosis of absence of the pericardium is suggested on chest radiographs by a contour abnormality in the cardiac silhouette (see Fig. 4). The appearance of lung interposed between the aorta and pulmonary artery and between the heart base and the diaphragm is also a radiographic sign of this entity. With cross-sectional imaging techniques, CT, and MRI, the focal defect in the pericardium and any associated herniation can be identified. As with chest radiography, lung surrounding the pulmonary outflow tract and interposed between the pulmonary outflow tract and the aorta is a sign of pericardial absence with cross-sectional imaging (26–29).

B. Pericarditis

Pericarditis is an inflammatory condition of the pericardium. The inflammatory process results in an increased vascularity of the pericardium. Pericardial effusion develops after the exudation of fluid, often with associated fibrin deposition. Pericardial effusions can be classified according to their time course as acute, chronic, or relapsing. The type of fluid within the pericardial sac may be serous, serofibrinous, hemorrhagic, suppurative, or complex. Cellular infiltrates may be present. In addition, effusions can be related to benign or malignant processes. Analysis of the pericardial fluid or sampling of the pericardium provides valuable information in determining the etiology.

Acute pericarditis is the rapid onset of inflammation of the pericardium.

Clinically, it may be associated with chest pain, and in some cases the pain may be positional. This condition is thought to be secondary to inflammation of the pericardium and adjacent pleura and may result in a pleuritic chest pain and associated dyspnea. On auscultation, either a two- or a three-component pericardial friction rub may be heard. Electrocardiography (ECG) changes have classically been grouped into four stages, with evolutionary changes noted in the ST segment and T-wave (6).

The etiologies of acute pericarditis are numerous. The most common cause is idiopathic, followed by viral; bacterial and uremic pericarditis are also common. Special mention should be made of tuberculous pericardial disease, which before successful public health intervention was a major cause of acute pericarditis, as well as chronic complications. Tuberculosis and atypical mycobacteria are a cause of pericarditis in the immunocompromised host. The resurgence of tuberculosis may make tuberculous pericarditis more common in years to come. Fungal infections and parasitic infestations also can result in an acute pericarditis. Trauma, myocardial infarction, and cardiac surgery can result in inflammation of the pericardium to varying degrees. Other causes of pericarditis include drugs, dissecting aortic aneurysms, and myxedema (6,10,30–32).

New approaches to treatment of pericardial disease include the use of thoracoscopes and pericardioscopes (30,32). These fiber-optic scopes allow direct visualization of the pericardial sac and epicardium. They also facilitate directed pericardial biopsies. In addition to these interventional techniques, with new methods of evaluating pericardial effusion, the etiologic diagnosis can be made more readily. The polymerase chain reaction has been used to identify both viral and tuberculous pericarditis (33,34).

Pericarditis after myocardial infarction is probably the most common cause of pericardial disease. Pericarditis was found in 20% of patients in the Multicenter Investigation of Limitation of Infarct Size (35) when diagnosed by the presence of pericardial friction rub at auscultation. A localized fibrinous reaction can be seen at autopsy after an infarction. This may be associated with serosanguineous fluid within the pericardial sac. Rupture of the ventricular free wall can lead to sudden death as a result of cardiac tamponade. Alternatively, a confined rupture can occur with development of a pseudoaneurysm (Fig. 5). After cardiac surgery, a combination of pericardial reactions may occur; these include fibrin deposition, development of pericardial effusion, focal and diffuse pericardial thickening, and cellular infiltrations (31). Enlarging serosanguineous effusions can lead to life-threatening cardiac tamponade (see discussion on cardiac tamponade). Congestive heart failure, endocarditis, and valvular heart disease are also associated with pericardial effusions (30).

Trauma to the thorax, either penetrating or nonpenetrating, can result in an associated pericarditis. Hemorrhage into the pericardial sac can lead to cardiac tamponade. Injuries caused by trauma can also lead to fibrinous deposits within

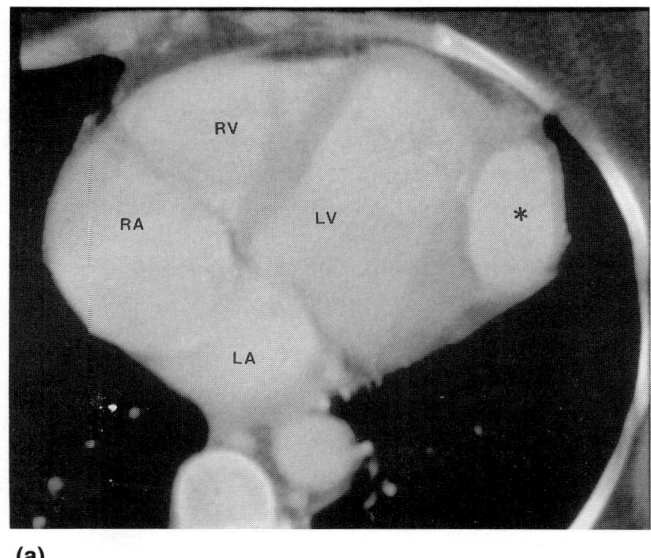

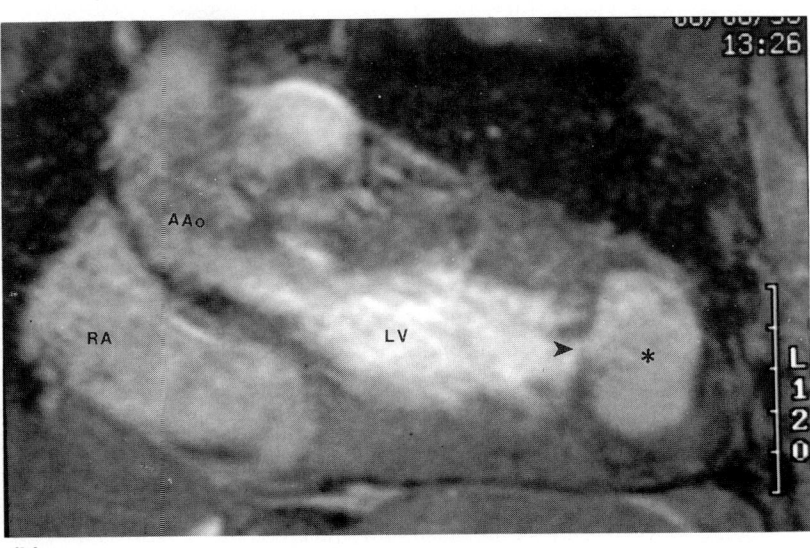

Figure 5 Pseudoaneurysm: (a) Contrast-enhanced CT demonstrates filling an oval cavity along the free wall of the left ventricle (*). (b) A single image of the cine MRI study in the coronal plane shows the communication of the pseudoaneurysm (*) with the chamber of the left ventricle (arrowhead). LV, left ventricle; RA, right atrium; AAO, ascending aorta; RV, right ventricle; LA, left atrium.

the pericardium. Iatrogenic injuries resulting from placement of transvenous cardiac pacing leads or catheter angiography are also reported causes of acute pericarditis.

In patients with renal disease, small pericardial effusions are common. A distinct and problematic entity is uremic pericarditis. In the acute phase, fibrinous pericardial deposits, with or without an associated pericardial effusion, may be seen. This may progress into a chronic form, with developed fibrous adhesions as well as chronic effusions. The mechanism of uremic pericarditis is not clearly defined, but it is believed to represent a chemical irritation of the pericardium. The diffuse fibrinous deposits associated with uremic pericarditis have classically been described as having a "bread-and-butter" appearance (6,31).

Systemic disease processes can also lead to pericarditis. Collagen-vascular diseases, including systemic lupus erythematosus, scleroderma, and rheumatoid arthritis, can have associated pericardial abnormalities. Pericarditis and pericardial effusion may occur as complications of numerous pharmacological agents. Hypersensitivity reactions may also include an inflammatory response in the pericardium.

The postmyocardial infarction (Dressler) syndrome and postpericardiotomy syndrome occur weeks to months after the initial event. The postmyocardial infarction syndrome is thought to be distinct from the acute pericarditis seen in the first week after myocardial infarction. An autoimmune response to the epicardium is hypothesized to be responsible for the syndromes, possibly in combination with a viral etiology (6).

Neoplastic infiltration of the pericardium is frequent in patients with malignancies (Fig. 6). It is reported that the heart is involved in 10% of all noncardiac malignancies. Of nonprimary tumors that involve the heart, more than 85% involve the pericardium in some manner. Even so, only 10% of patients with metastatic disease to the heart demonstrate overt clinical evidence of cardiac involvement (36). In addition, nonmalignant causes of pericardial effusions and pericarditis are common in patients with known malignancies (6). Complications of pericardial involvement include tamponade, which is secondary to rapid accumulation of pericardial effusion, and pericardial constriction. The constriction may be the result of thickening of the pericardium and direct tumor encasement. Neoplasms may directly invade the heart and lead to rupture and pericardial tamponade (6,31).

Radiation therapy to the mediastinum, most commonly for breast cancer, non-Hodgkin's lymphoma, and Hodgkin's lymphoma, can result in fibrous thickening of the parietal and visceral pericardial layers. Radiation-induced pericarditis may occur acutely, but a delayed reaction months to years later may present a more difficult diagnostic dilemma. It is often associated with pericardial effusions but may progress to an effusive-constrictive pericardial process. Differentiation from neoplastic recurrence may be difficult and may require histological evaluation (6,37).

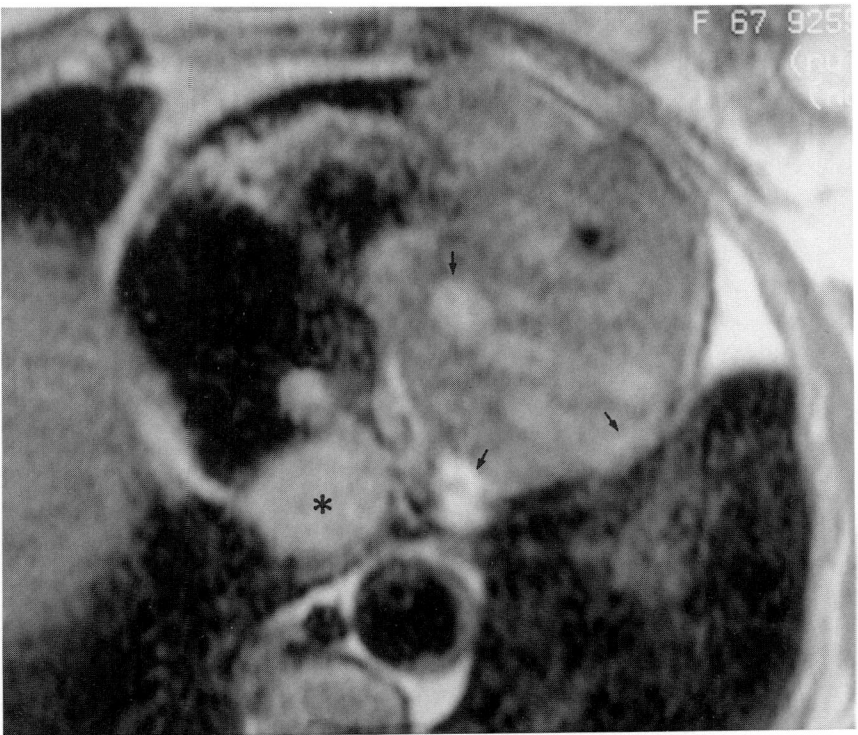

Figure 6 Metastatic melanoma: Enhancing myocardial and pericardial metastasis (arrows) are seen on this axial T1-weighted MRI scan acquired after IV administration of gadolinium DTPA through the apical region of the left ventricle. A larger metastasis is present in the posterior aspect of the right atrium (*).

Imaging in patients with pericarditis consists of identifying either abnormal thickness of the pericardium or pericardial effusions (Figs. 7 and 8). Chest radiographs are nonspecific, and an enlarged pericardial silhouette is generally identified only after 250 ml of fluid has accumulated (6). If the cardiac silhouette rapidly enlarges without development of associated pulmonary edema, then the possibility of a pericardial effusion should be considered. Both CT and MRI can demonstrate the normal and abnormal thickness of the pericardium. An MRI scan may better delineate the difference between pericardial effusion and thickened abnormal pericardium on long TR/TE (T2-weighted) images because of its higher contrast between fluid and tissue. A CT scan is superior to MRI and chest radiography for detecting calcifications within or around the pericardium. The mainstay of diagnosis of pericardial abnormalities is echocardiography. Real-time

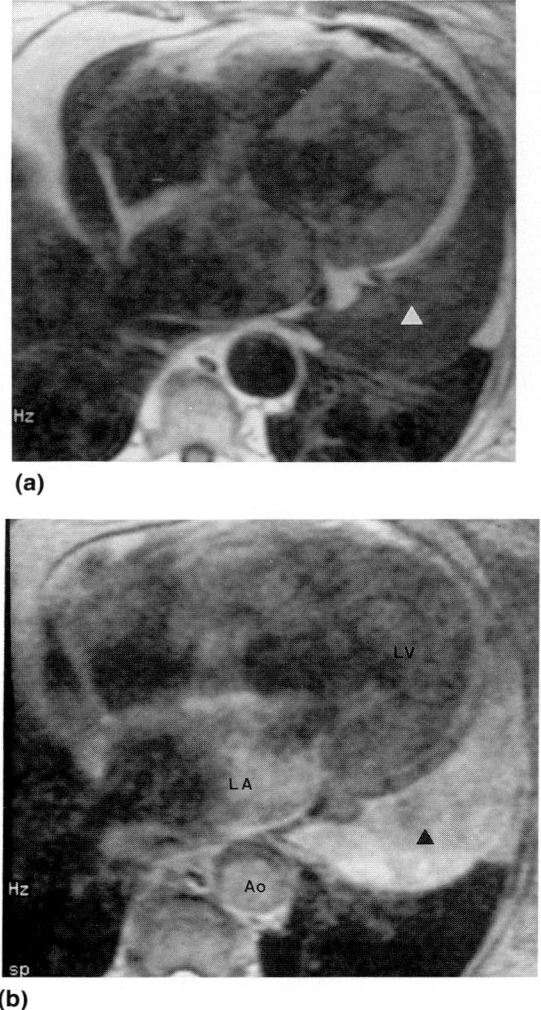

Figure 7 Pericardial effusion—MRI: (a) Transverse T1-weighted and (b) T2-weighted sequences with cardiac gating demonstrate the MR signal characteristics of pericardial effusions (triangles). The effusion has low signal intensity on T1- and high-signal intensity on T2-weighted sequences. Note that the largest amount of fluid is located posteriorly to the left ventricle, but smaller amounts of effusion can be seen anteriorly and adjacent to the right atrium. Ao, aorta; LA, left atrium; LV, left ventricle.

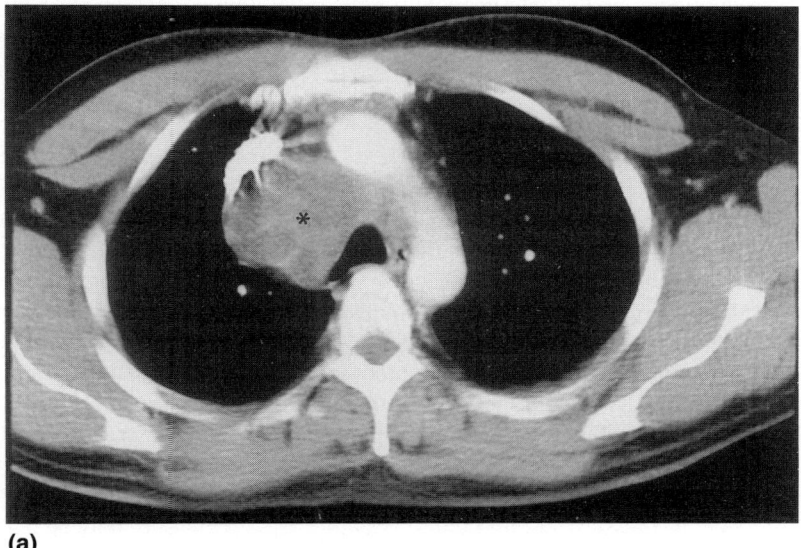

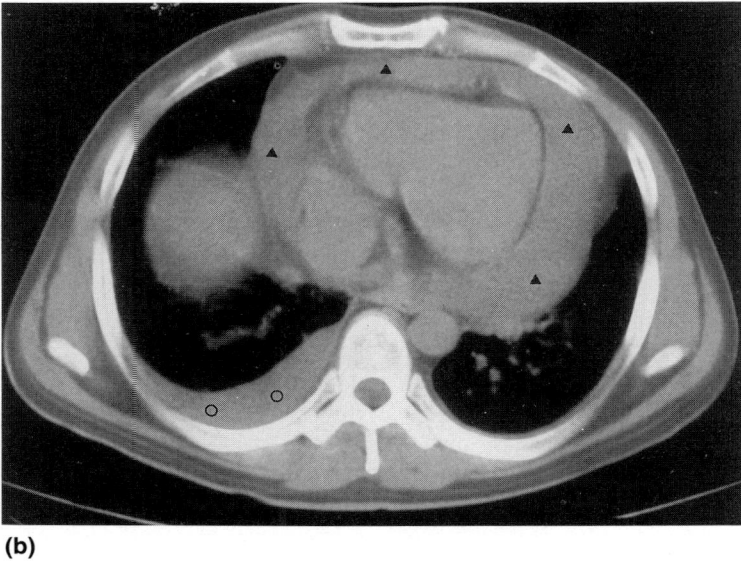

Figure 8 Pericardial effusions—CT: (a) The mediastinal germ cell tumor (*) was complicated by (b) the development of a large pericardial effusion (triangles) and right pleural effusion (circles).

echocardiography allows identification of pericardial fluid collections, as well as evaluation of the hemodynamics associated with the fluid accumulation. Echocardiography has, to a great extent, replaced the need for right-sided heart catheterization in this setting.

C. Cardiac Tamponade

Cardiac tamponade is a medical emergency. It represents compression of the heart by fluid or other substance within the pericardial sac and results in elevated intracardiac pressures, reduced ventricular diastolic filling, and reduced stroke volume. Rapid accumulation of even small volumes of fluid can result in the hemodynamic consequences of tamponade. Both the rate of fluid accumulation and the characteristics of the pericardium (compliance) are important in determining the manifestations of cardiac tamponade. Slow accumulations of volumes of 1–2 L can be tolerated without concomitant elevation of the intrapericardial pressure because of the compensatory and elastic nature of the pericardium (6).

Clinical signs of cardiac tamponade include tachycardia and evidence of elevated venous pressure. A rapid fall in systemic arterial pressure may be noted. Classically, the presence of pulsus paradoxus may serve as a clue to the diagnosis. Cardiac echocardiography has revolutionized the diagnosis of pericardial effusion and cardiac tamponade (30,38). The presence of fluid within the pericardial sac results in a rise in intrapericardial pressure. This may progress to right atrial compression and diastolic collapse of the right ventricle (Fig. 9). As with CT and MRI, the presence of dilation of the inferior vena cava and hepatic veins is an indicator of elevated central venous pressure. On chest radiographs the presence of cardiomegaly without evidence of pulmonary edema suggests the diagnosis (10).

Cardiac tamponade can be identified with echocardiography because of changes in cardiac physiology that occur as a result of the elevated intrapericardial pressure. Atrial compression, diastolic collapse of the right ventricle, and changes in cardiac morphology with the respiratory cycle are indicators of the effusion causing cardiac tamponade. When tamponade is present, during inspiration there is an increase in diastolic filling of the right ventricle, with corresponding reduction in the left ventricle (31,39). Doppler flow measurements that demonstrate an abnormal inspiratory increase of flow across the tricuspid valve or inspiratory decrease in velocity across the mitral valve are likewise indicators of tamponade. An abnormal cardiac motion, termed the "swinging heart" sign, may also be a clue to the diagnosis. Narrowing of the left ventricular outflow tract during inspiration and a dilated inferior vena cava are additional signs (30,38).

Both CT and MRI scans can demonstrate the presence of the pericardial effusion. To demonstrate cardiac tamponade, the imaging technique must be capable of showing wall motion abnormalities during the cardiac cycle or demonstrating velocity measurements with changes during inspiration and expiration. Currently, conventional CT cannot meet this requirement. An MRI scan has the potential to demonstrate wall motion abnormalities as well as flow velocities; however, in an urgent setting, echocardiography is more rapid and accessible. In addition, echocardiography can direct therapeutic procedures to relieve the elevated intrapericardial pressure through ultrasound-directed pericardiocentesis (30,38).

D. Constrictive Pericarditis

Constrictive pericarditis is an inflammatory process of the pericardium that alters cardiac physiology. The thickening of the pericardium decreases compliance of the pericardium and restricts ventricular diastolic filling. This reduced filling results in a reduced stroke volume. A key clinical distinction is that between constrictive pericardial disease and restrictive cardiomyopathy. As both conditions result in restriction to ventricular filling, the differential diagnosis is challenging (40). The presence of abnormally thickened pericardium is a key indicator of constrictive pericarditis; however, the absence of a thickened pericardium does not exclude the possibility of pericardial constriction. Constrictive pericarditis has been evaluated with both CT and MRI (8,41–43). A measurement of more than 4 mm with MRI has been used as a threshold for abnormally thickened pericardium. The pericardial thickness is most easily identified and measured anterior to the right ventricle (8,11,44). Echocardiography can also be helpful in distinguishing constrictive pericarditis from restrictive cardiomyopathy. Mitral valve Doppler inflow velocities vary with respirations, as with cardiac tamponade. These changes do not occur, or they occur to a much smaller degree, with a restrictive cardiomyopathy (45).

E. Paracardiac Masses

Masses that border the cardiac silhouette are often identified on the posteroanterior (PA) and lateral chest radiograph. Cross-sectional techniques, such as echocardiography, CT, and MRI, can provide valuable information on the location of a mass in relation to the pericardium and other cardiac structures. Information from these studies sometimes provides a definitive diagnosis of the etiology of the mass. In many instances, the information may be useful in planning further therapy or avoiding complications.

F. Pericardial Cysts

Pericardial cysts are benign masses that are typically identified as contour abnormalities on a chest radiograph. Pericardial cysts are generally asymptomatic. Symptoms that have been reported include chest pain, dystonia, cough, pneumo-

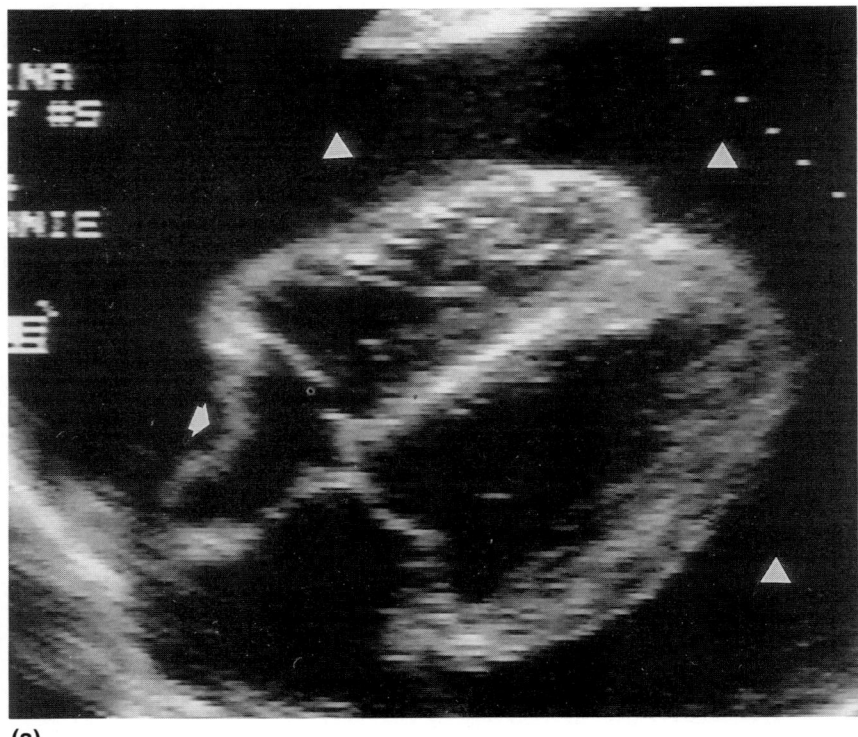

(a)

Figure 9 Cardiac tamponade—echocardiography: (a) The subcostal view demonstrates the cardiac structure surrounded by an anechoic fluid collection consistent with a large pericardial effusion (triangles). Note in this view the inversion of the right atrium (white arrow). (b) In the same patient in the parasternal long axis view, diastolic collapse of the right ventricle is identified (arrowhead). Both of these findings are indicators of cardiac tamponade.

thorax, hemoptysis, and fever. Pericardial cysts can be accurately characterized with echocardiography, MRI, or CT (Fig. 10). The mass should be contiguous with the pericardium. Classic pericardial cysts are anechoic to hypoechoic on echocardiograms. On CT, measurement of the Hounsfield values within the cysts should be consistent with fluid. An MRI scan demonstrates low signal intensity on short TR/TE sequences (T1-weighted images) and high signal intensity on long TR/TE sequences (T2-weighted images). Both MRI and CT can generally display the relation of the cyst to adjacent lung and to other structures. Some pericardial cysts may contain viscous or mucoid material. These cysts can demonstrate

Imaging of the Pericardium

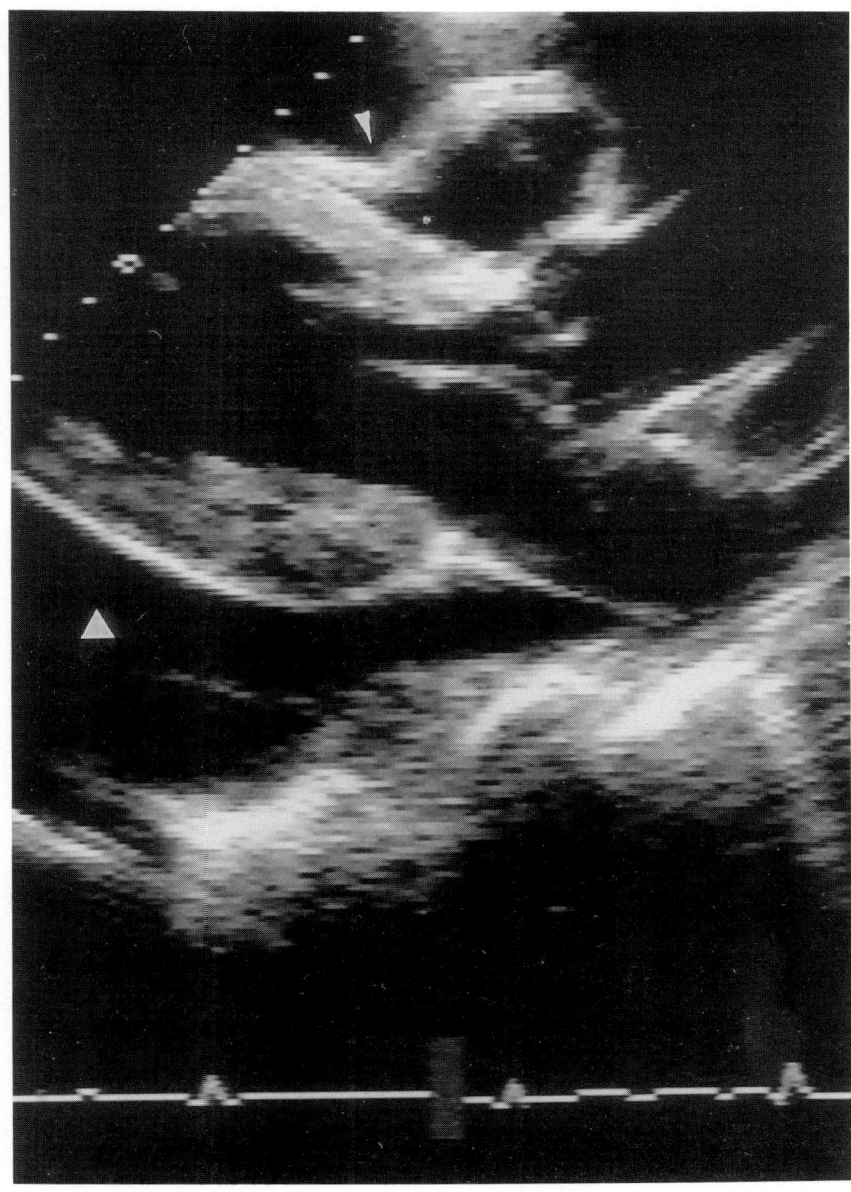

(b)

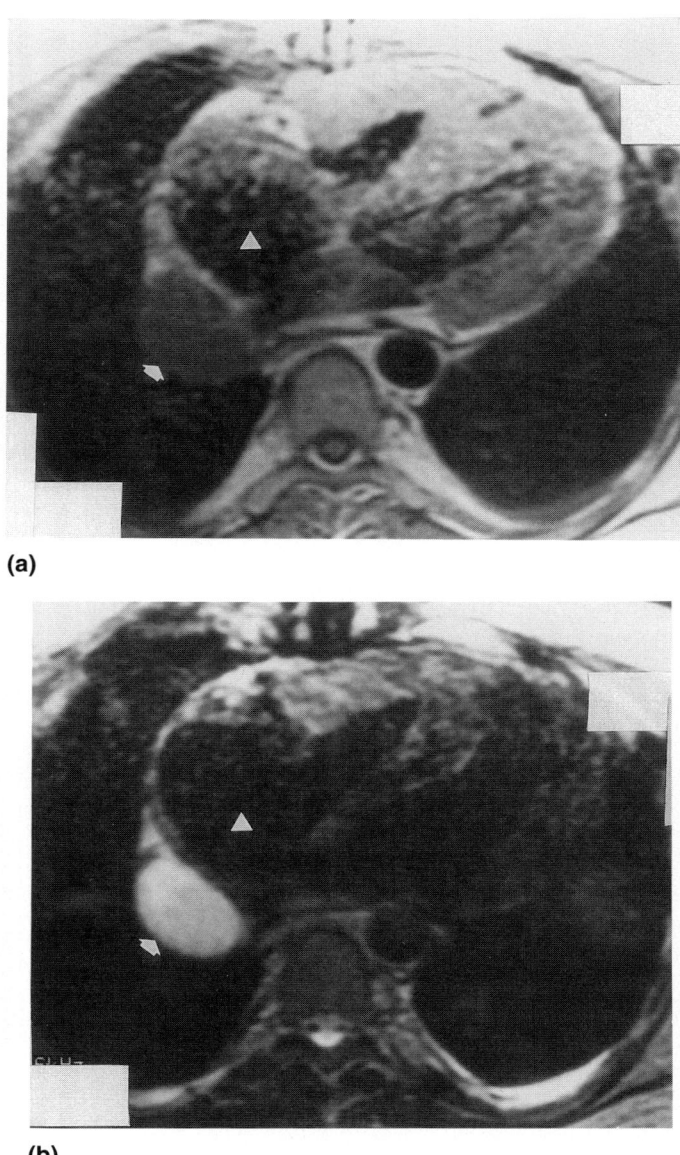

Figure 10 Pericardial cyst: (a) Transverse T1-weighted and (b) T2-weighted images demonstrate a mass (white arrow) adjacent to the right atrium (triangle). Note the low signal intensity on T1- and the high signal intensity on the T2-weighted sequence. These findings are consistent with the diagnosis of a pericardial cyst.

increased echogenicity, higher Hounsfield values, and higher signal intensity on the T1-weighted images. The most common location for pericardial cysts is in the right cardiophrenic angle (46). The successful identification and characterization of asymptomatic pericardial cysts precludes further workup, and conservative management is generally indicated.

Other paracardiac masses can present as abnormalities on the chest radiograph. Diaphragmatic hernias, resulting from a defect in the diaphragm, may be congenital or may be secondary to trauma or surgery (Fig. 11). Postoperative changes in the pericardium are also a common occurrence. Changes postoperatively include a diffuse thickening of the pericardium, as well as seromas and hematomas. These findings should be carefully correlated with the patient's surgical history and time course to exclude other considerations. Pseudoaneurysms can be a complication from prior myocardial infarction, surgery, or neoplastic involvement. The natural history of pseudoaneurysms is progressive enlargement with time. This process can lead to rupture and sudden death secondary to cardiac tamponade or exsanguination. Infections involving the mediastinum have numerous possible etiologies. Mediastinitis may progress to involve the pericardium. Further extension may result in a suppurative pericarditis with involvement of the pericardial sac (pericardiac abscess; 6,10,30,31).

G. Malignancy Involving the Pericardium

Although primary tumors of the pericardium are rare, numerous tumor types have been reported. In the series of cases compiled through the Armed Forces Institute of Pathology, the cell types of primary tumors of the pericardium include lymphoma, hemangioma, teratoma, thymoma, lymphangioma, mesothelioma, and liposarcoma (47,48).

Malignant pericardial mesotheliomas are rare and lethal primary tumors of the pericardium. Chest radiographs may demonstrate cardiac enlargement or irregularity of the cardiac silhouette. Echocardiography may demonstrate irregular thickening of the pericardium; however, at times it may be difficult to distinguish a homogeneous mass from the pericardial fluid (49). Both CT and MRI scans may be useful in evaluating the extent of disease (50). Cardiac catheterization through pressure readings may indicate changes caused by pericardial constriction. Although pericardial mesothelioma is a rare malignancy, it is the most common primary malignancy of the pericardium. In the past, the diagnosis was generally made at autopsy (51). No definite association between pericardial mesotheliomas and asbestos exposure has been demonstrated. Patients may present with constrictive pericarditis, cardiac tamponade, or mediastinal mass. Patients with malignant pericardial mesotheliomas have a poor prognosis. Of 27 patients, 24 were dead at the time of publication of the report in a recent review (52). Malignant mesotheliomas are difficult to resect surgically and respond poorly to

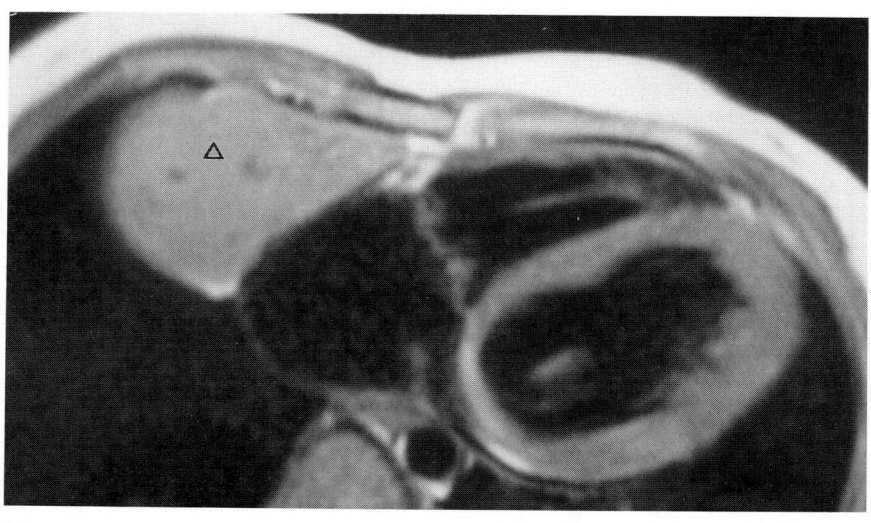

Figure 11 Congenital diaphragmatic hernia: A mass was seen adjacent to the right heart border on a prior chest radiograph. Further evaluation with an (a) axial and (b) coronal cardiac-gated T1-weighted MRI demonstrates herniation of the left lobe of the liver (triangles) through an anterior defect in the diaphragm (Morgagni hernia). Note that the herniated liver is directly adjacent to the right atrium.

chemotherapy and radiotherapy. A rare and presumed benign localized mesothelioma in the pericardial sac with associated effusion has been described (53).

Metastatic disease to the pericardium is common. Metastasis to the pericardium accounts for almost all cardiac metastases, and it is estimated that 10% of noncardiac neoplasms have cardiac metastases (36). Clinical evidence of metastatic involvement of the pericardium is infrequent, and the diagnosis is generally made at autopsy (54). Symptoms generally occur as a consequence of pericardial tamponade or pericardial constriction. The signs and symptoms are similar to those seen in nonneoplastic etiologies and include dyspnea, chest pain, chest discomfort, cough, elevated central venous pressures, and pulsus paradoxus. These signs and symptoms may be difficult to attribute to pericardial metastasis because of other findings in the patient with known metastatic disease.

Malignancies involving the mediastinum, the lung, and other sites can, through direct invasion, involve the pericardium. Malignant thymoma extends along pleural spaces and can extend into the pericardium (Fig. 12). Other tumors that can involve and breech the pericardium include lung, breast, and mesothelium (Fig. 13).

In patients who are immunocompromised secondary to human immunodeficiency virus (HIV) infection, pericardial and epicardial involvements by Kaposi's sarcoma, and non-Hodgkin's lymphoma have been noted (55,56). Pericardial involvement in this setting is generally associated with disseminated involvement by the malignancies throughout the body. These two malignancies are not mutually exclusive, and cardiac involvement with non-Hodgkin's lymphoma has been reported in patients with concurrent disseminated Kaposi's sarcoma in this population. Also, isolated non-Hodgkin's lymphoma of the pericardium resulting in cardiac tamponade has been reported (57).

H. Pneumopericardium

The pericardium can become distended with air if a communication exists between the pericardial sac and an air-containing structure. This condition is termed pneumopericardium. Because the pericardium is in direct contact with the esophagus posteriorly, the potential exists for formation of an esophageal-pericardial communication. Benign and malignant esophageal abnormalities can result in fistula formation with the pericardium. In a literature review of 60 published cases of acquired esophageal-pericardial fistulas, Miller et al. (58) found an 83% in-hospital mortality rate. In this series, 46 (77%) of 60 cases were due to benign esophageal conditions, and 14 (23%) of 60 cases were secondary to esophageal carcinoma. The most common etiology was esophageal ulceration in reflux esophagitis, which acccunted for 21 cases (35%). Ingestion of foreign objects and iatrogenic causes accounted for 13% and 10%, respectively (58). The presence of air in the pericardial sac on chest radiography or CT is diagnostic. In two

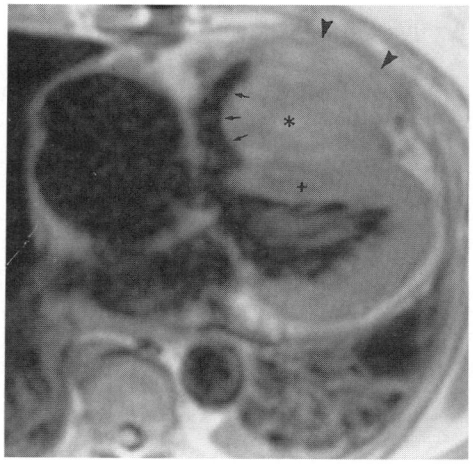

(a)

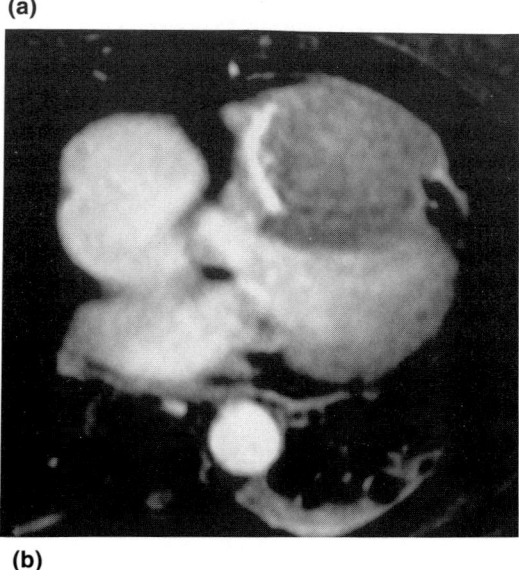

(b)

Figure 12 Metastatic thyroid carcinoma: A large mass (*) involves the pericardium (arrowheads) and extends into the pulmonary outflow tract and right ventricle, which is compressed (arrows). (a) The T1-weighted image demonstrates the abnormal pericardium (arrowheads), and (b) the single image from the cine gradient-echo sequence shows the high-signal blood flow in the compressed pulmonary outflow tract (+ = ventricular septum).

Imaging of the Pericardium

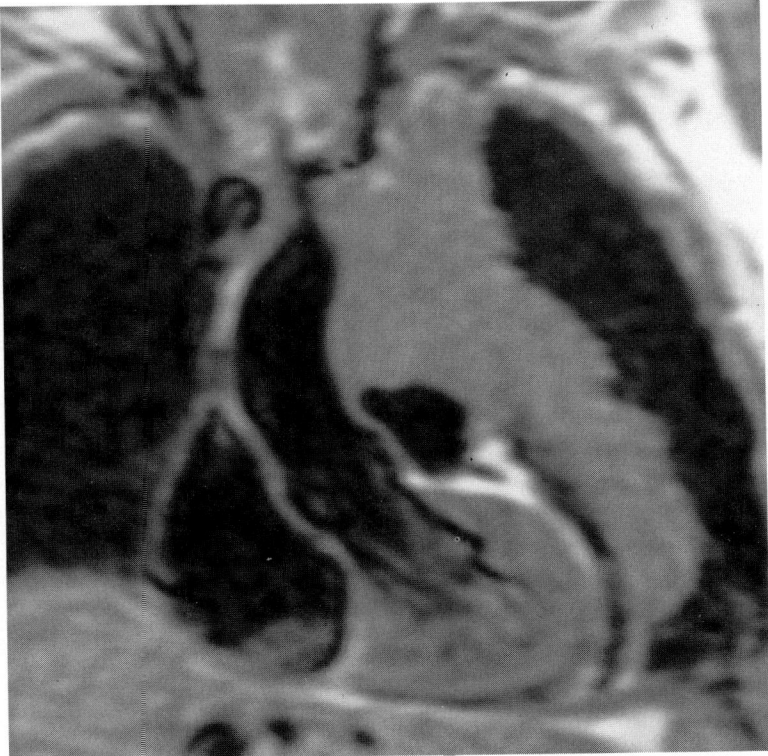

Figure 13 Invasive thymoma: Coronal T1-weighted MRI scan with cardiac gating demonstrates a mediastinal mass extending between the aorta and main pulmonary artery and along the pericardium. On the axial images, this invasive thymoma was seen to extend posteriorly to the paraspinal region. (From Ref. 19.)

previously reported cases, the chest radiograph was normal, and the diagnosis was made after barium swallow (59,60).

IV. Summary

This chapter has reviewed the anatomy and common pathological conditions of the pericardium; special emphasis has been placed on the imaging findings with echocardiography, CT, and MRI. The advances in imaging, minimally invasive procedures, and testing of pericardial fluid and biopsies are expanding our understanding of the pathological processes involving the pericardium. Continued progress will further our understanding of the pericardium and diseases that involve it.

References

1. Spodick DH. Medical history of the pericardium. The hairy hearts of hoary heroes. Am J Cardiol 1970; 26:447–454.
2. Moore KL. The developing human: clinically oriented embryology. 3d ed. Philadelphia: WB Saunders, 1982:479.
3. Ishihara T, Ferrans VJ, Jones M, et al. Histologic and ultrastructural features of normal human parietal pericardium. Am J Cardiol 1980; 46:744–753.
4. Spodick DH. Macrophysiology, microphysiology, and anatomy of the pericardium: a synopsis. Am Heart J 1992; 124:1046–1051.
5. Watkins MW, LeWinter MM. Physiologic role of the normal pericardium. Annu Rev Med 1993; 44:171–180.
6. Lorell BH, Braunwald E. Pericardial disease. In Braunwald E, ed. Heart disease: a textbook of cardiovascular medicine. Philadelphia: WB Saunders, 1988:1484–1534.
7. Silverman PM, Harell GS. Computed tomography of the normal pericardium. Invest Radiol 1983; 18:141–144.
8. Sechtem U, Tscholakoff D, Higgins CB. MRI of the normal pericardium, AJR 1986; 147:239–244.
9. Ferrans VJ, Ishihara T, Roberts WC. Anatomy of the pericardium. In: Reddy, PS, Leon DF, Shaver JA, eds. Pericardial disease. New York: Raven Press, 1982:77–92.
10. Miller SW. Imaging pericardial disease. Radiol Clin North Am 1989; 27:1113–1125.
11. Beache GM, Wedeen VJ, Dinsmore RE. Magnetic resonance imaging evaluation of left ventricular dimensions and function and pericardial and myocardial disease. Coron Artery Dis 1993; 4:328–333.
12. Roberts WC, Spray TL. Pericardial heart disease: a study of its causes, consequences, and morphologic features. Cardiovasc Clin 1976; 7:11–65.
13. Aronberg DJ, Peterson RR, Glazer HS, Sagel SS. The superior sinus of the pericardium: CT appearance. Radiology 1984; 153:489–492.
14. Glazer HS, Aronberg DJ, Sagel SS. Pitfalls in CT recognition of mediastinal lymphadenopathy. AJR 1985; 144:267–274.
15. Honda T, Yano K, Hamada M, et al. Usefulness of multiangle MRI in aortic arch dissection. J Comput Assist Tomogr 1992; 16:646–648.
16. Im J-G, Rosen A, Webb WR, Gamsu G. MR imaging of the transverse sinus of the pericardium. AJR 1988; 150:79–84.
17. Solomon SL, Brown JJ, Glazer HS, et al. Thoracic aorta dissection: pitfalls and artifacts in MR imaging. Radiology 1990; 177:223–228.
18. Levy-Ravetch M, Auh YH, Rubinstein W, et al. CT of the pericardial recesses. AJR 1985; 144:707–714.
19. Carr JJ, Hatabu H, Gefter WB. Thorax. In: Edelman RR, ed. Clinical magnetic resonance imaging. Philadelphia: WB Saunders, 1996:1615–1682.
20. Miller DL, Katz NM, Kulkarni PK, Green CE. Right congenital pericardial defects. Am Heart J 1993; 126:1235–1238.

21. van Son JAM, Danielson GK, Schaff HV, et al. Congenital partial and complete absence of the pericardium. Mayo Clin Proc 1993; 68:743–747.
22. Southworth H, Stevenson CS. Congenital defects of the pericardium. Arch Intern Med 1938; 61:223–240.
23. Jones JW, McManus BM. Fatal cardiac strangulation by congenital partial pericardial defect. Am Heart J 1984; 107:183–185.
24. Gehlmann HR, van Ingel GJ. Symptomatic congenital complete absence of the left pericardium. Case report and review of the literature. Eur Heart J 1989; 10:670–675.
25. Nassar WK, Helmen C, Tavel ME, et al. Congenital absence of the left pericardium. Clinical, electrocardiographic, radiographic, hemodynamic, and angiographic findings in six cases. Circulation 1970; 41:469–478.
26. Gutierrez FR, Shackelford GD, McKnight RC, et al. Diagnosis of congenital absence of left pericardium by MR imaging. J Comput Assist Tomogr 1985; 9:551–553.
27. Bank ER, Hernandez RJ. CT and MR of congenital heart disease. Radiol Clin North Am 1988; 26:241–262.
28. Moncada R, Baker M, Salinas M. Diagnostic role of computed tomography in pericardial heart disease: congenital defects, thickening, neoplasms, and effusions. Am Heart J 1982; 103:263–282.
29. Tabakin BS, Hanson JS, Tampas JP. Congenital absence of the left pericardium. AJR 1965; 94:122–128.
30. Maisch B. Pericardial diseases, with a focus on etiology, pathogenesis, pathophysiology, new diagnostic imaging methods, and treatment. Curr Opin Cardiol 1994; 9:379–388.
31. Waller BF, Taliercio CP, Howard J, et al. Morphologic aspects of pericardial heart disease: part II. Clin Cardiol 1992; 15:291–298.
32. Ferguson MK. Thoracoscopic management of pericardial disease. Semin Thorac Cardiovasc Surg 1993; 5:310–315.
33. Seino Y, Ikeda U, Kawaguchi K, et al. Tuberculosis pericarditis presumably diagnosed by polymerase chain reaction analysis. Am Heart J 1993; 126:249–251.
34. Satoh T, Kojima M, Ohshima K. Demonstration of the Epstein-Barr genome by the polymerase chain reaction and in situ hybridisation in a patient with viral pericarditis. Br Heart J 1993; 69:563–564.
35. Tofler GH, Muller JE, Stone PH. Pericarditis in acute myocardial infarction: characterization and clinical significance. Am Heart J 1989; 117:86–92.
36. Roberts WC, Spray TL. Pericardial heart disease. Curr Probl Cardiol 1977; 2:1–71.
37. Martin RG, Rickdeschel JC, Chang P, et al. Radiation-related pericarditis. Am J Cardiol 1975; 35:216–220.
38. Fowler NO. Cardiac tamponade: a clinical or an echocardiographic diagnosis? Circulation 1993; 87:1738–1741.
39. Feigenbaum H. Pericardial disease. In: Echocardiography. 4th ed. Philadelphia: Lea & Febiger, 1936:548–578.
40. Vaitkus PT, Kussmaul WG. Constrictive pericarditis versus restrictive cardiomyopathy: a reappraisal and update of diagnostic criteria. Am Heart J 1991; 122:1431–1441
41. Soulen RL, Stark DD, Higgins CB. Magnetic resonance imaging of constrictive pericardial disease. Am J Cardiol 1985; 55:480–484.
42. Sutton FJ, Whitley NO, Applefeld MM. The role of echocardiography and computed

tomography in the evaluation of constrictive pericarditis. Am Heart J 1985; 109: 350–355.
43. Isner JM, Carter BL, Bankoff MS, et al. Differentiation of constrictive pericarditis from restrictive cardiomyopathy by computed tomographic imaging. Am Heart J 1983; 105:1019–1025.
44. Masui T, Finck S, Higgins CB. Constrictive pericarditis and restrictive cardiomyopathy: evaluation with MR imaging. Radiology 1992; 182:369–373.
45. Hatle LK, Appleton CP, Popp RL. Differentiation of constrictive pericarditis and restrictive cardiomyopathy by Doppler echocardiography. Circulation 1989; 79: 357–370.
46. Feigin DS, Fenoglio JJ, McAllister HA, Madewell JE. Pericardial cysts: a radiologic–pathologic correlation and review. Radiology 1977; 125:15–20.
47. McAllister HAJ, Fenoglio JJ. Tumors of the cardiovascular system. In: Atlas of tumor pathology, f. 2d series. Washington DC: Armed Forces Institute of Pathology, 1978.
48. Pavlidis NA, Elisaf M, Bai M, et al. Primary lymphoma of the pericardium: report on a "cured" case and review of the literature. Med Pediatr Oncol 1994; 22:287–291.
49. Yilling FP, Schlant RC, Hertzler GL, Krzyaniak, R. Pericardial mesothelioma. Chest 1982; 81:520–523.
50. Gossinger HD, Siostrzonek P, Zangeneh M. Magnetic resonance imaging findings in a patient with pericardial mesothelioma. Am Heart J 1988; 115:1321–1322.
51. Kaul TK, Fields BL, Kahn DR. Primary malignant pericardial mesothelioma: a case report and review. J Cardiovasc Surg 1994; 35:261–267.
52. Thomason R, Schlegel W, Lucca M, et al. Primary malignant mesothelioma of the pericardium. Case report and literature review. Tex Heart Inst J 1994; 21:170–174.
53. Bortolotti U, Calabro F, Loy M, et al. Giant intrapericardial solitary fibrous tumor. Ann Thorac Surg 1992; 54:1219–1220.
54. Hanfling SM. Metastatic cancer to the heart: review of the literature and report of 127 cases. Circulation 1960; 22:474–483.
55. Silver MA, Macher AM, Reichert CM, et al. Cardiac involvement by Kaposi's sarcoma in acquired immune deficiency syndrome (AIDS). Am J Cardiol 1984; 53: 983–985.
56. Lewis W. AIDS: cardiac findings from 115 autopsies. Prog Cardiovasc Dis 1989; 32: 207–215.
57. Aboulafia DM, Bush R, Picozzi VJ. Cardiac tamponade due to primary pericardial lymphoma in a patient with AIDS. Chest 1994; 106:1295–1299.
58. Miller WL, Osborn MJ, Sinak LJ, Westbrook BM. Pyopneumopericardium attributed to an esophagopericardial fistula: report of a survivor and review of the literature. Mayo Clin Proc 1991; 66:1041–1045.
59. Maguire GP. Esophagopericardial fistulas. Mayo Clin Proc 1992; 67:913–914.
60. Cyrlak D, Cohen AJ, Dana ER. Esophagopericardial fistula: causes and radiographic features. AJR 1983; 141:177–179.

19

Adult Congenital Heart Disease

ROBERT J. OPTICAN

Baptist Memorial Hospital
Memphis, Tennessee

I. Introduction

Improvements in diagnosis, treatment, and follow-up care of patients with congenital heart disease (CHD) over the last several decades has led to an increasing number of patients who survive into adulthood, despite CHD (1). At the beginning of this decade, approximately 400,000 persons in the United States had surgically treated CHD, nearly one-fourth of whom were adults. At the same time, 150,000 more adults had unrecognized or unrepaired CHD (1). Each year, 25,000 infants are born with CHD, and 85% are expected to reach adulthood (2). As patients with CHD survive into reproductive age, the pool of patients with CHD is bound to increase (incidence of 5–15% in offspring of such parents versus 0.8% in general population; 3).

A wide variety of imaging methods are available to evaluate patients with CHD. These include standard chest radiography, cineangiography, echocardiography, magnetic resonance, computed tomography, and nuclear scintigraphy.

II. Techniques

A. Chest Radiography

The simplest imaging evaluation of adults with CHD is the standard chest radiograph (CXR). Differential diagnosis is derived from a combination of the following findings: heart size and configuration, pulmonary vasculature, great vessel anatomy, situs, and associated musculoskeletal findings. Heart configuration can help establish chamber size. The pulmonary vascular pattern can reflect shunts (left-to-right, right-to-left), pulmonary venous hypertension, or pulmonary artery hypertension. The initial CXR evaluation can narrow the differential diagnosis and, in combination with clinical findings, can direct any further workup needed. Follow-up CXR after initial diagnosis or following therapy can help define the course of disease. Pertinent findings include progressive chamber dilation or change in pulmonary vascularity (Fig. 1). The four-film "cardiac series," which included oblique views of the chest with barium in the esophagus, is no longer employed today with the advent of other noninvasive techniques to evaluate chamber size.

Adequate performance of plain chest radiography includes utilization of high-kilovolt peak (kVp) technique (140–160 kVp) and use of wide-latitude recording medium (film or digital phosphor plate) allowing adequate visualization of the heart and mediastinum, tracheobronchial tree, and pulmonary vasculature (4).

B. Cardiac Catheterization and Cineangiography

Cardiac catheterization and cineangiography are invasive techniques and, although supplanted in many instances by noninvasive studies, are still useful in a number of situations. They are indicated when data necessary to guide therapy cannot be obtained by noninvasive techniques alone (e.g., echocardiography or magnetic resonance). The appropriate performance of cardiac catheterization and cineangiography requires a team approach, including cardiology, radiology, anesthesiology, nursing, and technical support staff (4).

Patients with complex congenital heart disease pose particularly challenging problems, best addressed at large referral centers. Before performing a cardiac catheterization, as much detailed information as possible should be obtained from noninvasive procedures to allow appropriate planning. Optimal planning requires close consultation between cardiologist, radiologist, and surgeon.

Necessary equipment in the catheterization laboratory includes equipment for physiological monitoring and recording, imaging, and emergency resuscitation. Biplane equipment significantly reduces the number of necessary injections (5). In many centers, digital techniques have supplanted film (e.g., 35 mm). This reduces x-ray dosage, an especially important consideration in young patients.

Cardiac catheterization requires access to the heart and great vessels by a peripheral approach (usually femoral). In patients with congenital heart disease, many studies can be performed using a venous approach. This typically involves a flow-directed, balloon-tipped catheter that can be directed through the inferior vena cava into the right atrium, right ventricle, and pulmonary artery. In most patients, subsequent access to the left heart can be achieved by directing the catheter across the foramen ovale into the left atrium, left ventricle, and aorta. If necessary, peripheral arterial access can be used to study the left heart and aorta, using preformed torqueable (rather than flow-directed) catheters.

As the catheter is advanced under fluoroscopy through the great vessels and cardiac chambers, physiological information on chamber pressure and oxygen saturation provides important initial data about the congenital malformation. Cardiac output can be calculated by using the thermodilution method, or by the Fick principle. The latter is more accurate in the presence of a shunt (4). Shunt volumes can also be estimated by the Fick principle. Pulmonary vascular resistance, an often critical prognostic factor in patients with congenital malformations, is also calculated during the procedure.

Hemodynamic recordings are obtained, followed by angiocardiographic images. Proper interpretation depends on a systematic assessment of cardiac segments and great vessels. Problems with overlapping structures are partly overcome by angling the x-ray tube to provide optimal information about the structure in question (Fig. 2). A low-osmolar contrast medium, although more expensive than a conventional medium, can significantly decrease the risk for most patients undergoing cardiac cineangiography (5).

Therapeutic procedures can also be performed in the cardiac catheterization laboratory. These include balloon atrial septostomy (Rashkind procedure), balloon valvuloplasty (pulmonic and aortic valves), and balloon dilation of peripheral pulmonary stenoses, aortic coarctation, and stenotic Blalock-Taussig shunts (Fig. 3; 4). Clamshell devices have recently been used to close certain septal defects. In addition, embolotherapy provides a percutaneous method to close a patent ductus arteriosus, or to occlude unwanted aorticopulmonary collateral vessels.

C. Echocardiography

Echocardiography has provided a tremendous advance in noninvasive imaging of congenital heart disease. Currently available and applicable methods for evaluation of the heart include two-dimensional real-time, spectral Doppler, and color-flow Doppler echocardiography. Clinically useful routes of imaging include both transthoracic and transesophageal approaches. Endovascular techniques are, as yet, largely investigational.

Echocardiography (ultrasonography of the heart) employs reflected sound waves generated and detected by small transducers. The transducers contain piezoelectric crystals that convert mechanical energy into electrical impulses (and

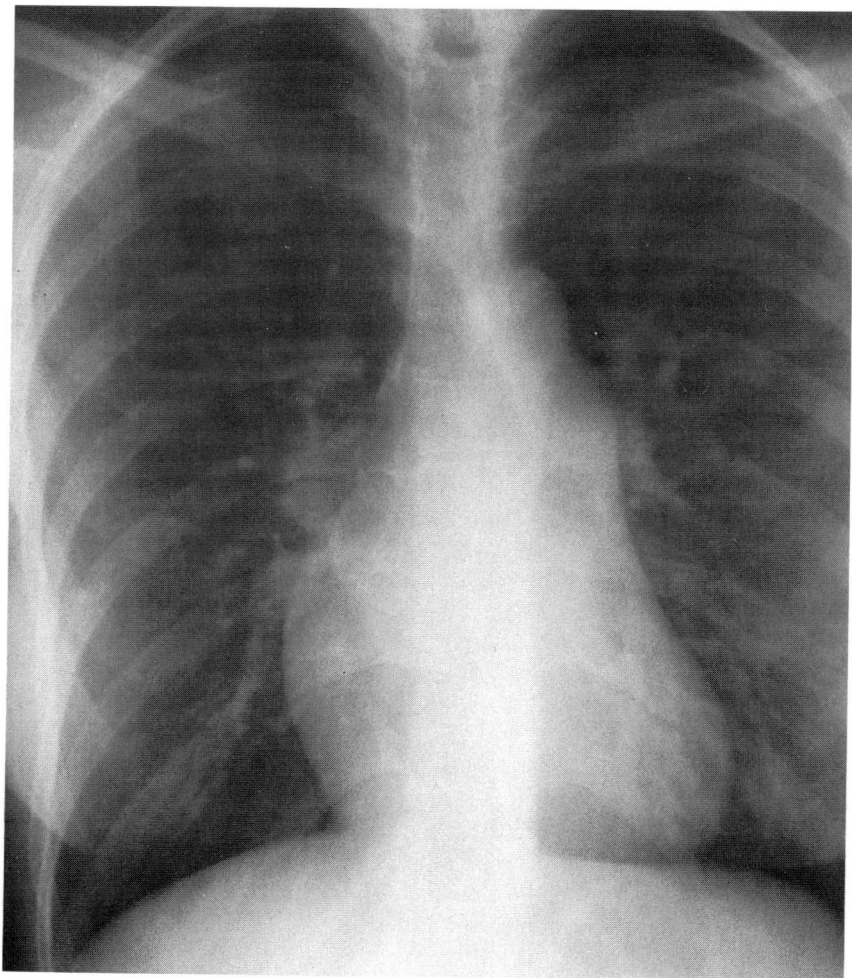

(a)

Figure 1 A 36-year-old woman (a) before and (b) 9 months after ASD repair. Note the reduction in caliber of the main pulmonary artery segment and normalization of the pulmonary vasculature. The right atrium remains enlarged, however. (Courtesy JTT Chen, Duke University Medical Center, Durham, NC.)

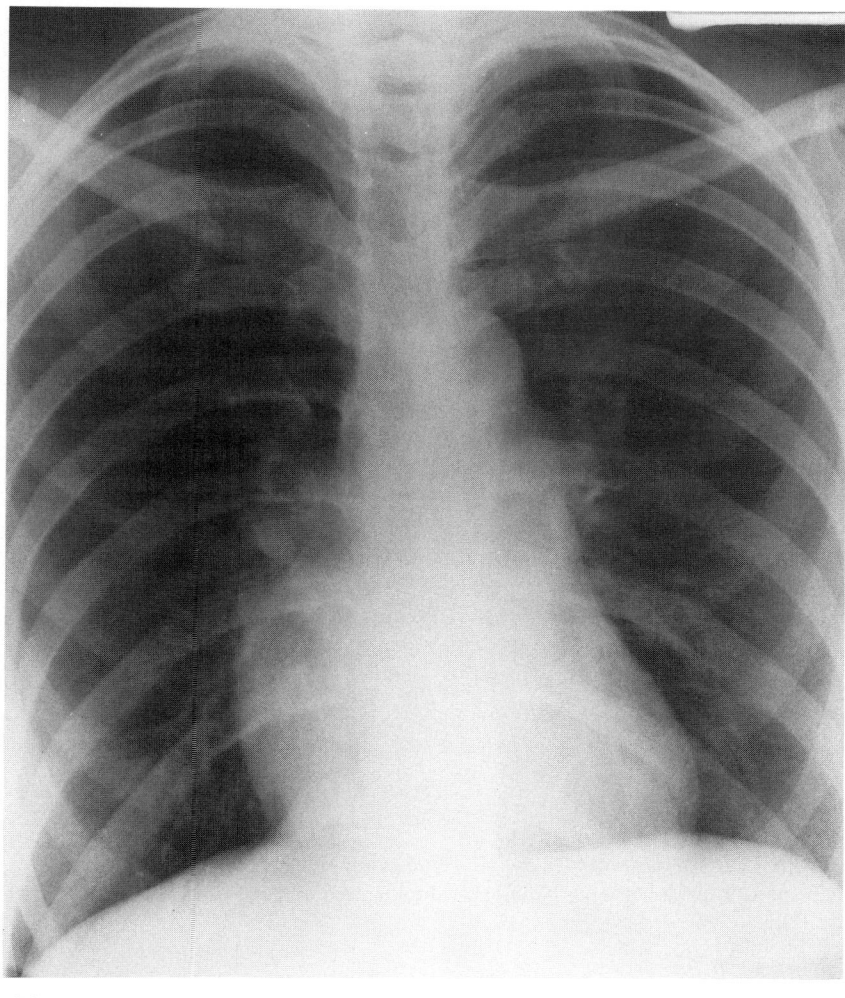

(b)

vice versa). M-mode examination provides an image consisting of a line of interrogation through the heart (on one axis) displayed over time (the second dimension) (6). This technique is still used for the analysis of motion of cardiac structures, but has largely been supplanted by two-dimensional techniques.

Two-dimensional (2-D) techniques allow definition of cardiac chamber anatomy and evaluation of ventricular function and wall motion. This type of echocardiography displays a cross-sectional plane of anatomy generated from sets

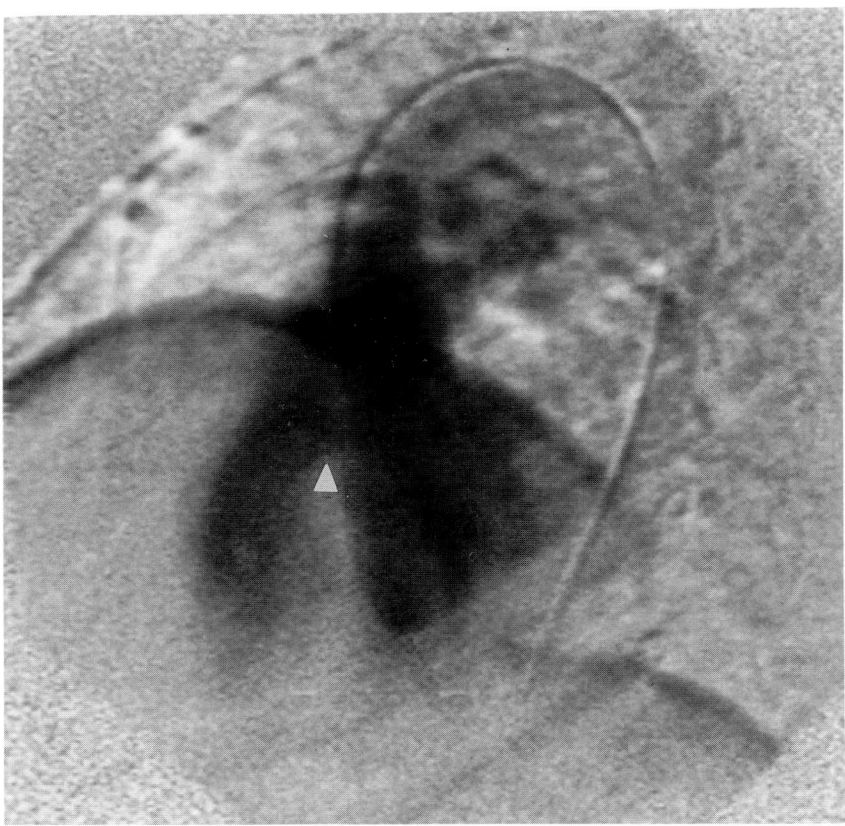

Figure 2 LAO projection of a digital subtraction angiogram in a patient with a perimembranous VSD (arrowhead). (Courtesy I. Tonkin, LeBonheur Childrens Hospital, Memphis, TN.)

of multiple individual "lines" of information. These real-time images are acquired so rapidly that the resulting display appears continuous (6).

Because ultrasound waves do not travel well through bone or lung, transthoracic imaging "windows" are somewhat limited. Conventional transthoracic-imaging windows include parasternal, apical, subcostal, and suprasternal. Each of these windows can be used in concert with any number of imaging axes. Certain anatomical structures are better seen with certain windows or axes.

Doppler echocardiography (both spectral and color-flow) allows determination of the velocity of a moving structure along the course of the ultrasound beam.

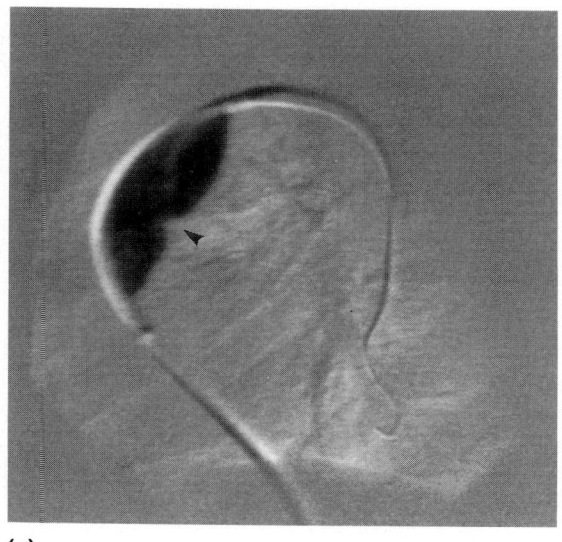

Figure 3 Balloon valvuloplasty of a congenitally stenotic pulmonic valve at (a) the initiation and (b) termination of balloon inflation. Note effacement of the impression on the balloon (arrowhead) caused by the stenotic pulmonic valve. (Courtesy I. Tonkin, LeBonheur Childrens Hospital, Memphis, TN.)

The two basic modes of spectral Doppler interrogation are continuous-wave, and pulsed-wave. Continuous-wave instruments use two separate piezoelectric crystals: one for emission and the other for detection. This allows detection of very large Doppler shifts along a line of interrogation, but cannot resolve depth along the line. Pulsed-Doppler scanning provides both velocity and positional information. The transmitter emits short bursts at precise rates of repetition. The receiver then listens for short periods at the same rate. The depth of the returning signal is a function of the time of flight and the velocity of sound in tissue. The visual display of conventional spectral Doppler imaging plots time along the x-axis and velocity along the y-axis (6).

Spectral Doppler examination (pulsed and continuous wave) allows estimation of flow velocities. This permits quantitation of valvular regurgitation and stenosis. Pressure gradients can be approximated, using the Bernoulli equation, which allows approximation of gradients across stenotic lesions, and also (in certain conditions) allows estimation of right ventricular systolic pressures (and pulmonary artery systolic pressures). Analysis of flow velocities in the aorta and pulmonary artery can also help estimate shunt ratios (3).

Color-flow Doppler combines 2-D echocardiography with pulsed-Doppler (using multiple gates), creating an anatomical gray-scale image, with superimposed velocity information encoded by a color scale. Color-Doppler evaluation combines the structural information of 2-D real-time examination with the flow information of Doppler. Color-flow allows detection of small defects that would otherwise be difficult to detect by 2-D echocardiography.

Contrast echocardiography involves the use of agitated saline solution injected intravenously to produce an echogenic blood pool that is detectable on 2-D real-time images. This technique has largely been supplanted by color-flow imaging, but still has occasional application (e.g., detection of low-velocity shunts, intracardiac baffle leaks, or extracardiac shunts; 3).

Transesophageal echocardiography (TEE) is a semiinvasive technique that uses the esophagus as a window for the sonographic examination. The ultrasound transducer is incorporated into the tip of a flexible endoscope that can be introduced into the esophagus of a sedated patient. This approach allows exquisite evaluation of the heart, particularly with attention to more posteriorly positioned structures. In adults with CHD, this includes evaluation of atrial septal defects (ASD), anomalous pulmonary venous return, ventricular outflow tract lesions, and aortic coarctation. Intraoperative TEE has been used successfully to help better-define known lesions as repair is initiated, to evaluate the adequacy of surgical repair as it is completed, and to detect postoperative complications (7). Transesophageal echocardiography can also be used as a guide for interventional catheter-based procedures, such as aortic and pulmonic balloon valvuloplasty, balloon dilation of aortic coarctation, balloon atrial septostomy, and clamshell device atrial septal defect closure (7).

D. Magnetic Resonance Imaging

During the past 10 years, magnetic resonance imaging (MRI) has become an important clinical tool in the assessment of patients with congenital heart disease. Although echocardiography remains the workhorse for the noninvasive evaluation of most intracardiac defects (e.g., uncomplicated ASD or ventricular septal defect, VSD), MRI plays an important complementary role, especially for the evaluation of extracardiac anatomy. Such instances include aortic or pulmonary artery anomalies, abnormal situs, anomalous venous connections, detection of systemic-to-pulmonary collaterals, and evaluation of postoperative anatomy, including surgically created systemic-to-pulmonary artery conduits. In addition, MRI can play an important role in the evaluation of complex intracardiac lesions, especially for atrioventricular and ventriculoarterial connections (Fig. 4).

Most MRI scanners in clinical use are capable (with the appropriate software) of executing the necessary scan sequences to achieve diagnostic examination. Much information can be obtained with spin-echo techniques gated to the patient's electrocardiogram (or peripheral pulse). Spin-echo techniques optimally display regional anatomy, and can be tailored to the individual patient by appropriately selecting the slice plane, thickness, and field of view appropriate for the anatomy in question. With spin-echo techniques, flowing blood usually appears as a signal void.

When physiological information about blood flow and myocardial dynamics is desired, cine-gradient echo imaging can be an important adjunct. This technique provides images at multiple (e.g., 16) phases of the cardiac cycle at one or several locations that can then be displayed in a continuous loop (or "movie"). With this technique, laminar blood flow appears bright, whereas areas of disturbed flow (turbulence) appear dark. Such turbulence can be detected as blood flows through septal defects, across regurgitant or stenotic heart valves, and through areas of vascular stenosis. When indicated, ventricular volumes, ejection fractions, regurgitant volumes, and shunt volumes can be estimated with these techniques (8).

The nature of the MRI examination (with multiple potential sequences, scan variables, and imaging planes) dictates that the examination be tailored to answer specific questions in advance. This requires knowledge of pertinent clinical and surgical information and of previous imaging findings. Thus, close collaboration between radiologist, cardiologist, and surgeon is required before, during, and after the examination. It is essential that the radiologist closely supervise the examination as it progresses, to ensure that each pertinent question has been addressed.

Because of limitations of the static and gradient magnetic fields, a few patients cannot be evaluated with MRI. The most important contraindications are the presence of implanted pacemakers and of cerebral aneurysm clips. Contrary to popular belief, almost all prosthetic heart valves are compatible with the MRI

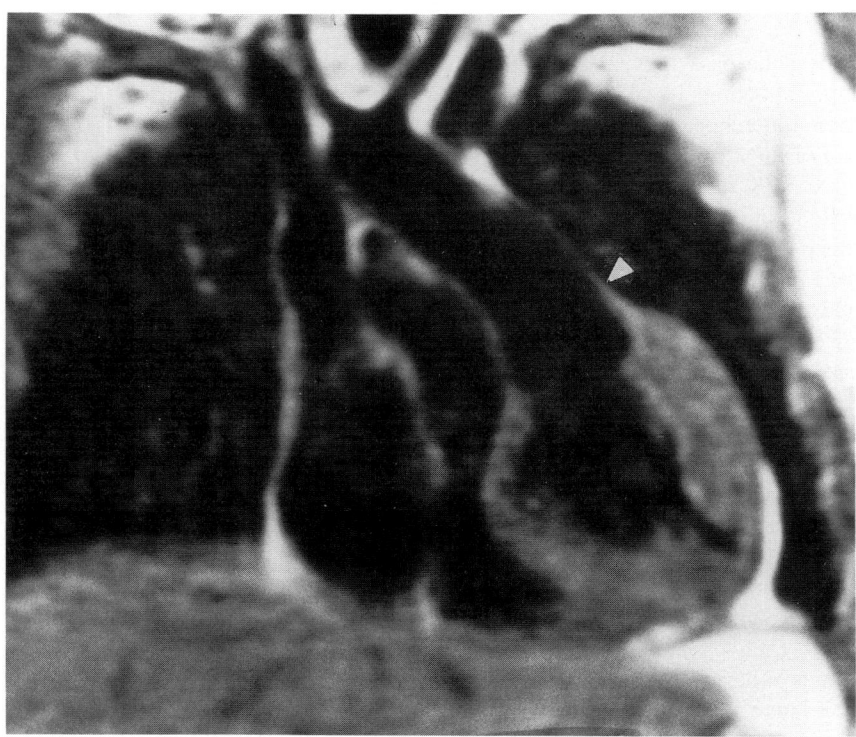

Figure 4 Congenitally corrected L-transposition of the great vessels. Coronal-gated spin-echo MRI. Note the position of the ascending aorta (arrowhead). Ventricular inversion is also present. (Courtesy T. Poulton, Canton, OH.)

scanner. If concerns about MRI compatibility of surgically implanted devices arise, reference should be made to the latest review on the subject (9).

Although sedation is often used for children undergoing examination, it is typically not necessary for most adolescents and adults. When used, it is important that these patients be continuously monitored with MRI-compatible equipment (e.g., pulse oximetry) and supplemental oxygen be administered when necessary (10,11).

The advantages of MRI relative to electron beam computed tomography (EBCT; see following section) for the evaluation of CHD include the following: lack of ionizing radiation, no need for IV contrast administration, ability to directly image in an infinite number of planes, no need for breath-holding, and wider availability. The disadvantages of MRI relative to EBCT are the inability to scan patients with absolute contraindications, incompatibility with certain monitoring devices, and longer acquisition times.

E. Computed Tomography

Computed tomography (CT) employs x-rays, receptors, and computer reconstructions to generate cross-sectional images. Nearly all CT scanners in clinical use today use a conventional x-ray tube that revolves around the patient. This revolution may be continuous (i.e., helical or spiral CT) or incremental (i.e., conventional CT). Both of these modalities are limited in the speed at which an image is generated (usually on the order of 1–2 sec/image). Therefore, motion artifact limits the analysis of intracardiac structures. However, these techniques are quite useful for the evaluation of great vessel anatomy, and may also be used to evaluate the patency of surgically created systemic-to-pulmonary shunts. In fact, commercially available software can allow creation of potentially useful three-dimensional images with CT-generated data.

Analysis of intracardiac structure and function may be obtained with CT, but requires a unique scanner. This technology has been called ultrafast CT or electron beam CT (EBCT). An EBCT scan uses an electron beam, focused and deflected by electromagnetic coils, directed at an arc of tungsten targets positioned under the patient. The x-rays then emitted are received by detectors positioned above the patient. Since no moving parts are present, scan times are very rapid, on the order of 50–100 msec. This allows excellent temporal resolution (Figs. 5a,b). In addition, significantly smaller amounts of IV contrast are necessary than with conventional CT (12).

The EBCT scanners can operate in three different modes: volume, flow, and cine. Volume mode operates similarly to conventional CT, but is faster. Flow mode allows serial slices to be performed in rapid succession at several contiguous levels to generate time–density curves following a bolus of IV contrast. These curves can provide estimates of shunt volume and cardiac output. Cine mode allows the acquisition of multiple slices in rapid succession (up to 17 images per second) at a few levels. This information can be played back in a continuous loop and can be used to analyze stroke volumes and ejection fractions. Cine mode may also help define complex intracardiac anatomy (13).

The primary difficulty in the use of EBCT to analyze CHD is its lack of availability. Currently, only a few centers in this country have the equipment. Other disadvantages of EBCT (especially in contrast with MRI) include the requirement for IV contrast, need for breath-holding, limited slice orientations, and use of ionizing radiation (14).

F. Radionuclide Imaging

Radionuclide imaging can provide useful physiological information in the evaluation of congenital heart disease. These techniques require nuclear medicine train-

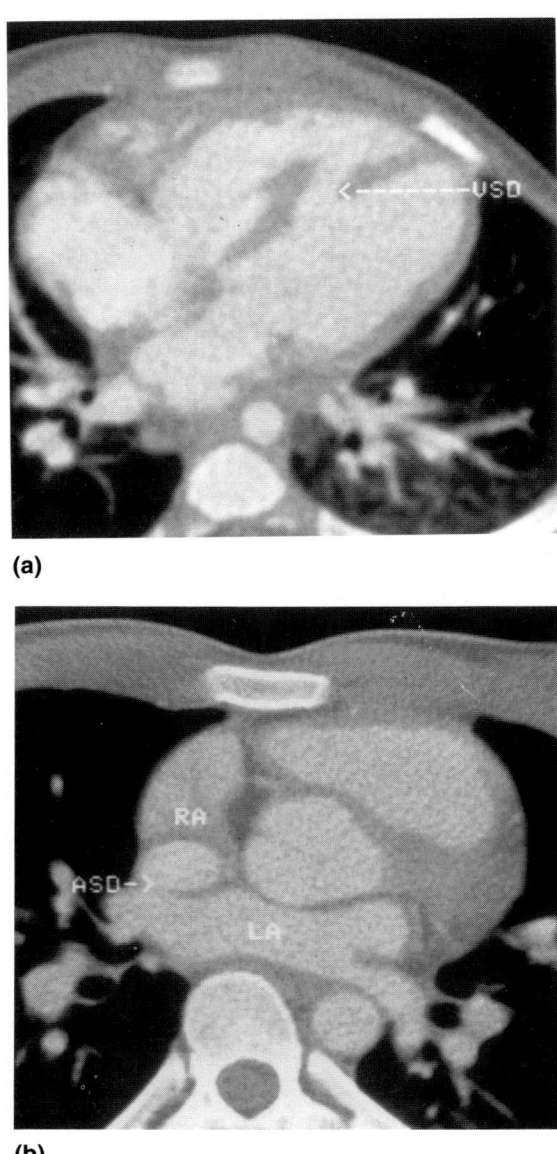

Figure 5 (a) Cine CT (EBCT) of muscular ventricular septal defect (VSD). (b) Cine CT (EBCT) of a sinus venosus atrial septal defect (ASD): RA, right atrium; LA, left atrium. (Courtesy L. Wexler, Stanford University, Stanford, CA.)

ing, certification, and licensure from the Nuclear Regulatory Commission, or its state equivalent, for the handling of radioactive materials (15).

All these techniques involve the intravascular administration of radiopharmaceuticals that emit photons detectable by special cameras placed near the body. Studies used in evaluation of congenital heart disease primarily utilize technetium Tc-99m or thallium Tl-201-labeled radiopharmaceuticals. Positron techniques are as yet not useful for the evaluation of CHD unless superimposed ischemia is present.

The most common use of radionuclide imaging from the evaluation of CHD is for the quantification of shunt lesions. Radionuclide imaging can also be used to evaluate ventricular function and myocardial perfusion.

Left-to-right shunts are usually evaluated by a first-pass method. This method requires the rapid intravenous injection of a small bolus of radiopharmaceutical (e.g., ^{99m}Tc-pentitates DTPA). The patient is imaged dynamically with a camera situated over the anterior chest. Because multiple frames of data are acquired per second, the bolus of tracer can be followed from the right atrium and right ventricle, into the pulmonary arteries and lungs, back into the left atrium and left ventricle, and then into the aorta. Time–activity curves drawn from regions of interest over the lung periphery allow shunt quantification. Computer approximations can then calculate Q_p/Q_s (16).

Right-to-left shunts may be detected and quantified by various scintigraphic methods. The simplest method involves the IV administration of ^{99m}Tc-labeled macroaggregated albumin (MAA) particles, the same radiopharmaceutical used in perfusion lung scans for pulmonary embolism. Because the size of the MAA particles is greater than the diameter of capillary beds, all of the injected tracer should deposit within pulmonary capillaries during its first pass through the lung. In patients with right-to-left shunts, some particles will bypass the pulmonary capillary bed and deposit instead in systemic capillary beds. The percentage of right-to-left shunting can then be calculated based on the ratio of extrapulmonary activity to whole-body activity (16,17).

Ventricular function can be evaluated using gated–equilibrium techniques or first-pass studies. The gated–equilibrium technique employs labeling of patient red blood cells with ^{99m}Tc. The test is essentially identical with that used in patients with acquired heart disease, allowing evaluation of left ventricular (LV) ejection fraction and regional wall motion (with or without exercise). Unfortunately, the technique is inadequate for the evaluation of right heart function and is not helpful for shunt evaluation.

First-pass studies (described in the foregoing) enable evaluation of right heart function and shunt analysis. The technique is rapid, and a smaller radiation dose is administered. First-pass techniques, however, require more sophisticated cameras and computers and require the administration of a tight bolus (typically through an external jugular vein).

Myocardial perfusion imaging plays a smaller role in the evaluation of CHD, but can be used to assess the functional significance of coronary anomalies, should they exist. In most center, perfusion imaging is accomplished with 201 Tl or ^{99m}Tc-MIBI.

III. Specific Lesions

A. Great Vessel Anomalies

Aortic Coarctation

Coarctation represents congenital narrowing of the thoracic aorta at the level of the aortic isthmus. Presentation is variable, depending on the degree of LV outflow obstruction and other associated lesions. Presentation in adolescence and adulthood is not uncommon.

The characteristic adult plain film demonstrates mild cardiomegaly. The upper left mediastinal border shows a characteristic "three" configuration: the dilated distal arch and left subclavian, followed by the coarctation itself, and then a segment of poststenotic aortic dilation. Rib notching is present in most adults and is caused by internal mammary–intercostal collaterals. Although bicuspid aortic valve is present in most patients with coarctation, symptoms of aortic stenosis usually occur later in adulthood.

Magnetic resonance imaging is now the gold standard for noninvasive imaging of coarctation (11). An MRI scan can reliably identify important associated structures that can impinge on surgical treatment of coarctation, including transverse arch hypoplasia, bicuspid aortic valve with ascending aortic dilation, and collateral vessels (Fig. 6). Additional, MRI is very important in postsurgical assessment (see Sec. IV). Echocardiography can supply some information, but often requires a transesophageal approach in adults. Cardiac catheterization may be reserved to directly measure pressure gradients, if necessary preoperatively. It can also be used as a guide for balloon angioplasty of recurrent stenosis after surgery.

Vascular Rings

Patients with arch anomalies that encircle the trachea and esophagus may be symptomatic or asymptomatic, depending on the "tightness" of the ring. If these patients do not present in childhood (e.g., stridor), they may develop into asymptomatic adults. However, as the adult aorta undergoes elongation and atherosclerotic change with aging, symptoms may develop in adulthood (e.g., dysphagia).

Although many anatomical combinations are possible, the most common vascular rings are due to a double aortic arch or a right-sided arch, with an aberrant left subclavian artery and short left ligamentum arteriosum.

Some surgeons believe plain film and barium esophagram are sufficient for

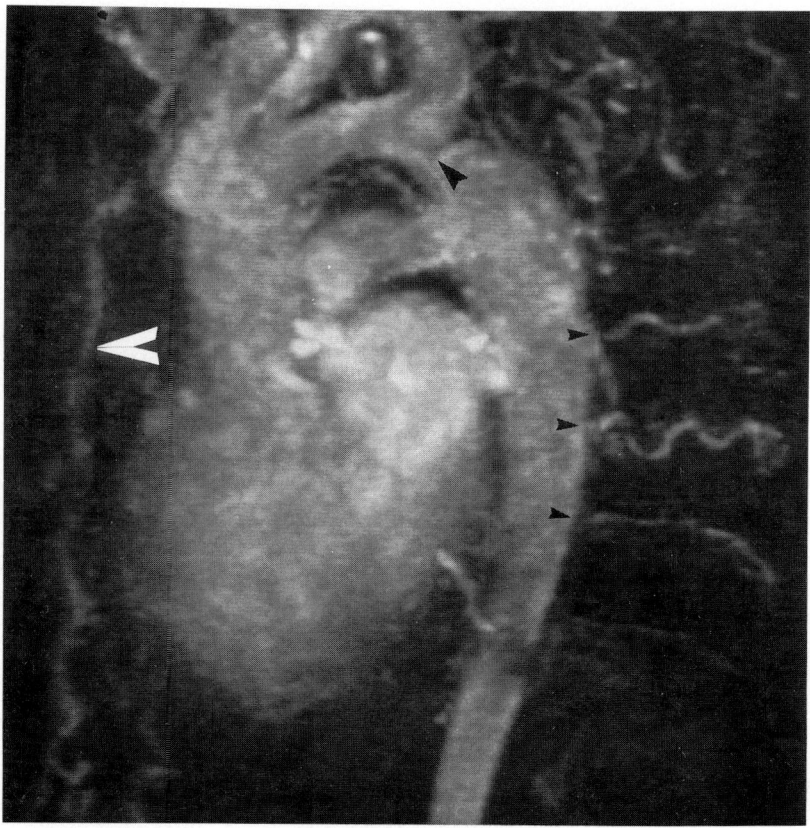

Figure 6 Two-dimensional time-of-flight MRA of a tight coarctation (black arrowhead). Note intercostal collaterals (small arrowheads) and internal mammary collaterals (white arrowhead).

the preoperative evaluation of these patients because the surgical approach is usually the same (4). However, MRI is an extremely accurate noninvasive method of defining anatomy and has become the preoperative-imaging modality of choice (over angiography) in most centers (Figs. 7a,b) (11).

B. Left-to-Right Shunts

Atrial Septal Defect

Atrial septal defect (ASD) is the most common left-to-right shunt that presents in adulthood. Three major types exist. Ostium secundum defects, the most common,

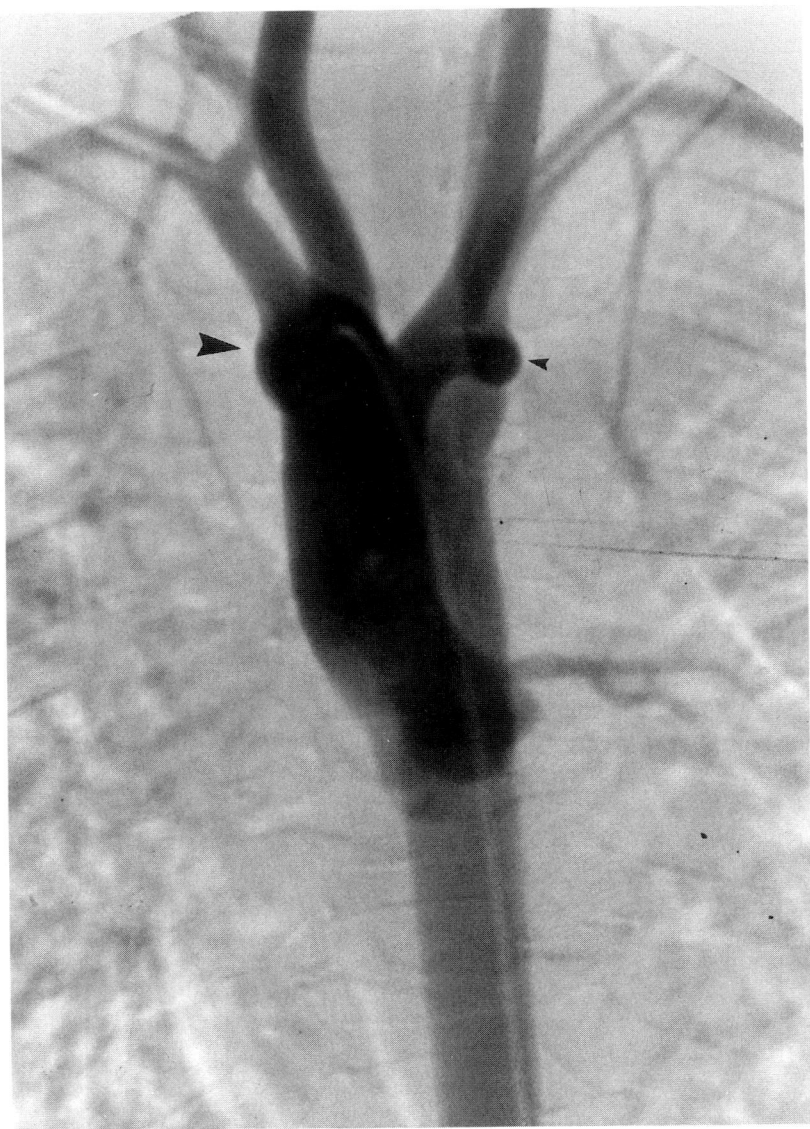

(a)

Figure 7 (a) Digital subtraction angiogram of a double aortic arch (anterior projection). Right-sided component (large arrowhead) is larger and more cephalad than left-sided component (small arrowhead). (b) Coronal-gated spin-echo MRI of another patient with double aortic arch. Note large right arch (large arrowhead), and smaller left arch giving rise to the left common carotid artery (small arrowhead).

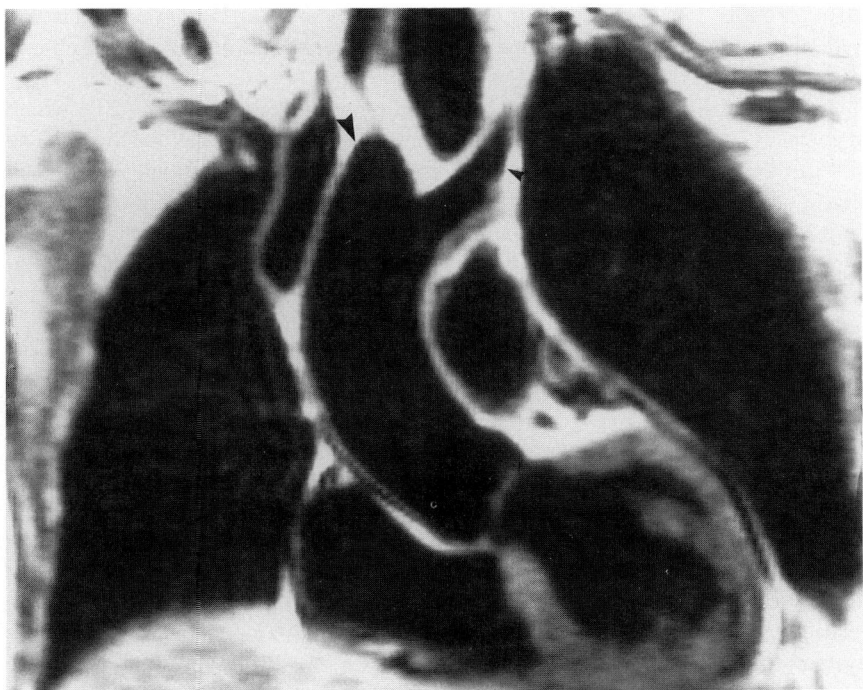

(b)

occur in the midportion of the atrium septum. Ostium primum defects occur in the most inferior portion of the septum, and are commonly associated with abnormalities of the atrioventricular (AV) valves and inlet ventricular septum. Sinus venosus defects occur high in the posterior portion of the septum, near the entrance of the superior vena cava (SVC), and are commonly accompanied by anomalous drainage of the right upper and middle lobe pulmonary veins to the SVC. (Isolated partial anomalous pulmonary venous return may also occur, causing a hemodynamic picture similar to uncomplicated ASD.)

The magnitude of shunting in ASD is dependent on the size of the ASD and the relative compliance of the right and left ventricles. Symptoms commonly present (or progress) during adulthood. The progression of symptoms in adulthood is usually due to one of three problems: decreasing LV compliance, leading to increasing left-to-right shunting; development of atrial arrhythmias (e.g., atrial fibrillation); and development of pulmonary artery hypertension (18).

The plain radiograph in ASD classically shows diffusely increased ("shunt") pulmonary vascularity accompanied by right atrial and right ventricular enlargement (see Fig. 1.) The size of left atrium is usually normal. If pulmonary arterial hypertension ensues, there will be concomitant centralization of the pulmonary vascular pattern (19).

Echocardiography clearly delineates the presence and type of ASD, which appears as an echo-free region in the appropriate location. Color-Doppler can confirm the direction and estimate the size of the associated shunt. An MRI or EBCT scan, although not typically used to evaluate isolated ASDs, is effective in demonstrating them (see Fig. 5b). In most institutions, cineangiography has been supplanted by echocardiography in the evaluation of ASD. Instead, cardiac catheterization is reserved to confirm pulmonary artery pressure is cases of suspected pulmonary artery hypertension.

Ventricular Septal Defect

Although ventricular septal defect (VSD) is one of the most common congenital defects, most are either treated in childhood or spontaneously close; thus, it accounts for a small proportion of left-to-right shunts in the adult. The VSDs are classified by their location (perimembranous, muscular, inlet, or supracristal), size (restrictive or nonrestrictive), and alignment (malalignment or alignment). Most adult survivors with uncorrected VSDs have small, restrictive defects. These restrictive defects may prevent the pulmonary vascular tree from exposure to systemic pressures, thereby preventing the development of abnormal pulmonary vascular resistance. If shunt flow is large enough (i.e., 2:1 or greater), these patients will exhibit shunt vascularity on plain film, with enlargement of the right ventricle, left atrium, and sometimes left ventricle. Patients with very small shunts may have normal chest radiographs (19).

Adults with nonrestrictive VSDs typically develop pulmonary artery hypertension from long-standing exposure of the pulmonary vascular tree to systemic pressures. This leads to diminution of the left-to-right shunt, which eventually reverses, causing cyanosis (Eisenmenger's complex). A plain radiograph will demonstrate centralization of the pulmonary vasculature superimposed on the other findings of VSD.

Echocardiography should easily confirm the presence, size, and location of most VSDs. Although large defects are easily seen on 2-D imaging, smaller defects may require color flow for detection. Doppler techniques can also be used to estimate shunt size and right-sided heart pressures (3).

Although not usually required to make the diagnosis, cineangiography can be useful in demonstrating small, muscular VSDs, especially if multiple (see Fig. 2). In addition, the hemodynamic data derived from cardiac catheterization is often essential in planning surgical treatment. Use of MRI or EBCT can usually detect the presence of VSD (see Fig. 5a), but they are not often used in the setting of isolated VSD, particularly if echocardiography is diagnostic.

Patent Ductus Arteriosus

Although patent ductus arteriosus (PDA) is among the most common lesions in infancy, it is relatively uncommon in adults. However, if the ductus does not close spontaneously by 2 months of age, it often remains patent into adulthood (20). Adults with small (restrictive) PDAs are usually asymptomatic, although they carry a significant risk of developing endocarditis. Patients with large (nonrestrictive) defects either develop congestive heart failure or, if pulmonary resistance rises high enough, shunt reversal, with the subsequent development of differential cyanosis (toes > fingers) (18).

By far, the most common configuration of PDA is a connection between the inferior aspect of the aortic arch, just beyond the origin of the left subclavian artery, and the superior surface of the proximal left pulmonary artery (3,18). A chest radiograph classically shows shunt vascularity in the presence of left atrial, left ventricular, ascending aortic, and pulmonary trunk enlargement. In older adults, the ductus can calcify, causing a characteristic appearance on plain film (19).

Noninvasive confirmation can be obtained in several ways. Although echocardiography (transthoracic or transesophageal) does not easily display the ductus in adult patients, it can detect its presence by identifying the color-flow jet from the aorta into the pulmonary artery at the typical location (3,7). Direct imaging of the PDA and direction of shunt flow can be accurately obtained with MRI (Fig. 8). CT scan is helpful in identifying calcium in the wall of the ductus, but offers no other advantage to MRI or echo. Cardiac catheterization is typically not required to establish the diagnosis, but may be necessary to quantify pulmonary vascular resistance before repair in patients with significant pulmonary artery hypertension.

C. Right-to-Left Shunt: Tetralogy of Fallot

The tetralogy of Fallot (TOF) includes infundibular stenosis. VSD (malalignment type), overriding aorta, and secondary right ventricular hypertrophy. Tetralogy of Fallot, the most common cause of cyanotic CHD, most commonly presents in childhood, but approximately 11% of untreated patients survive into adulthood (18).

Plain CXR in these patients typically demonstrates a normal-sized cardiac silhouette with RV hypertrophy suggested on the lateral film. Pulmonary vascularity is typically normal or low-normal (19). Confirmation of the diagnosis is usually readily made with echocardiography, cineangiography, or MRI (Fri. 9).

As in many other cyanotic conditions, evaluation of the size of the central pulmonary arteries is often helpful before surgical repair. Size and configuration of the central pulmonary arteries often dictates the type of surgical repair that can be performed. An MRI scan is the only noninvasive modality that can consistently define the morphology of the central pulmonary arteries (Fig. 10; 10).

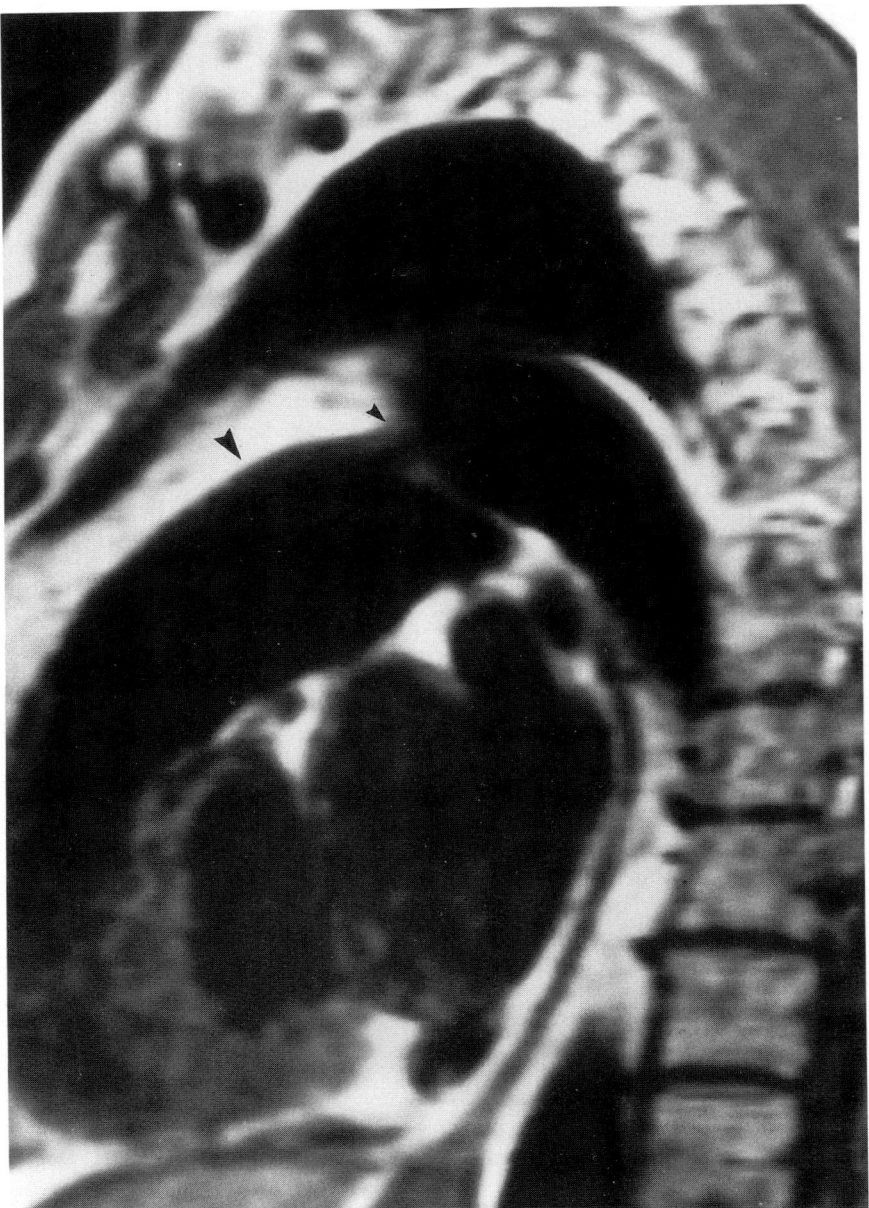

Figure 8 Oblique sagittal-gated spin-echo MRI of a patent ductus arteriosus (small arrowhead). Note enlarged main pulmonary trunk (large arrowhead).

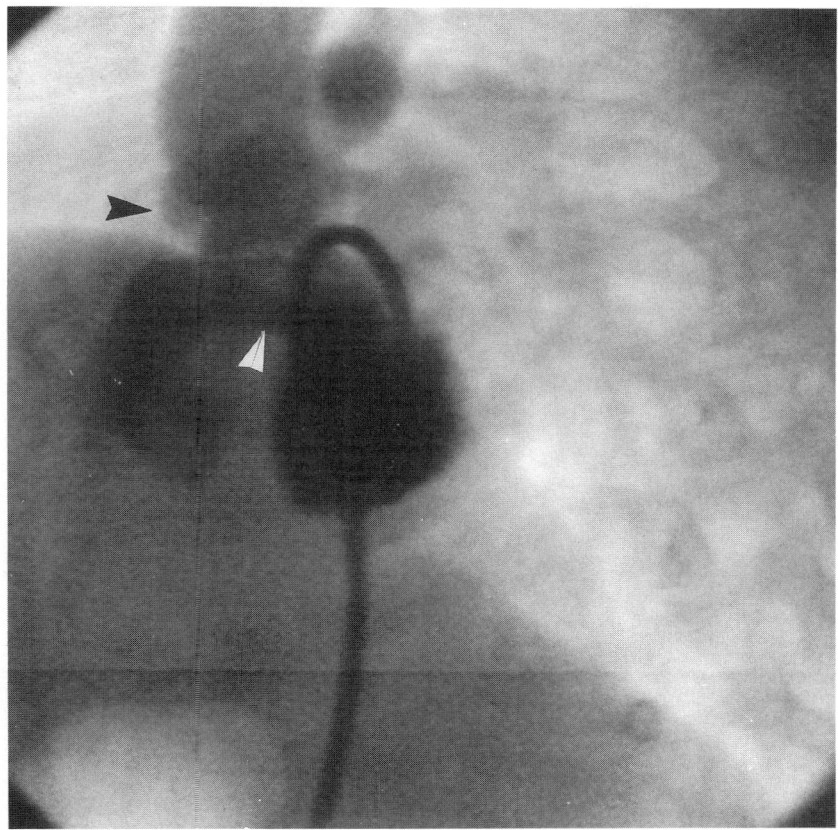

Figure 9 Digital subtraction angiogram with left anterior oblique orientation of TOF. A balloon-tipped catheter has been positioned in the LV from a transeptal approach. Note the aortic root (black arrowhead) overriding a malalignment VSD (white arrowhead). (Courtesy I. Tonkin, LeBonheur Childrens Hospital, Memphis, TN.)

D. Valvular Disease

Bicuspid Aortic Valve

Congenital bicuspid aortic valve is the most common congenital heart defect, occurring in 2% of the general population (18). Typically, the left and right coronary cusps are fused and situated opposite an enlarged noncoronary cusp. Some patients with bicuspid aortic valve remain asymptomatic throughout life. Others develop symptomatic aortic stenosis during adulthood, caused by gradual

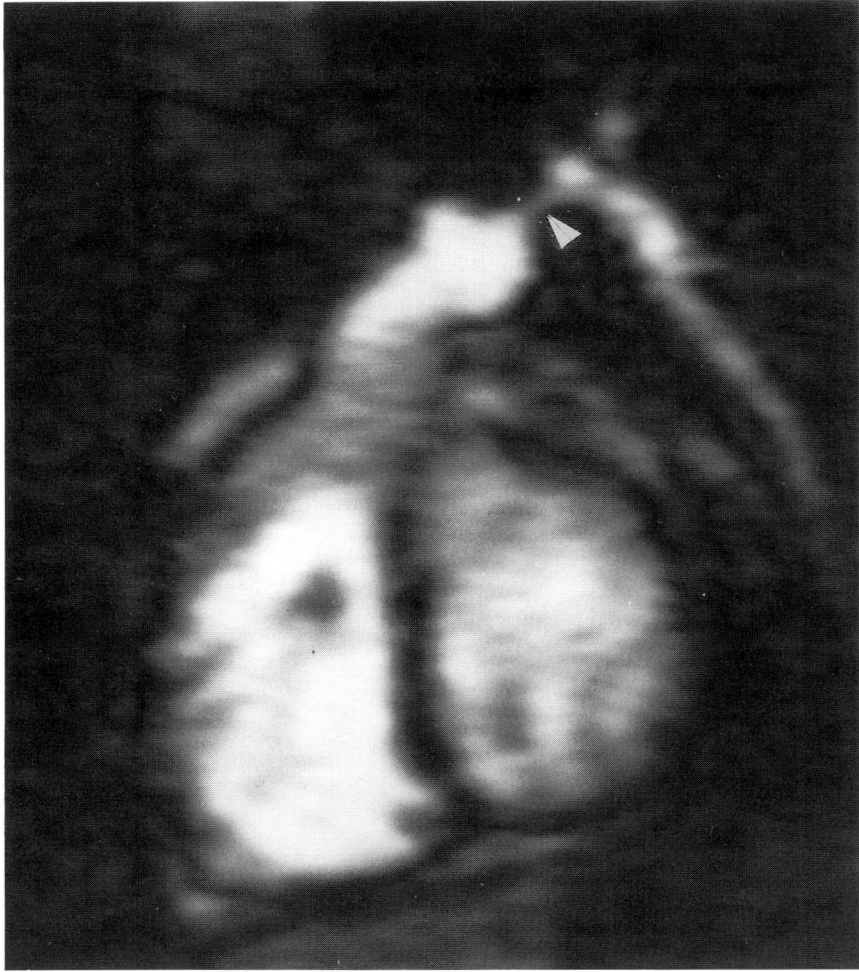

Figure 10 Oblique sagittal cine-gradient echo image of branch stenosis of the proximal left pulmonary artery (arrowhead) in a patient after TOF repair.

fibrocalcific thickening of the bicuspid valve. A significant proportion of patients with a bicuspid aortic valve have associated disease of the thoracic aorta, the most common being coarctation (21).

Standard chest radiograph in patients with bicuspid aortic valve and aortic stenosis demonstrates poststenotic dilation of the ascending aorta. The left ventricle is typically normal in size radiographically, unless aortic insufficiency coexists. Calcification of the aortic valve leaflets can often be seen (Fig. 11; 19,21).

Echocardiography easily confirms the diagnosis of aortic stenosis and can usually demonstrate the thickened bicuspid aortic valve. The transvalvular pressure gradient and aortic valve area can be estimated using continuous-wave Doppler techniques. Although MRI can detect the presence of aortic stenosis and image the bicuspid valve, its major use is the assessment of the thoracic aortic abnormalities that commonly accompany this condition (e.g., aneurysmal poststenotic dilation and coarctation). Cardiac catheterization is typically reserved for more accurately assessment of cardiac hemodyanamics preoperatively, or as an adjunct to balloon valvuloplasty.

Valvular Pulmonic Stenosis

Valvular pulmonic stenosis (PS) is usually isolated, typically presenting in asymptomatic adults, with a characteristic ejection murmur detecting on physical examination. In most instances, the valve is normally formed, but is fused at the commissures.

The plain radiograph characteristically shows enlargement of the pulmonary trunk and left pulmonary artery, owing to the direction of the poststenotic jet (Fig. 12; 19,21). The overall heart size may be normal, or it may demonstrate mild right-sided enlargement.

Echocardiography easily confirms the presence of valvular PS and can estimate the severity of the transvalvular gradient. Percutaneous transluminal valvuloplasty, using balloon dilation has become the treatment of choice for patients with isolated valvular PS (see Fig. 3).

Ebstein's Anomaly

Ebstein's anomaly is a relatively uncommon condition, characterized by congenital tricuspid insufficiency owing to a malformed and malpositioned tricuspid valve. Typically, the septal and posterior leaflets are partially fused with the inlet portion of the right ventricle. This results in tricuspid insufficiency, which may be severe. A patent foramen ovale or ASD frequently coexist, thereby allowing right-to-left shunting and cyanosis (18).

Patients may develop symptoms at a wide range of ages, usually dictated by the degree of tricuspid insufficiency and right-to-left shunt. Occasionally, these patients experience tachyarrhythmias caused by coexistent accessory conduction pathways (18).

The classic radiographic appearance is that of an enlarged, globular cardiac silhouette, a narrow vascular pedicle, and decreased pulmonary vascularity (Fig. 13; 19,21). The anatomy of the malformed tricuspid valve and associated tricuspid insufficiency can be readily assessed by echocardiography. The characteristic abnormalities may also be imaged with MRI, cineangiography, or CT.

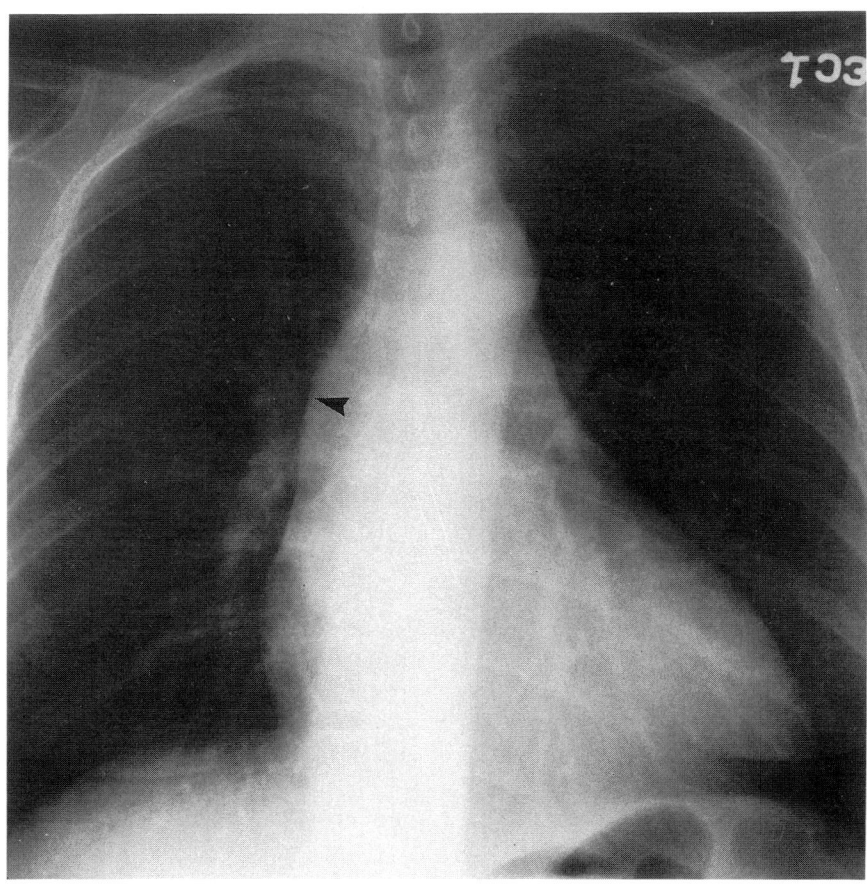

(a)

Figure 11 (a) PA and (b) lateral radiograph of a patient with bicuspid aortic valve and associated aortic stenosis. Note the dilation of the ascending aorta on the frontal film (arrowhead) and calcification of the aortic valve on the lateral film (arrowheads). (Courtesy JTT Chen, Duke University Medical Center, Durham, NC.)

E. Uncommon Conditions: Congenitally Corrected L-Transposition of the Great Vessels

Although a relatively uncommon condition, most of these patients present in adulthood. Embryonically, these hearts form with a left (rather than right) ventricular loop. The ventricles are thus inverted, with the morphological left ventricle situated anterior and to the right, receiving blood from the right atrium and

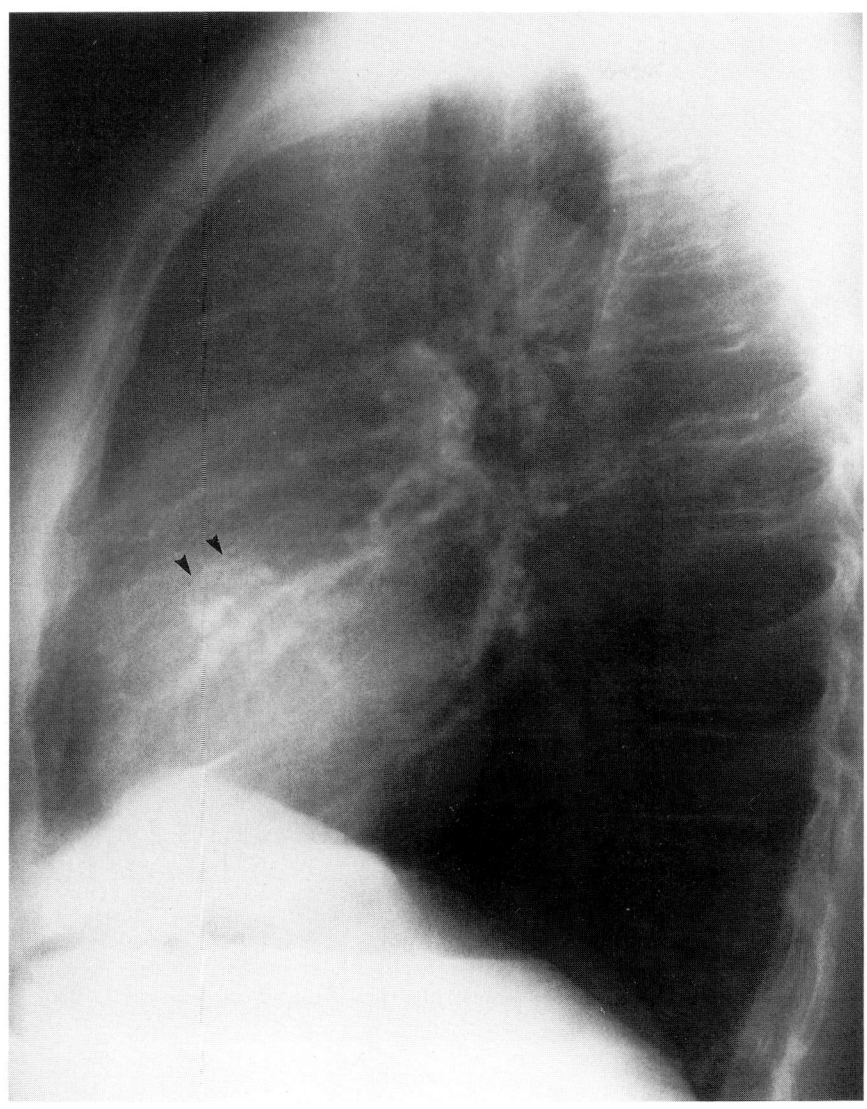

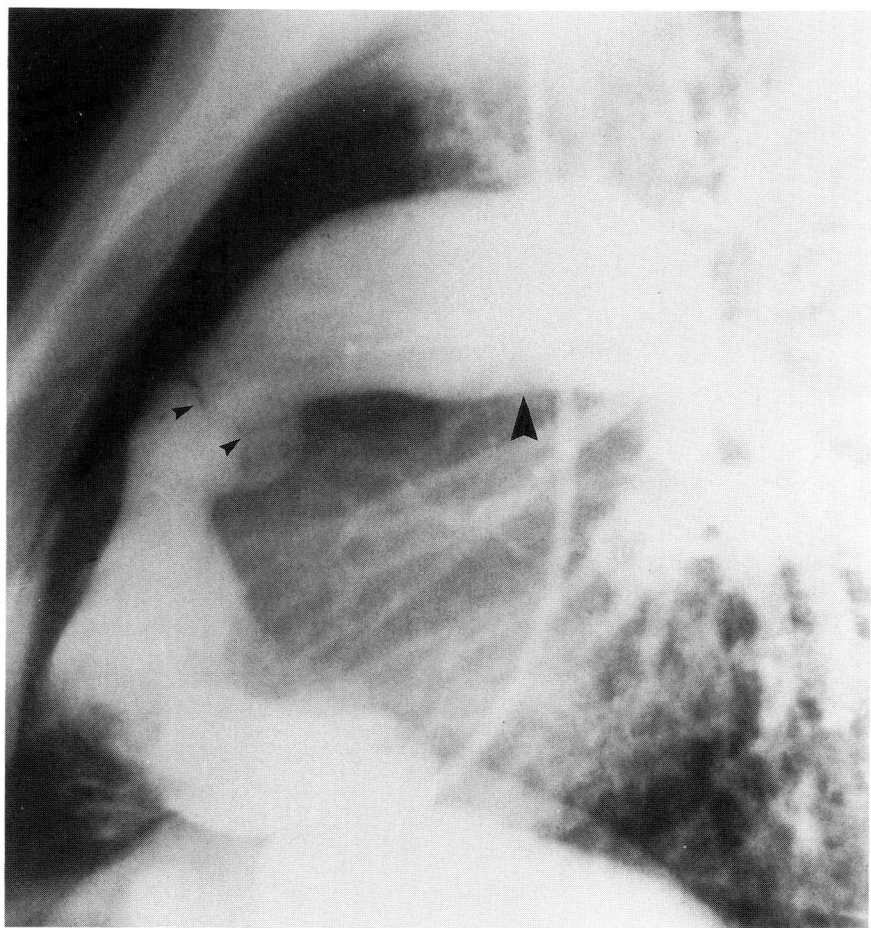

Figure 12 Lateral cine angiogram of valvular pulmonic stenosis. Note domed pulmonic valve (small arrowheads) with poststenotic dilation of the main and proximal left pulmonary artery (large arrowhead).

emptying into the pulmonary artery. The morphological right ventricle is situated posteriorly and to the left, receiving blood from the left atrium and emptying into the aorta. The ascending aorta and pulmonary artery are transposed, with the ascending aortic root situated anterior and to the left of the pulmonary artery origin (4).

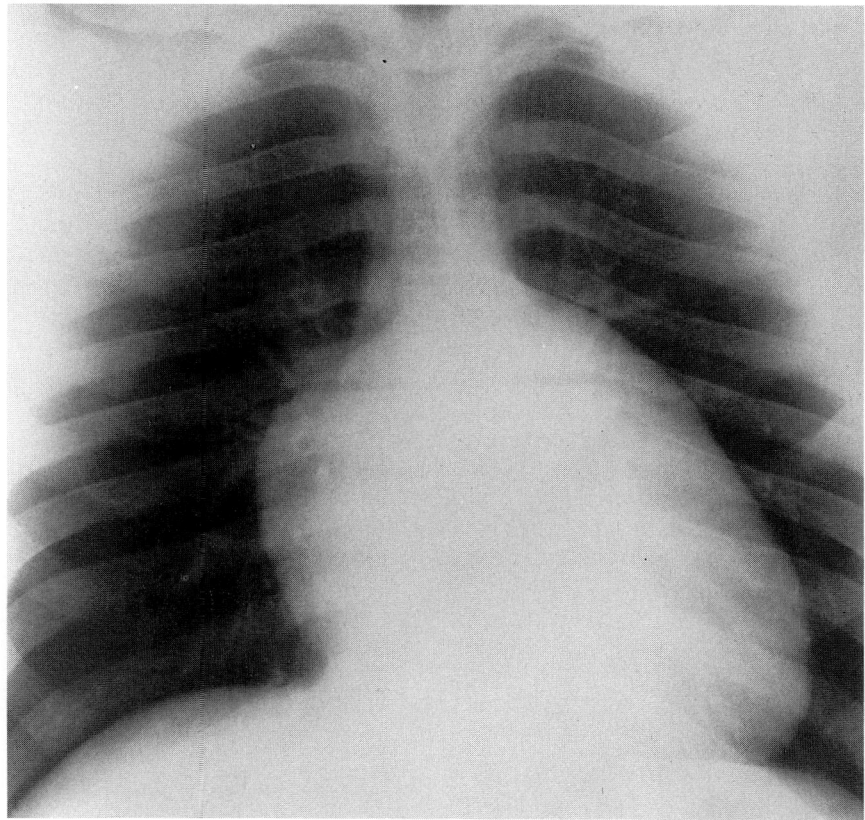

Figure 13 Frontal radiograph of Ebstein's anomaly shows globular cardiac silhouette, from right heart enlargement, and decreased pulmonary vascularity.

In the absence of associated defects, the direction of blood flow is physiologically correct; however, these patients are at risk of developing problems in adulthood, including premature failure of the right (systemic) ventricle, tricuspid insufficiency, and heart block (18,21).

Plain CXR is most remarkable for the broad convex curve of the upper left mediastinal border formed by the leftward ascending aorta. Although often not a straightforward diagnosis, the anatomical defects can be confirmed with echo, MRI, cineangiography, or CT (see Fig. 4).

IV. Postoperative Imaging of Congenital Heart Disease

Plain CXR analysis after surgical palliation or repair often provides clues to the nature of the surgical procedure and helps analyze the physiological changes that result. For instance, the nature of the approach (thoracotomy vs. median sternotomy) is dictated by the nature of the procedure.

Pulmonary vascularity subsequent to palliation or repair of shunts provides important physiological information. For example, pulmonary vascularity should increase after palliative shunt placement for TOF. Conversely, pulmonary vascularity and cardiac chamber enlargement should decrease after repair of left-to-right shunts, although this process is extremely slow in older adults who undergo repair (see Fig. 1; 19).

Long-term residua and sequelae of intracardiac repair for CHD are often well evaluated with echocardiography. Examples include residual septal defects, ventricular outflow obstruction, and residual valvular insufficiency. The integrity of intracardiac prostheses and conduits are also well evaluated by echocardiogra-

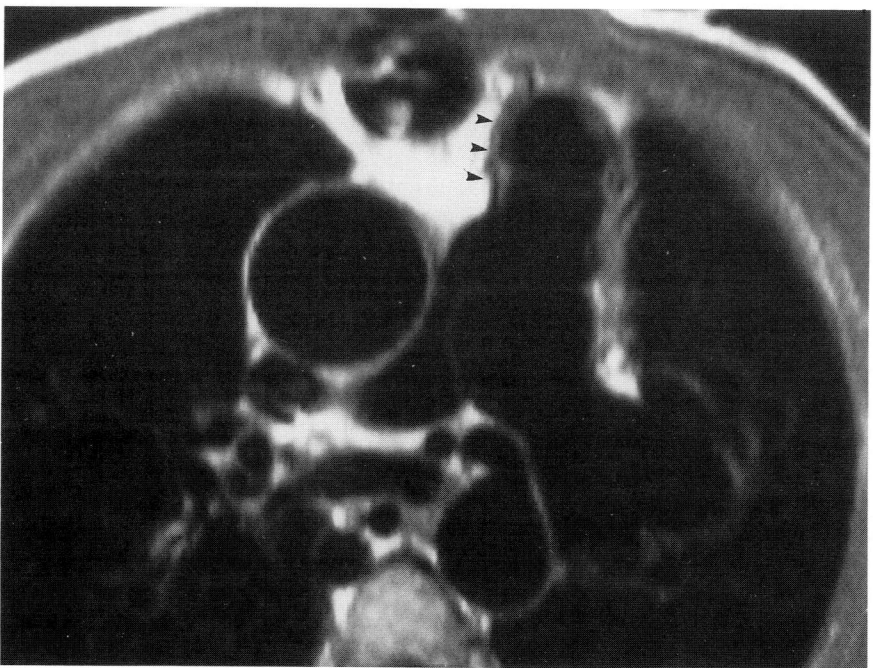

Figure 14 Axial-gated spin-echo MRI of a patent Rastelli conduit (arrowheads) in a patient following TOF repair.

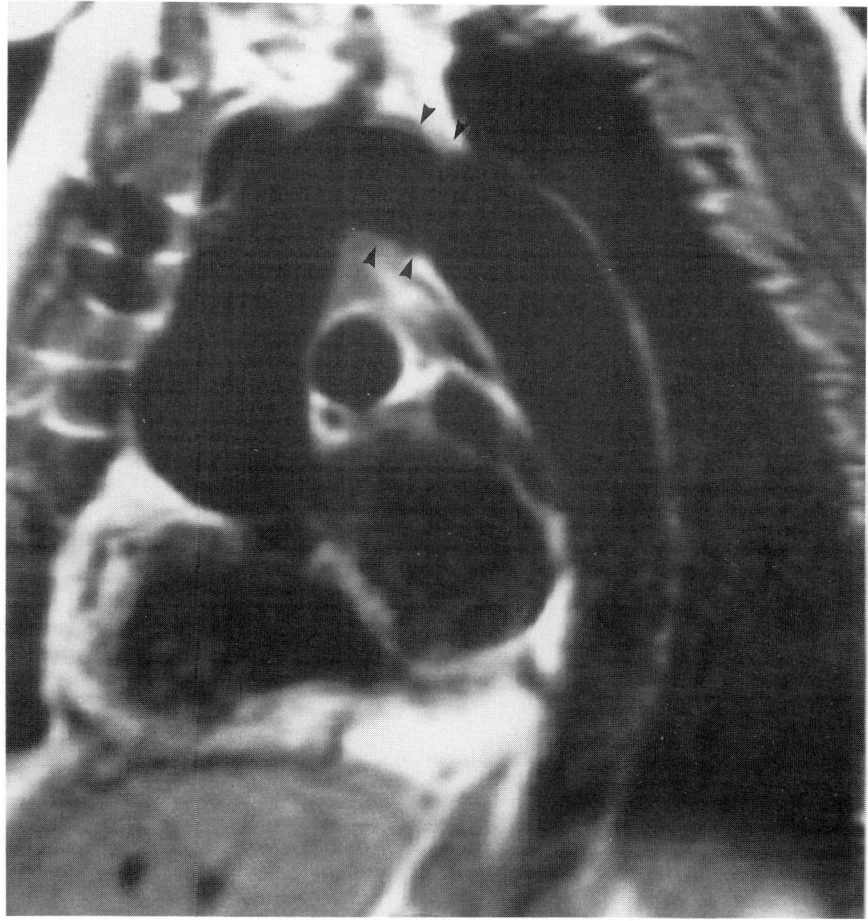

Figure 15 Sagittal oblique spin-echo MRI in a patient after coarctation repair. The site of repair (arrowheads) is widely patent, with no evidence of recurrent stenosis.

phy. If echocardiography is difficult postoperatively because of limited acoustic window, MRI or cineangiography may be required (Fig. 14).

Evaluation of extracardiac anatomy postoperatively is usually well suited to MRI. The status of coarctation repair and presence of restenosis can be easily studied (Fig. 15). In addition, MRI can noninvasively evaluate the condition of palliative systemic–pulmonary shunts and follow the growth of pulmonary arteries in anticipation of subsequent repair (10,11).

Table 1 Relative Comparison[a] of Advantages and Disadvantages of Different Imaging Modalities for Congenital Heart Disease

	Availability	Noninvasiveness	Lack of ionizing radiation	Lack of IV contrast	Intracardiac anatomy	Extracardiac anatomy	Cost[b] ($)
Standard chest film	++++	++++	+++	++++	+	++	68
Angiocardiography	++++	−	−	−	++++	++++	5000
Echocardiography	++++	++++	++++	++++	++++	++	768
Transesophageal	+++	+/−				+++	878
Magnetic resonance	++	++++	++++	++++	++++	+++	790
EB computed tomography	+/−	++++	++	−	+++	++++	854
Radionuclide imaging	+++	++++	++	++++	++	+	500

[a]++++, excellent; +++, good; ++, fair; +, poor; − very poor.
[b]Cost reflects typical 1995 changes in the greater Memphis, Tennessee area.

V. Summary

A wide variety of imaging options are available to study adults with congenital heart disease. Analysis should always begin with proper evaluation of the plain CXR. Subsequent imaging choices depend on various factors, including cost, invasiveness, ability to answer the questions at hand, and the available expertise to perform and interpret the studies (Table 1). Although cardiac catheterization and cineangiography remain important tools in diagnosis, emphasis continues to move toward noninvasive techniques, such as echocardiography (for intracardiac abnormalities) and MRI (for extracardiac abnormalities), with CT and nuclear scintigraphy helpful for certain specific situations.

References

1. McNamara DG. The adult with congenital heart disease. Curr Probl Cardiol 1989; 14: 59–114.
2. Perloff JK, Child JS, eds. Congenital heart disease in adults. Philadelphia: WB Saunders, 1991.
3. Child JS. Echo-Doppler and color flow imaging in congenital heart disease. Cardiol Clin 1990; 8:289–313.
4. Soto B, Kassner EG, Baxley WA, eds. Imaging of cardiac disorders. Vol. 1. Philadelphia: JB Lippincott, 1992.
5. Boxt LM, Reagan K, Katz J. Angiocardiography in the diagnosis of congenital heart disease. Radiol Clin North Am 1994; 32:435–460.
6. Curry TS, Dowdey JE, Murry RC, eds. Christensen's physics of diagnostic radiology. 4th ed. Philadelphia: Lea & Febiger, 1990.
7. Marelli AJ, Child JS, Perloff JK. Transesophageal echocardiography in congenital heart disease in the adult. Cardiol Clin 1993; 11:505–520.
8. Mohiaddin RH, Longmore DB. Functional aspects of cardiovascular nuclear magnetic resonance imaging. Circulation 1993; 88:264–281.
9. Shellock FG, Morisoli S, Kanai E. MR procedures and biomedical implants: 1993 update. Radiology 1993; 189:587–599.
10. Bissett GS. Magnetic resonance imaging of congenital heart disease in the pediatric patient. Radiol Clin North Am 1991; 29:279–291.
11. Bank ER. Magnetic resonance of congenital cardiovascular disease. Radiol Clin North Am 1993; 31:553–572.
12. Flicker S, Naidech HJ, Altin RS, et al. Ultrafast computed tomography techniques in cardiac disease. J Thorac Imaging 1989; 4:42–49.
13. Steiner RM, Flicker S, Eldridge WJ, et al. Clinical experience with rapid acquisition cardiovascular CT imaging (cine CT) in the adult patient. Radiographics 1989; 9: 283–305.
14. MacMillan RM. Magnetic resonance imaging vs ultrafast computed tomography for cardiac diagnosis. Int J Cardiac Imaging 1992; 8:217–227.

15. Mettler FA, Guiberteau MJ. Essentials of nuclear medicine imaging. 3rd ed. Philadelphia: WB Saunders, 1991.
16. Dea MW. Nuclear imaging of congenital heart disease. In: Higgins CB, ed. Essentials of cardiac radiology and imaging. Philadelphia: JB Lippincott, 1992; 397–403.
17. Dogan AS, Rezai K, Kirchner PT, et al. A scintigraphic sign for detection of right-to-left shunts. J Nucl Med 1993; 34:1607–1611.
18. Perloff JK. Congenital heart disease in adults. In: Braunwald E, ed. Heart disease. 4th ed. Philadelphia: WB Saunders, 1992.
19. Gross GW, Steiner RM. Radiographic manifestations of congenital heart disease in the adult patient. Radiol Clin North Am 1991; 29:293–317.
20. McManus BM. Patent ductus arteriosus. In: Roberts WC, ed. Adult congenital heart disease. Philadelphia: FA Davis, 1987:443–462.
21. Chen JTT. Essentials of cardiac roentgenology. Boston: Little, Brown & Co, 1987.

20

The Thoracic Aorta

JOHN R. MAYO

University of British Columbia
and Vancouver Hospital and Health Sciences Centre
Vancouver, British Columbia, Canada

I. Introduction

In the last 20 years, the introduction of computed tomography (CT), magnetic resonance imaging (MRI), and transesophageal echocardiography (TEE) has greatly facilitated the assessment of the thoracic aorta. These new modalities have augmented and, in certain instances, supplanted the earlier investigational tools of chest radiography and angiography. However, specific technical limitations associated with each one of these imaging techniques creates various diagnostic approaches, depending on the clinical problem. Therefore, although technical advances have improved preoperative diagnosis, the imaging algorithm has become more complicated.

The purpose of this chapter is to outline the strengths and weaknesses of the available thoracic aortic-imaging techniques. Suggested imaging algorithms for thoracic aortic aneurysm, dissection, traumatic rupture, and aortic stenosis will be presented.

II. Imaging Techniques

A. Chest Radiography

The chest radiograph is the most commonly performed imaging procedure in North America (1) and is often the first indication of thoracic aortic abnormality. Unfortunately the primary x-ray photons that contain the information necessary to generate the image account for only 10% of the photons that darken the film (2). The remaining 90% of x-ray photons are scattered rays and contribute only to image noise. For this reason, only large differences in tissue density (i.e., air–soft tissue, bone–soft tissue) are visualized. Consequently, the right lateral aspect of the ascending thoracic aorta and the left lateral aspect of the descending thoracic aorta are usually seen adjacent to an air-filled lung. However, the left side of the ascending aorta, the transverse aorta, and the right side of the descending aorta all lie adjacent to soft tissues and are not routinely seen. A nasogastric tube may be passed to identify the position of the esophagus, allowing one to infer the position of the right side of the descending aorta.

In the absence of complete visualization, aortic abnormality can be suspected on the chest radiograph when the superior mediastinum is enlarged. Eight centimeters is usually quoted as the upper limit of normal for the superior mediastinum (superior vena cava to aortic arch; 3). Unfortunately, mediastinal widening is not specific for aortic disease and may be due to other abnormalities, including anterior mediastinal masses, excessive mediastinal fat, mediastinal hematoma caused by venous bleeding, or cardiac disease. In addition, technical factors in film exposure can also affect the mediastinal outline, with increasing mediastinal width on anteroposterior (AP), portable, and supine studies.

As a result of the limited visualization of the aorta, chest radiography is useful only as a screening study. An abnormality in the region of the aorta may be due to other structures, and a normal chest radiograph does not preclude a substantial aortic abnormality.

B. Angiography

In thoracic angiography, injection of iodine-containing contrast material allows assessment of the lumen of the aorta and the interface between flowing blood and the interior of the vessel. However, because the intima, media, and adventitia of the vessel wall are not identified, mural thrombus within an aneurysm, or a nonopacified false channel of a dissection, may not be appreciated. Therefore, angiography has limitations in the assessment of thoracic aortic aneurysms and dissections. Other limitations include the invasive nature of the examination and the toxicity of radiopaque contrast material. However, no other technique offers the combination of a large field of view, submillimeter spatial resolution, rapid image acquisition, and temporal resolution up to four frames per second.

The Thoracic Aorta

To perform aortic angiography, a high-flow pigtail catheter is placed in the mid-ascending aorta, usually through the femoral artery. Then 60–90 ml of 60% ionic or nonionic contrast material is injected at 25–30 ml/sec, while filming at two to four frames per second. Ten to 15 images are obtained either in biplane (anteroposterior and lateral) or 40°-left–anterior oblique projections. If only a single plane is initially obtained, a second orthogonal projection (50°-right–anterior oblique) may be necessary to detect abnormalities parallel to the first-imaging plane. The ascending, transverse, and descending thoracic aorta and proximal great vessels are well visualized with this technique. Selective injection of the great vessels can be performed, if necessary. Digital subtraction angiography may also be used, with excellent results in cooperative patients.

C. Computed Tomography

Compared with the plain film techniques of chest radiography and angiography, CT provides much greater contrast resolution. This improved contrast resolution arises as a consequence of three unique features (4): First, the image is a transverse cross-sectional view, eliminating overlap of structures. Second, the x-ray beam that produces the image is highly collimated, with minimal scatter radiation. Third, because CT is a digital technique, image acquisition and display are independent functions. Therefore, the display parameters of window and level can be manipulated, allowing regions with subtle differences in tissue density to be isolated and displayed over the entire gray scale. As a result CT allows visualization of density differences of only 0.5%, approximately 20 times more sensitive than the plain radiograph. In aortic imaging this permits separation of contrast-enhanced flowing blood from mural thrombus and surrounding mediastinal fat.

The limitations of CT are the relatively long acquisition times and limited spatial resolution. Whereas chest radiography and angiography acquire an image in less than 0.1 sec, conventional CT requires at least 1 sec. Electron beam CT scanners are available with scan times of 0.08 sec (5). However, this equipment is not yet widely available and will not be addressed in this chapter. The in-plane (xy) spatial resolution of conventional CT (approximately 0.5 mm) is approximately five times lower than the plain radiograph (approximately 0.1 mm). Spatial resolution is further degraded by section thickness of 5–10 mm.

For thoracic aortic imaging, contrast-enhanced CT scanning is usually employed: 90–150 ml of iodinated 60% contrast material is injected through an arm vein at 2–5 ml/sec. Sections through the thoracic aorta are rapidly acquired during maximum opacification of contrast, allowing differentiation of rapidly flowing blood (i.e., true lumen of a dissection), slowly flowing blood (i.e., false lumen of a dissection), mural thrombus, and vessel wall. Three different techniques of data acquisition can be used, depending on the CT equipment available. The dynamic, static technique obtains multiple images at one level every 4–8 sec, following a small bolus of approximately 50 ml of contrast at 2 ml/sec. Usually, this approach is used at three levels in the aorta; aortic root, mid-ascending aorta, and transverse aortic arch. The dynamic incremental technique uses the full 150 ml of contrast injected at 2–3 ml/sec and scans with progressive table motion from the aortic arch to the diaphragm, or lower, as required. In the spiral technique, 150 ml of contrast is injected at 2–5 ml/sec, with spiral scanning from the transverse aortic arch to the diaphragm or lower. These three techniques differ in both the time taken to obtain the scan and in the maximum contrast enhancement obtained in the aorta. In general, the spiral and dynamic incremental techniques offer better contrast enhancement and a more rapid examination, in comparison with the dynamic static technique. However, in both the spiral and dynamic incremental techniques the entire contrast volume is injected in one bolus; therefore, the timing of the scans relative to the injection is critical. To account for variations in cardiac output, which can affect the timing delay with spiral and dynamic incremental techniques, many centers use timing bolus. Twenty milliliters of contrast material is injected and images are obtained at a single level (right pulmonary artery) every 4 sec for a total of eight to ten images. Observing the time of maximum contrast enhancement in the aorta with this small test injection allows optimal time of the scan delay for the spiral or dynamic image acquisition. In all three techniques, 5- to 10-mm–section thickness is employed. Scans are obtained during suspended respiration to minimize motion artifact. If possible nasogastric tube and central lines should be withdrawn from the region of interest to minimize spray artifacts. A motion artifact, simulating aortic dissection, may be seen on spiral acquisitions (6,7). This artifact can usually be recognized, as it changes orientation or disappears from section to section (Fig. 1).

Computed tomography allows excellent assessment of the ascending and descending thoracic aorta, where the aorta is perpendicular to the transverse-imaging plane. Unfortunately, owing to the effect of slice thickness and resultant volume averaging, the junction of the transverse and descending aorta is often poorly visualized on transverse CT images. Sagittal and coronal reformatting of thin transverse sections (5 mm) may be useful in this region (Fig. 2).

D. Magnetic Resonance Imaging

In contrast with x-ray techniques (chest radiograph, angiography, and CT), which are sensitive to only one parameter (tissue density), magnetic resonance imaging (MRI) detects the effects of four tissue parameters (proton density, T1 relaxation, T2 relaxation, and flow; 8). Images are formed by the application of radiofrequency pulses and manipulation of an external magnetic field. The advantages of MRI include intrinsic flow contrast; multiplanar capacity, with direct sagittal-, coronal-, and oblique-imaging planes; large field of view; and the absence of ionizing radiation. However, on current equipment, image acquisition is very slow

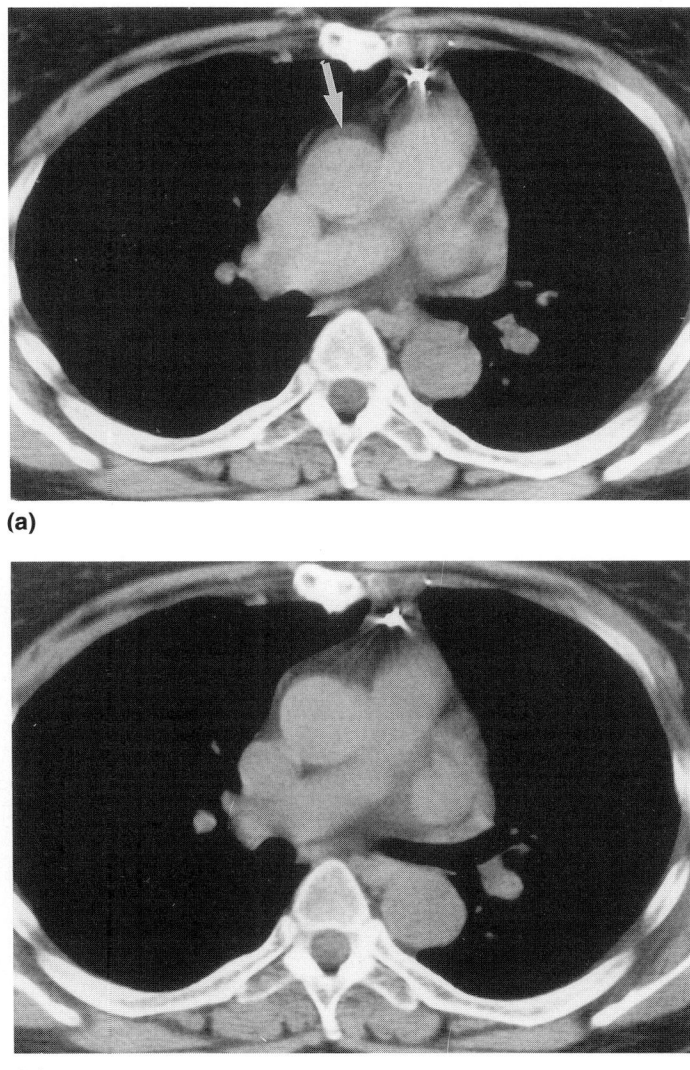

(a)

(b)

Figure 1 (a) Contrast-enhanced CT section through the ascending aorta using a 10-mm–collimation spiral technique showing a crescentic area of low density on the anterior aspect of the ascending aorta (arrow), suggestive of aortic dissection. However, (b) failure to visualize the suspected dissection on the adjacent slice indicates the presence of a motion artifact.

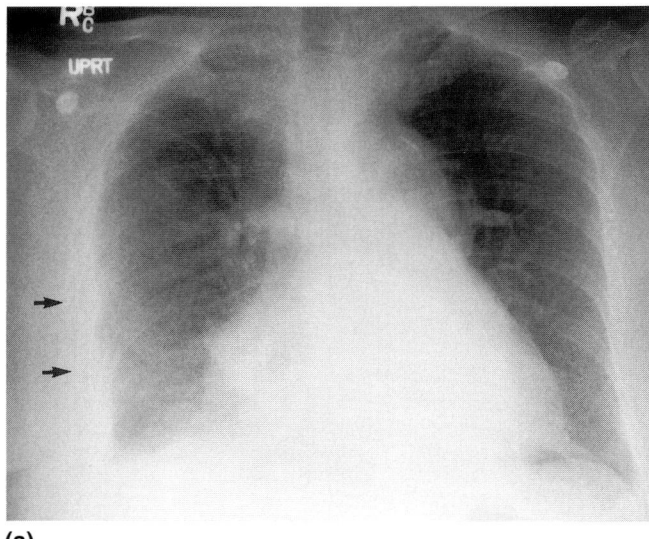

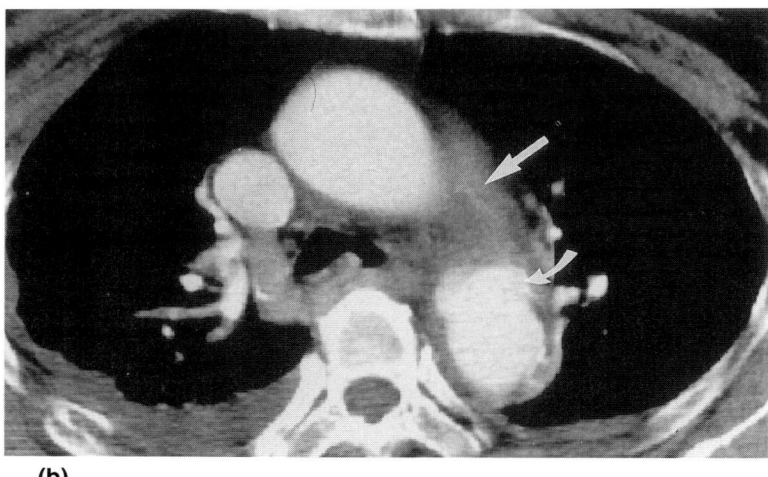

Figure 2 (a) Portable, upright chest radiograph in a 64-year-old woman motor vehicle accident victim shows right-sided rib fractures (arrows), mild cardiac failure, and a tortuous aorta. (b) Contrast enhanced 5-mm–thick spiral section at the junction of the transverse and descending thoracic aorta, demonstrates soft-tissue density within mediastinal fat, consistent with mediastinal hematoma (arrow). An abnormal contour of the aorta is also noted (curved arrow). (c) Sagittal reconstruction of the CT sections and (d) an arch aortogram both demonstrate a focal disruption of the aorta (arrow) diagnostic of a traumatic rupture of the thoracic aorta. These findings were confirmed at surgery.

The Thoracic Aorta

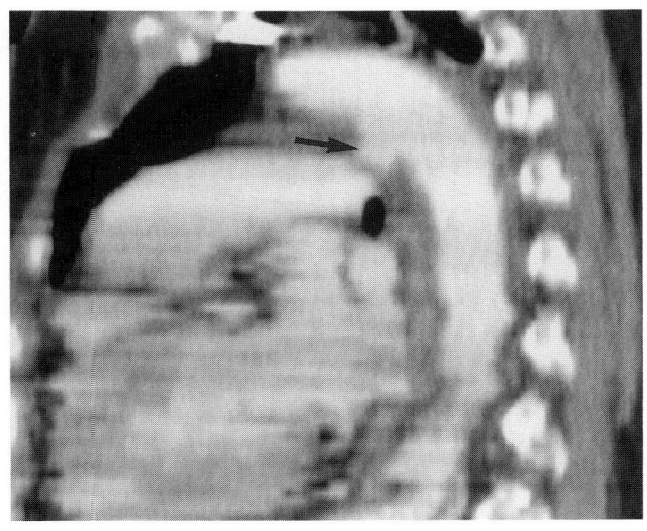

(c)

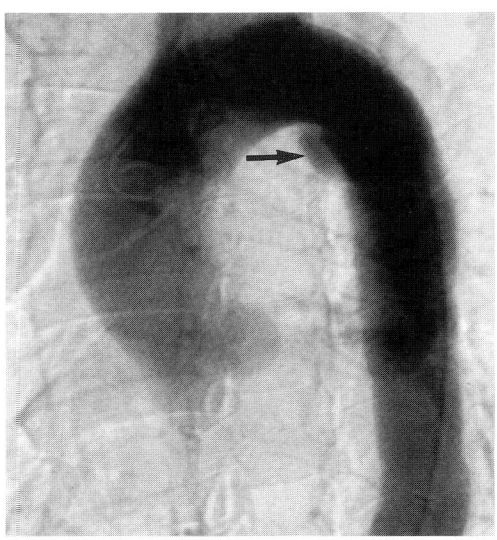

(d)

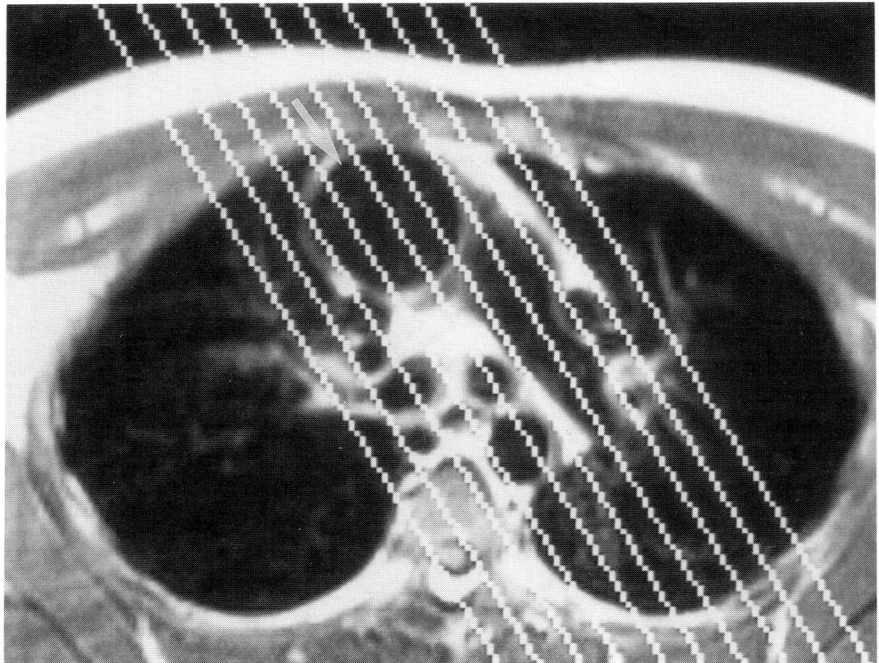

(a)

Figure 3 (a) Transverse T1-weighted (TR 800, TE 20) MR image at the level of the left pulmonary artery in a patient with a 5-cm–diameter ascending aortic aneurysm (arrow). The superimposed lines on the transverse image indicate the orientation of the oblique sagittal section. (b) Oblique sagittal T1-weighted (TR 800, TE 20) MR image demonstrates aneurysmal dilation of the proximal and mid-ascending aorta (arrow).

(minimum 10 sec/section), making cardiac synchronization, or gating, mandatory to minimize cardiac motion artifact.

For the assessment of the aorta, cardiac-gated T1-weighted spin-echo sequences are usually used in orthogonal- and oblique-imaging planes (Fig. 3). Respiratory compensation and spatial presaturation are employed to minimize motion artifact. To maximize contrast differences between flowing blood and stationary vessel walls, flow compensation is not used. Even with this protocol, slowly flowing blood can mimic thrombus. This slow-flow effect can be reduced by acquiring the sections during a period of high blood flow (e.g., systole). With appropriate technical factors, cine-gradient echo or velocity-encoded cine sequences can be used to evaluate for high-velocity jets in stenotic regions and, with appropriate calibrations, pressure gradients can be inferred (9,10).

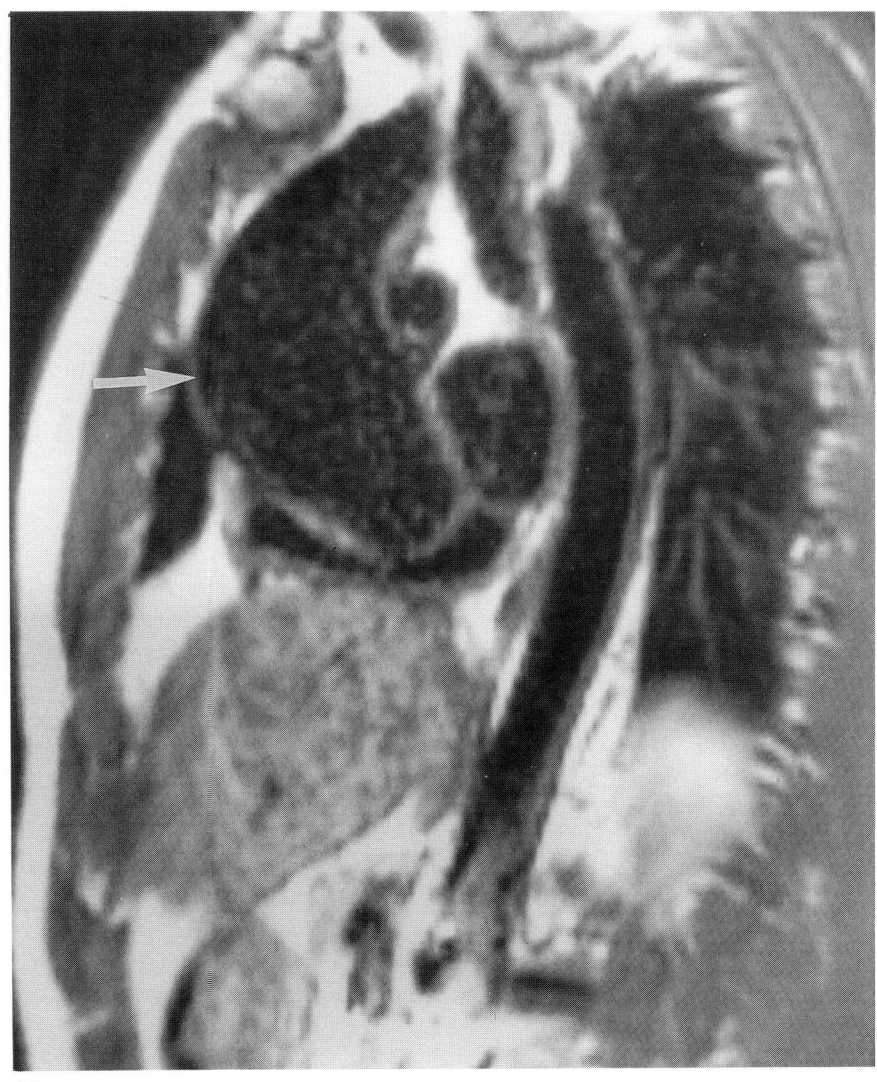
(b)

The spatial resolution of MRI is inferior to CT, with in-plane resolution of approximately 1 mm and slice thickness of 3–10 mm. However, this limitation is partially offset by the multiplanar capacity of MRI, allowing superior spatial resolution in the sagittal- and coronal-imaging planes in comparison with reformatted CT sections. Similar to CT, angiography is sometimes necessary to further evaluate small or tortuous branch vessels.

E. Echocardiography

In the last 10 years, ultrasound has become an accepted modality to image the thoracic aorta (11). Echocardiography provides high contrast between flowing blood and the vessel wall. Doppler echocardiography can provide real-time direct measurement of blood velocity and with temporal integration, blood volume. Temporal resolution is excellent, with up to 30 frames per second (0.03 sec/image). With the high-frequency transducers utilized (3.5–7.0 MHz) submillimeter spatial resolution is obtained, allowing visualization of the vessel intima, media, and adventitia. Echocardiography can be performed quickly at the bedside, facilitating diagnosis in the emergency setting.

Initially, transthoracic ultrasound was performed, using parasternal-, suprasternal notch-, and apical-imaging windows. With these limited-imaging windows, visualization of the entire thoracic aorta is often suboptimal, especially the descending thoracic aorta, which is in the far field. Physical factors, such as obesity, chest deformity, emphysema, recent chest surgery, and mechanical ventilation can also compromise the transthoracic examination.

The introduction of transesophageal echocardiography has been a significant advance for thoracic aortic imaging. With biplane or omniplane transducers, the esophageal-imaging position provides excellent visualization of virtually all the ascending, transverse, and descending thoracic aorta. The aortic valve is well seen, allowing assessment of valvular competence. Although the proximal abdominal aorta is seen through the stomach wall, the mid- and distal abdominal aorta is not reliably seen. Contraindications to transesophageal echocardiography include esophageal disorders (varices, obstruction, diverticulum), perforated viscus, active upper gastrointestinal bleeding, and severe cervical arthritis. The procedure is moderately invasive, usually requiring benzodiazepine anesthesia. Limitations include a small field of view, poor visualization of aortic branch vessels and, in some centers, limited local expertise.

III. Aortic Diseases and Imaging Algorithms

A. Thoracic Aortic Aneurysm

In normal subjects, the thoracic aorta decreases in diameter from the aortic root (mean diameter 3.7 SD 0.3 cm), through the ascending (mean diameter 3.3 SD

0.6), to the descending aorta (mean diameter 2.4 SD 0.3) (12). A gradual increase in size occurs with increasing age, but any measurement over 4 cm is considered aneurysmal. However, many older individuals with systemic hypertension will have aortic diameters larger than 4 cm, without intrinsic aortic abnormality. Surgery is usually not indicated if the diameter of the aorta is smaller than 5 cm in diameter. As a result of the high mortality (95%; 13,14) associated with thoracic aneurysm rupture, surgery is indicated for symptomatic aortic aneurysms and aneurysms larger than 6 cm in diameter (15–17). Because most thoracic aneurysms enlarge over time, periodic assessment of patients with known aneurysms is recommended (18). Coronal or sagittal reconstructions can be useful in tortuous aortas.

The wall of true aneurysms contains all three layers: intima, media, and adventitia. True aneurysms of the thoracic aorta are usually due to atherosclerosis. These are most common in the transverse and descending aorta, reflecting the lower incidence of atherosclerosis in the ascending aorta (19). Atherosclerotic aneurysms tend to be fusiform, with long segments of involvement, often extending into the abdomen. With extensive aortic involvement, the thoracoabdominal junction is usually the least involved region, possibly owing to the buttressing effect of the diaphragmatic crus. Although less common, aneurysms of the ascending aorta are seen secondary to atherosclerosis, cystic medial necrosis, and rarely, syphilis.

False aneurysms do not contain all elements of the aortic wall and are usually eccentric or saccular in shape, often with narrow entry sites. False aneurysms may result from trauma (high-speed motor vehicle, penetrating trauma, or surgical; Fig. 4), or from infection (mycotic aneurysms).

Symptoms of thoracic aneurysms, especially in the ascending and descending aorta, are often nonspecific: vague chest pain, transient ischemic attacks, and syncope. In comparison, aneurysms of the transverse aorta produce more symptoms owing to compression of neighboring structures: stridor, hoarseness, and dysphagia. In general, symptomatic presentation is associated with a 5-year survival of only 27%, compared with 58% in those discovered incidentally on chest radiography (16). True and false aneurysms can rupture into the pleural space, pericardium, mediastinum, atria, or airways. Rupturing thoracic aneurysms have a worse outcome than those in the abdomen because of the more-limited ability of thoracic tissues to tamponade the bleeding.

Once aortic enlargement is either suspected or identified, definitive assessment of aortic size is necessary. Contrast-enhanced CT (20), MRI (21), or echocardiography (22) can be used for this purpose. Equipment availability and local expertise influence the specific modality chosen. Assessment of involvement of the transverse aorta and great vessels is important for the surgeon to plan cross clamp sites and extent of resection. We have found sagittal or oblique sagittal T1-weighted thin section (3–5 mm) MRI very useful for this purpose (see Fig. 3).

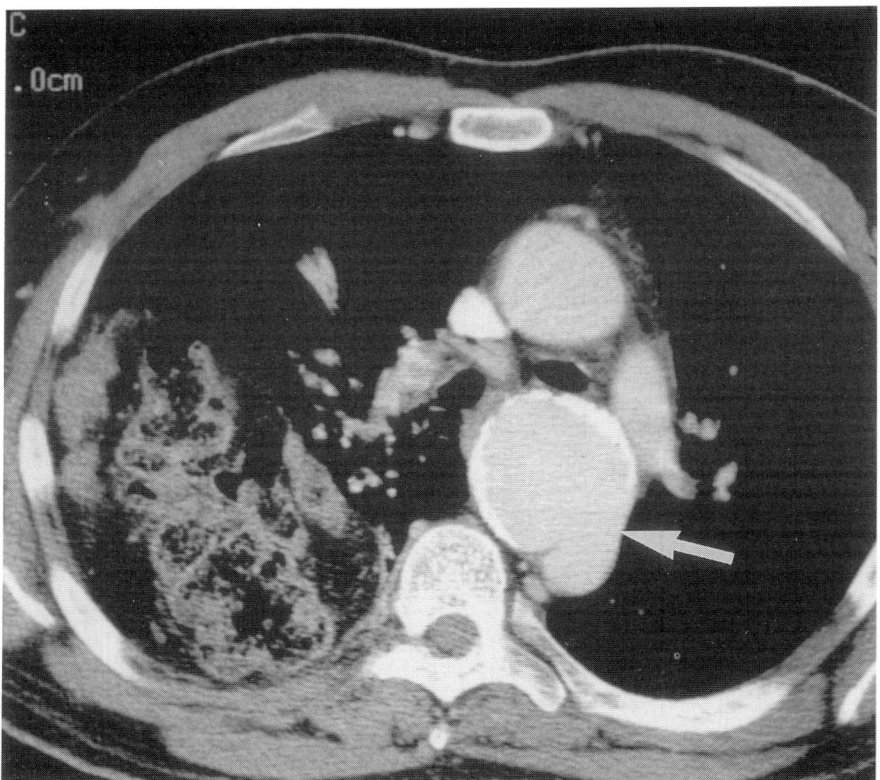

Figure 4 Contrast-enhanced CT section showing an eccentric calcified aneurysm of the descending thoracic aorta at the level of the insertion of the ligamentum arteriosum (arrow). A rupture of the right hemidiaphragm resulting in herniated large bowel within the right hemithorax is also seen. These injuries were ascribed to severe trauma that occurred 32 years previously.

However, in patients with markedly tortuous or stenotic branch vessels, angiography may be necessary.

Postoperative fluid collections persisting after 3 months between the graft and the native aorta wrap may indicate perigraft infection in the appropriate clinical setting. T1- and T2-weighted MRI sequences, which differentiate fibrotic perigraft scarring from fluid collections, may be helpful (23). Pseudoaneurysms can form owing to suture dehiscence at anastomotic sites. These can be detected with CT; however, MRI or angiography may be required to identify the site of origin and extent of the false aneurysm.

In summary, CT and MRI provide excellent delineation of thoracic aortic aneurysms. Angiography may underestimate the size of aneurysms owing to the presence of mural thrombus and is reserved for more accurate anatomical delineation of tortuous branch vessels. The exact role of echocardiography remains to be determined.

B. Thoracic Aortic Dissection

In aortic dissection, an intimal tear occurs, with formation of a false lumen within the media of the aortic wall (24). The false lumen can dissect both proximal and distal to the entry site. Entry sites are most common either in the ascending aorta (Stanford type A, DeBakey type I and II; Fig. 5), or in the proximal descending aorta, just distal to the left subclavian artery (Stanford type B, DeBakey type III; 25). Often, as the dissection progresses, multiple tears are formed in the intima, with resultant multiple entry and exit sites (26,27). Commonly, although not invariably, dissections involve the right anterior aspect of the ascending aorta and the posterior left lateral aspect of the descending aorta. As a result of this orientation, ischemia of the left kidney may accompany aortic dissection. The goal of imaging is to visualize the true and false channels separated by a thin intimal flap and to identify involvement of the ascending aorta.

Untreated dissections of the ascending aorta carry a poor prognosis, with 62% mortality at 1 week and 95% by 1 year (28). Fatal complications of ascending aortic dissections include rupture into the pericardium, with resultant cardiac tamponade, occlusion of coronary artery ostia or interference with aortic valvular structure, with resultant acute aortic regurgitation. Dissections of the descending aorta have a much lower morbidity and mortality. The classification of dissections centers on involvement of the ascending aorta, as a result of the markedly poorer associated prognosis. In the Stanford classification, type A dissections involve the ascending aorta and type B dissections involve the descending aorta, distal to the left subclavian artery (25). A second system, the DeBakey classification, differentiates type A lesions into DeBakey I, which involve both the ascending and descending aorta, and DeBakey II, which involve only the ascending aorta (29).

In type A or DeBakey I or II lesions surgical replacement of the ascending aorta and, if indicated, the aortic valve, is the procedure of choice (30). Uncomplicated type B or DeBakey III dissections are treated medically with pharmacological control of high blood pressure. Both surgically treated type A and medically treated type B dissections require ongoing imaging surveillance. Disease progression with eventual surgical treatment of type B dissections is indicated for aneurysmal enlargement, recurrent or persistent pain, development of significant left pleural effusion, vascular compromise, or rupture (31). In surgically treated type A dissections, imaging follow-up is required because complications, including aneurysm and pseudoaneurysm formation, occur in 19–30% of patients (32,33).

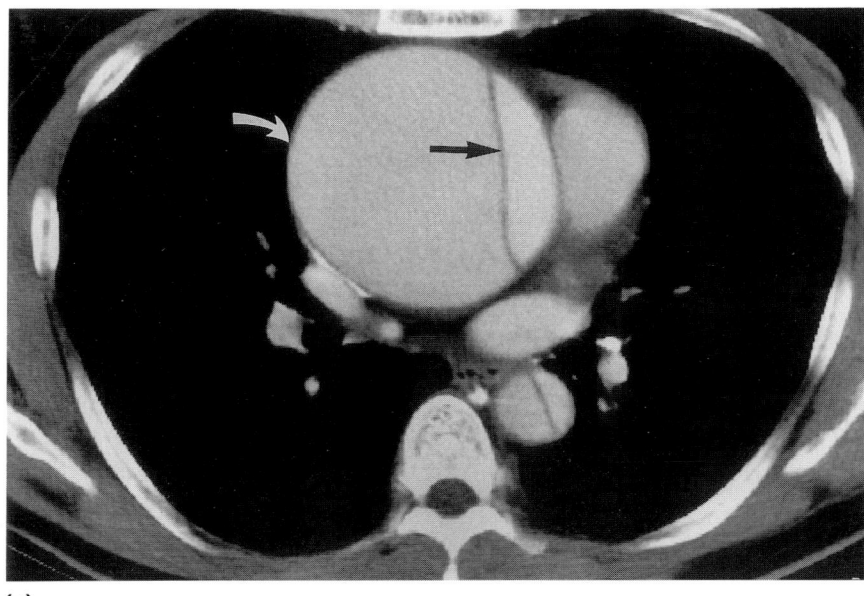

(a)

Figure 5 (a) Contrast-enhanced CT scan through the upper chest demonstrates a type A dissection, with an intimal flap (arrow) and aneurysmal dilatation (8 cm) of the ascending aorta (curved arrow). (b) Coronal T1-weighted (TR 779, TE 16) MRI scan through the ascending aorta shows a focal defect in the intimal flap suggestive of the entry site (arrow). (c) The entry site (curved arrow) is confirmed on a coronal cine MR (TR 40, TE 3.4, FASTCARD) sequence.

Clinically, aortic dissection is characterized by the presence of ripping chest or back pain in hypertensive patients. However, chronic dissections (more than 2 weeks old; 34) can be found in asymptomatic individuals on chest radiography or echocardiography. Predisposing factors for dissection include Marfan's and Ehler-Danlos' syndrome, aortitis, or vascular catheterization (35). Dissection can occasionally be seen in association with traumatic aortic rupture. Previous reports suggested that, in women younger than 40 years of age, aortic dissection was associated with pregnancy (36). However, a more recent study concluded that there was no association and proposed that this may be an artifact of selective reporting (37).

Two other entities, aortic dissection without intimal rupture (38) and penetrating atherosclerotic ulcer (19,39,40), can be clinically indistinguishable from classic aortic dissection. In aortic dissection without intimal rupture, there is thickening of the aortic wall in a crescentic fashion suggestive of dissection, but

The Thoracic Aorta

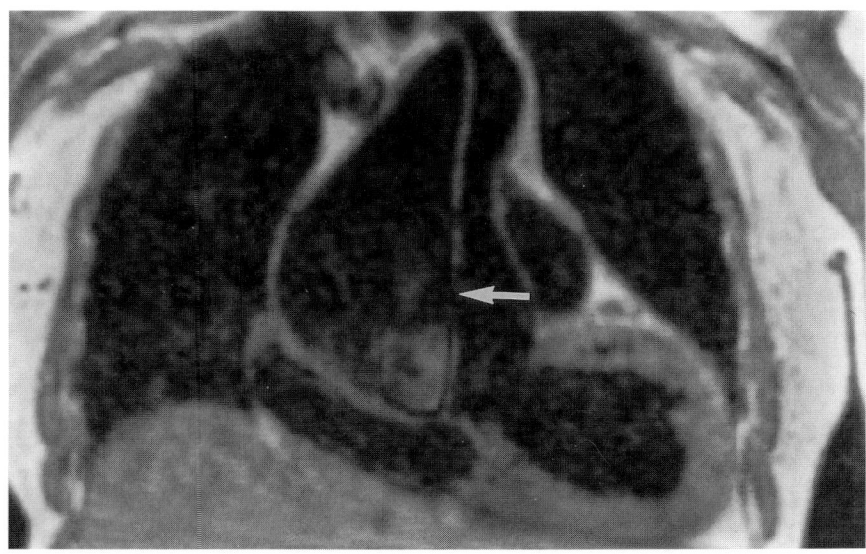

(b)

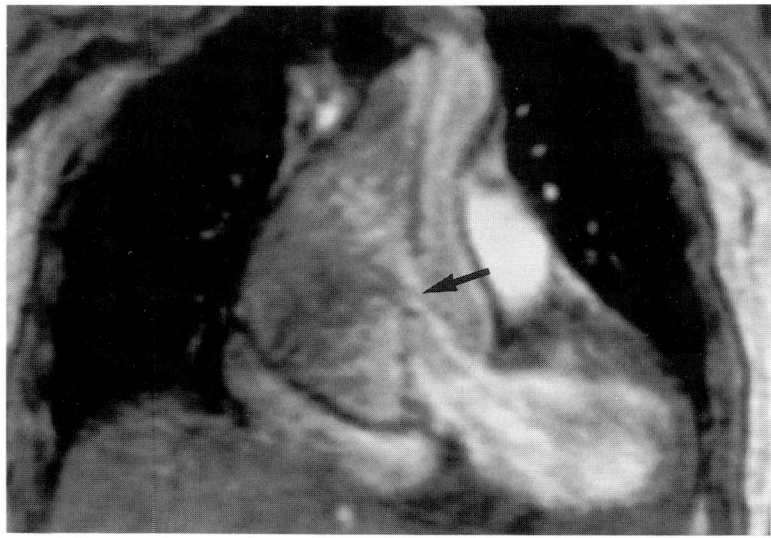

(c)

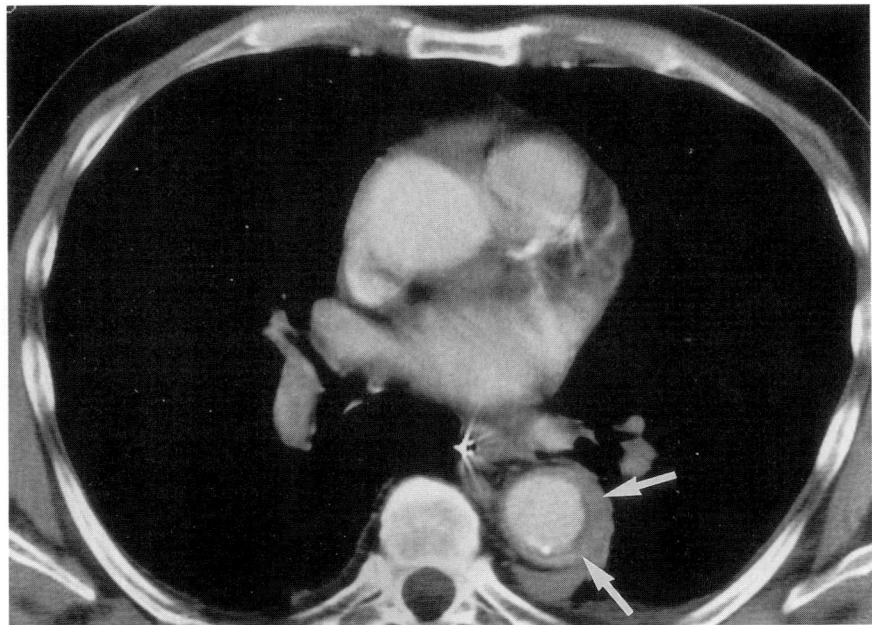

Figure 6 Contrast-enhanced CT scan showing crescentic thickening (arrows) in the wall of the descending thoracic aorta, consistent with aortic dissection, without intimal rupture. There is associated pleural effusion and atelectasis in the left hemithorax.

there is no flow in a false lumen and no detectable intimal tear (Fig. 6). Some authors have suggested this is due to spontaneous rupture of the vasa vasorum, with a contained hematoma in the media (38). This presentation is seen in 5–15% of dissections and occurs in both the ascending and descending aorta.

Penetrating atherosclerotic ulcer is an ulcerating atheromatous lesion that extends through the intima to form a hematoma within the media. Affected patients present with severe chest or back pain and hypertension, symptoms indistinguishable from aortic dissection. The differentiation of penetrating ulcer from dissection is important for surgical management, because more extensive resection of the aorta is required in cases of penetrating ulcer owing to severe, associated atherosclerotic disease (19). The hematoma in penetrating ulcer usually is more localized than in dissection, owing to fibrosis of the vessel media by extensive atherosclerosis. Occasionally, penetrating ulcer can perforate through the media to form an adventitial false aneurysm, or can rupture into the mediastinum (41; Fig. 7). The diagnosis of penetrating ulcer rests on identifying the ulcer crater in the vicinity of the localized hematoma (42,43).

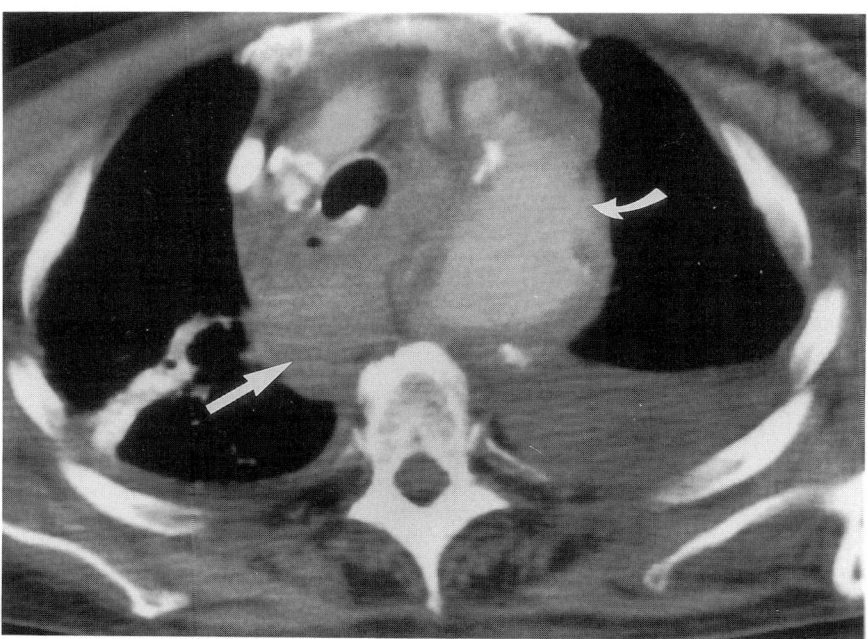

Figure 7 Contrast-enhanced CT scan at the level of the aortic arch showing extensive hematoma in the mediastinum (arrow). A focal irregularity consistent with a penetrating ulcer is seen on the lateral aspect of the transverse aorta (curved arrow). At autopsy, this penetrating atherosclerotic ulcer was the source of the mediastinal hematoma.

In most centers, imaging of patients with suspected aortic dissection is performed with contrast-enhanced CT (44–47). Bolus injection of contrast with rapid acquisition of sections through the aorta is performed with either a dynamic static, dynamic incremental, or a spiral protocol. Differential enhancement of the true and false lumen, with identification of the intimal flap, is necessary to confirm the diagnosis. Identification of the dissection within the ascending or transverse aorta is necessary to differentiate surgically treated type A from medically treated type B dissections. The presence of pericardial fluid must also be assessed to evaluate for possible rupture into the pericardial sac. A limitation of the CT technique is that aortic regurgitation and coronary artery involvement cannot be assessed. The CT images may be degraded by spray artifact from nasogastric tubes, electrocardiography (ECG) leads, or central lines. Poor cardiac output, caused by aortic regurgitation, may also limit the study.

Recent studies have suggested that MRI and transesophageal echocardiography (TEE) may be more accurate in aortic dissection than CT (48–50). An MRI scan is more sensitive to flow abnormalities, potentially offering improved visualization of the intimal flap and entry site as a result of sagittal and coronal imaging. With cine sequences, MRI can detect aortic regurgitation. The increased spatial resolution, temporal resolution, and flow sensitivity of transesophageal echocardiography are highly useful in detecting the mobile intimal flap, differential blood flow in the true and false channels, involvement of the coronary ostia, and aortic regurgitation.

Angiography may be misleading in dissection, if the false lumen is not opacified, if equal flow occurs in both true and false channels, or if the separating intimal flap is not seen in profile. In addition, inadvertent injection of the false channel may cause rapid extension of the dissection and exacerbate cardiac tamponade. However, angiography is indicated if surgical technique is influenced by the relation between poorly visualized branch vessels and the true and false lumen.

C. Traumatic Rupture of the Aorta

Traumatic rupture of the aorta can occur secondary to either blunt or penetrating trauma. In North America, this injury occurs most commonly following severe deceleration in high-speed motor vehicle collisions. Other mechanisms include falls and explosions. Penetrating trauma is most commonly due to gunshot and knife wounds. Autopsy studies in blunt trauma have shown approximately 50% of aortic tears occur at the junction of the transverse and descending aorta (aortic isthmus) just distal to the left subclavian artery (51). Most of the remaining aortic ruptures occur in the ascending aorta. However, ascending aortic ruptures are virtually universally fatal; therefore, most patients who present for aortography will have traumatic aortic tears at the aortic isthmus (52). Patients who have experienced the necessary level of trauma for aortic injury present with a myriad of signs and symptoms, none of which are specific for an aortic tear. Unrecognized and untreated, this injury carries a dismal prognosis, with 90% mortality at 4 months. The most common surgical procedure for traumatic aortic tear is a Dacron interposition graft. Although the procedure is associated with some morbidity (paraplegia 9.9%) and mortality (21.3%, including injury-associated mortality; 53), once treated, there is minimal ongoing morbidity or mortality related to the aortic repair. With these facts and the recognition that many of the patients are healthy before the traumatic event, prompt and accurate diagnosis is essential.

The exact mechanism of this injury is controversial. Since the injury is most often located in either the proximal ascending aorta or at the aortic isthmus, it has been suggested that the combination of local pressure, traction, and water hammer tears the vessel wall (54). Recently, an alternative mechanism, the osseous pinch, has been suggested. It is postulated that the sternum is displaced posteriorly by the acute deceleration force and impacts the anterolateral aspect of the vertebral body, pinching the aorta (55,56). Given the forces involved in high-speed motor vehicle trauma, it is likely that both of these mechanisms may cause this injury.

Because clinical findings are nonspecific, aortic injury is suggested by the mechanism of injury and findings on the chest radiograph. Widening of the mediastinum is the most sensitive finding (67–100%); however, it has associated low specificity (10–52%; 3,57–59). Other findings include indistinctness of the aortic contour, obscuration of the aorticopulmonary window, widening of the right or left paratracheal stripes, rightward deviation of the trachea, inferior deviation of the left main stem bronchus, left apical cap, fracture of the first and second ribs, clavicular fracture, pulmonary contusion, and left pleural effusion (60). This large list highlights the nonspecificity of the plain film in this diagnosis, for the aorta is not directly visualized owing to lack of contrast. In addition, although uncommon (7.3%; 61), a normal chest radiograph does not exclude an aortic tear. Consequently, aortography, with direct visualization of the aortic lumen has been the only reliable diagnostic test However, only 5–15% of patients with abnormal chest radiograph have positive arch aortograms.

In an attempt to decrease the rate of negative angiography, the use of contrast-enhanced chest CT has been investigated as an additional screening examination (62–58). Unfortunately, the junction of the transverse and descending aorta creates significant volume-averaging problems for transverse section CT, even with 5-mm collimation. Therefore, direct visualization of the aortic rupture on CT cannot be relied on to make the diagnosis. As a result, in clinically stable patients who has a moderate or low index or suspicion for aortic injury, CT has been used as a more-sophisticated screening examination to identify mediastinal hematoma as a marker of force sufficient to injure the aorta. Aortography would then be performed in all patients with mediastinal hematoma to make the definitive diagnosis of aortic injury. This approach has created considerable controversy in the literature (69). Authors have questioned whether too many patients which high probability of aortic injury might receive chest CT, with resultant delay in definitive diagnosis by aortography, increase in contrast-associated morbidity, and increased cost (70). This controversy has been further fueled by data indicating that chest CT may falsely indicate no aortic trauma in the presence of aortic transection and great vessel injury (71). In light of this controversy, we believe that chest CT plays a limited role in the diagnosis of aortic rupture.

Angiographically, traumatic rupture most often demonstrates focal discontinuity of the aorta (Fig. 8). In more subtle cases, a lucent band may be seen across the aorta (Fig. 9), with delayed clearing of contrast adjacent to this, secondary to turbulent flow. Although the angiographic findings in traumatic aortic rupture have been described as "unmistakable and characteristic" (72), confusion can arise with an atypical ductus diverticulum or an unusual ulcerating atherosclerotic plaque (73). Normally, the ductus diverticulum forms obtuse angles with the aortic wall. However, occasionally, an acute angle is seen on its superior aspect,

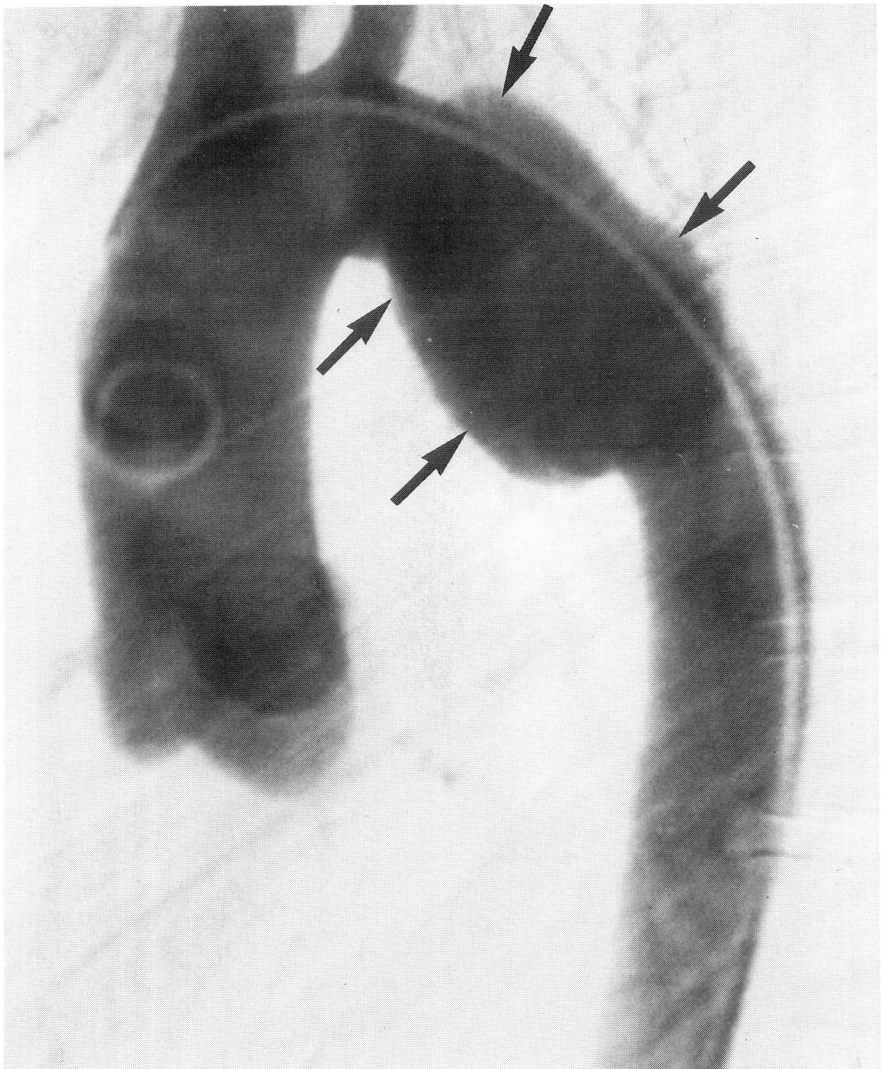

Figure 8 Arch aortogram in the left anterior oblique projection, demonstrating a pseudoaneurysm at the junction of the transverse and descending thoracic aorta (arrows).

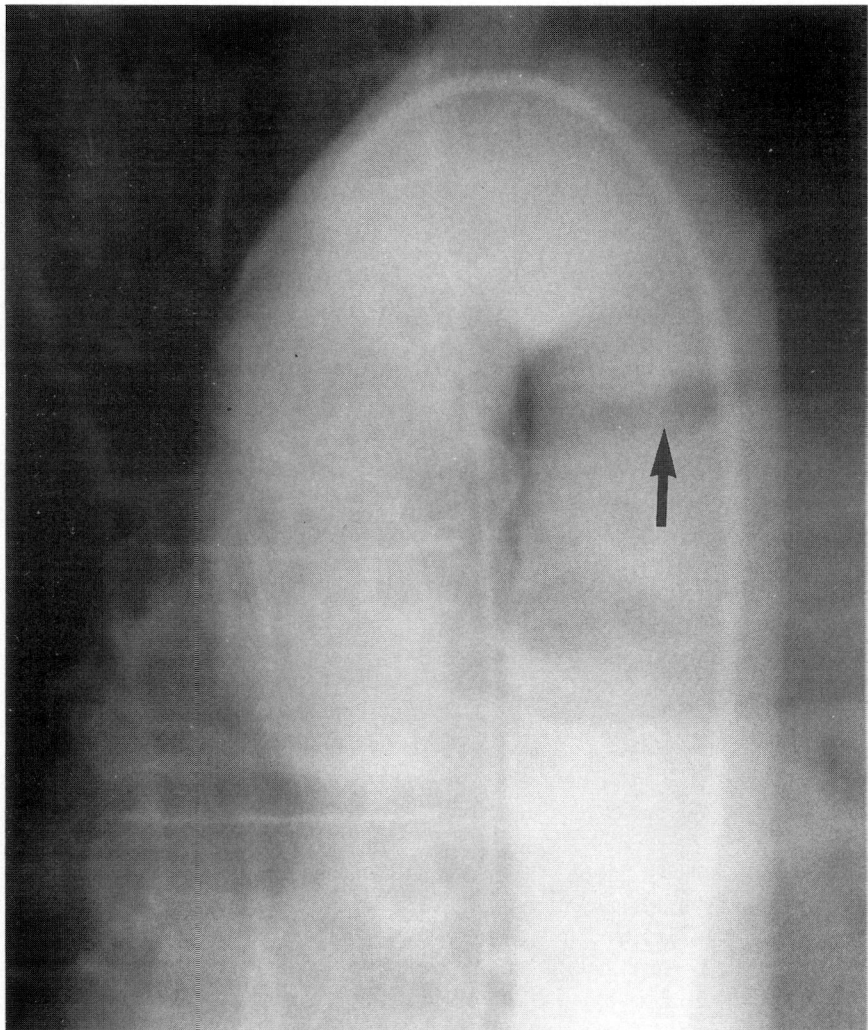

Figure 9 Arch angiogram in the AP projection, demonstrating a subtle filling defect at the junction of the transverse and descending thoracic aorta, corresponding to a focal intimal flap (arrow) in a patient with a traumatic rupture of the aorta.

mimicking a focal tear. The absence of an intimal flap may help distinguish the atypical ductus diverticulum from an aortic tear.

At our institution, we perform arch angiography when there is either a high clinical suspicion of aortic rupture caused by mechanism of injury, or two or more abnormalities on chest radiography. In patients for whom clinical suspicion is low, we perform chest CT if the patient is undergoing CT for abdominal, pelvic or neurological assessment. We obtain chest CT in all patients for whom there is minimal clinical suspicion because of inadequate mechanism of action, but an abnormal mediastinum seen on chest radiography. Angiography is always performed if mediastinal blood or abnormal contour of the aorta is identified.

Clearly, assessment of arch injuries with CT is suboptimal. Use of MRI may be superior to CT as a result of the superior spatial resolution in the coronal- and sagittal-imaging planes. However, the logistics of placing critically injured patients within the magnet, currently precludes this approach. Recent studies using transesophageal echocardiography have been encouraging (74,75). Transesophageal echocardiography has significant advantages, including direct sagittal and coronal imaging, excellent temporal and spatial resolution, allowing direct visualization of intimal injury, and the ability to rapidly perform the procedure at the bedside. Although further experience is necessary to substantiate these early reports, this technique may emerge as the modality of choice.

D. Aortic Stenosis

Stenotic lesions of the aorta are uncommon and are usually due to either congenital coarctation or Takyasus's arteritis. These two entities are usually differentiated on the basis of site and extent of involvement. Other, less common, congenital arch abnormalities have been described (76), but are beyond the scope of this chapter.

Congenital coarctation is a narrowing of the aortic isthmus in the vicinity of the ligamentous arteriosus. A focal shelf of abnormal fibromuscular tissue is seen. This lesion is often associated with diffuse narrowing of the aortic arch (arch hypoplasia) and bicuspid aortic valve. Commonly, it presents in childhood with a bruit heard over the back and differential blood pressure between either the right and left arms or between arms and legs. The classic plain radiograph findings include aortic deformity, with interruption of the normally continuous lateral margin of the "aortic knob" and descending thoracic aorta (three sign); retrosternal soft-tissue density; rib notching (usually ribs 4 and 8), which may be unilateral, depending on the site of coarctation; and less commonly, a prominent ascending aorta (77). Rib notching is common in adults, but unusual in patients younger than 5 years of age.

The diagnosis of coarctation may be confirmed with sagittal and coronal T1-weighted MRI (78,79). An MRI scan can also identify associated transverse arch hypoplasia. Aortography may be necessary to measure pressure gradients and identify the origin of tortuous great vessels.

In comparison, Takyasus's arteritis usually shows more diffuse involvement of the aorta, or focally involves sites other than the aortic isthmus (80). There is a female preponderance, and this disease is more common in Orientals. The pulmonary arteries may be involved (81). With current MRI scanners, involvement of the aorta and proximal great vessels is usually identifiable (Fig. 10). However, angiography may be necessary to augment suboptimal MRI studies, or to delineate involvement of medium-sized vessels in the neck and proximal arms (82).

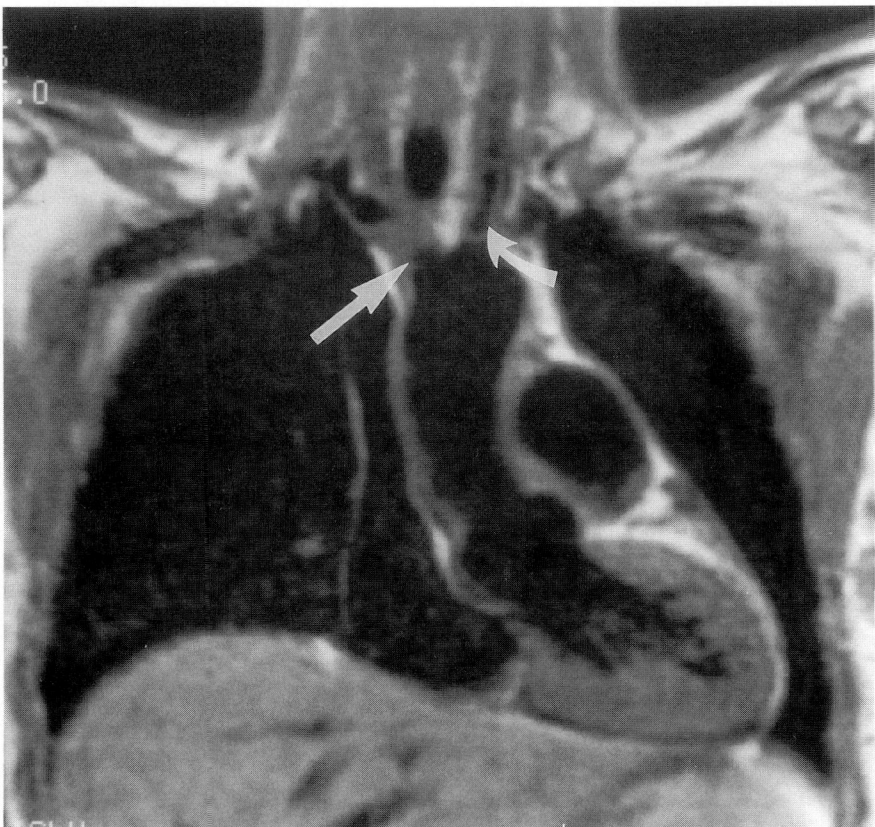

Figure 10 Coronal T1-weighted MRI scan (TR 800, TE 20), demonstrating focal thickening of the wall of the proximal innominate (straight arrow) and left carotid (curved arrow) arteries in a patient with Takayasu's arteritis.

IV. Summary

The introduction of CT, MRI, and transesophageal echocardiography has greatly improved our imaging assessment of the thoracic aorta. However, owing to current limitations in each of these techniques, angiography remains an essential tool in aortic assessment.

References

1. Gurney JW. Historical perspective. Why chest radiography became routine. Radiology 1995; 195:245–246.
2. Curry TS III, Dowdey JE, Murry RC. Christensen's introduction to the physics of diagnostic radiology. 3rd ed. Philadelphia: Lea & Febiger, 1984: 73.
3. Mirvis SE, Bidwell JK, Buddemeyer EU, Diaconis JN, Pais SO, Whitley JE, Goldstein LD. Value of chest radiography in excluding traumatic aortic rupture. Radiology 1987; 163:487–493.
4. Sprawls P Jr. Physical principles of medical imaging. 2nd ed. Gaithersburg, MD: Aspen, 1993:361–363.
5. Boyd DP, Farmer DW. Cardiac computed tomography. In: Collin SM, Skorton DJ, eds. Cardiac imaging and imaging processing. New York: McGraw-Hill, 1986:68–87.
6. Burns MA, Molina PL, Gutierrez FR, Sagel SS. Motion artifact simulating aortic dissection on CT. AJR 1991; 157:465–467.
7. Posniak HV, Olson MC, Demos TC. Aortic motion artifact simulating dissection on CT scans: elimination with reconstructive segmented images. AJR 1993; 161:557–558.
8. Mayo JR. Magnetic resonance imaging of the chest: where we stand. Radiol Clin North Am 1994; 32:795–809.
9. Sechtem U, Pflugfelder PW, White RD, et al. Cine MR imaging: potential for the evaluation of cardiovascular function. AJR 1987; 148:239–246.
10. Suzuki J, Caputo GR, Kondo C, et al. Cine MR imaging of valvular heart disease: display and imaging parameters affect the size of the signal void caused by valvular regurgitation. AJR 1990; 155:723–727.
11. Goldstein SA, Mintz GS, Lindsay J Jr. Aorta: comprehensive evaluation by echocardiography and transesophageal echocardiography [review]. J Am Soc Echocardiogr 1993; 6:634–659.
12. Guthaner DF, Wexler L, Harell G. CT demonstration of cardiac structures. AJR 1979; 133:75–81.
13. Bickerstaff LK, Pairolero PC, Hollier LH, Melton LJ, Van Peenen HJ, Cherry KJ, Joyce JW, Lie JT. Thoracic aortic aneurysms: a population-based study. Surgery 1982; 12:1103–1108.
14. Crawford ES, DeNatale RW. Thoracoabdominal aortic aneurysm: observations regarding the natural course of the disease. J Vasc Surg 1986; 3:578–582.
15. Pressler V, McNamara JJ. Thoracic aortic aneurysm: natural history and treatment. J Thorac Cardiovasc Surg 1980; 79:489–498.

16. Joyce JW, Fiarbairn JF, Kincaid OW, et al. Aneurysms of the thoracic aorta: a clinical study with special reference to prognosis. Circulation 1964; 29:176–181.
17. Friedman SA. The evaluation and treatment of patients with arterial aneurysms. Med Clin North Am 1981; 65:83–103.
18. Hirose Y, Hamade S, Takamiya M, Imakita S, Naito H, Nishimura T. Aortic aneurysms: growth rates measured with CT. Radiology 1992; 185:249–252.
19. Cooke JP, Kazmier FJ, Orszulak TA. The penetrating aortic ulcer: pathologic manifestations, diagnosis, and management. Mayo Clin Proc 1988; 63:718–725.
20. Godwin JD, Herfkens RL, Sklöldebrand CG, Federle MP, Lipton MJ. Evaluation of dissections and aneurysms of the thoracic aorta by conventional and dynamic CT scanning. Radiology 1980; 136:125–133.
21. Dinsmore RE, Liberthson RR, Wismer GL, Miller SW, Liu P, Thompson R, McLoud TC, Marshall J, Saini S, Stratemeier EJ, Okada RD, Brady TJ. Magnetic resonance imaging of thoracic aortic aneurysms: comparison with other imaging methods AJR 1986; 146:309–314.
22. Kamp O, van Rossum AC, Torenbeek R. Transesophageal echocardiography and magnetic resonance imaging for the assessment of saccular aneurysm of the transverse thoracic aorta. Int J Cardiol 1991; 33:330–333.
23. Auffermann W, Olofsson PA, Rabahie GN, Tavares NJ, Stoney RJ, Higgins CB. Incorporation versus infection of retroperitoneal aortic grafts: MR imaging features. Radiology 1989; 172:359–362.
24. Roberts WC. Aortic dissection: anatomy, consequences, and causes. Am Heart J 1981; 101:195–214.
25. Daily PO, Trueblood HW, Stinson EB, Wuerflein RD, Shumway NE. Management of acute aortic dissection. Ann Thorac Surg 1970; 10:237–247.
26. Stein HL, Steinberg I. Selective aortography, the definitive technique for diagnosis of dissecting aneurysm of the thoracic aorta. Am J Radiol 1968; 102:333–347.
27. Shuford WH, Sybers RG, Weens HS. Problems in aortographic diagnosis of dissecting aneurysm of the aorta. N Engl J Med 1969; 280:225–231.
28. Hirst AE, Johns VJ, Kime SW. Dissecting aneurysm of the aorta: a review of 505 cases. Medicine 1958; 37:217–279.
29. DeBakey ME, Henly WS, Cooley DA, et al. Surgical management of dissecting aneurysms of the aorta. J Thorac Cardiovasc Surg 1965; 49:130–149.
30. Wolfe WG, Oldham HN, Rankin JS, Moran JF. Surgical treatment of acute ascending aortic dissection. Ann Surg 1983; 197:738–742.
31. Crawford ES, Svensson LG, Coselli JS, Safi HJ, Hess KR. Aortic dissection and dissecting aortic aneurysm. Ann Surg 1988; 208:254–272.
32. Yamaguchi T, Guthaner DF, Wexler L. Natural history of the false channel of type A aortic dissection after surgical repair: CT study. Radiology 1989; 170:743–747.
33. DeBakey ME McCollum CH, Crawford ES, et al. Dissection and dissecting aneurysms of the aorta: twenty-year follow-up of five hundred twenty-seven patients treated surgically. Surgery 1982; 92:1118–1134.
34. Doroghazi RM, Slater E, Desanctis RW, et al. Long term survival of patients with treated aortic dissection. J Am Coll Cardiol 1984; 3:1026–1034.

35. Sakamoto I, Hayashi K, Matsunaga N, Matsuoka Y, Uetani M, Fukuda T, Fujisawa H. Aortic dissection caused by angiographic procedures. Radiology 1994; 191:467–471.
36. Melville Williams G, Gott VL, Brawley RK, Schauble JF, Labs JD. Aortic disease associated with pregnancy. J Vasc Surg 1988; 8:470–475.
37. Oskoui R, Lindsay J. Aortic dissection in women < 40 years of age and the unimportance of pregnancy. Am J Cardiol 1994; 73:821–823.
38. Yamada T, Tada S, Harada J. Aortic dissection without intimal rupture: diagnosis with MR imaging and CT. Radiology 1988; 168:347–352.
39. Hussain S, Glover JL, Bree R, Bendick PJ. Penetrating atherosclerotic ulcers of the thoracic aorta. J Vasc Surg 1989; 9:710–717.
40. Harris JA, Bis KG, Glover JL, et al. Penetrating atherosclerotic ulcers of the aorta. J Vasc Surg 1994; 19:90–99.
41. Primack SL, Mayo JR, Fradet G. Case report: penetrating atherosclerotic ulcer presenting with airway obstruction. Can Assoc Radiol J 1995; 46:209–211.
42. Kazerooni EA, Bree RL, Williams DM. Penetrating atherosclerotic ulcers of the descending thoracic aorta: evaluation with CT and distinction from aortic dissection. Radiology 1992; 183:759–765.
43. Yucel EK, Steinberg FL, Egglin TK, Geller SC, Waltman AC, Athanasoulis CA. Penetrating aortic ulcers: diagnosis with MR imaging. Radiology 1990; 177:779–781.
44. Demos TC, Posniak HV, Marsan RE. CT of aortic dissection. Semin Roentgenol 1989; 24:22–37.
45. Fisher ER, Stern EJ, Godwin JD, Otto CM, Johnson JA. Acute aortic dissection: typical and atypical imaging features. Radiographics 1994; 14:1263–1271.
46. Tarver RD. What does the surgeon want to know? Radiographics 1994; 14:1271–1274.
47. Petasnick JP. Radiologic evaluation of aortic dissection. Radiology 1991; 180:297–305.
48. Nienaber CA, von Kodolitsch Y, Nicolas V, Siglow V, Piepho A, Brockhoff C, Koschyk DH, Spielmann RP. The diagnosis of thoracic aortic dissection by noninvasive imaging procedures. N Engl J Med 1993; 328:1–9.
49. Cigarroa JE, Isselbacher EM, DeSanctis RW, Eagle KA. Diagnostic imaging in the evaluation of suspected aortic dissection. N Engl J Med 1993; 328:35–43.
50. Deutsch HJ, Sechtem U, Meyer H. Theissen P, Schicha H, Erdmann E. Chronic aortic dissection: comparison of MR imaging and transesophageal echocardiography. Radiology 1994; 192:645–650.
51. Parmley LF, Mattingly TW, Manion WC, Jahnke EJ. Nonpenetrating traumatic injury of the aorta. Circulation 1958; 17:1086–1101.
52. Fisher RG, Hadlock F, Ben-Menachem Y. Laceration of the thoracic aorta and brachiocephalic arteries by blunt trauma: report of 54 cases and review of the literature. Radiol Clin North Am 1981; 19:91–109.
53. von Oppell UO, Dunne TT, De Groot MK, Zilla P. Traumatic aorta rupture: twenty-year metaanalysis of mortality and risk of paraplegia. Ann Thorac Surg 1994; 58:585–593.
54. Lundevall J. The mechanism of traumatic rupture of the aorta. Acta Pathol Microbiol Scand 1964; 62:34–46.

55. Crass JR, Cohen AM, Motta AO, Tomashefski JF, Wiesen EJ. A proposed new mechanism of traumatic aortic rupture: the osseous pinch. Radiology 1990; 176: 645–649.
56. Cohen AM, Crass JR, Thomas HA, Fisher RG, Jacobs DG. CT evidence for the "osseous pinch" mechanism of traumatic aortic injury. AJR 1992; 159:271–274.
57. Barcia TC, Livoni JP. Indications for angiography in blunt thoracic trauma. Radiology 1983; 147:15–19.
58. Sefczek DM, Sefczek RJ, Deeb ZL. Radiographic signs of acute traumatic rupture of the thoracic aorta. AJR 1983; 141:1259–1262.
59. Kram HB, Appel PL, Wohlmuth DA, Shoemaker WC. Diagnosis of traumatic thoracic aortic rupture: a 10-year retrospective analysis. Ann Thorac Surg 1989; 47: 282–286.
60. Marnocha KE, Maglinte DDT. Plain-film criteria for excluding aortic rupture in blunt chest trauma. AJR 1985; 144:19–21.
61. Woodring JH. The normal mediastinum in blunt traumatic rupture of the thoracic aorta and brachiocephalic arteries. J Emerg Med 1990; 8:467–476.
62. Heiberg E, Wolverson MK, Sundaram M, Shields JB. CT in aortic trauma. AJR 1983; 140:1119–1124.
63. Ishikawa T, Nakajima Y, Kaji T. The role of CT in traumatic rupture of the thoracic aorta and its proximal branches. Semin Roentgenol 1989; 24:38–46.
64. Richardson P, Mirvis SE, Scorpio R, Dunham CM. Value of CT in determining the need for angiography when findings of mediastinal hemorrhage on chest radiographs are equivocal. AJR 1991; 156:273–279.
65. Madayag MA, Kirshenbaum KJ, Nadimpalli SR, Fantus RJ, Cavallino RP, Crystal GJ. Thoracic aortic trauma: role of dynamic CT. Radiology 1991; 179:835–855.
66. Morgan PW, Goodman LR, Aprahamian C, Foley WD, Lipchik EO. Evaluation of traumatic aortic injury: does dynamic contrast-enhanced CT play a role? Radiology 1992; 182:661–666.
67. Raptopoulos V, Sheiman RG, Phillips DA, Davidoff A, Silva WE. Traumatic aortic tear: screening with chest CT. Radiology 1992; 182:667–673.
68. Fisher RG, Chasen MH, Lamki N. Diagnosis of injuries of the aorta and brachiocephalic arteries caused by blunt chest trauma: CT vs aortography. AJR 1994; 162: 1047–1052.
69. Raptopoulos V. Chest CT for aortic injury: maybe not for everyone. AJR 1994; 162: 1053–1055.
70. Wills JS, Lally JF. Use of CT for evaluation of possible traumatic aortic injury [letter]. AJR 1991; 157:1123–1124.
71. Miller FB, Richardson JD, Thomas HA, Cryer HM, Willing SJ. Role of CT in diagnosis of major arterial injury after blunt thoracic trauma. Surgery 1989; 105: 596–603.
72. Kirsh MM, Behrenot DM, Orringer MB, et al. The treatment of acute traumatic rupture of the aorta: a ten year experience. Ann Surg 1976; 184:300–316.
73. Morse SS, Glickman MG, Greenwood LH, Denny DF, Strauss EB, Stavens BR, Yoselevitz M. Traumatic aortic rupture: false-positive aortographic diagnosis due to atypical ductus diverticulum. AJR 1988; 150:793–796.

74. Smith MD, Cassidy JM, Souther S, Morris EJ, Sapin PM, Johnson SB, Kearney PA. Transesophageal echocardiography in the diagnosis of traumatic rupture of the aorta. N Engl J Med 1995; 332:356–362.
75. Vlahakes GJ, Warren RL. Traumatic rupture of the aorta [editorial]. N Engl J Med 1995; 332:389–390.
76. Shuford WH, Sybers RG. The aortic arch and its malformations with emphasis on the angiographic features. Springfield: Charles C Thomas, 1974.
77. Figley MM. Accessory roentgen signs of coarctation of the aorta. Radiology 1954; 62:671–686.
78. von Schulthess GK, Higashino SM, Higgins SS, Didier D, Fisher MR, Higgins CB. Coarctation of the aorta: MR imaging. Radiology 1986; 158:469–474.
79. Rees S, Somerville J, Ward C, Martinez J, Johiaddin RH, Underwood R, Longmore DB. Coarctation of the aorta: MR imaging in late postoperative assessment. Radiology 1989; 173:499–502.
80. Yamada I, Numano F, Suzuki S. Takayasu arteritis: evaluation with MR imaging. Radiology 1993; 188:89–94.
81. Yamada I, Shibuya H, Matsubara O, Omehara I, Makino T, Numano F, Suzuki S. Pulmonary artery disease in Takayasu's arteritis: angiographic findings. AJR 1992; 159:263–269.
82. Miller DL, Reinig JW, Volkman DJ. Vascular imaging with MRI: inadequacy in Takayasu's arteritis compared with angiography. AJR 1986; 146:949–954.

21

Interventional Techniques in Cardiac Diagnosis and Treatment

GEORGE G. HARTNELL

Deaconess Hospital
and Harvard Medical School
Boston, Massachusetts

I. Introduction

Since the first percutaneous, transluminal coronary angioplasty (PTCA), was performed by Andreas Gruentzig in 1976 (1), the use of PTCA has grown exponentially. PTCA is now performed more often than coronary artery bypass grafting (CABG). The growth of PTCA fueled, and financed, an explosion of developments in related interventional techniques. These include diagnostic techniques for intravascular imaging (angioscopy, ultrasound) and percutaneous cardiac interventions (balloon valvuloplasty, laser recanalization, mechanical atherectomy). By far the greatest workload has been generated by interventional therapeutic techniques. The interventional diagnostic techniques of angioscopy and intravascular ultrasound (IVUS) are currently used much less frequently.

The enthusiasm with which many of these new technologies were introduced was often misplaced. Initial device design, based on theoretical considerations, was frequently suboptimal, but this was often ignored, and objective evaluation was delayed. This chapter attempts to put the proper role of these techniques and devices into perspective, knowing that designs and applications are constantly changing.

II. Interventional Diagnostic Techniques

For many years, coronary angiography was the only reliable method for diagnosing coronary artery disease and for assessing its severity. Intravascular imaging by angioscopy or IVUS has increased knowledge about coronary artery disease, and has shown that angiography often provides an incomplete picture of the extent and nature of coronary artery disease. Angioscopy and IVUS have also been used, to a very limited extent, to examine intracardiac anatomy. Although these techniques have improved understanding of vascular disease and have allowed some monitoring of therapeutic procedures, their clinical use is still limited by costs, potential risks, and lack of demonstrated benefit for most individual patient's management.

A. Coronary Angioscopy

Early angioscopy devices were difficult and potentially hazardous to use. Either single fibers, with very limited steerability, or much larger 5-F or 6-F angioscopes, more suited to peripheral angioscopy, were used (2). Steering the angioscope was difficult, as was providing a bloodless field of view. However, even these early devices showed that angiography frequently failed to show complex plaques or thrombi in patients with unstable angina. Early studies confirmed that angioscopy (and IVUS) accurately detect thrombus and stable atheroma when compared with histopathology (3).

The development of smaller systems (3-F or less) that can pass over a PTCA guidewire, with a coaxial balloon occlusion catheter, allows assessment of coronary lesions before and after intervention. These devices are relatively safe (Table 1) and, in most patients, are not excessively difficult to use, although their introduction and use is time-consuming.

Coronary angioscopy is used with increasing frequency to characterize stenoses before interventions and provides extra useful information not obtainable by angiography (2). Coronary angioscopy shows that angiography frequently fails to show the full extent of intraluminal disease (4) and cannot reliably differentiate between different types of lesion (5). In patients with unstable angina or acute

Table 1 Safety of Coronary Angioscopy

Procedures	1746	Patients	1076
Death	1 (0.09%)	Acute MI	2 (0.019%)
Dissection	31 (2.88%)	Urgent CABG	5 (0.46%)
Dissection needing stent	5 (0.46%)		
Significant VF	18 (1.67%)		

Source: Ref. 106.

Interventional Techniques in Cardiac Diagnosis

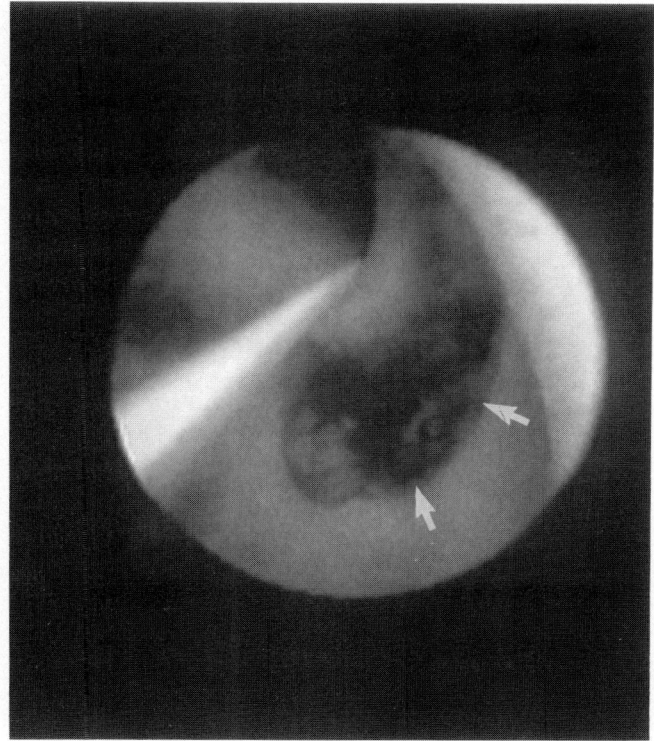

Figure 1 Angioscopic image from a patient with recent myocardial infarction shows an irregular, ulcerated plaque (arrowheads). This was found in the culprit vessel and represents the plaque that ruptured, causing myocardial infarction. The color image showed that this had a dark red surface. (Courtesy Drs. R. Nesto and S. Waxman, Deaconess Hospital, Boston MA.)

myocardial infarction, angioscopy has confirmed in vivo that there is usually coronary thrombus associated with the responsible lesions (Fig. 1). In unstable angina, the thrombus is usually gray-white (suggesting it is composed of aggregated platelets). In acute myocardial infarction the thrombus is usually reddish, suggesting a fibrin-rich clot with numerous erythrocytes (2,6). In patients with stable angina the responsible plaque is usually smooth, with a yellow surface (Fig. 2). These findings have been indirectly confirmed by histopathological studies (3) and may explain the difference in behavior of patients with unstable angina, compared with patients with myocardial infarction (especially differences in response to thrombolysis).

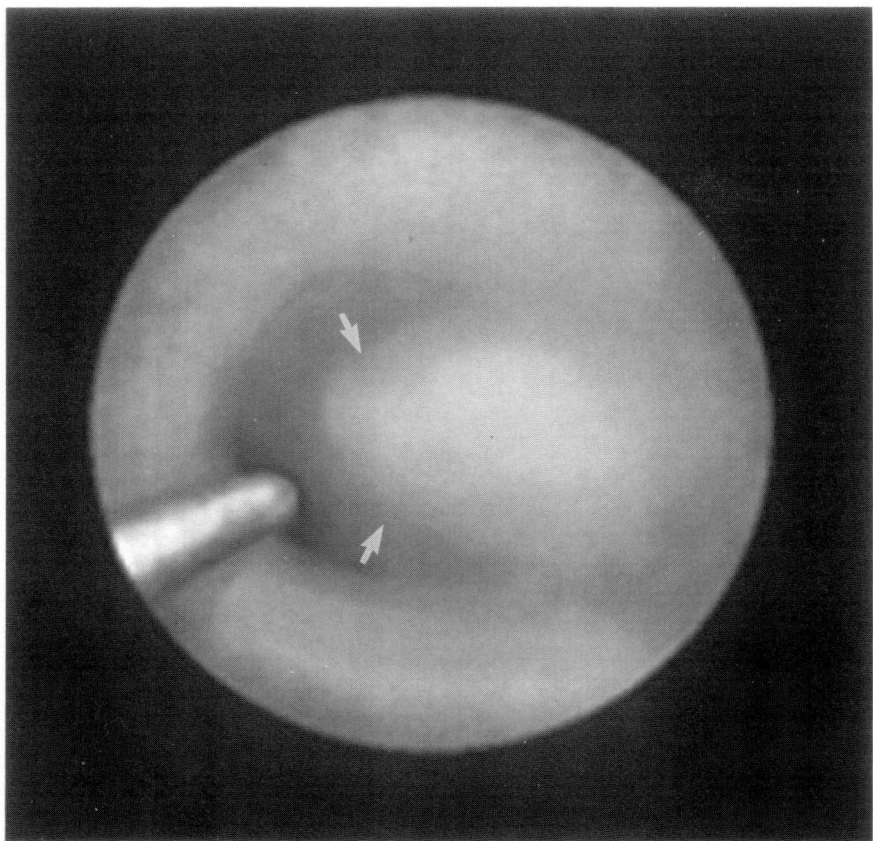

Figure 2 Angioscopic image from a patient with chronic, stable angina shows a smooth plaque (arrowheads). This appearance suggests stable plaque morphology. The color image showed that this lesion had an even, yellow surface. (Courtesy Drs. R. Nesto and S. Waxman, Deaconess Hospital, Boston MA.)

Angioscopy shows that angiography frequently fails to show thrombus and dissection before and after PTCA. This is not surprising, as the limitations of angiography for showing thrombus and dissection, especially after PTCA, are well known from pathological studies. However, the magnitude of the difference is remarkable (angioscopy detects thrombus in up to 50% before and > 90% after PTCA, whereas angiography showed thrombus in < 20%; 7). In the same study, angioscopy detected dissection in 44% before and 100% after PTCA (compared with 0 and 44%, respectively by angiography). Others report similar results with angiographic features of dissection seen in only one-third of patients in whom dissection is seen by angioscopy (8). The magnitude of this difference emphasizes the need for more accurate intravascular diagnosis to assess the immediate effects of PTCA and related interventions, which are poorly characterized by angiography.

Angioscopy may be useful in patients who have abrupt occlusion following PTCA, the major cause of mortality and morbidity after this procedure. Reintervention is usually empirical and may fail to address the major cause of reocclusion in a particular patient. Angioscopy allows more accurate diagnosis of post-PTCA occlusion, when compared with angiography, and more appropriate selection of treatment for occlusion (9). In patients with restenosis after PTCA, angioscopy shows that this is generally due to development of a fibrotic lesion, rather than progression of atherosclerosis (4).

The evaluation of CABG stenosis is another area in which angioscopy provides more accurate information than angiography concerning the presence of dissection and intraluminal thrombus (10). This may also be useful for selecting appropriate interventions for treating CABG stenosis.

Data on the effect of angioscopy to select different treatments is limited, although the ability to provide in vivo images of the response to PTCA, stenting, and other interventions may be useful for modifying interventional devices or changing the way in which they are used (4,11). Angioscopy can also evaluate the response to different anticoagulation regimens (12).

Intracardiac angioscopy is a more difficult imaging problem than coronary angioscopy, owing to the difficulty in replacing a larger volume of blood by transparent fluid, which is required for angioscopy. Several methods have been tried, mainly in animal studies, but they may soon have human applications (13,14). These could include guiding interventions for arrhythmias and for diagnosis of intracardiac masses. It has already been possible to use angioscopy to guide radiofrequency ablation in dogs (Fig. 3), with a fair degree of accuracy (15).

B. Intravascular Ultrasound

Coronary intravascular ultrasound (IVUS) catheters use very high-frequency transducers ($\geqslant$ 20 MHz) on 5-F or smaller catheter systems. Current IVUS devices provide only a side view of the vessel wall, but forward, or at least oblique, viewing devices will become available soon. The size of the larger devices (systems under 3-F diameter are available) may prevent passage through tight stenoses, so that IVUS has mainly been used to assess stenosis in larger vessels or after intervention. Passage of even 2.9-F IVUS catheters can have a measurable Dotter effect (16) and cause plaque disruption (Fig. 4), although coronary IVUS appears to be very safe (Table 2). Thus, although IVUS has been described as a new gold standard for assessing coronary artery disease (17), there remain limitations to its routine use. Further miniaturization is likely to increase

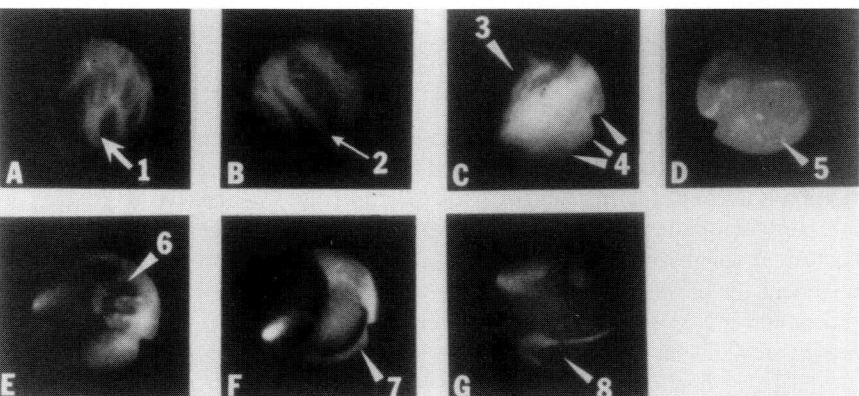

Figure 3 (A) Normal right heart endoscopy in a canine experiment shows right atrial free wall pectinate muscles (arrow 1). (B) Right atrial free wall showing different pattern of pectinate muscles (arrow 2). (C) Area of the right atrial wall near the atrioventricular (AV) node (arrow 3). Branches of the AV nodal artery (arrows 4) are visible on the color image. (D) Septal leaflet of the tricuspid valve (arrow 5). (E) Dorsal leaflet of the tricuspid valve (arrow 6). (F) Ostium of the coronary sinus (arrow 7). (G) Right ventricular view showing papillary muscles and chordae tendinae (arrow 8). (From Ref. 15.)

the applicability of IVUS, especially as part of interventional therapeutic procedures (18). Developments in three-dimensional image reconstruction, to more clearly represent plaque and vessel wall morphology, may also increase the usefulness of this technique (19).

The use of IVUS provides more information on coronary artery wall morphology and composition than does coronary angiography (3,20), as well as more accurately detecting stenosis calcification and determining wall thickness (21,22). One of the most important findings from IVUS is that in vessels with a stenosis there is hardly any segment of the affected artery that is free of plaque (23). Even in angiographically normal coronary arteries, IVUS can show extensive plaque and plaque calcification in a vessel that has a true media-to-media diameter that is significantly larger than the diameter of the lumen (24,25). These findings may help explain why acute coronary events develop as a result of occlusion or thrombus in what were previously thought to be normal coronary arteries. Angiographically, the arteries may be normal, but IVUS has shown that extensive plaque, as a substrate for plaque rupture (Fig. 5), may be present (23,25). In patients with intermediate lesions on angiography, IVUS helps identify which lesions require intervention and which can be safely left untreated (26).

Underestimation of the true size of an angiographically normal artery could explain some of the unsatisfactory results of intervention. Undiagnosed disease, causing nonfocal luminal narrowing in reference segments used to determine the size of balloons or depth of atherectomy, could cause undertreatment of a lesion. This may explain why the plaque burden in the reference segment is related to the likelihood of restenosis after PTCA (27). There are also differences in post-PTCA plaque morphology (such as detection of deep, plaque fissuring) and vessel diameter, as shown by IVUS compared with angiography, which may affect the outcome of PTCA (28).

Along with angioscopy, IVUS has provided extra information, which is not obtainable from angiography, concerning the effects of therapeutic interventional procedures. This may allow a better directed approach to different types of lesion and more accurate diagnosis of complications (see Fig. 4), also allowing more appropriate treatment (29). Angioscopy has provided some insight into the poor midterm performance of directional atherectomy (DCA; discussed in Sec. IV.B). Angiographically directed DCA is unable to accurately remove plaque and, frequently, media and adventitia are also removed. IVUS can be used to direct DCA to increase the removal of plaque and to reduce inappropriate subintimal atherectomy (Fig. 6). IVUS also shows that following DCA, what looks like angiographically adequate debulking, in fact, may leave a large part of the cross-sectional area of the vessel filled with plaque and a very irregular surface (30,31).

High-speed, rotational atherectomy (Rotablator, described in Sec. IV.A) has been advocated for the treatment of calcified stenoses, in which the atherectomy burr is thought to preferentially ablate calcified plaque; IVUS confirms that this is true (32). Because IVUS has greater sensitivity to calcification than angiography, it may be the best method for choosing suitable lesions for rotablation and monitoring the response to this type of atherectomy.

One of the most immediate practical applications of IVUS may be to optimize stent deployment (Fig. 7). Passing an IVUS transducer through a stent is relatively quick, safe, and the area of interest is readily apparent (without angiography). In spite of apparently good deployment on angiography, IVUS shows that a substantial proportion of stents are not fully expanded and may benefit from further dilation (33). This allows a greater postprocedure lumen and may reduce restenosis and acute occlusion, although, as with all other applications of intravascular imaging, further experience is required.

III. Interventional Therapeutic Techniques

A. Percutaneous Transluminal Coronary Angioplasty

Percutaneous transluminal coronary angioplasty (PTCA) is the most common cardiovascular intervention, in spite of its high restenosis rate (30%, or more at 6 months) and procedural risks. So far, newer devices have had only limited success

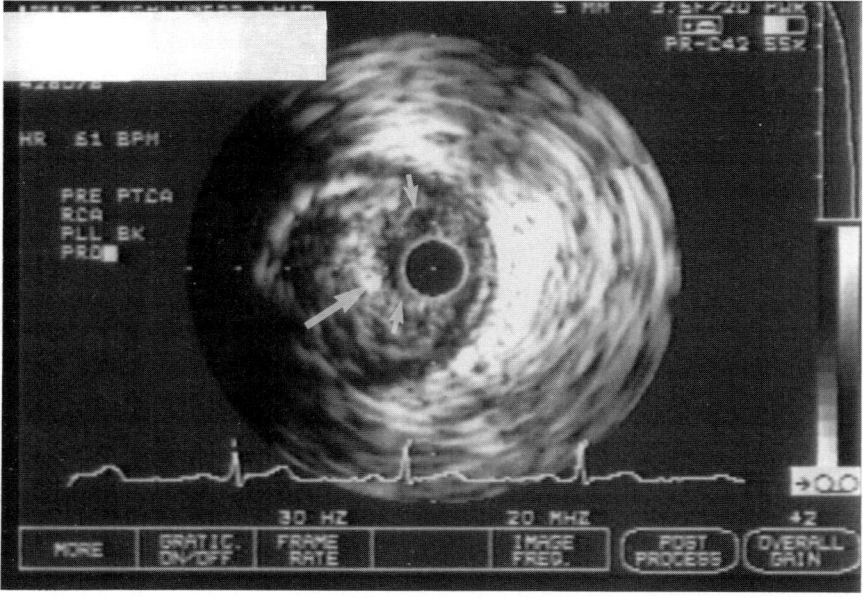

(a)

Figure 4 (a) IVUS shows an eccentric, partly calcified complicated plaque (arrow indicates calcification). Note the patent lumen of the vessel (between arrowheads) is very small, although the vessel itself is large, but filled with complicated atheroma. (b) Following passage of the IVUS catheter through the tight stenosis, on pullback, IVUS imaging showed a linear split (arrow). This demonstrates the effect that passage of an IVUS catheter can have in causing a Dotter effect and disrupting the stenosis. (c) Following balloon dilation, there is a large dissection flap (arrow), not well shown angiographically. (Courtesy Dr. S. Zarich, Deaconess Hospital, Boston MA.)

in improving on the results of conventional PTCA, and in most situations balloon angioplasty remains the most appropriate technique. Numerous technical improvements have allowed continuing progress in the application of conventional balloon PTCA.

Catheter design and construction has improved, providing better balloon and wire support than the original guide catheters (34), and this is probably the most important single factor when attempting to cross difficult stenoses. Balloons have lower profiles, more flexible shafts, and smoother or more slippery (i.e., hydrophilic) surfaces, which increase the ability to cross tighter and more distal lesions. Noncompliant plastics produce reliable inflation to the designed diameter (to within 10%) and tolerate higher pressures. Noncompliant balloons can be

Interventional Techniques in Cardiac Diagnosis 543

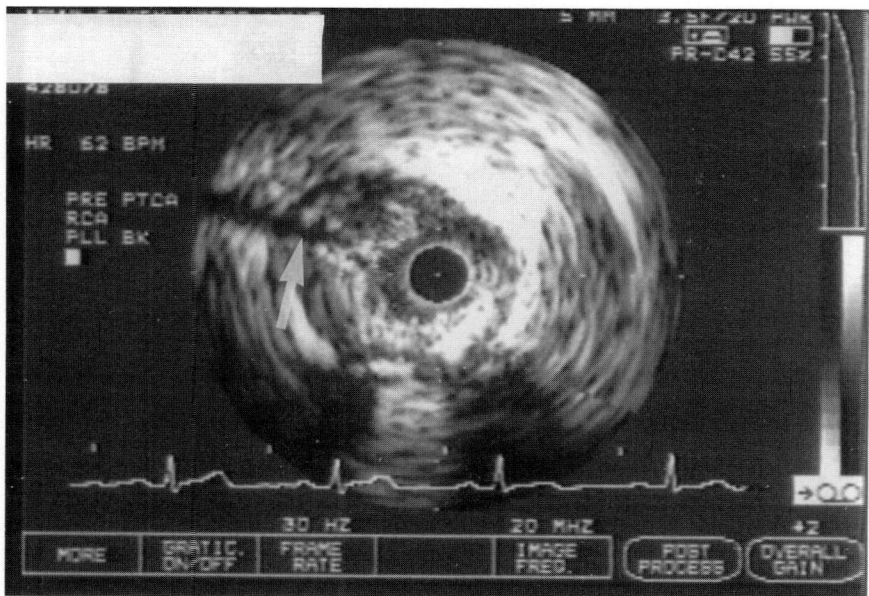

(b)

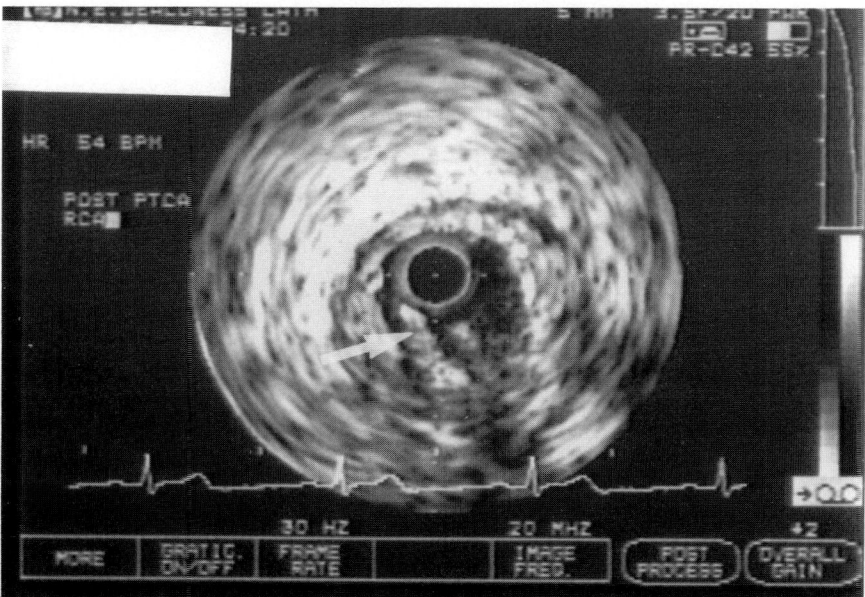

(c)

Table 2 Safety of Coronary IVUS

Procedures	718	Patients	708
Total complication	8	Guidewire entrapment	2
Spasm	4	Dissection	2
Significant adverse clinical outcome		0	

Source: Ref. 106.

inflated to varying, but relatively predictable, diameters at different pressures, allowing graded dilation, until a good result is obtained, although overdilation, especially at the ends of the balloon, may increase the risk of occlusive dissection and restenosis (35). Maximum inflation pressures have also increased (up to 20 atm with polyethylene terephthalate or PET balloons). Longer balloons allow more successful treatment of long stenoses or long dissections (36).

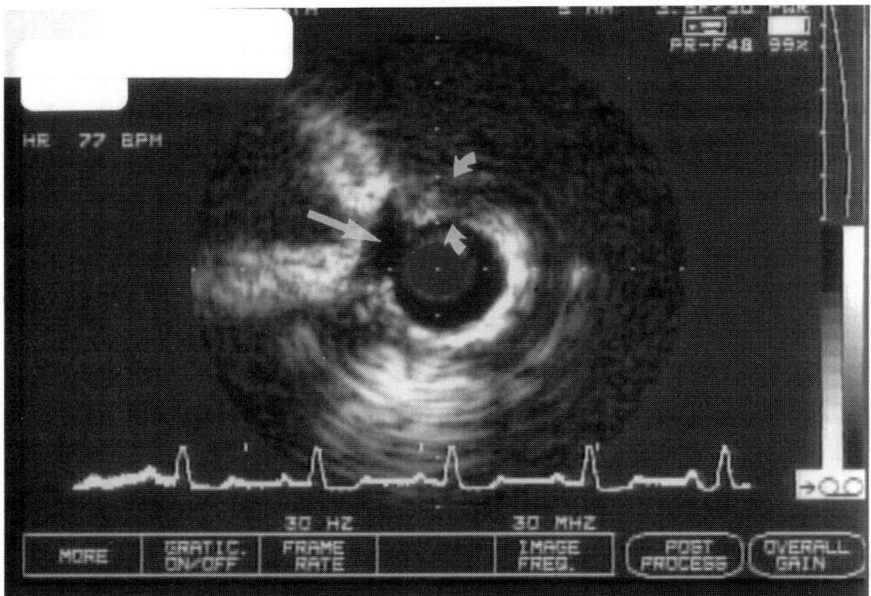

Figure 5 IVUS shows generalized wall thickening (between curved arrows) with a low reflectivity segment of arterial wall (arrow). This patient had a recent myocardial infarction, and it was thought that the low-signal area represented an unstable lipid pool in the thickened wall of the coronary artery. (Courtesy Dr. S. Zarich, Deaconess Hospital, Boston MA.)

Guidewires with appropriate flexibility, torque control, and stiffness can be chosen to suit the lesions being treated. These give better support crossing tight stenoses or occlusions, although recanalization of occlusions is more difficult and has more complications (37). Individual technical improvements in guidewire or balloon design usually have small effects, but the aggregate effect of multiple technical changes has been considerable.

Increased operator skill and improved technology have improved PTCA primary success rates and reduced complication rates in patients with classically indicated lesions. PTCA is increasingly used in unstable patients with poor cardiac function and in those with multivessel disease (38). More recent indications for PTCA include unstable angina (to prevent myocardial infarction), to salvage myocardium after myocardial infarction, as primary treatment for myocardial infarction, or for residual stenosis after thrombolysis.

For patients with stable angina, PTCA relieves symptoms, with low risk and an expectation of restenosis in about 30%. There is no significant effect on mortality when PTCA is compared with medical therapy for stable angina. One study found fewer symptoms after PTCA, but less myocardial infarction with medical therapy. In the randomized intervention treatment in angina (RITA) trial, during which PTCA was compared with CABG, there were more interventions (38 vs. 11% at 2 years) and more symptoms (32 vs. 11% at 6 months) in the PTCA group, although there was no survival difference at 2 years (40).

The expected primary success rates for PTCA continue to improve. Most patients should expect a primary success rate of 90% for PTCA of nonoccluded arteries (41). For chronically occluded arteries, the success rate falls to 65–70%. The greatest problem following PTCA remains the high incidence of restenosis, varying from 30–60%, depending on the nature of the lesion and length of follow-up (Table 3). Clinical follow-up tends to underestimate restenosis rates, as angiographic restenosis may be asymptomatic. Although restenosis can be treated by repeat PTCA, recurrent restenosis occurs in a similar proportion.

In spite of extensive experimental work, little improvement in restenosis rates has been achieved after PTCA. Various drug regimens have been tried, and some preliminary studies suggested that restenosis could be reduced pharmacologically (i.e., by giving calcium channel blockers). Unfortunately, when larger studies with better follow-up have been performed no drug regimen has had a significant effect; the same applies to atherectomy (discussed in Sec. IV.B). The only technique that has had a significant effect on restenosis is stenting, and even this has serious limitations (discussed in Sec. IV.E).

The use of PTCA in acute myocardial infarction has advantages over intravenous thrombolysis in suitable high-risk patients. Overall, the advantages are small and the circumstances in which skilled PTCA is readily available are limited. PTCA produces higher patency rates (up to 95%) than conventional thrombolysis, improves prognosis, reduces recurrent ischemia, and inhospital stay

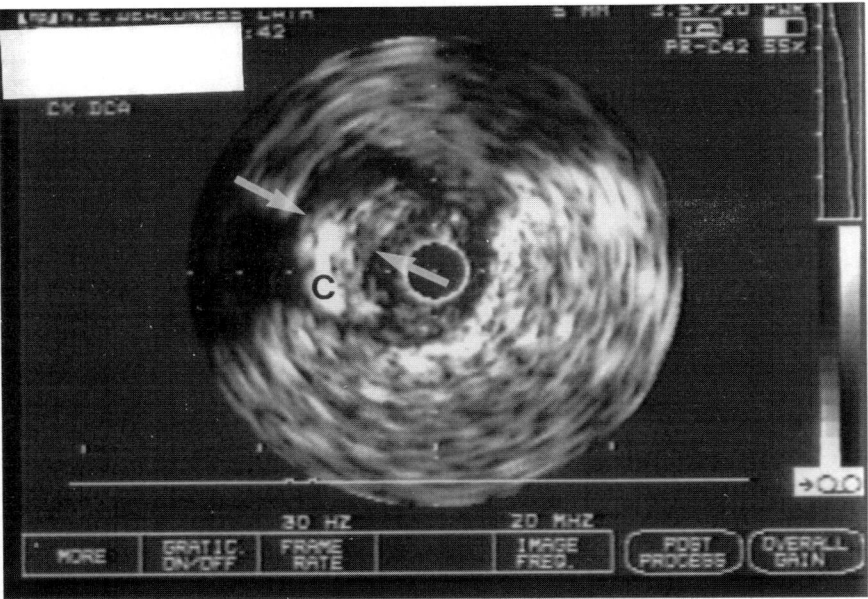

(a)

Figure 6 (a) An eccentric complicated plaque (between arrows) with an area of calcification (C) is demonstrated by IVUS in the circumflex coronary artery. (b) Following directional atherectomy (DCA), a large part of the atheromatous material has been removed (arrow indicates site of DCA cut), but the lumen of the vessel remains irregular, and part of the wall is still thickened with echogenic, calcified material within it. (Courtesy Dr. S. Zarich, Deaconess Hospital, Boston MA.)

is shorter (42,43). PTCA is probably indicated for patients with suitable anatomy (preferably single-vessel disease), large infarctions, cardiogenic shock, when there are contraindications to thrombolysis, with persisting ischemia, or if there has been previous CABG (43,44).

B. Laser Assisted Percutaneous Transluminal Coronary Angioplasty

It was originally hoped that laser-assisted PTCA would improve the results of PTCA by allowing easier recanalization of occluded arteries and reducing restenosis rates. Although hot-tip and hybrid probes could recanalize occluded arteries, early and late results were no better than for PTCA. There is no indication

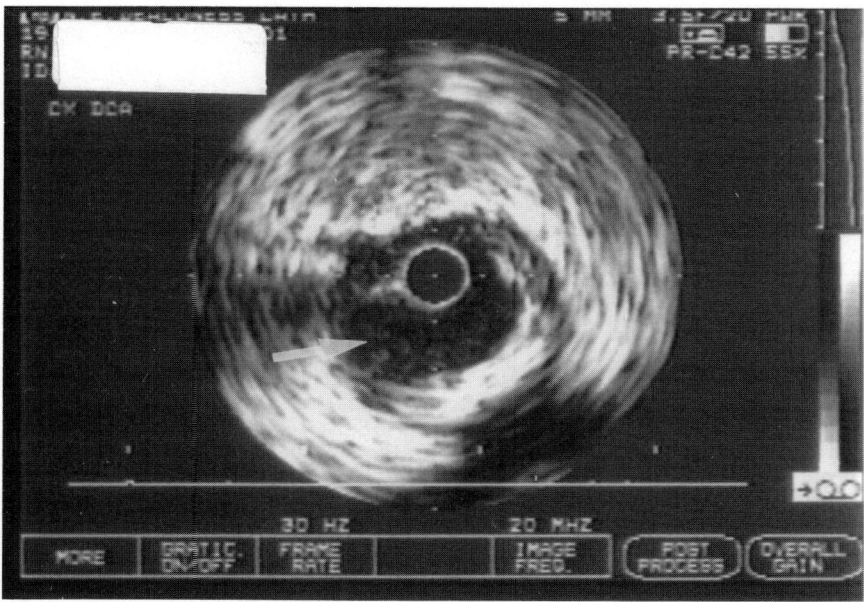

(b)

for the use of hot-tip and hybrid lasers. In spite of a perforation rate higher than for PTCA (near 2%; 45), there is probably a role for excimer lasers.

Results from a registry of patients treated with the Spectranetics xenon chloride excimer laser show that, although it may have some benefits over balloon PTCA, adjunctive balloon angioplasty is usually required ($> 80\%$). The primary success rate (with adjunctive PTCA as required) is reported to be 89%, with major complications in about 7%, and restenosis in about 50% (45,46). There may be benefit from using excimer laser to treat saphenous vein graft stenosis (Fig. 8), ostial stenoses, short occlusions, and calcified lesions. There was no benefit in complete occlusions or long stenoses, and success is reduced when thrombus is present (47).

The AIS excimer laser (Advanced Interventional Systems, Inc.) has a procedural success rate of about 90% (using balloon PTCA after laser if judged to be necessary). In the first 3000 patients, there was an acceptable complication rate; mortality 0.5%; Q-wave MI 2.1%; urgent CABG 3.8%; angiographic dissection 13%; sustained occlusion 3.1% (48). Coronary perforation was initially a problem, but declined in frequency with time, presumably owing to an increase in operator skill and judgment. The angiographic restenosis rate was the same as

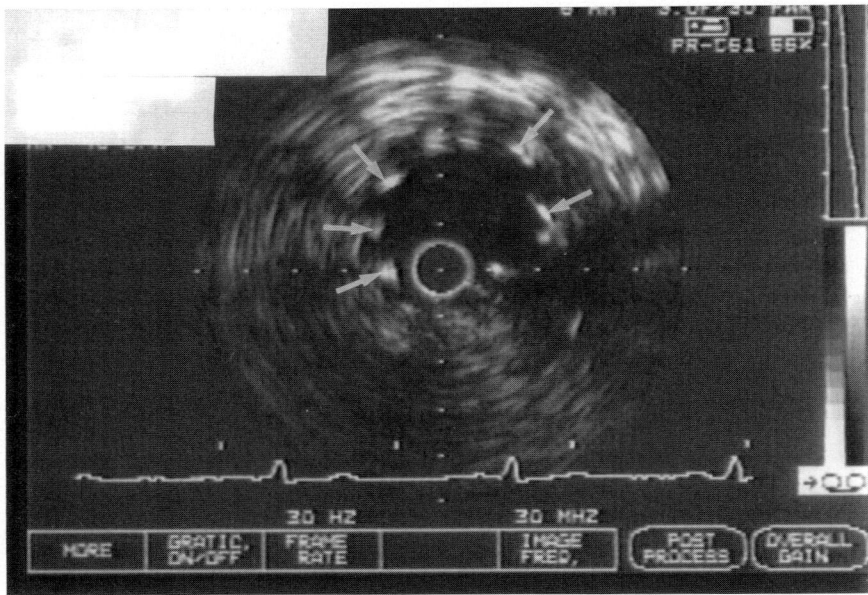

(a)

Figure 7 (a) Following insertion of a Palmaz stent across a CABG stenosis, IVUS shows acoustic shadowing (arrows) by the stent lattice. The stent is well seated, with no gap between the stent lattice and the CABG wall. (b) IVUS image of CABG above the stent at a level that appeared normal on angiography. In spite of this, IVUS shows diffuse wall thickening (between curved arrows). (Courtesy Dr. S. Zarich, Deaconess Hospital, Boston MA.)

expected for other PTCA approaches. When using the AIS system specifically in lesions that are not ideal for PTCA, a procedural success rate of 94% was reported, in spite of a high proportion of type C lesions (49). There may be a niche for treating difficult ostial or CABG stenosis (50).

IV. Mechanical Coronary Recanalization

Many types of cutting, drilling, and pulverizing devices have been designed to overcome problems of PTCA in recanalizing occluded arteries and reducing restenosis. Most have failed to demonstrate significant benefit when compared with conventional PTCA, although some have limited applications.

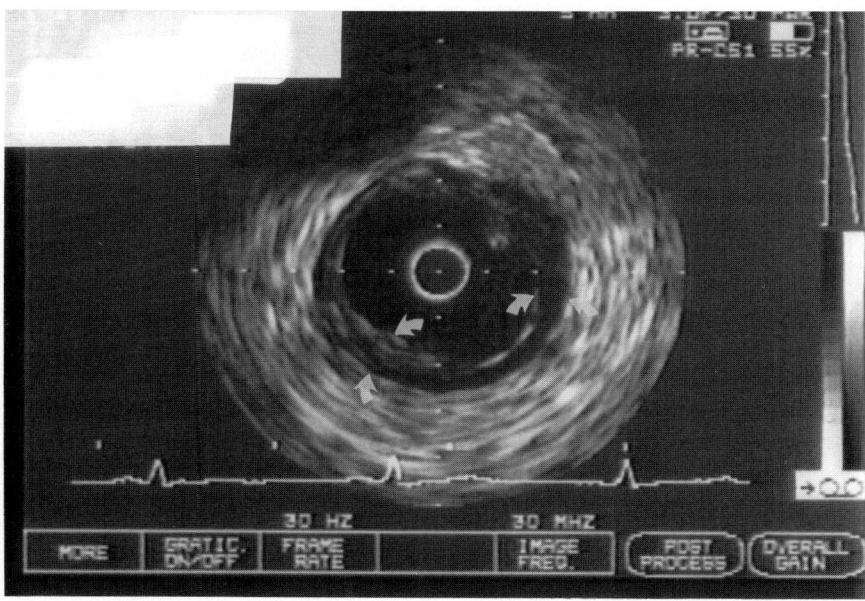

(b)

A. Rotablator

The Rotablator (Heart Technology Inc.) is a high-speed (190,000 rpm) cutting device powered by compressed air. A diamond chip covered burr (Fig. 9), introduced over a 0.009-in. guidewire, cuts a channel a little smaller than the burr diameter (1.25–2.5 mm). Because of the small channel produced, adjunctive low-pressure PTCA is usually required. The procedural success rate varies from 57

Table 3 Predictors of Recurrent Restenosis after PTCA

Short interval between PTCAs (< 3 or 5 mo)
Presentation with unstable symptoms
Male gender
Lesions >15 mm long
Diabetes mellitus
Large number of inflations
Need for high-inflation pressure

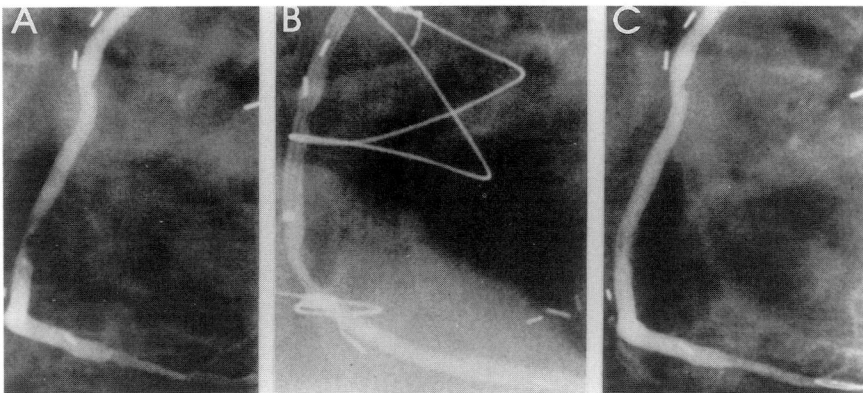

Figure 8 (A) Selective CABG angiogram shows severe distal stenosis (arrow) above the distal anatomosis. (B) Selective angiogram shows passage of an excimer laser catheter (arrows) through the distal stenosis. (C) Selective angiogram after laser ablation shows minimal irregularity at the site of the previous stenosis. (From Ref. 108.)

(86% with PTCA) to 95% (51,52). The primary success rate for some lesions is superior to that expected for conventional PTCA, but overall, is not significantly better (51). In spite of producing a cleaner lumen (see Fig. 9), there is little or no effect on restenosis rates (ranges 30–55%), depending on the lesions being treated (52,53).

B. Directional Coronary Atherectomy

The only available directional coronary atherectomy (DCA) device is the Simpson Atherocath (DVI, Inc.). The aim of this approach in treating stenosis is to remove plaque completely from the arterial wall, leaving a larger lumen, with less extensive wall damage than that with PTCA (see Fig. 6). DCA was thought to be useful for treating restenoses, eccentric lesions, and possibly, complex lesions. More recently, large studies have shown that DCA has limited short-term benefits and no significant effect on midterm restenosis rates (54,55). Primary success rates range from 88 up to 98% (when PTCA is used for DCA failure; 56), with sudden closure in 4.3% (55). In spite of the larger initial lumen produced by DCA, there is no improvement in the incidence of restenosis (6-month angiographic restenosis is seen in 32–50%; 55–57). Early cardiac and vascular complications are more common with DCA, and procedural costs are increased (inhospital costs for DCA are 11,904 dollars vs. 10,637 dollars for PTCA; 54). The probability of death or myocardial infarction is also increased (DCA event rate, 8.5 vs. 4.6% for PTCA; Table 4; 54).

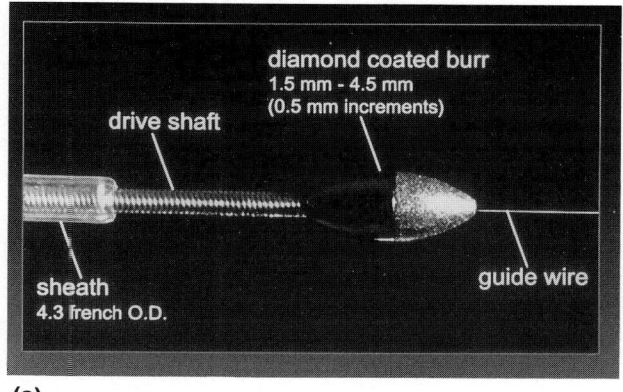

(a)

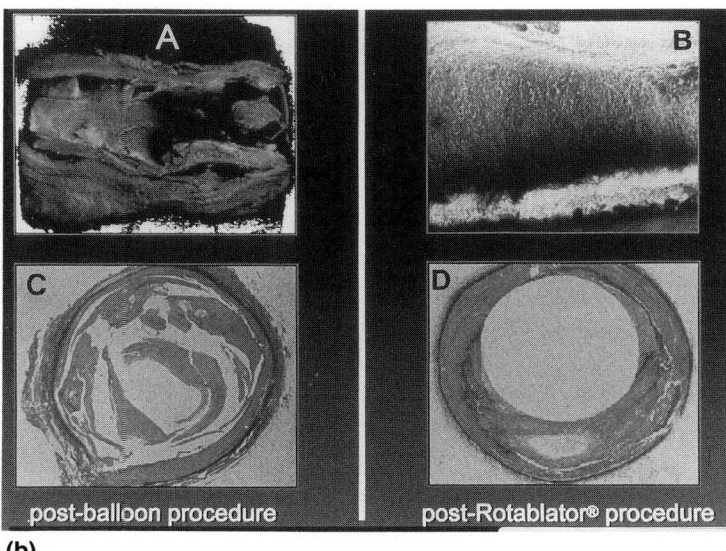

(b)

Figure 9 (a) Magnified image showing the burr of the Rotablator device (Heart Technology, Inc., Redmond WA) over its introducing guidewire. (b) Comparison of effect of balloon PTCA (images A and C) and Rotablator (images B and D) on the gross appearance (images A and B) and cross-sectional histological appearance (images C and D) of a treated artery. The Rotablator leaves a much smoother inner lumen. (Courtesy G. F. Janko, Heart Technology, Inc., Redmond WA.)

Table 4 Summary of Findings of the CAVEAT Study: Randomized Comparison of DCA vs. PTCA[a]

Finding	DCA	PTCA
1° success (< 50% stenosis)	89%	80%
Increase vessel diameter	1.05 mm	0.86 mm[b]
Inhospital death/clinical MI	6%	3.4%
Total adverse events (MI, death, urgent CABG, vessel closure)	11%	5%
6-mo restenosis	50%	57%[b]
6-mo death/MI	8.6%	4.7%[b]
6-mo CABG	8.2%	6.8%[b]

[a]1012 patients in study.
[b]Significant difference: $p > 0.05$.
Source: Ref. 54.

The failure of DCA to reduce restenosis is not surprising. Up to 50% or more of the effect of DCA is due to dilation, rather than plaque removal. Also more than plaque is removed, with media retrieved in up to 67% and adventitia in up to 27% of procedures (58). This predisposes to iatrogenic ectasia (10–13%; 59) and occasionally coronary artery aneurysms (60). Some authors have argued that DCA is very operator-dependent and that the poor results from large studies are due to suboptimal DCA, and may be improved by limiting DCA to larger vessels (57). Better intravascular imaging during DCA may also improve its results, by allowing more complete initial debulking of stenoses (11,30).

C. Rotacs

Various rotating wires have been evaluated for recanalizing occluded coronary arteries as a prelude to PTCA. None are widely used, and there is very limited published experience. Of these, the coronary Rotacs wire (Dr Osypka GMBH) is available in Europe. This is a noncutting, large-diameter wire that rotates slowly (up to 200 rpm) and has been used to recanalize occluded coronary arteries (61). Success rates can be good (93% occlusions < 3 months old; 52% occlusions 6–12 months old), but others have reported poor results (62). As with other innovative devices, there is a significant learning curve. In one comparative study, Rotacs was more effective than PTCA (63) for recanalizing occluded coronary arteries, and was just as safe.

D. Ultrasonic Devices

Ultrasound can recanalize chronically or acutely occluded arteries, rapidly ablating thrombus, while producing little heat. Peripheral arterial and animal coronary studies show that ultrasound debulks stenoses and occlusions with low risk (64). Human coronary studies have begun, with variable early results, but there appears to be a role in treating lesions with visible thrombus, although conventional PTCA is usually still required (65).

E. Coronary Stents

Stents provide mechanical support after PTCA, which can reduce the effects of elastic recoil, keep open occlusive dissection flaps (66,67) and, by achieving a larger post-PTCA lumen, reduce restenosis rates (68,69). The most important drawback of coronary stents is the need for vigorous and prolonged anticoagulation to prevent acute thrombosis, which leads to a high incidence of vascular complications (with transfusion required in up to 16%) (68–70).

Stents currently available for cardiac use (although not approved in all countries) include the Palmaz, Wallstent, Strecker, and Wiktor stents. The current approved indications in the United States are for rescue of occlusive dissection during balloon PTCA and for CABG stenosis. Stents are widely used for treating acute closure during or following PTCA (66,67), although the acute thrombosis rate following stenting for acute occlusion is higher (21%) than that for elective use (3.4%) (69). A direct comparison with the alternative bail-out option of 15-min inflation with an autoperfusion catheter, suggests that prolonged inflation may be as good or even a superior alternative (71). Angiographic restenosis rates after stenting for dissection are similar (38%) to those of uncomplicated PTCA (72).

Stents achieve lower restenosis rates from their ability to produce the largest initial lumen diameter, rather than to reduce intimal hyperplasia (compared with PTCA, laser-assisted balloon angioplasty, and DCA; 66,68). The reduced restenosis rate (about 18 vs. 31%) is outweighed in many patients by the increased risks of stent use (peripheral vascular complications requiring surgery, 9%; transfusion, 5%; other bleeding complications 3%; 68). Vascular complications are likely to remain a problem until nonthrombogenic stents become available. Although still in an early stage of development, heparin-coated stents used in the Benestent II study reduce the need for intensive anticoagulation, which causes the vascular complications of conventional stent deployment (73).

The Palmaz stent (Johnson and Johnson Interventional Systems) is a balloon-expandable stainless steel lattice with restenosis rates from 13 to 25% (de novo uses; 74). In the randomized Benestent study the 6-month stent restenosis rate was 22%, compared with a PTCA restenosis rate of 32% (68). In an uncontrolled study of stenting native coronaries, de novo restenosis to 50% reduction in diameter occurred in only 14% (compared with 39% when there had been previous PTCA) (75). The Palmaz stent is approved for use in treating CABG stenosis, for which it has a high immediate success rate and a low (17%) restenosis rate (76). Restenosis rates are lowest when there is a large residual lumen (about

20% for residual lumens > 3.2 mm, about 34% for lumens < 3.2 mm; 68,74). Palmaz stenting for occlusive dissection complicating PTCA, restores flow, improves angiographic appearance, and reduces the acute occlusion rate. As with all coronary stents, access site complications are common and lead to increased hospitalization times, mainly owing to vascular complication related to intensive anticoagulation (68,74,77).

The Gianturco-Roubin Flex-Stent (Cook, Inc.) is a stainless steel balloon-expandable coil made up of multiple loops of wire. This makes it very flexible, and it does not shorten when expanded. Stainless steel is more thrombogenic than tantalum, but only 10% of the surface of the stented region is covered by stent material. The Flex-Stent has a restenosis rate of about 30% (77), suggesting a limited effect on restenosis compared with PTCA. It is used mainly for treating acute occlusion complications, and reduces the need for CABG (78).

Although there is a clear role for stenting in the treatment of sudden closure complicating PTCA the value of elective stenting is still unclear. Short-term restenosis rates are reduced at the expense of a substantial vascular complication rate. There is a paucity of long-term data, and more widespread use of primary stenting should wait until these are available.

F. Autoperfusion Catheters

There are several strategies for dealing with acute or threatened closure complicating PTCA. There is limited data on whether surgery, stenting, or prolonged inflation of an autoperfusion catheter is most appropriate. Although many cardiologists prefer to stent for threatened closure, there are data that suggest that prolonged (15- or if that fails 60-min) inflation of an autoperfusion catheter may have advantages (71,79). Autoperfusion balloon catheters allow distal artery perfusion, while maintaining pressure on the site of occlusion. Although the best results of bailout using an autoperfusion catheter are good, results are variable (reported success ranging from 40 to 97%; large series report about 70% inhospital success). If there is no response to prolonged inflation, the perfusion catheter can be used to maintain flow while awaiting surgery.

G. Intracoronary Thrombolysis

Intravenous thrombolysis is well established for early treatment of acute myocardial infarction, but in some patients, systemic thrombolytic agents are contraindicated, or thrombolysis is unsuccessful or too slow. Alternative methods are being developed to achieve rapid thrombolysis with little systemic effect by using selective-delivery systems, such as porous balloon or selective microcatheterization.

The success rate of selective coronary thrombolysis in early reports was about 60% for recanalizing occlusions (80). Although somewhat overshadowed by the introduction of systemic thrombolysis, small-bore infusion catheters allow infusion of thrombolytic agents directly into the thrombus, with improved immediate success rates (81). Thrombolysis as an adjunct to PTCA for chronic or acute occlusion usually achieves patency, but makes little difference to immediate success, complication rates, or restenosis. A porous balloon system, which produces high local concentrations of thrombolytic agent at the site of PTCA, has been used to achieve local thrombolysis in patients with unstable angina, but experience is limited (82).

V. Balloon Valvuloplasty

Balloon valvuloplasty was developed as a potential alternative to valve replacement. Although valvuloplasty is less invasive, has lower costs, and avoids general anesthesia and surgery, early enthusiasm for valvuloplasty has not been justified for all valves (83).

A. Pulmonary Valvuloplasty

Balloon pulmonary valvuloplasty is the treatment of choice for most patients older than 1 year of age with pulmonary valve stenosis, when the valve is well formed (84). Balloon valvuloplasty of dysplastic pulmonary valves is usually satisfactory, although results are not as satisfactory as for well-formed valves (gradients reduced by 50–100%; 85). Residual gradients may continue to fall after valvuloplasty as infundibular hypertrophy subsides (86). The long-term results are good, with improvements maintained for 3–5 years or more (87), and restenosis in less than 10% cases. Balloon valvuloplasty is more difficult in neonates with critical pulmonary stenosis who have more complications and poorer results (88).

B. Mitral Valvuloplasty

Various types of balloon valvuloplasty have been tried for mitral valvuloplasty. The most common methods use a transeptal approach and either two, conventional large-diameter balloons or the Inoue balloon (Toray, Inc., Tokyo). The Inoue balloon is a compliant balloon, with a shape specifically designed for balloon mitral valvuloplasty (Fig. 10), which allows incremental dilation until a good result has been achieved. This is more difficult with the double-balloon technique. The two techniques have similar immediate results when used by experienced operators, but complications (especially myocardial perforation in up to 4%) and procedure times are reduced with the Inoue balloon (89). Long-term results are probably better with the Inoue balloon.

Balloon mitral valvuloplasty is generally very successful, especially when there is minimal calcification and distortion of the subvalvar apparatus. Valve

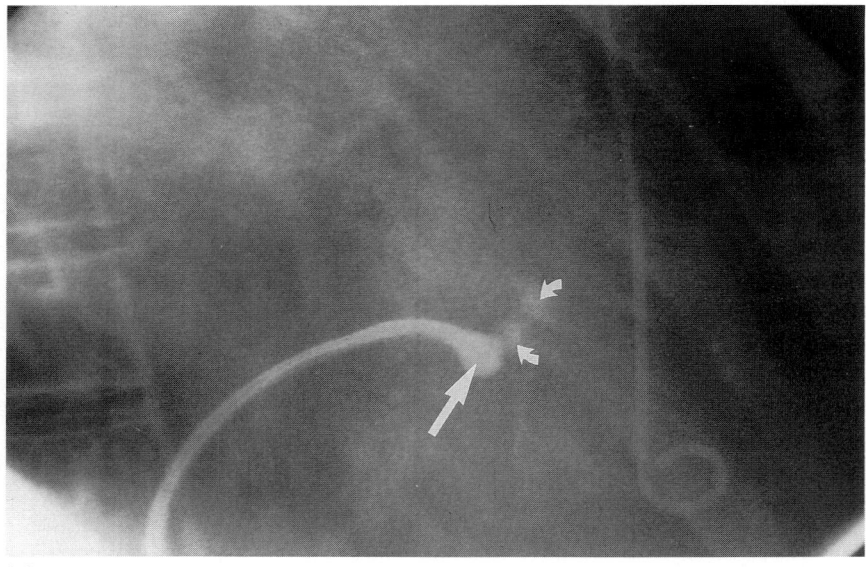

(a)

Figure 10 (a) Inoue balloon mitral valvuloplasty: After transeptal puncture, the balloon (arrow) is passed over stiff, coiled guidewire (in the left atrium), across the interatrial septum, and into the left atrium. Calcification (curved arrows) indicates the position of the mitral valve in this patient. (b) The partly inflated balloon is indented by the calcified mitral valve (arrows). (c) Further inflation of the Inoue balloon fully across the mitral valve led to the balloon reaching its maximum diameter. This procedure increased mitral valve area by over 100%.

calcification or severe distortion produce poorer results, although even with scores of less than 8, acceptable results can be achieved with the Inoue technique (90). Following balloon mitral valvuloplasty, restenosis is slow, in most patients becoming serious only after 3 years, and severe restenosis is uncommon (7/294 lost > 50% of the increase in valve area; 91).

C. Aortic Valvuloplasty

Balloon aortic valvuloplasty was introduced for use in patients unsuitable for, or at high risk for, aortic valve replacement. Improvements in surgical technique have reduced the need for valvuloplasty.

Balloon aortic valvuloplasty can be performed through a transarterial approach (92) or a transeptal, transvenous approach (93). The transvenous approach is used if the valve cannot be crossed retrogradely or the femoral arteries are too

Interventional Techniques in Cardiac Diagnosis 557

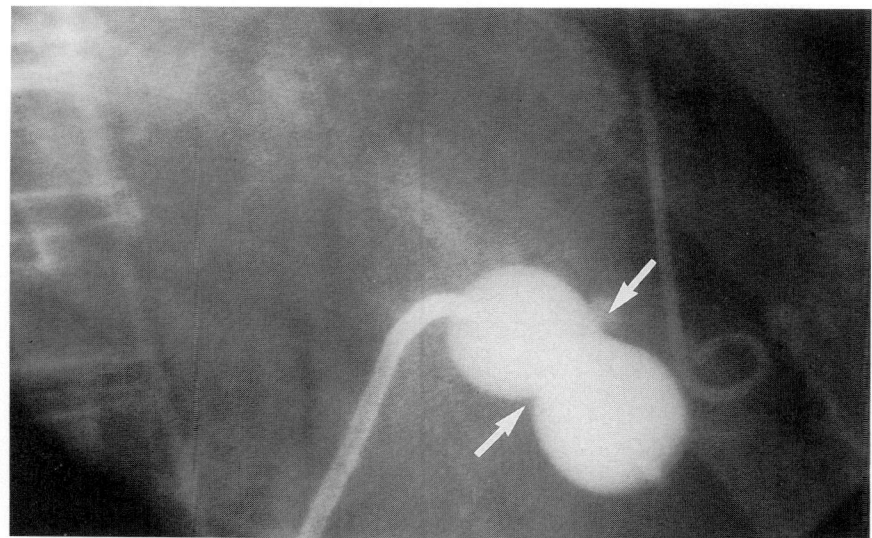
(b)

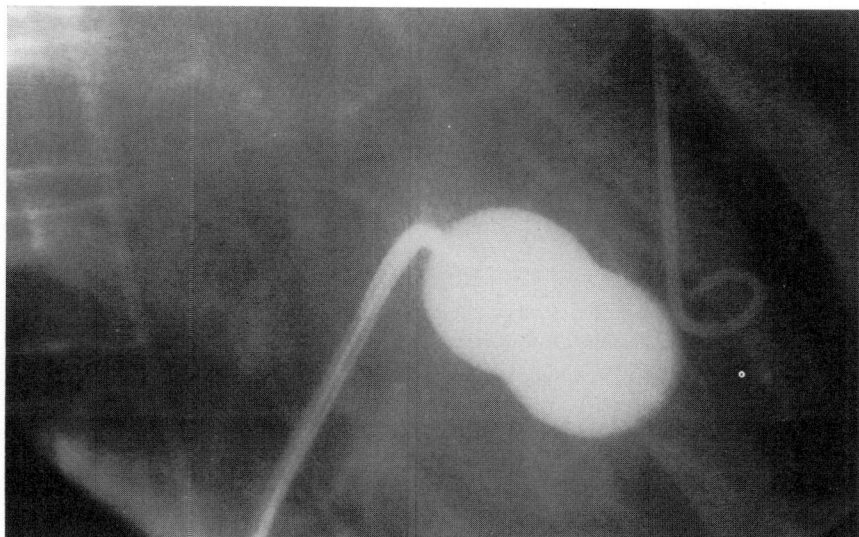
(c)

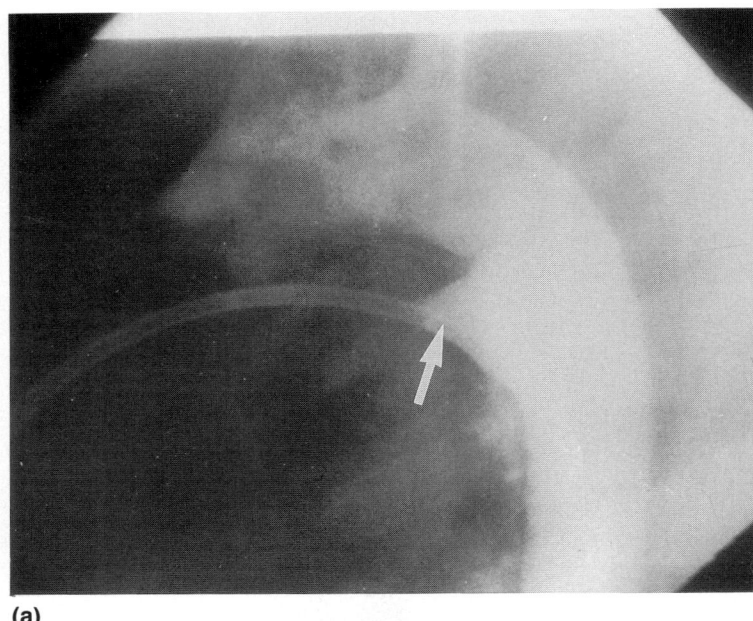

Figure 11 (a) Aortogram showing position of PDA (arrow). An introducer catheter has been passed from the pulmonary artery, through the PDA into the descending aorta. (b) Aortogram shows USCI PDA, umbrella (arrow) deployed in PDA but still attached to deployment catheter (curved arrow). Aortogram confirms satisfactory position of the umbrella. (c) Aortogram following release of the umbrella (arrow) in the PDA, shows satisfactory position and no residual shunt.

small for safe insertion of the large sheaths used (15-F) (94). Most patients have symptomatic improvement after aortic valvuloplasty, but increases in valve area are usually modest (50% reduction in valve gradient, 0.2–0.4 cm^2 increase in valve area) and transient (95). Persisting symptomatic improvement may be the result of improved left ventricular function, in spite of a return of valve area to prevalvuloplasty values (94,96).

Complications are common, with vascular complications requiring surgery in up to 13%, amputation in 0.6%, other complications (death, stroke, severe aortic regurgitation) in 6.3% (97).

Aortic valvuloplasty for congenital aortic stenosis is controversial, but has results similar to surgery. Substantial reductions in valve gradients can be achieved (from mean 77 mmHg to 30 mmHg; 98), with an acceptable increase in aortic regurgitation, which is usually well tolerated (99).

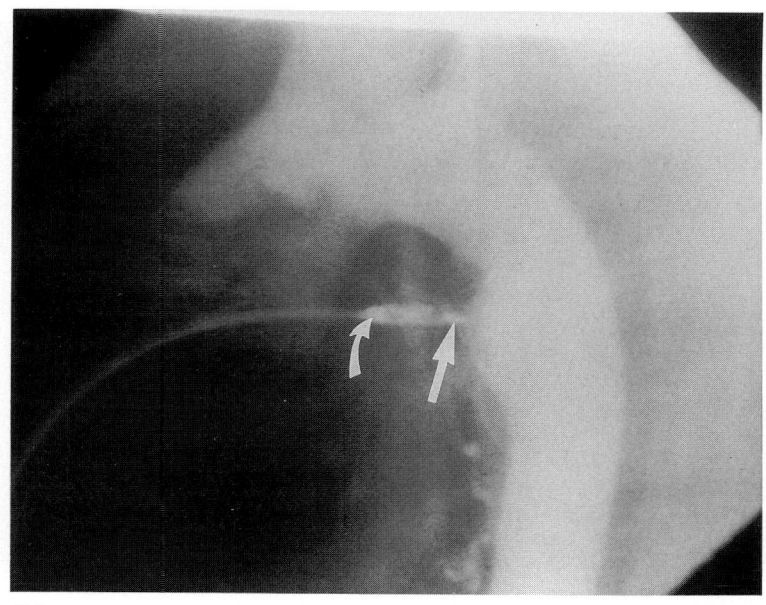

(b)

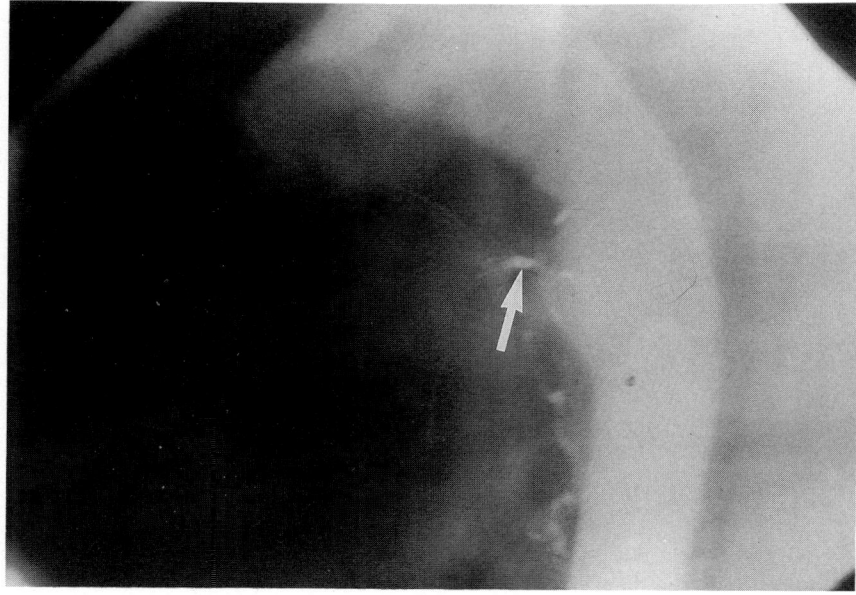

(c)

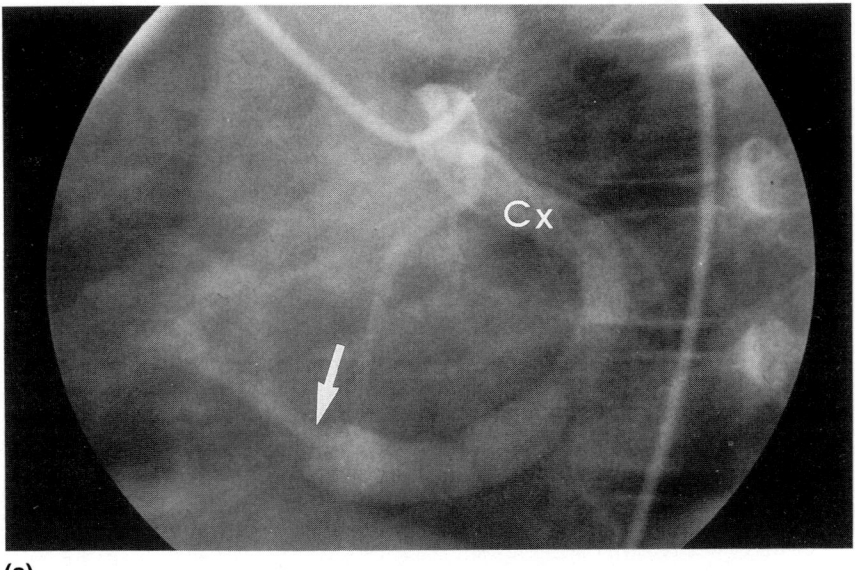

(a)

Figure 12 (a) Selective coronary arteriogram, in a 3-year-old child, shows a circumflex coronary artery (Cx) to right atrium fistula (arrow). (b) An inflatable embolization balloon was deployed in the aneurysmal segment immediately proximal to the fistula. (c) After the release of the embolization balloon, there is no residual shunt.

D. Dilation of Coarctation

Native coarctation can be treated by balloon dilation, but its value is limited as, compared with surgery, the balance of improvement to risks does not justify routine use (17% incidence of complications and late aneurysm formation up to 43%; 100). Balloon dilation of coarctation after surgery is safer and more successful, with gradients reduced to less than 20 mmHg in about 80% of patients and a mortality of 2–3% (101).

E. Embolization

Persistent ductus arteriosus (PDA) can be closed by embolization, most commonly using the USCI PDA umbrella (Fig. 11). There are limitations imposed by the diameter of the introducer sheaths and the size of PDAs that can be occluded safely. Results are generally satisfactory, although 6–31% may have a residual shunt; and a few need a second embolization (102).

Coronary artery fistulae are a rare cause of left-to-right shunt endocarditis

Interventional Techniques in Cardiac Diagnosis

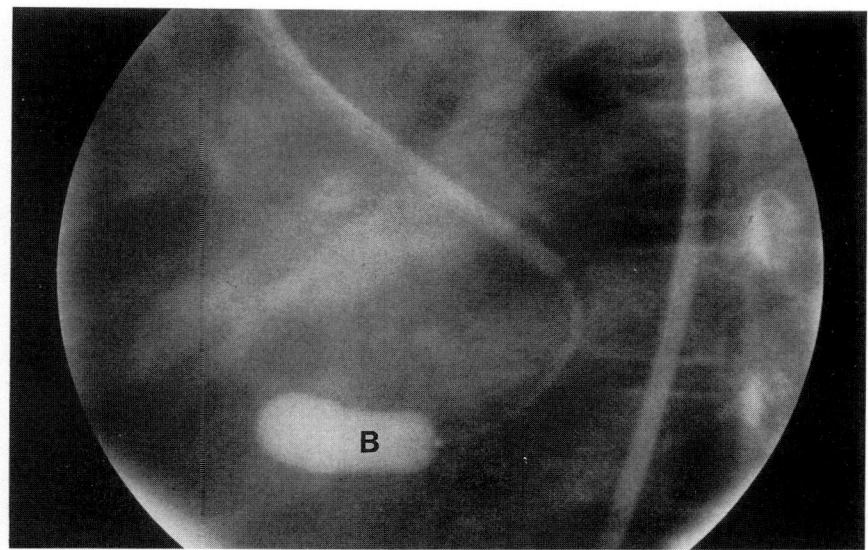
(b)

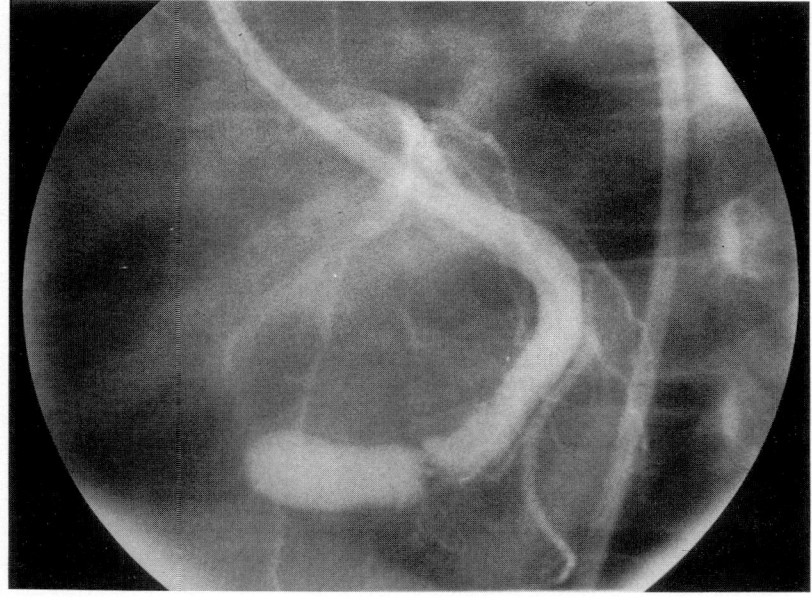
(c)

(5%) and ischemia owing to coronary steal. Coils or balloons (Fig. 12) can be used to embolize fistulae, while sparing adjacent normal vessels, which may not be possible with surgery (103).

Systemic–pulmonary collaterals or palliative surgical shunts can be occluded by balloons or coils in patients with cyanotic congenital heart disease (104). Other devices have been developed for percutaneous closure of atrial and ventricular septal defects (105). These devices are still evolving and experimental.

Acknowledgments

I would like to thank my colleagues Drs. R. Nesto, S. Waxman and S. Zarich in the Cardiovascular Division at the Deaconess Hospital for providing Figures 1, 2, 4–7; Dr. G. A. Abela, Figure 8; Dr. O. Fujimura, Figure 3; and Mr. G. F. Janko, Figure 9.

References

1. Gruentzig A. Transluminal dilatation of coronary artery stenosis. Lancet 1978; 1:263.
2. Sherman CT, Litvack F, Grundfest W, et al. Coronary angioscopy in patients with unstable angina pectoris. N Engl J Med 1986; 315:913–919.
3. Siegel RJ, Ariani M, Fishbein MC, et al. Histopathologic validation of angioscopy and intravascular ultrasound. Circulation 1991; 84:109–117.
4. White CJ, Ramee SR, Mesa JE, Collins TJ. Percutaneous coronary angioscopy in patients with restenosis after coronary angioplasty. J Am Coll Cardiol 1991; 17: 46B–49B.
5. White CJ, Ramee SR, Collins TJ, Mesa JE, Jain A. Percutaneous angioscopy of saphenous vein coronary bypass grafts. J Am Coll Cardiol 1993; 21:1181–1185.
6. Mizuno K, Satomura K, Miyamoto A, et al. Angioscopic evaluation of coronary-artery thrombi in acute coronary syndromes. N Engl J Med 1992; 326:287–291.
7. Ramee SR, White CJ, Collins TJ, Mesa JE, Murgo JP. Percutaneous angioscopy during coronary angioplasty using a steerable microangioscope. J Am Coll Cardiol 1991; 17:100–105.
8. den Heijer P, Foley DP, Escaned J, et al. Angioscopic versus angiographic detection of intimal dissection and intracoronary thrombus. J Am Coll Cardiol 1994; 24: 649–654.
9. White CJ, Ramee SR, Collins TJ, Jain SP, Escobar A. Coronary angioscopy of abrupt occlusion after angioplasty. J Am Coll Cardiol 1995; 25:1681–1684.
10. Ramee SR, White CJ, Collins TJ, Mesa JE, Murgo JP. Percutaneous angioscopy during coronary angioplasty using a steerable microangioscope. J Am Coll Cardiol 1991; 17:100–105.
11. Leon MB, Kuntz RE, Popma JJ, et al. Acute angiographic, intravascular ultrasound and clinical results of directional atherectomy in the optimal atherectomy restenosis

study. Presented at 44th Annual Scientific Sessions, American College Cardiology 1995. J Am Coll Cardiol 1995; 137A.
12. Guagliumi G, Valsecchi O, Tespili M, et al. Serial angioscopic assessment of coronary stent lining with antiplatelet or anticoagulant therapy. Presented at 44th Annual Scientific Sessions, American College Cardiology 1995. J Am Coll Cardiol 1995; 154A.
13. Uchida Y, Tomaru T, Nakamura F, Sonoki H, Sugimoto T. Fiberoptic angioscopy of cardiac chambers, valves, and great vessels using a guiding balloon catheter in dogs. Am Heart J 1988; 115:1297–1302.
14. Fujimura O, Lawton MA, Koch CA. Direct in vivo visualization of right cardiac anatomy by fiberoptic endoscopy: observation of radiofrequency-induced acute lesions around the ostium of the coronary sinus. Eur Heart J 1994; 15:534–540.
15. Fujimura O, Lawton MA, Koch CA. Direct in vivo visualization of right cardiac anatomy by fiberoptic endoscopy: hemodynamic effects and image validation. Angiology 1995; 46:201–209.
16. Weissman NJ, Foster GP, Allen J, et al. Dotter effect of intravascular ultrasound catheters. Presented at 44th Annual Scientific Sessions, American College Cardiology 1995. J Am Coll Cardiol 1995; 119A.
17. de Man F, de Scheerder I, Herregods MC, Piessens J, de Geest H. Role of intravascular ultrasound in coronary artery disease: a new gold standard? An overview. Acta Radiol 1994; 49:223–231.
18. Yock PG, Mullen WL, Fitzgerald PJ. Intravascular ultrasound: an inside view. Br Heart J 1994; 72:97–98.
19. Roelandt JRTC, di Mario C, Pandian NG, et al. Three-dimensional reconstruction of intracoronary ultrasound images. Rationale, approaches, problems, and directions. Circulation 1994; 90:1044–1055.
20. St Goar FG, Pinto FJ, Alderman EL, Fitzgerald PJ, Stadius ML, Popp RL. Intravascular ultrasound imaging of angiographically normal coronary arteries: an in vivo comparison with quantitative angiography. J Am Coll Cardiol 1991; 18:952–958.
21. Mintz GS, Douek P, Pichard AD, et al. Target lesion calcification in coronary artery disease: an intravascular ultrasound study. J Am Coll Cardiol 1992; 20:1149–1155.
22. Willard JE, Netto D, Demian SE, et al. Intravascular ultrasound imaging of saphenous vein grafts in vitro: comparison with histologic and quantitative angiographic findings. J Am Coll Cardiol 1992; 19:759–764.
23. Mintz GS, Painter JA, Pichard AD, et al. Atherosclerosis in angiographically "normal" coronary artery reference segments: an intravascular ultrasound study with clinical correlations. J Am Coll Cardiol 1995; 25:1479–1485.
24. Ge J, Erbel R, Gerber T, et al. Intravascular ultrasound imaging of angiographically normal coronary arteries: a prospective study in vivo. Br Heart J 1994; 71:572–578.
25. Porter TR, Sears T, Xie F, et al. Intravascular ultrasound study of angiographically mildly diseased coronary arteries. J Am Coll Cardiol 1993; 22;1858–1865.
26. Mintz GS, Bucher TA, Kent KM, et al. Clinical outcomes of patients not undergoing coronary artery revascularization as a result of intravascular ultrasound imaging. Presented at 44th Annual Scientific Sessions, American College Cardiology 1995. J Am Coll Cardiol 1995; 61A.

27. Nissen SE, de Franco AC, Raymond RE, Franco I, Eaton G, Tuzcu M. Angiographically unrecognized disease at "normal" reference sites: a risk factor for suboptimal results after coronary intervention. Circulation 1993; 88:I-412.
28. Nakamura S, Mahon DJ, Meheswaran B, Gutfinger DE, Colombo A, Tobis JM. An explanation for discrepancy between angiographic and intravascular ultrasound measurements after percutaneous transluminal coronary angioplasty. J Am Coll Cardiol 1995; 25:633–639.
29. Baptista J, di Mario C, Escaned J, et al. Intracoronary two-dimensional ultrasound imaging in the assessment of plaque morphologic features and the planning of coronary interventions. Am Heart J 1995; 129:177–187.
30. Thieme T, Felix SB, Meyer R, et al. Angioscopy guided Simpson atherectomy—new insights into directional coronary atherectomy results. Presented at 44th Annual Scientific Sessions, American College Cardiology 1995. J Am Coll Cardiol 1995; 137A.
31. Leon MB, Kuntz RE, Popma JJ, et al. Acute angiographic, intravascular ultrasound and clinical results of directional atherectomy in the optimal restenosis trial. Presented at 44th Annual Scientific Sessions, American College Cardiology 1995. J Am Coll Cardiol 1995; 137A.
32. Kovach JA, Mintz GS, Pichard AD, et al. Sequential intravascular ultrasound characterization of the mechanisms of rotational atherectomy and adjunct balloon angioplasty. J Am Coll Cardiol 1993; 22:1024–1032.
33. Goldberg SL, Colombo A, Nakamura S, Almagor Y, Maiello L, Tobis JM. Benefit of intracoronary ultrasound in the deployment of Palmaz-Schatz stents. J Am Coll Cardiol 1994; 24:996–1003.
34. Nesto RW. Performance characteristics of a new shape of guiding catheter for PTCA of the left coronary artery. Cathet Cardiovasc Diagn 1991; 24:144–148.
35. Roubin GS, Douglas JS, King SB, et al. Influence of balloon size on initial success rate, acute complications, and restenosis after PTCA. Circulation 1988; 78:557–565.
36. Tenaglia AN, Zidar JP, Jackman JD, et al. Treatment of long coronary artery narrowings with long coronary angioplasty balloon catheters. Am J Cardiol 1993; 71:1274–1277.
37. Stewart JT, Denne L, Bowker TJ, et al. Percutaneous transluminal coronary angioplasty in chronic coronary artery occlusion. J Am Coll Cardiol 1993; 21:1371–1376.
38. Holmes DR, Holubkov R, Vliestra RE, et al. Comparison of complications during percutaneous transluminal coronary angioplasty from 1977 to 1981 and from 1985 to 1986: the National Heart, Lung and Blood Institute Percutaneous Coronary Angioplasty Registry. J Am Coll Cardiol 1988; 12:1149–1155.
39. Parisi AF, Folland ED, Hartigan P. A comparison of angioplasty with medical therapy in the treatment of single vessel coronary artery disease. N Engl J Med 1992; 326:10–16.
40. RITA trial participants. Coronary angioplasty versus coronary artery bypass surgery: the randomized intervention treatment in angina (RITA) trial. Lancet 1993; 341: 573–580.
41. Landau C, Lange RA, Hillis LD. Percutaneous transluminal coronary angioplasty. N Engl J Med 1994; 330:981–993
42. Ribeiro EE, Silva LA, Carneiro R, et al. Randomized trial of direct coronary

angioplasty versus intravenous streptokinase in acute myocardial infarction. J Am Coll Cardiol 1993; 22:376–380.
43. Simari RD, Berger PB, Bell MR, Gibbons RJ, Holmes DR. Coronary angioplasty in acute myocardial infarction: primary, immediate adjunctive, rescue, or deferred adjunctive approach? Mayo Clin Proc 1994; 69:346–358
44. Muller DWM, Topol EJ. Thrombolytic therapy: adjuvant mechanical intervention for acute myocardial infarction. Am J Cardiol 1992; 69:60A–70A.
45. Baumback A, Bittl JA, Fleck E, et al. Acute complications of excimer laser coronary angioplasty: a detailed analysis of multicenter results. J Am Coll Cardiol 1994; 23:1305–1315.
46. Bittl JA, Kuntz RE, Estella P, Sanborn TA, Baim DS. Analysis of late lumen narrowing after excimer laser-facilitated coronary angioplasty. J Am Coll Cardiol 1994; 23:1314–1320.
47. Estella P, Ryan TJ, Landzberg JS, Bittl JA. Excimer laser-assisted coronary angioplasty for lesions containing thrombus. J Am Coll Cardiol 1993; 21:1550–1556.
48. Litvack F, Eigler N, Margolis J, et al. Percutaneous excimer laser coronary angioplasty: results in the first consecutive 2000 patients. J Am Coll Cardiol 1994; 23: 323–329.
49. Cook SL, Eigler NL, Shefer A, Goldenberg T, Forrester JS, Litvack F. Percutaneous excimer laser coronary angioplasty of lesions not ideal for balloon angioplasty. Circulation 1991; 84:632–643.
50. Diethrich EB. Has excimer laser angioplasty finally found a niche? Circulation 1991; 84:939–940.
51. Borrione M, Hall P, Almagor Y, Maiello L, Khlat B, Colombo A. Treatment of simple and complex coronary stenosis using rotational ablation followed by low pressure balloon angioplasty. Cathet Cardiovasc Diagn 1993; 30:131–137.
52. Stertzer SH, Rosenblum J, Shaw RE, et al. Coronary rotational ablation: initial experience in 302 procedures. J Am Coll Cardiol 1993; 21:287–295.
53. Bertrand ME, Lablanche JM, Leroy F, et al. Percutaneous transluminal coronary rotary ablation with Rotablator (European experience). Am J Cardiol 1992; 69: 470–474.
54. Topol EJ, Leya F, Pinkerton CA, et al. A comparison of directional atherectomy with coronary angioplasty in patients with coronary artery disease. N Engl J Med 1993; 329:221–227.
55. Adelman AG, Cohen EA, Kimball BP, et al. A comparison of directional atherectomy with balloon angioplasty for lesions of the left anterior descending coronary artery. N Engl J Med 1993; 329:228–233.
56. Fishman RF, Kuntz RE, Carroza JP, et al. Long-term results of directional coronary atherectomy: predictors of restenosis. J Am Coll Cardiol 1992; 20:1101–1110.
57. Umans VA, Hermans W, Foley DP, et al. Restenosis after directional coronary atherectomy and balloon angioplasty: comparative analysis based on matched lesions. J Am Coll Cardiol 1993; 21:1382–1390.
58. Safian RD, Gelbfish JS, Erny RE, Schnitt SJ, Schmidt DA, Baim DS. Coronary atherectomy: clinical, angiographic and histological findings and observations regarding potential mechanisms. Circulation 1990; 82:69–79.
59. DeCesare NB, Popma JJ, Holmes DR, et al. Clinical, angiographic and histologic

correlates of ectasia after directional coronary atherectomy. Am J Cardiol 1992; 69:314–319.
60. Bell MR, Garratt KN, Bresnahan JF, Edwards WD, Holmes DR. Relation of deep arterial resection and coronary artery aneurysms after directional coronary atherectomy. J Am Coll Cardiol 1992; 20:1474–1481.
61. Kaltenbach M, Valbracht C, Hartmann A. Recanalization of chronic coronary occlusions by low speed rotational angioplasty (Rotacs). J Int Cardiol 1991; 4:155–165.
62. Anderson MH, Ward DE. Early experience with low speed rotational angioplasty. Br Heart J 1991; 66:130–133.
63. Danchin N, Julliere Y, Cassagnes J, et al. Randomized multicenter study of low speed rotational angioplasty versus standard angioplasty for total coronary occlusion [abst]. Circulation 1992; 86:I-782.
64. Steffen W, Fishbein MC, Luo H, et al. High intensity, low frequency catheter-delivered ultrasound dissolution of occlusive coronary artery thrombi: an in vitro and in vivo study. J Am Coll Cardiol 1994; 24:1571–1579.
65. Hamm CW, Bertrand ME, de Scheerder I, et al. Initial multicenter experience with therapeutic ultrasonic coronary angioplasty in patients. Presented at 44th Annual Scientific Sessions, American College Cardiology 1995. J Am Coll Cardiol 1995; 268A.
66. Lincoff AM, Topol EJ, Chapekis AT, et al. Intracoronary stenting compared with conventional therapy for abrupt vessel closure complicating coronary angioplasty: a matched case–control study. J Am Coll Cardiol 1993; 21:866–875.
67. Herrmann HC, Buchbinder M, Clemen MW, et al. Emergent use of balloon expandable coronary stenting for failed percutaneous transluminal coronary angioplasty. Circulation 1992; 86:812–819.
68. Serruys PW, Macaya C, de Jeagere P, et al. Interim analysis of the Benestent trial. Circulation 1993; 88:I-594.
69. Fishman D, Savage M, Leon MB, et al. Acute and late angiographic results from the stent restenosis study (STRESS) [abst]. J Am Coll Cardiol 1994; 60A.
70. George BS, Voorhees WD, Roubin GS, et al. Multicenter investigation of coronary stenting to treat acute or threatened closure after percutaneous transluminal coronary angioplasty. Clinical and angiographic outcomes. J Am Coll Cardiol 1993; 22:135–143.
71. DeMuinck ED, Hillege HL, van Dijk RB, et al. Perfusion balloon versus stent for acute or threatened closure: equal efficacy but significantly higher costs after stenting [abst]. J Am Coll Cardiol 1994;103A.
72. Schomig A, Kastrati A, Dietz R, et al. Emergency coronary stenting for dissection during percutaneous transluminal coronary angioplasty: angiographic follow-up after stenting and after repeat angioplasty of the stented segment. J Am Coll Cardiol 1994; 23:1053–1060.
73. Serruys P. Should all PTCA's be stented. Data presented at Angioplasty '95, London, January 1995.
74. Carrozza JP, Kuntz RE, Levine MJ, et al. Angiographic and clinical outcome of intracoronary stenting: immediate and long-term results from a large single-center experience. J Am Coll Cardiol 1992; 20:328–337.

75. Savage MP, Fischman DL, Schatz RA, et al. Long-term angiographic and clinical outcome after implantation of a balloon-expandable stent in the native coronary circulation. J Am Coll Cardiol 1994; 24:1207–1212.
76. Piana RN, Moscucci M, Cohen DJ, et al. Palmaz-Schatz stenting for treatment of focal vein graft stenosis: immediate results and long term outcome. J Am Coll Cardiol 1994; 23:1296–1304.
77. Macander PJ. Agrawa SK, Roubin GS. The Gianturco-Roubin balloon expandable intracoronary flexible coil stent. J Invest Cardiol 1991; 3:85–94.
78. George BS, Voorhees WD, Roubin GS, et al. Multicenter investigation of coronary stenting to treat acute or threatened closure after percutaneous transluminal coronary angioplasty: clinical and angiographic outcomes. J Am Coll Cardiol 1993; 22: 135–143.
79. Van der Linden LP, Bakx ALM, Sedney MI, et al. Prolonged dilatation with an autoperfusion balloon catheter for refractory acute occlusion related to percutaneous transluminal coronary angioplasty. J Am Coll Cardiol 1994; 22:1016–1023.
80. Tennant SN, Dixon J, Venable TC, et al. Intracoronary thrombolysis in patients with acute myocardial infarction: comparison of the efficacy of urokinase with streptokinase. Circulation 1984; 69:756–760.
81. Gurbel PA, Davidson CJ, Ohman EM, Smith JE, Stack RS. Selective infusion of thrombolytic therapy in the acute myocardial infarct-related coronary artery as an alternative to rescue percutaneous transluminal coronary angioplasty. Am J Cardiol 1990; 66:1021–1023.
82. Cumberland DC, Gunn J, Tsikaderis D, et al. Initial clinical experience of local drug delivery via a porous balloon during percutaneous coronary angioplasty [abst]. J Am Coll Cardiol 1994; 186A.
83. Isom OW, Rosengart TK. Percutaneous aortic valvuloplasty: off the bandwagon, again. J Am Coll Cardiol 1992; 20:804–805.
84. Kan JS, White RI, Mitchell SE, et al. Percutaneous balloon valvuloplasty: a new method for treating congenital pulmonary stenosis. N Engl J Med 1982; 307:540–542.
85. McCrindle BW, Kan JS. Long-term results after balloon pulmonary valvuloplasty. Circulation 1991; 83:1915–1922.
86. Fontes VF, Esteves CA, Sousa EMR, Virginia M, Bembom MCB. Regression of infundibular hypertrophy after pulmonary valvuloplasty for pulmonic stenosis. Am J Cardiol 1988; 62:977–979.
87. Masura J, Burch M, Deanfield JE, Sullivan ID. Five-year follow-up after balloon pulmonary valvuloplasty. J Am Coll Cardiol 1993; 21:32–136.
88. Stanger P, Cassidy SC, Girod DA, Kan JS, Lababidi Z, Shapiro SR. Balloon pulmonary valvuloplasty: results of valvuloplasty and angioplasty of congenital anomalies registry. Am J Cardiol 1990; 65:775–783.
89. Bassand J-P, Schiele F, Bernard Y, et al. The double-balloon and Inoue techniques in percutaneous mitral valvuloplasty: comparative results in a series of 232 cases. J Am Coll Cardiol 1991; 18:982–989.
90. Hung J-S, Chern M-S, Wu J-J, et al. Short- and long-term results of catheter balloon percutaneous transvenous mitral commissurotomy. Am J Cardiol 1991; 67:854–862.

91. Babic UU, Grujicic S, Popovic Z, Djurisic Z, Pejcic P, Vucinic M. Percutaneous transarterial balloon dilatation of the mitral valve: five year experience. Br Heart J 1992; 67:185–189.
92. Letac B, Cribier A, Koning R, Bellefleur J-P. Results of percutaneous transluminal valvuloplasty in 218 adults with valvular aortic stenosis. Am J Cardiol 1988; 62: 598–605.
93. Block PC, Palacios IF. Comparison of results of anterograde versus retrograde percutaneous balloon aortic valvuloplasty. Am J Cardiol 1987; 60:659–662.
94. Crook R, Weston M, Wilde RPH, Hartnell GG. Aortic valvuloplasty: comparison of the techniques and results of transeptal and retrograde methods. Clin Radiol 1990; 42:110–113.
95. Bernard Y, Etievent J, Mourand J-L, et al. Long-term results of percutaneous aortic valvuloplasty compared with aortic valve replacement in patients more than 75 years old. J Am Coll Cardiol 1992; 20:796–801.
96. Safian RD, Warren SE, Berman AD, et al. Improvement in symptoms and left ventricular performance after balloon aortic valvuloplasty in patients with aortic stenosis and depressed left ventricular ejection fraction. Circulation 1988; 78:1181–1191.
97. Isner JM, the Mansfield Scientific Aortic Valvuloplasty Registry Investigators. Acute catastrophic complications of balloon aortic valvuloplasty. J Am Coll Cardiol 1991; 17:1436–1444.
98. Rocchini AP, Beekman RH, Shachar GB, Benson L, Schwartz D, Kan KS. Balloon aortic valvuloplasty: results of valvuloplasty and angioplasty of congenital anomalies registry. Am J Cardiol 1990; 65:784–789.
99. O'Connor BK, Beekman RH, Rocchini AP, Rosenthal A. Intermediate-term effectiveness of balloon valvuloplasty for congenital aortic stenosis: a prospective follow-up study. Circulation 1991; 84:732–738.
100. Tynan M, Finley JP, Fontes V, Hess J, Kan J. Balloon angioplasty for the treatment of native coarctation: results of valvuloplasty and angioplasty of congenital anomalies registry. Am J Cardiol 1990; 65:790–792.
101. Hellenbrand WE, Allen HD, Golinko RJ, Hagler DJ, Lutin W, Kan J. Balloon angioplasty for aortic recoarctation: results of valvuloplasty and angioplasty of congenital anomalies registry. Am J Cardiol 1990; 65:793–797.
102. Transcatheter occlusion of persistent arterial duct: report of the European Registry. Lancet 1992; 340:1062–1066.
103. Reidy JF, Anjos RT, Qureshi SA, Baker EJ, Tynan MJ. Transcatheter embolization in the treatment of coronary artery fistulas. J Am Coll Cardiol 1991; 18:187–192.
104. Mitchell SE, Kan JS, White RI. Interventional techniques in congenital heart disease. Semin Roentgenol 1985; 20:290–311.
105. Lock JE, Cockerham JT, Keane JF, Finley JP, Wakely PE, Fellows KE. Transcatheter umbrella closure of congenital heart defects. Circulation 1987; 75:593–599.
106. Lablanche JM, Geschwind H, Cribier A, et al. Coronary angioscopy safety survey: European multicenter experience. Presented at 44th Annual Scientific Sessions, American College Cardiology 1995. J Am Coll Cardiol 1995; 154A.

107. Batkoff BW, Linker DT. The safety of intracoronary ultrasound: data from a multi-center European registry. Presented at 44th Annual Scientific Sessions, American College Cardiology 1995. J Am Coll Cardiol 1995; 143A.
108. Abela GA, Comti CR. The use of the laser in the treatment of coronary and peripheral arterial obstruction. In: Schlant RC, Alexander RW, eds. The heart. New York: McGraw-Hill, 1994:1363.

22

Advances in Cardiac Imaging

LEWIS WEXLER, H. WILLIAM STRAUSS, NAEEM MERCHANT, and BOB HU

Stanford University School of Medicine
Stanford, California

I. Introduction

The ability to diagnose specific cardiac abnormalities using newer-imaging modalities far surpasses that achieved by taking a history and performing a physical examination. The demonstration of morphological and functional abnormalities in both acquired and congenital heart disease affecting adults, children, and fetuses is largely accomplished today by noninvasive-imaging methods, such as echocardiography and nuclear medicine. Some conditions, particularly coronary artery disease, still require catheterization and angiography for specific evaluation, but considerable information is provided by noninvasive diagnostic modalities. This chapter describes the current state of cardiac imaging and discusses recent advances that promise to increase our ability to evaluate structure and function, emphasizing noninvasive techniques.

II. Brief History of Cardiac-Imaging Modalities and Current Indications

A. Chest Radiography

Within a year of Roentgen's discovery of the X-ray, Francis H. Williams described the fluoroscopic findings in patients with cardiomegaly and pericardial effusion (1). Shortly thereafter, chest radiographs were published with cardiac mensuration and descriptions of several cardiac and aortic conditions. It was clear that the heart could be studied using x-ray devices; the field of cardiac imaging was born (2). Today, the chest roentgenograph is used to assess heart size and configuration, but individual cardiac structures are more accurately defined by other techniques. Pulmonary vascular pressures and flows are altered in various ways by specific cardiac abnormalities, and this important physiologic information is reflected in the appearance of the pulmonary vessels on a radiograph of the chest (3,4). The chest film is particularly useful in detecting pulmonary abnormalities that confound or contribute to cardiac symptoms, such as dyspnea or chest pain. Evaluation of patients in postoperative intensive care and coronary care units requires high-quality chest radiography (5).

B. Angiocardiography

Angiocardiography was introduced by Castellanos during the 1930s primarily to study patients with congenital heart disease (6). Relatively safe intravascular contrast agents were developed in the 1960s, and further improvements were achieved in the 1980s, with the introduction of low-osmotic iodinated contrast agents. Additional technical developments included rapid film changers, image intensifiers, cineradiography, contrast injectors, and cardiac catheterization methods that facilitated selective opacification of the coronary arteries, the cardiac chambers, and the great arteries. Thus, the groundwork for modern invasive cardiac diagnostic and interventional techniques began about 100 years ago, reaching its present level of sophistication with the introduction of computed image acquisition and digital image manipulation during the past 10 years. Today, diagnostic angiocardiography and coronary arteriography are performed for detailed anatomical description, particularly in the setting of an expected intervention, such as surgery or angioplasty. Chapter 21 describes currently used interventional techniques in more detail.

C. Radionuclide Cardiac Imaging

The first application of radioactive isotopes to the study of cardiac function was Blumgart's use of a tracer to measure circulation time in 1943. Subsequent advances, particularly during the decades of the 1970s and 1980s, include development of safer radiopharmaceuticals, single-photon emission computed tomography (SPECT), and positron emission computed tomography (PET), techniques that provide assessment of myocardial perfusion and ventricular performance. In the 25 years since their introduction, these techniques have found major applications in the evaluation of patients with coronary artery disease and heart failure. The repertoire of tests has grown to encompass determinations of metabolism, receptor occupancy, and the detection of necrosis (7,8) (Table 1). Decisions about the need for revascularization, the success of the revascularization procedure, and the efficacy of medical therapy are often made based on the data provided by these images. The imaging and radiopharmaceutical technology used to make these determinations has advanced from rectilinear scanners to the enhanced resolution now available with digital scintillation cameras. Radiopharmaceuticals have evolved from potassium-43 to thallium-201 to the technetium-labeled radiopharmaceuticals that offer combined measurements of perfusion and function. Right and left ventricular contraction and diastolic function are evaluated, usually with a technetium-labeled radio tracer ($^{99m}TcO_4$ or ^{99m}Tc-labeled red blood cells). Rapid sequence imaging with a gamma camera or cine display provides information about regional wall motion. Similar information can be obtained by gating image acquisition to the electrocardiographic (ECG) signal over several hundred cardiac cycles (Fig. 1). Myocardial perfusion is regularly measured using thallium-201 (^{201}Tl) or ^{99m}Tc sestamibi, both at rest and after exercise, to determine flow reserve, infarcted and ischemic myocardium, and in the acute setting, differentiating infarcted, hibernating, and stunned myocardium (Fig. 2).

Table 1 Radionuclide Measurements of the Heart

Measurement	Radiopharmaceutical	Application
Perfusion	^{201}Tl-thallous chloride ^{99m}Tc-sestamibi ^{99m}Tc-tetrofosmin ^{99m}Tc-teboroxime [^{81}Rb] rubidium chloride	Define the presence, location, and extent of myocardial ischemia and scar; can also be used to determine left ventricular volumes, ejection fraction, and regional wall thickening.
Function	^{99m}Tc-labeled red blood cells ^{99m}Tc-labeled albumin	Measure ejection fraction, ventricular volumes, regional wall motion, ejection and filling rates
Necrosis	^{99m}Tc-pyrophosphate ^{111}In-antimyosin	Identify the site and extent of acute infarction, transplant rejection, and acute myocarditis
Metabolism	^{18}F-deoxyglucose	Define ischemia by increased metabolism by glucose
Receptors	[^{123}I]monoiodobenzylguanidine	Sympathethic innervation

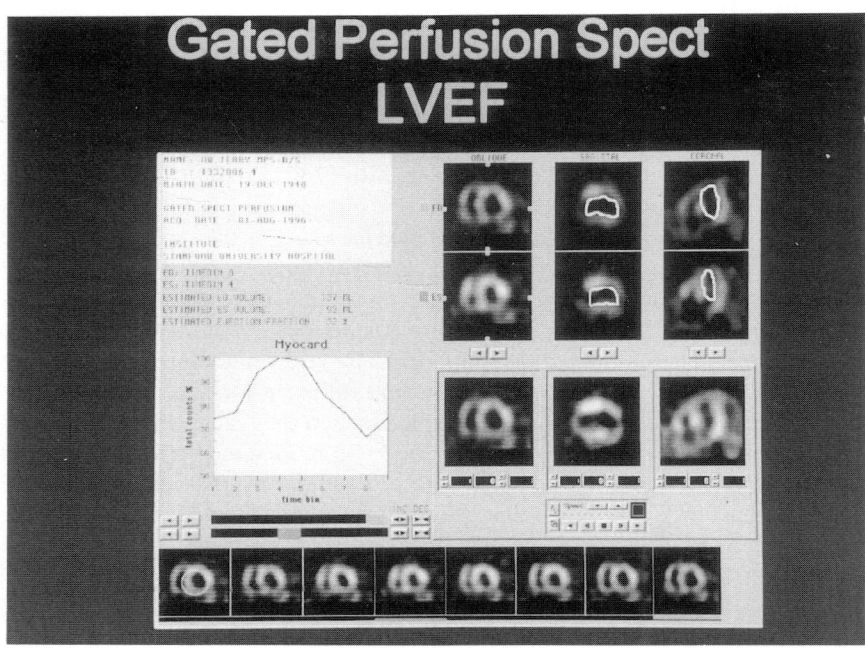

Figure 1 Gated cardiac SPECT images of a patient with apical inferior infarction in diastole (top row) and systole (second row). Ventricular short axis (left column), vertical long axis (center column), and horizontal long axis (right column) images are shown. Note the change in cavity size and wall thickness on these slices. The bottom row depicts the eight images collected throughout the cardiac cycle in a mid-short axis plane. LVEF = left ventricular ejection fraction. In this patient, the estimated ejection fraction is 32%.

D. Echocardiography

During the 1950s, Keidel (9) and Edler and Hertz (10) were among the first to recognize that reflected high-frequency ultrasonic waves could be used to evaluate cardiac anatomy. By the late 1950s and early 1960s, M-mode pulsed ultrasound was in use for assessing mitral valve stenosis, pericardial effusion, and cardiac chamber size (11,12). Subsequently, two-dimensional echocardiography, pulsed and continuous wave Doppler techniques, transesophageal echocardiography (TEE), fetal echocardiography, intravascular ultrasound, and the use of digitization, quantitation, and stress echo studies, have expanded the clinical range of echocardiography so that, currently, it is the primary noninvasive method of cardiac diagnosis.

Echocardiography is the most frequently used cardiac-imaging modality

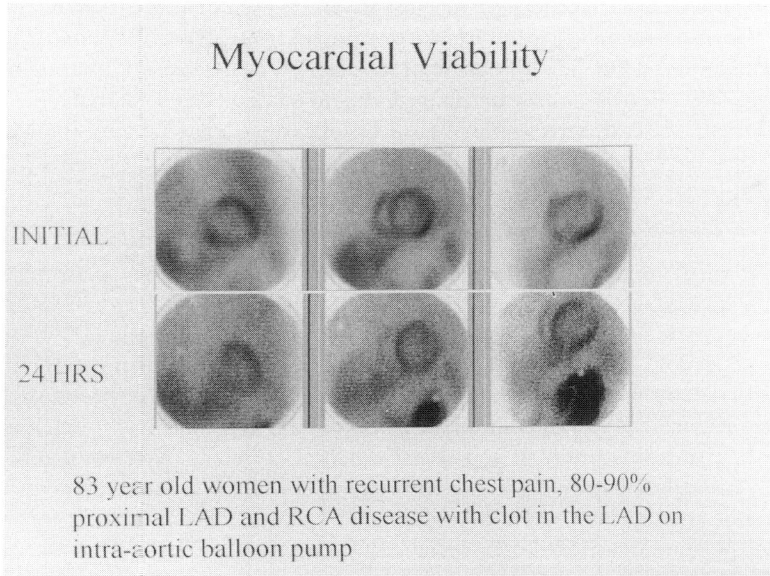

Figure 2 Planar perfusion images in a patient with severe coronary disease in the anterior view (left panels), LAO 45-degree view (center panels), and left lateral view (right panels). Note the change in the relative intensity of tracer concentration in the septum (best seen in the LAO view) from the initial to the 24-h images, indicating that the myocardium is viable. LAD = left anterior descending coronary artery. RCA = right coronary artery.

because the technology is almost ubiquitously available in inpatient and outpatient settings; is portable and can be applied at the bedside during acute episodes; is only moderately expensive and requires only a modicum of skill to perform; and is noninvasive, with no known significant complication rate. Over 3 million echocardiographic examinations are performed annually in the United States. It can very accurately evaluate aortic and mitral valve stenosis and insufficiency, left ventricular wall motion abnormalities, and pericardial effusion. Pulmonary artery pressure is reliably estimated (13) and the anatomical relationships in complex congenital anomalies are routinely deciphered.

Transesophageal echocardiography is more reliable in evaluating mitral valve morphology and function and detecting intracardiac shunts and aortic dissection, particularly when standard transthoracic echocardiography (TTE) is hindered by body habitus or emphysema. Considerable improvements in diagnostic accuracy were achieved with the introduction of biplane and multiplanar probes with mechanically driven annular array transducers. Echocardiography has limited application in coronary artery disease and is used mainly to detect regional wall motion abnormalities after exercise or pharmacological stress (dipyridamole or dobutamine) which identify areas of myocardial ischemia and infarction. The strength of echocardiography lies in its ability to qualitatively and, in many cases, to quantitatively assess the important aspects of cardiac anatomy, physiology, and pathology. New indications for echocardiography are expanding rapidly.

Ventricular Function

Evaluation of ventricular size and function is most commonly performed by echocardiography. Compared with x-ray angiography, echocardiography provides cross-sectional anatomical images that depict ventricular morphology and segmental function. Segmental wall function can be ascertained using a variety of pharmaceuticals to stress the heart by increasing the heart rate or decreasing peripheral resistance (vasodilatation), or by combining the echo study with a treadmill exercise test. Abnormal segmental function correlates well with ischemia, usually caused by narrowing of the coronary artery supplying that segment of the myocardium. Echocardiographic assessment of ventricular flow patterns provides a clinically noninvasive tool for evaluating diastolic dysfunction, an important cause of the symptoms of congestive heart failure, particularly in hypertensive hearts, in the absence of systolic dysfunction.

Valvular Morphology and Function

Detailed examination of valvular morphology and function requires high spatial (< 1 mm) and temporal resolution. Currently, echocardiography is the one method that is capable of achieving the necessary resolution in a real-time fashion to allow detailed interrogation of valvular and subvalvular structures. High-resolution real-time images are routinely obtained in the operating room for the repair of valvular lesions. Echocardiography is often the first and, frequently, the only assessment of valvular stenosis or regurgitation before a therapeutic intervention is entertained. Valvular regurgitation remains difficult to quantify and still represents a fertile area of research.

Myocardial Ischemia

The indications for stress echocardiography have steadily expanded since the introduction of exercise and pharmacological stress studies. Echocardiography has proved to be equivalent to other image-based stress studies, such as thallium perfusion scintigraphy, and also provides information on ventricular and valvular function that are important for evaluating the diseased heart. An important question to answer after coronary artery occlusion is whether the affected myocardium has the potential for function after revascularization by thrombolysis, angioplasty, or surgery. Echocardiography may have greater usefulness to predict the return of mechanical function than nuclear studies that are based on myocardial metabolism.

Aortic Disease

Transesophageal echocardiography is a sensitive and specific technique for the detection of acute and chronic dissections of the thoracic aorta. Because it is readily available and can be used in acutely ill patients, it is the primary modality for evaluating potential aortic dissection. It has some limitations compared with spiral computed tomography (CT) or magnetic resonance imaging (MRI) in detecting extension into the brachiocephalic vessels and in the infradiaphragmatic portions of the aorta. Dissecting hematoma, or intramural hemorrhage, is more easily appreciated on MR studies (14). Atheromatous disease of the aortic arch is related to the incidence of strokes, and screening of the aorta has been advocated for its potential predictive value.

Congenital Heart Disease

Transthoracic echocardiography is the method of choice for evaluating cardiac morphology and function in infants and children. Simple shunts and aortic anomalies are generally evaluated only with echocardiography before correction. The more complex anomalies may require catheterization and angiocardiography, particularly to evaluate structures that are difficult to visualize on an echo study, such as the central and hilar pulmonary arteries, the pulmonary veins, and the systemic venous drainage.

E. Computed Tomography

Godfrey Hounsfield and Allan Cormack received the Nobel Prize in Physiology and Medicine in 1979 for their contributions to the development of computed tomography (CT) (15,16). An English company, EMI Ltd., was the first to introduce CT to diagnostic medicine in 1973. Although the earliest images took several minutes to generate, and the spatial resolution was considerably poorer than film-screen radiography, rapid technological advances during the past 25 years have established CT as a major diagnostic tool for noninvasive evaluation of most body parts. CT technology has continued to advance and currently enjoys wide popularity for the evaluation of the pericardium and the aorta (see Chaps. 18 and 20). Spiral CT technology is a recent development that has extended the usefulness of CT for studies of the aorta (17). Because of the continuous, unalterable motion of the heart, electron beam CT (EBCT or ultrafast CT; 18), with exposure times in the 50–100 ms range, has become the primary CT device for cardiac imaging. It has been used, primarily, to detect coronary artery calcification, which is a marker for coronary atherosclerosis (see Chap. 17). Epidemiological studies (19) suggest that the absence of coronary calcium indicates a low probability of significant coronary artery narrowing and for subsequent cardiac events. There is an increase in calcium with age and after menopause. A relatively linear relation exists between increasing calcium scores and severity of coronary artery disease, although it is not site-specific in identifying flow-limiting coronary lesions. EBCT detection of coronary artery calcification is a non–exercise-dependent test, with a high sensitivity for predicting the presence of obstructive coronary artery disease, particularly in younger patients and when present in multiple vessels. Because EBCT technology is available in relatively few centers in the United States, it has not enjoyed wide use as a clinical-imaging modality.

F. Magnetic Resonance Imaging

Lauterbur, in 1973, described image formation using the differential response of protons and chemical structures in high magnetic fields when stimulated with radiofrequency waves (20). Bloch and Purcell had received the Nobel Prize in Physics in 1952 for their description of this property; nuclear magnetic resonance (21,22). Magnetic resonance imaging (MRI) was introduced into clinical practice in 1981, largely for the study of the central nervous system. However, its potential for cardiac imaging was recognized, awaiting the introduction of technical developments in both hardware and software.

Currently, MRI is the medium of choice for evaluating disease of the thoracic aorta (see Chap. 20). MRI studies of cardiac anatomy, particularly in congenital malformations (see Chap. 19), three-dimensional morphology, motion, functional parameters, and myocardial perfusion measurements have also become routine in many centers; however, only a small number of physicians with sufficient knowledge of the technology and cardiac pathology, morphology, and physiology have active clinical cardiac-imaging services. Newer advances promise to further exploit this noninvasive technology to obtain unique diagnostic information. Techniques for imaging the heart vary from institution to institution and even from magnet to magnet. In general, gated T1-weighted spin-echo imaging is used for morphological imaging, usually obtained in the coronal and axial planes, with sagittal and oblique planes optional. T2-weighted images are generally used only when assessing for neoplasm, infection, adenopathy, or ischemia. In these situations, administration of gadolinium with fat-suppressed T1-weighted images, may also be helpful.

Cine, gradient-echo, and velocity-encoded, phase-contrast images are helpful to evaluate flow and to distinguish slow flow from a thrombus. These techniques are also indispensable for functional cardiac assessment; for example, measuring cardiac output, shunt flow, regurgitant volumes, ventricular volumes, and ejection fractions.

Specific indications for cardiovascular MRI include the study of pericardial (see Chap. 18 for a detailed discussion) and valvular disease, the assessment of aortic dissection and aneurysms (see Chap. 20), characterization of certain types of myocardial disease, the identification of specific mediastinal vessels, such as the central pulmonary arteries, and both systemic and pulmonary venous structures in congenital heart disease (see also Chap. 19), and the identification and characterization of cardiac tumors. Brief descriptions of these entities follow.

Pericardial Disease

The pericardium consists of a fibrous outer (parietal) and a thick inner (visceral) membrane. The pericardial space exists between these two layers and normally contains 20–60 ml of fluid. Normal (parietal) pericardium appears as a relatively thin, uniform band of low-signal intensity, 1–3 mm thickness.

MRI can detect the presence of as little as 30 ml of pericardial fluid. Clear pericardial fluid demonstrates low T1 signal intensity. Hemorrhagic effusions may display increased T1 signal because of the presence of reduced hemoglobin, although cardiac contraction will often create sufficient motion of a hemorrhagic effusion to produce low-signal intensity of the fluid. Inflammatory exudates with high protein or cellular content also produce an increased T1 signal.

Acute pericarditis may demonstrate a thickened pericardium (4 mm or greater) of increased signal intensity. The pericardium may thicken to the point of impeding ventricular diastolic filling or may fibrose, resulting in constrictive pericarditis. This condition is clinically difficult to distinguish from restrictive cardiomyopathy (23). MRI is of benefit in distinguishing between the two by delineating the presence of a thickened or nodular pericardium, which favors the diagnosis of constrictive pericarditis.

Aortic Disease

There have been numerous studies describing the efficacy of MRI in the diagnosis of aortic dissection (24). Spin-echo images demonstrate an intimal flap, identified as a thin line of intermediate signal intensity within the signal void of the aorta, separating true from false lumen. Detection of the intimal flap and false lumen may be difficult if the tear is small. The distinction between slow flow and mural thrombus on spin-echo images may be problematic, because both produce a higher signal than flowing blood. Cine phase-contrast images can be very helpful in distinguishing thrombus from slow flow because slow flow will produce a signal and mural thrombus will not. In addition, the signal is direction-sensitive, with flow in the cranial direction typically depicted in black and flow in the caudal direction in white.

MRI can also identify some of the complications of aortic dissection, such as pericardial, pleural, or mediastinal hemorrhage, as well as aortic insufficiency. Aortic ulceration, intramural hematomas, and false aneurysms of the aorta can be elucidated with the combination of spin-echo imaging in transverse and sagittal planes and phase-contrast imaging to depict flow or hematomas.

Ischemic Heart Disease

T2-weighted, gated spin-echo images have demonstrated regions of increased signal intensity corresponding to acutely infarcted myocardium. The increase in signal is thought to be a result of an increase in the water content of the tissue, as well as an increase in the ratio of free to bound water in infarcted myocardium (25). Care must be taken in defining the region of increased T2 signal, as motion artifacts may result in a heterogeneous myocardial signal. Volume averaging of myocardium with adjacent epicardial fat may also result in a region of myocardium demonstrating spuriously increased T2 signal. Cine, as well as segmented breath-held gradient-echo techniques, can demonstrate wall motion abnormalities and thinning of the infarcted segment in both the acute and chronic settings (Fig. 3).

Although MRI has limited current clinical use in the setting of ischemic heart disease, ongoing research investigation with fast-imaging techniques, such as echo-planar imaging and segmented breath-held gradient imaging, in combination with new MRI contrast agents and pharmacological stress, may, in the future, offer accurate assessment of residual, viable myocardium and regional myocardial perfusion.

Cardiomyopathy

The cardiomyopathies are generally divided into dilated, restrictive, and hypertrophic categories. The primary modality for evaluation of cardiomyopathy is echocardiography and, although data on the use of MR in the assessment of the various cardiomyopathies are continuing to grow, hypertrophic cardiomyopathy (HCM) and the unusual entity called arrhythmogenic right ventricular dysplasia (ARVD) have received the greatest attention.

MRI can accurately depict the severity, extent, and specific location of myocardial hypertrophy in patients with HCM (Fig. 4). Although myocardial hypertrophy affects primarily the interventricular septum, only a portion of the septum or only the LV apex may be involved. MRI can also be used to assess wall thickness and muscle mass as well as the presence and severity of LV outflow tract obstruction or mitral valve regurgitation, which is frequently associated with this disease (26). In addition, the diastolic restriction or loss of diastolic compliance, which is a cardinal feature of HCM, has been studied using cine MRI techniques (27).

Arrhythmogenic right ventricular dysplasia (ARVD) is a condition in which the right ventricle is focally or completely replaced with fatty or fibrous tissue (Fig. 5). This is associated with ventricular tachycardia, originating from the right

Advances in Cardiac Imaging

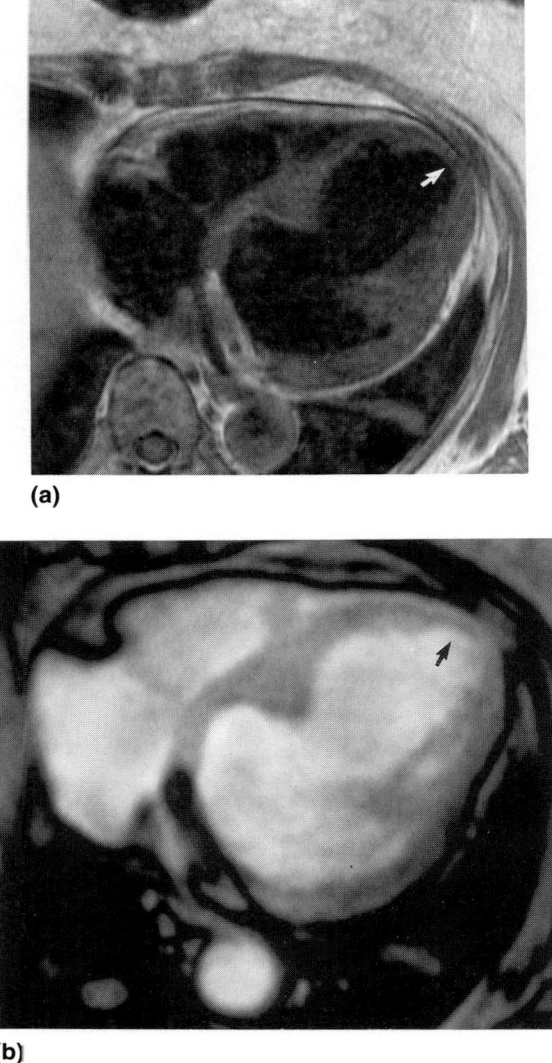

(a)

(b)

Figure 3 Spin-echo image in a 70-year-old woman with an anterior and apical myocardial infarction. Thinning of the apical myocardium (arrow) extends to involve the septum. The lateral wall myocardium is normal. (b) Gradient echo (cine) study showed that the apical portion of the ventricle (arrow) bulged outward during systole, indicating the presence of an aneurysm.

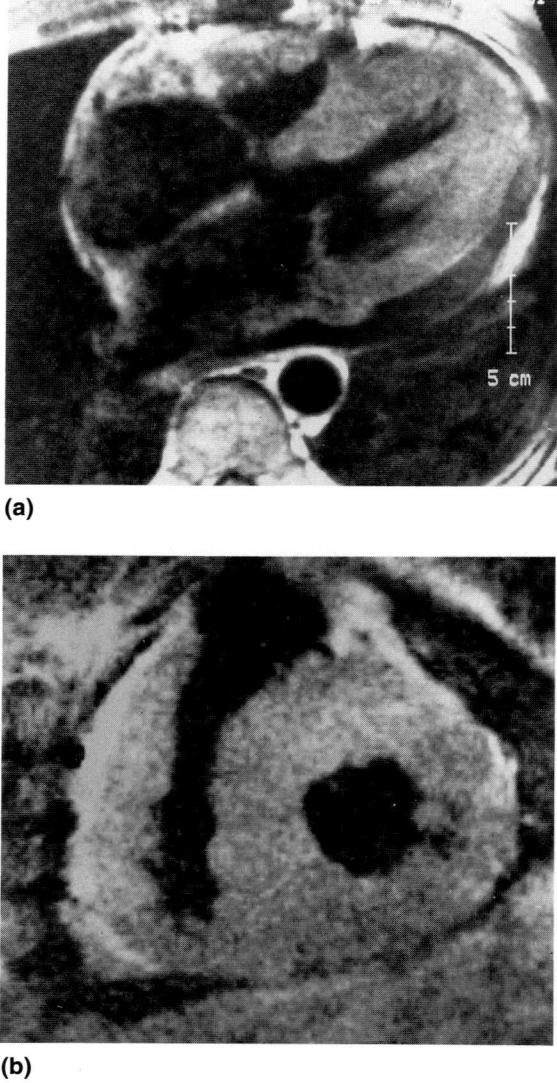

Figure 4 Hypertrophic cardiomyopathy. (a) Transverse image depicts marked symmetrical thickening of the left ventricular myocardium. Both right and left ventricular chambers are small. (b) Oblique sagittal slice in the left anterior oblique at the level of the right ventricular outflow tract shows symmetrical hypertrophy that also involves the right ventricular free wall.

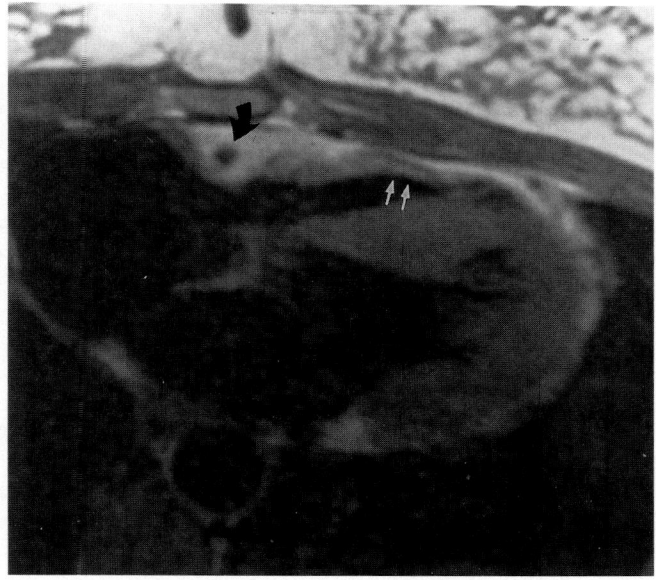

Figure 5 Arrhythmogenic right ventricular dysplasia. Fatty replacement of the right ventricular myocardium is seen as a thin white line (arrows) beneath the epicardial fat. The epicardial fat extends into the atrio-ventricular groove to surround the right coronary artery (curved arrow).

ventricle. Because of MRI's ability to distinguish fat from myocardium, it has been proposed that MRI may be the imaging modality of choice in the diagnosis of ARVD (28). In addition, cine—gradient-echo techniques can demonstrate wall motion abnormalities of the right ventricle associated with the fibrofatty replacement of myocardium (29).

Valvular Disease

The assessment of valvular disease by MRI has been aided greatly by the advent of cine–gradient-echo and phase–contrast-imaging techniques. These methods allow a semiquantitative measurement of valvular stenosis or insufficiency when viewed in a cine mode, as well as an accurate and reproducible quantitative assessment of stenosis and regurgitation when using phase-contrast velocity data (30). Nevertheless, echocardiography, with Doppler flow measurements, remains the modality of choice for the study of valvular disease.

The MR studies of valvular stenoses (31) demonstrate a triangular zone of signal loss distal to the diseased valve as a result of turbulent flow caused by the stenotic lesion. Because of MRI's ability to calculate peak velocities across the valve, a transvalvular pressure gradient can be calculated using a modified Bernoulli equation: $\Delta P = 4V^2$ (ΔP = pressure gradient in mmHg (torr), and V = velocity in mm/s).

Valvular insufficiency results in a similar triangular region or cloud of signal loss proximal to the diseased valve. A quantitative measurement of regurgitation can be applied to any valve if isolated valvular insufficiency is present. Aortic insufficiency would be measured from velocity-encoded phase-contrast images of the ascending aorta, for example, by calculating the forward and backward components of flow during the cardiac cycle (32). Normally, there is only a small component of backward flow into the coronary arteries.

Cardiac Tumors

Cardiac tumors are rare entities. Metastatic disease to the heart is found at autopsy 20–40 times more commonly than primary cardiac tumors. MRI is helpful in assessing cardiac tumors, because it provides an accurate definition of the tumor location, size, and its relation to important structures, such as the pericardium bronchi, cardiac valves, great vessels, and the coronary arteries and veins (Figs. 6, 7).

In general, the signal characteristics and morphology of malignant primary and secondary cardiac tumors are nonspecific. Most tumors demonstrate low T1 and increased T2 signal relative to normal myocardium. Most malignant tumors also demonstrate enhancement with gadolinium (33) (Fig. 8), with no identifiable tissue-specific enhancement pattern, although vascular metastases and primary vascular tumors, such as angiosarcoma, may demonstrate more pronounced enhancement. The most common primary sources for metastatic disease to the heart and pericardium include lung carcinoma, breast carcinoma, lymphoma, malignant melanoma, and leukemia.

Atrial myxoma is the most common benign primary cardiac tumor most frequently found in the left atrium, arising from the interventricular septum or posterior left atrial wall. It may be difficult to distinguish myxoma from clot, based on MR signal intensity and morphology. The administration of gadolinium has been advocated in this situation, because tumor enhances and clot does not.

Cardiac lipomas and lipomatous hypertrophy of the atrial septum (Fig. 9) are conditions that can greatly benefit from MRI's ability to define fatty elements (29). T1-weighted images, in which fat demonstrates increased signal, as well as fat suppression techniques, such as chemical saturation, inversion recovery, and 2- or 3- point Dixon techniques, can be used to further define the fatty content of a lesion.

Congenital Heart Disease

The role of MRI in the evaluation of congenital heart disease continues to evolve as newer MRI technologies are developed. Chapter 19 discusses imaging of adult

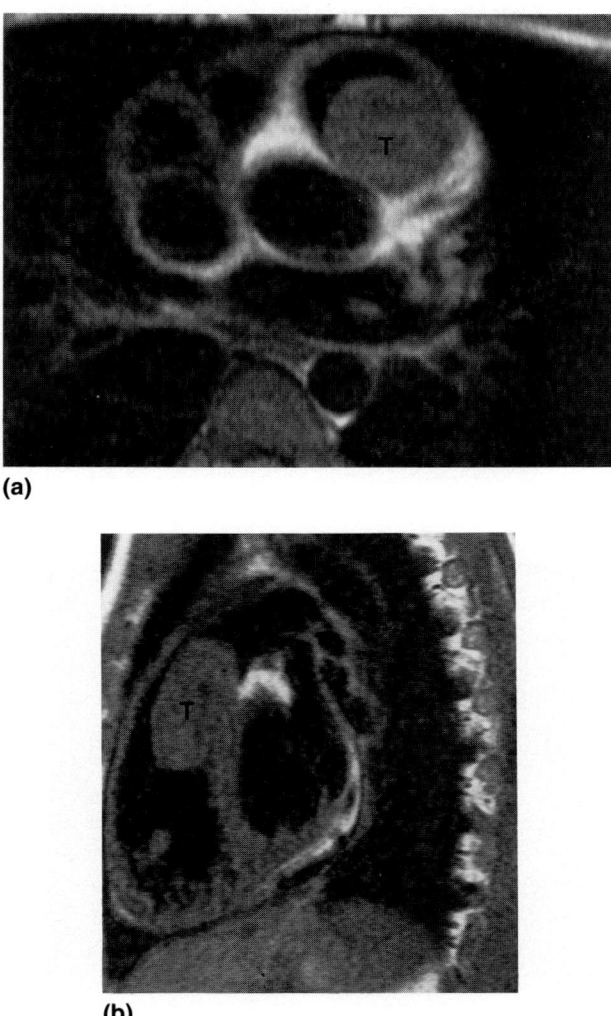

Figure 6 Twenty-two-year-old woman who presented with fatigue, chest pain, and mild exertional dyspnea. Echocardiography suggested pulmonary stenosis. (a) Transverse spin-echo image depicts tumor mass (T) partially obstructing the right ventricular outflow tract. (b) Sagittal image shows dilated right ventricle with tumor (T) attached to the septum almost completely obstructing the outflow tract below the level of the pulmonary valve. A fibrohistiocytic neoplasm of low-grade malignancy was removed.

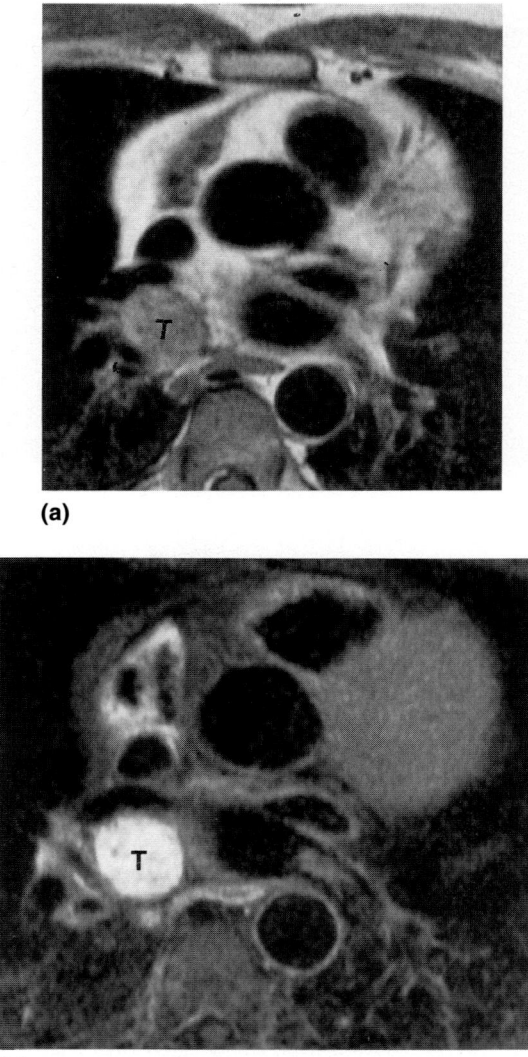

Figure 7 Forty-nine-year-old man with history of carotid body tumor removed in the past. Abnormality seen on CT scan. (a) Transverse spin-echo image shows medium signal in mass (T) located posterior to the left atrium and pulmonary vein. (b) Post-gadolinium T_1-weighted fat saturated image shows high signal in mass (T) which is separate from the heart. An extracardiac paraganglioma was removed.

congenital heart disease in detail. Echocardiography and cardiac angiography are the primary-imaging modalities for congenital heart defects. MRI is used when these modalities fail to provide adequate definition of complex cardiac chamber and great vessel anatomy. MRI's larger field-of-view and multiplanar capability provides some advantage here. Recent work suggests that MRI may be the modality of choice in the evaluation of anomalous pulmonary venous return and for the central pulmonary vessels (34). Potential uses include assessment of surgically corrected shunts and conduits and pre- and postsurgical assessment of right and left ventricular function.

III. Recent Advances and Potential Applications of Newer Imaging Modalities

A. Radionuclide Cardiac Imaging

Technical Enhancements

Function and Perfusion

The technetium-labeled perfusion agents can be administered in doses of 10–30 mCi/injection. The resultant photon flux is sufficient to permit recording high-quality, first-pass studies. Data are recorded at the time of radiopharmaceutical administration, usually in the anterior view, at 25–50 msec/frame for about 1 min (35). When patients are injected while exercising on a treadmill or bicycle, motion correction should be used to optimize data analysis. Right and left ventricular ejection fraction and regional wall motion can be assessed from these data. This information serves as a cross-check on the perfusion data recorded on subsequent planar and tomographic acquisitions.

Regional Wall Thickening

Technetium Tc^{99m} sestamibi and technetium Tc^{99m} tetrofosmin have relatively long half-lives in the myocardium, allowing SPECT perfusion data to be recorded with gating to evaluate regional thickening. Thickening can separate attenuation artifacts from ischemia and helps differentiate ischemic myocardium from scar (36). This information is particularly powerful when combined with first-pass data obtained at the peak of stress, because transient ischemia produces a change in regional and global function from the stress-injected study to the gated perfusion scan (usually recorded 15–30 min later).

Gated myocardial perfusion data usually divide the cardiac cycle into 8 frames (rather than the minimum of 16 frames usually employed for blood pool imaging). Although 16 frames can be recorded for each cycle at each detector position, the volume of data lengthens reconstruction time and does not add materially to the quality of the resultant information. Because the goal of gated perfusion imaging is to define thickening of each segment, 8 frames per cycle are

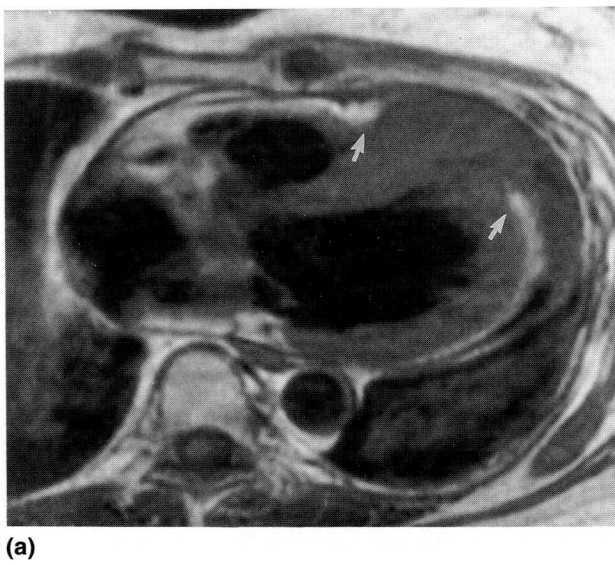

(a)

Figure 8 Forty-five-year-old woman with a primary cardiac sarcoma. (a) Standard spin-echo image with disruption of the pericardium (arrows) and tissue extending into the pericardial sac. A small pericardial effusion is present. (b) Second echo image distinguishes between normal myocardium and tumor, which has an slightly increased signal. (c) Gadolinium enhanced scan clearly depicts the increased signal in the tumor which extends through the pericardium into the pericardial sac.

sufficient. The low temporal resolution means that end-systole will not be properly sampled and ejection fraction will be underestimated. In addition, definition of the endocardial borders is relatively poor, compared with that obtained with blood pool imaging. In spite of these limitations, these studies allow categorization of ventricular function into good, impaired, and poor.

Regional thickening is estimated from regional change in myocardial counts during the cardiac cycle. SPECT resolution is insufficient to depict true wall thickness; but even with this poor resolution, a change in thickness is reflected as a change in regional counts (37). Viewing the tomographic cine sequence of multiple slices on the screen provides additional information about ischemia and attenuation. An ischemic area has a decrease in regional count density on the diastolic images, but has a relative increase in counts during systole that is similar to the adjacent functioning tissue. When the rest data are reviewed in a similar fashion, the zone has a normal (or near-normal) distribution of activity and a comparable increase in counts during systole. A zone of attenuation will appear to have decreased counts on both sets of images with normal thickening.

Advances in Cardiac Imaging 589

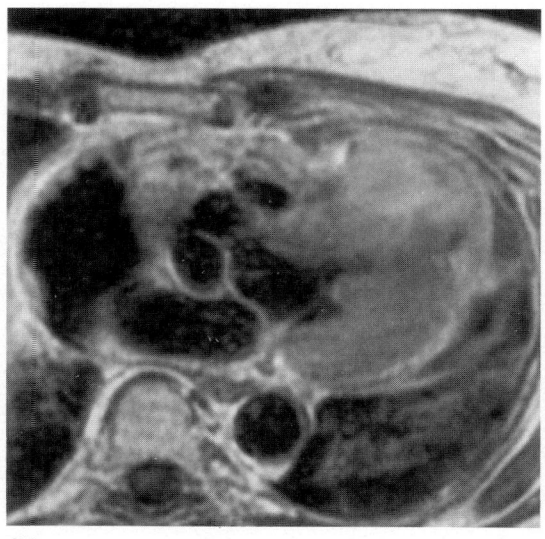

(b)

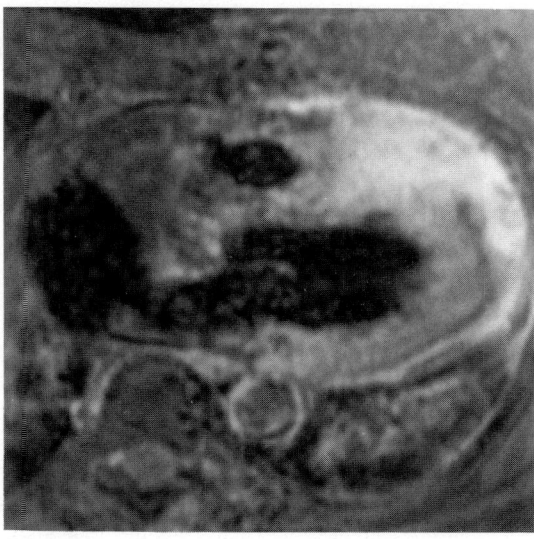

(c)

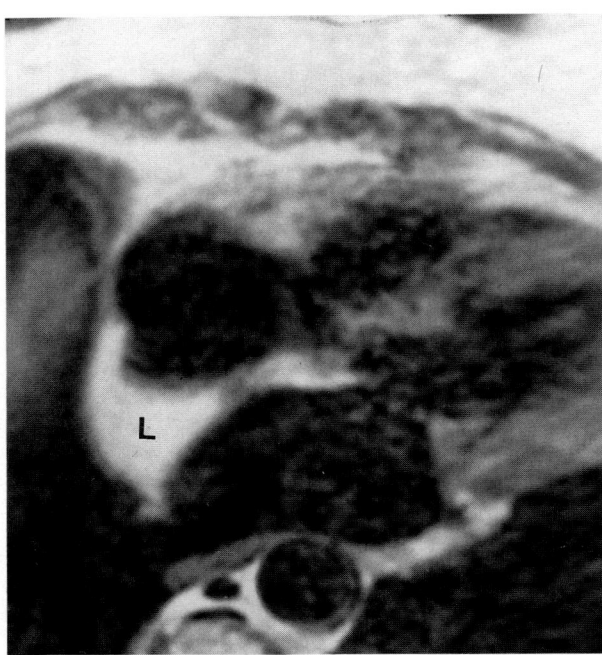

Figure 9 Lipoma of the atrial septum (L). This accumulation of fat in the septum is benign, but may simulate a tumor on echocardiography. Fat suppression causes a decrease in signal similar to that of the epicardial fat and breast tissue.

Selecting the Perfusion Agent

Selecting the most appropriate radiopharmaceutical for perfusion imaging can also be challenging. Four agents with markedly different imaging properties are approved for single photon imaging. Thallium 201(^{201}Tl) has the best-defined properties and is considered to be the most sensitive of the single-photon agents for identifying ischemic viable tissue in patients with severe ventricular dysfunction (38). Of the technetium agents, teboroxime (39,40) has remarkably different properties than sestamibi or tetrofosmin. Teboroxime has the highest myocardial extraction of the technetium-labeled perfusion agents, but also the most rapid clearance. Images of regional perfusion must be recorded within 5 min of administration to identify the regional distribution of perfusion. Although this is challenging to accomplish, the high contrast between ischemic and normally perfused areas makes this agent extremely useful for detecting coronary disease. Recent studies suggest that recording data during the 5- to 20-min–poststress injection clearance phase will allow detection of ischemic areas from a single injection of this tracer (41). Although this approach is intriguing, few investigators routinely employ teboroxime because of the major logistical changes required from the typical practice employed for thallium imaging.

Sestamibi (^{99m}Tc-MIBI) has substantial myocardial retention, which allows useful images to be recorded within the first hour after injection. One potential problem with sestamibi imaging is the relative insensitivity of this agent for the differentiation of ischemic myocardium from scar in patients with very severe coronary artery disease. This problem can be reduced by administering a short- or long-acting nitroglycerin preparation before MIBI administration (42). Tetrofosmin, the newest tracer approved for perfusion imaging, seems to share many of the properties of MIBI but has the advantage of lower liver uptake immediately after administration.

To take full advantage of perfusion imaging, a combination of the redistribution properties of thallium and the high photon flux of the technetium agents is desirable. If thallium is used for the rest-injected portion of the study and MIBI for the stress, this can be accomplished (43). Dual-tracer imaging allows more flexibility in patient scheduling and permits the entire examination to be completed within 3 hr. Typically, thallium data are recorded immediately after the rest injection and ^{99m}Tc immediately after the stress injection. If patients weigh less than 82 kg (180 lb), and the dose of MIBI or tetrofosmin is 10 mCi and thallium 3 mCi, both thallium and the technetium tracer can be imaged simultaneously. As a result, a more precise assessment of the extent of ischemia is possible. In heavier patients, the attenuation and scatter of the 80-keV x-ray from thallium, superimposed on the scatter from technetium, make the thallium image recorded in this fashion very difficult to interpret. The technetium data can be recorded as a combined first-pass and gated perfusion scan to maximize the value of the perfusion examination. If review of the data raises a question about viability, delayed redistribution images of the thallium distribution can be recorded at 24 hr. At that time, the residual amount of technetium in the myocardium will be less than 5% of the administered dose, whereas the residual amount of thallium will be approximately 25% of the administered dose.

Opportunities on the Horizon

Specific Markers of Hypoxia and Necrosis

Two new agents under development may add substantially to the value of perfusion imaging. One, the technetium nitroimidazole markers of hypoxia (44), identify ischemic but viable myocardium. The other, ^{99m}Tc-glucarate, localizes specifically in acutely necrotic (less than 10 hr old) myocardium (45). If the preclinical studies with the nitroimidazole and the early human studies with glucarate are borne out in larger clinical trials, these agents will provide markers for key decisions in the management of patients with acute coronary syndromes.

Potential clinical applications of these agents include evaluation of patients following revascularization or after the administration of drugs designed to decrease the extent of ischemia or necrosis. Glucarate imaging may be particularly useful in the emergency room when patients are seen with acute chest pain syndromes. When the etiology of chest pain is unclear, the agent could be administered and images recorded 2–3 hr later. Focal localization provides a definitive answer to the question of whether myocyte necrosis is present and additional information about the site and extent of the lesion within a few hours of onset of symptoms. Thus, this imaging procedure may result in a substantial reduction in the number of patients hospitalized to rule out infarction.

Direct Clot Imaging

Several technetium 99m-labeled peptides directed against the GpIIb/IIIa receptor expressed on activated platelets have been tested in animal models. These agents localize well in zones of preformed clots in experimental animals. In preliminary human studies, one of these agents demonstrates definite localization in venous thrombi and possibly in pulmonary emboli. A potential application of these agents in patients with coronary disease is the detection of residual clot in the coronary arteries following thrombolysis (46,47).

B. Echocardiography

Detection of Embolic Source

The indications for echocardiography continue to expand. Although the heart is seemingly remote from the brain, several potential causes of stroke can be identified using echocardiography. Emboli can originate either from atheromatous plaques in the aorta (48) or from the left atrium (49,50), mitral valve (51), or left ventricle (52). Cardiac arrhythmias are commonly associated with stroke (53).

Intervention Guidance

Echocardiography has long been used in the operating room during surgery to monitor cardiac function. More recently, the availability of expertise in transesophageal and intravascular ultrasound has greatly expanded the use of image-guided therapy in a variety of settings, particularly catheter-based techniques to ablate aberrrant electrical pathways that cause arrhythmias (54,55) and during percutaneous transluminal coronary angioplasty (56) and stent placement (57).

Flow and Volumetric Quantification

Each new technical development in echocardiography has led to new applications. The ability to depict anatomy and function has progressed from M-mode graphic displays, through two-dimensional representations in a variety of projections, to transesophageal devices that improve the acoustic window and, hence, the resolution of structures deep within the chest. Most recently, three-dimensional volumetric assessment of ventricular function (58), valvular regurgitation, and ventricular mass (59), and the complex congenital cardiac malformations (60,61), promise to improve the visualization of cardiac morphology and pathology.

Research packages endowed with three-dimensional acquisition and analysis tools are now available on commercial machines. Animal studies show that these approaches offer a high degree of quantitative accuracy (62,63). Flow quantitation appears highly reproducible, and several techniques are currently undergoing extensive clinical testing (64–66).

Contrast Echocardiography

Distinguishing among the various tissues of the heart has been a major goal of echocardiography. If viable myocardium could be separated from nonviable myocardium, or if a sarcoma of the myocardium could be separated from normal myocardium based on a characteristic echo signal, then echocardiography would provide a noninvasive approach to the myocardium, similar to that provided by ultrasound in the abdomen. However, this potential has not been realized, and attention has been directed to a variety of echocardiographic contrast agents that might enhance the differentiation of tissue (67,68). A major obstacle to the success of these agents is that they lose their properties during passage through the lungs when delivered by intravenous injection. Newer agents that provide improved integrity during transpulmonary passage offer the promise of expanded application and indications (69–71). Their highly nonlinear acoustic properties have made feasible the use of second-harmonic–imaging studies that isolate the blood pool more clearly and may result in improved coronary artery visualization (72,73).

Further developments in image quality that will enhance the diagnostic value of echocardiography and its potential applications are likely based in new transducer technology and image-processing techniques. The development of less expensive and more portable ultrasound-imaging systems will empower primary care physicians to perform ultrasound diagnostics, a phenomenon that has already begun in Germany and Japan, and is likely to result in more widespread application of echocardiography in patient management.

C. Spiral Computed Tomography

Recent advances in CT technology permit continuous volume acquisition of axial sections with reconstruction in both the traditional transverse plane and in various three-dimensional formats, including surface rendering, maximum intensity projections, and curved planar reconstructions. With these techniques the thoracic aorta and its branches have been imaged with information that is comparable with, and in some cases, superior to, that obtained by angiography. Further manipulation of the three-dimensional data sets affords "fly-through" perspectives similar to those obtained at endoscopy. This "virtual endoscopy" has been applied to the aorta and tracheobronchial tree and may have a future role in exploring intracardiac anatomy, particularly to define the relations of the great vessels to the ventricles and the inflow pathways in complex congenital cardiac anomalies.

D. Electron Beam Computed Tomography

Three-dimensional reconstruction techniques have also been applied to images obtained with electron beam (EB) technology, using a continuous acquisition mode with the patient moving through the gantry. Preliminary results show that the coronary arteries can be visualized in considerable detail with a surface-rendering technique (74). Clinical studies to demonstrate the sensitivity and specificity of this approach are in progress. Physiological studies using pharmacological stress can produce images of the beating heart with excellent definition of areas of wall motion abnormality and differential wall thickening. These studies are comparable or better than those obtained using radionuclear or echocardiographic techniques. Attempts to define myocardial blood flow after intravenous contrast injection have been frustrated by beam-hardening artifacts caused by the adjacent contrast pool in the left ventricle.

E. Magnetic Resonance Imaging

Studies of Myocardial Motion

Myocardial motion analysis with MRI is a relatively new, unique noninvasive method initially introduced by Zerhouni et al. (75). The technique of myocardial tagging and its subsequent modifications involve placing multiple squares during diastole in a grid-like pattern across the myocardium. Assessment of the motion of these "tagged" segments during the cardiac cycle permits evaluation of myocardial wall thickening and dynamics (76). Regional myocardial strain can be estimated by measuring the fractional change in the length of the tagged segments during systole (77).

Phase velocity mapping is an alternative approach for assessing circumferential shortening and myocardial strain (78). This technique takes advantage of phase shifts, related to motion, that can be used to determine myocardial velocities at sequential points and specific phases during the cardiac cycle.

Myocardial Infarct Sizing

The identification and quantification of myocardial infarct size has been extensively investigated using gadolinium-enhanced spin-echo MRI (79–81). These studies report good correlation with enzymatic indices and histochemical staining for the area of myocardial necrosis. This technique, combined with assessment of myocardial motion, may prove useful for evaluating ventricular function and myocardial viability in the region of the infarct.

Estimation of Oxygen Saturation

A preliminary report in 1991 suggested the possibility that the oxygen saturation of human blood (%HbO$_2$) could be measured *in vivo* (82). With use of specially modified sequences, the T2 of blood varies predictably from about 30 to 250 msec as %HbO$_2$ varied from 30 to 96%. Although this concept has been applied to measuring changes in the oxygen saturation of visceral arteries in a variety of circumstances (83), it has not been systematically applied to measuring oxygen saturation in the various cardiac chambers and central vessels, or for determining intracardiac shunts or other cardiac abnormalities.

Coronary Artery Visualization

The development of ultrafast-echo gradient techniques and "K"-space segmentation has permitted the morphological assessment of coronary arteries by MRI. This topic will be extensively covered in Chapter 18. Although considerable interest and excitement was generated by the early descriptions of coronary artery visualization using MR techniques (84), the current status suggests that the technique is still incapable of accurately guiding treatment decisions or defining accurately the extent of coronary atherosclerosis (85).

Functional Imaging of the Coronary Arteries

The MR flow quantification of coronary arteries is also a field with potential future applications. Breath-hold techniques, with time of flight, and phase contrast cine MRI have both been used (86,87) to quantify flow in the left anterior descending artery (LAD). A recent study (88) has suggested that these techniques can be used to assess coronary flow reserve when coronary flow velocity measurements are assessed pre- and postintravenous dipyridamole administration. This information may be used noninvasively to assess for the presence of a significant stenotic lesion within the LAD.

IV. Conclusion

Cardiac imaging consists of many modalities, including radiography and fluorography of the chest, angiocardiography, radionuclide cardiography, echocardiography, computed tomography, and magnetic resonance imaging. Sophisticated cardiac imaging underlies the modern advances in interventional cardiology and cardiac surgery. Exquisite depiction of cardiac morphology and the changes that occur during the cardiac cycle or after stress is performed daily, not only in catheterization laboratories, but at the bedside and in office practices. An understanding of disease processes and the relation between symptoms, pathological anatomy, and pathophysiology; and the ability to predict outcome and to develop treatment strategies, are greatly enhanced by modern cardiac imaging. In the near future, technical improvements that are under study promise to propel noninvasive imaging even farther and to provide precise tissue morphology and metabolic functional data that likely will create opportunities for therapeutic advances heretofore unrecognized.

References

1. Williams FH. A method for more fully determining the outline of the heart by means of the fluoroscope together with other uses of this instrument in medicine. Boston Med Surg J 1896; 135:335–337.
2. Abrams HL. History of Cardiac Radiology. AJR 1996; 167:431–438.
3. Kostuk WJ, Barr JW, Simon AL, et al. Correlation between the chest film and hemodynamics in acute myocardial infarction. Circulation 1973; 48:624.
4. Milne ENC. Physiological interpretation of the plain radiograph in mitral stenosis, including a review of criteria for the radiological estimation of pulmonary arterial and venous pressures. Br J Radiol 1963; 36:902.
5. Milne ENC. A physiological approach to reading critical care unit films. J Thorac Imaging 1986; 1:60.
6. Castellanos A, Pereiras R, Garcia A, et al. On the factors intervening in the obtention of perfect angiocardiograms. Bol Soc Cubana Pediatr 1938; 10:217.
7. Berman DS, Mason DT. Introduction to clinical nuclear cardiology. In: Berman DS, Mason DT, eds. Clinical Nuclear Cardiology. New York: Grune & Stratton, 1981:1–27.
8. Gerson MC. Cardiac Nuclear Medicine, 2nd ed. New York: McGraw-Hill, 1991.
9. Keidel WD. Uber eine neue Methode zur Registrierung der Voluman-derungen des Herzen am Menschen. Kreisl-Forschung 1950; 39:257–271.
10. Edler I, Hertz CH. The use of ultrasonic reflectoscope for the continuous recording of movement of heart walls. Kungl Fysiogr Sallski Fund Forhandl 1954; 24:40–45.
11. Feigenbaum H, Waldhausen JA, Hyde PP. Ultrasound diagnosis of pericardial effusion. JAMA 1965; 191:711–714.
12. Joyner CR, Reid JM, Bond JP. Reflected ultrasound in the assessment of mitral valve disease. Circulation 1963; 27:503–509.
13. Courtois M, Fattal PG, Kovacs SJJ, et al. Anatomically and physiologically based reference level for measurement of intracardiac pressures. Circulation 1995; 92:1994–2000.
14. Nienaber CA, von Kodolitsch Y, Petersen B, et al. Intramural hemorrhage of the thoracic aorta. Diagnostic and therapeutic implications. Circulation 1995; 92:1465–1472.
15. Hounsfield GN. A method of an apparatus for examination of the body by radiation such as X or gamma radiation. British patent 1283915. United Kingdom: 1972.

16. Cormack AM. Representation of a function by its line integrals with some radiological applications. J Appl Physiol 1963; 34:2722.
17. Rubin GD, Beaulieu CF, Argiro V, et al. Perspective volume rendering of CT and MR images: applications for endoscopic imaging. Radiology 1996; 199:321–330.
18. Boyd DP, Gould RG, Quinn JR, et al. A proposed dynamic cardiac 3-D densitometer for early detection and evaluation of heart disease. IEEE Trans Nucl Sci 1979; 26: 2724–2727.
19. Detrano R, Hsai T, Wang S, et al. Prognostic value of coronary calcification and angiographic stenosis in patients undergoing coronary arteriography. J Am Coll Cardiol 1996; 27:285–290.
20. Lauterbur PC. Image formation by induced local interactions: examples employ nuclear magnetic resonance. Nature 1973; 242:190–191.
21. Bloch FR, Hansen WW, Packard ME. Nuclear induction. Phys Rev 1946; 69:127.
22. Purcell EM, Torrey HC, Pound RV. Resonance absorption by nuclear magnetic moments in a solid. Phys Rev 1946; 69:37–38.
23. Masui T, Finck S, Higgins CB. Constrictive pericarditis and restrictive cardiomyopathy: evaluation with MR imaging. Radiology 1992; 182:369–373.
24. Nienaber CA, Spielman RP, von Kodolitsch Y, et al. Diagnosis of thoracic aortic dissection. Magnetic resonance imaging versus transesophageal echocardiography. Circulation 1992; 85:434–447.
25. Fisher MR, McNamara MT, Higgins CB. Acute myocardial infarction: MR evaluation in 29 patients. AJR 1987; 148:247–251.
26. Park JH, Kim YM, Chung JW, et al. MR imaging of hypertrophic cardiomyopathy. Radiology 1992; 185:441–446.
27. Suzuki J, Chang JM, Caputo GR, et al. Evaluation of right ventricular early diastolic filling by cine nuclear magnetic resonance imaging in patients with hypertrophic cardiomyopathy. J Am Coll Cardiol 1991; 18:120–126.
28. Auffermann W, Wichter T, Breithardt G, et al. Arrhythmogenic right ventricular disease: MR imaging vs angiography. AJR 1993; 161:549–555.
29. Kriegshauser JS, Julsrud PR, Lund JT. MR imaging of fat in and around the heart. AJR 1990; 155:271–274.
30. Fujita N, Chazouilleres AF, Hartiala JJ, et al. Quantification of mitral regurgitation by velocity-encoded cine nuclear magnetic resonance imaging. J Am Coll Cardiol 1994; 23:951–958.
31. Kilner PJ, Manzara CC, Mohiaddin RH, et al. Magnetic resonance jet velocity mapping in mitral and aortic valve stenosis. Circulation 1993; 87:1239–1248.
32. Dulce M, Mostbeck G, O'Sullivan M, et al. Severity of aortic regurgitation: interstudy reproducibility of measurements with velocity-encoded cine MR imaging. Radiology 1992; 185:235–240.
33. Funari M, Fugita N, Peck WW, et al. Cardiac tumors; assessment with Gd-DTPA-enhanced MR imaging. J Comput Assist Tomogr 1991; 15:953–958.
34. Duerinckx AJ, Wexler L, Banerjee A, et al. Postoperative evaluation of pulmonary arteries in congenital heart surgery by MR imaging: comparison with echocardiography. Am Heart J 1994; 128:1139–1146.
35. Jones RH, Borges-Neto S, Potts JM. Simultaneous measurement of myocardial

perfusion and ventricular function during exercise from a single injection of technetium-99m sestamibi in coronary artery disease. Am J Cardiol 1990; 66:68E–71E.
36. Maddahi J, Rodrigues E, Berman DS, et al. State-of-the-art myocardial perfusion imaging. Cardiol Clin 994; 12:199–222.
37. Shirakawa S, Hattori N, Tamaki N, et al. Assessment of left ventricular wall thickening with gated 99mTc-MIBI SPECT—value of normal file. Kaku Igaku Jpn J Nucl Med 1995; 32:643–650.
38. Patterson RE, Horowitz SF, Eisner RL. Comparison of modalities to diagnose coronary artery disease. Semin Nucl Med 1994; 24:286–310.
39. Hendel RC, Dahlberg ST, Weinstein H, et al. Comparison of teboroxime and thallium for the reversibility of exercise-induced myocardial perfusion defects. Am Heart J 1993; 126:856–862.
40. Dahlberg ST, Leppo JA. Physiologic properties of myocardial perfusion tracers. Cardiol Clin 1994; 12:169–185.
41. Chiao PC, Ficaro EP, Dayanikli F, et al. Compartmental analysis of technetium-99m-teboroxime kinetics employing fast dynamic SPECT at rest and stress. J Nucl Med 1994; 35:1265–1273.
42. Galli M, Marcassa C, Imparato A, et al. Effects of nitroglycerin by technetium-99m sestamibi tomoscintigraphy on resting regional myocardial hypoperfusion in stable patients with healed myocardial infarction. Am J Cardiol 1994; 74:843–848.
43. Kiat H, Germano G, Friedman J, et al. Comparative feasibility of separate or simultaneous rest thallium-201/stress technetium-99m-sestamibi dual-isotope myocardial perfusion SPECT. J Nucl Med 1994; 35:542–548.
44. Nunn A, Linder K, Strauss HW. Nitroimidazoles and imaging hypoxia. Eur J Nucl Med 1995; 22:265–280.
45. Ohtani H, Callahan RJ, Khaw BA, et al. Comparison of technetium-99m-glucarate and thallium-201 for the identification of acute myocardial infarction in rats. J Nucl Med 1992; 33:1988–1993.
46. Knight LC, Radcliffe R, Maurer AH, et al. Thrombus imaging with technetium-99m synthetic peptides based upon the binding domain of a monoclonal antibody to activated platelets. J Nucl Med 1994; 35:282–288.
47. Muto P, Lastoria S, Varrella P, et al. Detecting deep venous thrombosis with technetium-99m-labeled synthetic peptide P280. J Nucl Med 1995; 36:1384–1391.
48. Montgomery DH, Ververis JJ, McGorisk G, et al. Natural history of severe atheromatous disease of the thoracic aorta: a transesophageal echocardiographic study. J Am Coll Cardiol 1996; 27:95–101.
49. Benjamin EJ, D'Agostino RB, Belanger AJ, et al. Left atrial size and the risk of stroke and death. The Framingham Heart Study. Circulation 1995; 92:835–841.
50. Collins LJ, Silverman DI, Douglas PS, et al. Cardioversion of nonrheumatic atrial fibrillation. Reduced thromboembolic complications with 4 weeks of precardioversion anticoagulation are related to atrial thrombus resolution. Circulation 1995; 92:160–163.
51. Orsinelli DA, Pearson AC. Detection of prosthetic valve strands by transesophageal echocardiography: clinical significance in patients with suspected cardiac source of embolism. J Am Coll Cardiol 1995; 26:1713–1718.

52. Stoddard MF, Prince CR, Dillon S, et al. Exercise-induced mitral regurgitation is a predictor of morbid events in subjects with mitral valve prolapse. J Am Coll Cardiol 1995; 25:693–699.
53. Manning WJ, Silverman DI, Keighley CS, et al. Transesophageal echocardiographically facilitated early cardioversion from atrial fibrillation using short-term anticoagulation: final results of a prospective 4.5-year study. J Am Coll Cardiol 1995; 25:1354–1361.
54. Lee RJ, Kalman JM, Fitzpatrick AP, et al. Radiofrequency catheter modification of the sinus node for "inappropriate" sinus tachycardia. Circulation 1995; 92:2919–2928.
55. Kalman JM, Lee RJ, Fisher WG, et al. Radiofrequency catheter modification of sinus pacemaker function guided by intracardiac echocardiography. Circulation 1995; 92:3070–3081.
56. Mintz GS, Popma JJ, Pichard AD, et al. Intravascular ultrasound predictors of restenosis after percutaneous transcatheter coronary revascularization. J Am Coll Cardiol 1996; 27:1678–1687.
57. Hall P, Nakamura S, Maiello L, et al. Clinical and angiographic outcome after Palmaz-Schatz stent implantation guided by intravascular ultrasound. J Invasive Cardiol 1995; 7(suppl A):12A-22A.
58. Gopal AS, Shen Z, Sapin PM, et al. Assessment of cardiac function by three-dimensional echocardiography compared with conventional noninvasive methods. Circulation 1995; 92:842–853.
59. Jiang L, Vazquez de Prada JA, Handschumacher MD, et al. Quantitative three-dimensional reconstruction of aneurysmal left ventricles. In vitro and in vivo validation. Circulation 1995; 91:222–230.
60. Marx GR, Fulton DR, Pandian NG, et al. Delineation of site, relative size and dynamic geometry of atrial septal defects by real-time three-dimensional echocardiography. J Am Coll Cardiol 1995; 25:482–490.
61. Salustri A, Spitaels S, McGhie J, et al. Transthoracic three-dimensional echocardiography in adult patients with congenital heart disease. J Am Coll Cardiol 1995; 26:759–767.
62. Shiota T, Jones M, Teien DE, et al. Dynamic change in mitral regurgitant orifice area: comparison of color Doppler echocardiographic and electromagnetic flowmeter-based methods in a chronic animal model. J Am Coll Cardiol 1995; 26:528–536.
63. Shiota T, Jones M, Yamada I, et al. Evaluation of aortic regurgitation with digitally determined color Doppler-imaged flow convergence acceleration: a quantitative study in sheep. J Am Coll Cardiol 1996; 27:203–210.
64. Evangelista A, Garcia-Dorado D, Garcia del Castillo H, et al. Cardiac index quantification by Doppler ultrasound in patients without left ventricular outflow tract abnormalities. J Am Coll Cardiol 1995; 25:710–716.
65. Kim WY, Poulsen JK, Terp K, et al. A new Doppler method for quantification of volumetric flow: in vivo validation using color Doppler. J Am Coll Cardiol 1996; 27:182–192.
66. Enriquez-Sarano M, Miller FA Jr, Hayes SN, et al. Effective mitral regurgitant orifice area: clinical use and pitfalls of the proximal isovelocity surface area method. J Am Coll Cardiol 1995; 25:703–709.

67. Cheirif J, Narkiewicz-Jodko JB, Hawkins HK, et al. Myocardial contrast echocardiography: relation of collateral perfusion to extent of injury and severity of contractile dysfunction in a canine model of coronary thrombosis and reperfusion. J Am Coll Cardiol 1995; 26:537–546.
68. Perchet H, Dupouy P, Duval-Moulin AM, et al. Improvement of subendocardial myocardial perfusion after percutaneous transluminal coronary angioplasty. A myocardial contrast echocardiography study with correlation between myocardial contrast reserve and Doppler coronary reserve. Circulation 1995; 91:1419–1426.
69. Porter TR, Xie F. Visually discernible myocardial echocardiographic contrast after intravenous injection of sonicated dextrose albumin microbubbles containing high molecular weight, less soluble gases. J Am Coll Cardiol 1995; 25:509–515.
70. von Bibra H, Sutherland G, Becher H, et al. Clinical evaluation of left heart Doppler contrast enhancement by a saccharide-based transpulmonary contrast agent. The Levovist Cardiac Working Group. J Am Coll Cardiol 1995; 25:500–508.
71. Ismail S, Jayaweera AR, Goodman NC, et al. Detection of coronary stenoses and quantification of the degree and spatial extent of blood flow mismatch during coronary hyperemia with myocardial contrast echocardiography. Circulation 1995; 91:821–830.
72. Mulvagh SL, Foley DA, Aeschbacher BC, et al. Second harmonic imaging of an intravenously administered echocardiographic contrast agent: visualization of coronary arteries and measurement of coronary blood flow. J Am Coll Cardiol 1996; 27:1519–1525.
73. Porter TR, Xie F, Kricsfeld D, et al. Improved myocardial contrast with second harmonic transient ultrasound response imaging in humans using intravenous perfluorocarbon-exposed sonicated dextrose albumin. J Am Coll Cardiol 1996; 27:1497–1501.
74. Moshage WE, Achenbach S, Seese B, et al. Coronary artery stenoses: three-dimensional imaging with electrocardiographically triggered, contrast agent-enhanced, electron-beam CT. Radiology 1995; 196:707–714.
75. Zerhouni EA, Parrish DM, Rogers WJ, et al. Human heart tagging with MRI—a method for non-invasive assessment of myocardial motion. Radiology 1988; 169:59–63.
76. Clark N, Reicheck N, Bergey P, et al. Circumferential myocardial segment shortening in the normal human left ventricle using spatial modulation of magnetization. Circulation 1991; 84:67–74.
77. McVeigh ER, Zerhouni EA. Non-invasive measurement of transmural gradient in myocardial strain with MR imaging. Radiology 1991; 180:667–683.
78. van Dijk P. Direct cardiac NMR imaging of heart wall and blood flow velocity. J Comput Assist Tomogr 1984; 8:429–436.
79. Saeed M, Wendland MF, Takehara Y, et al. Reperfusion and irreversible myocardial injury: identification with nonionic MR imaging contrast medium. Radiology 1992; 182:625–683.
80. Mathejssen NA, de Roos A, Van der Wall EE, et al. Acute myocardial infarction: comparison of T_2 weighted and T_1 weighted gadolinium-DTPA enhanced MR imaging. Magn Reson Imaging Med 1991; 17:460–469.

81. Dulce MC, Deurinckx AJ, Hartiala JJ, et al. MR imaging of the myocardium using nonionic contrast medium: signal intensity changes in patients with subacute myocardial infarction. AJR 1993; 160:963–970.
82. Wright GA, Hu B, Mackovski A. Estimating oxygen saturation of blood in vivo with MR imaging at 1.5T. J Magn Reson Imaging 1991; 1:447–457.
83. Li KC, Wright GA, Pelc LR, et al. Oxygen saturation of blood in the superior mesenteric vein: in vivo verification of MR imaging measurements in a canine model. Work in progress. Radiology 1995; 194:321–325.
84. Manning WJ, Li W, Edelman RR. A preliminary report comparing magnetic resonance coronary angiography with conventional angiography. N Engl J Med 1993; 323:828–832.
85. Pennell DJ, Bogren HG, Keegan J, et al. Assessment of coronary artery stenosis by magnetic resonance imaging. Heart 1996; 75:127–133.
86. Poncelot BP, Weisskoff RM, Wedeen VJ, et al. Time of flight quantification of coronary flow with echoplanar MRI. Magn Reson Med 1993; 30:447–457.
87. Clarke GD, Eckles R, Chaney C, et al. Measurement of absolute epicardial coronary artery flow and flow reserve with breath-hold cine phase-contrast magnetic resonance imaging. Circulation 1995; 91:2627–2634.
88. Sakuma H, Blake L, Amidone T, et al. Coronary flow reserve: noninvasive measurement in humans with breath-hold velocity encoded cine MR imaging. Radiology 1996; 198:745–750.

AUTHOR INDEX

Italic numbers give the page on which the complete reference is listed.

A

Aarnio, P., 304, *317*
Abboud, R., 200, *215*
Abboud, R. T., 284, *296*
Abd, A. G., 43, *66*
Abdallah, P. S., 28, *38*
Abdullah, A. K., 253, *271*
Abela, G. A., 550, *569*
Aberle, D. R., 33, *39,* 202, 212, *216, 218,*
  270, *274,* 331, 335, *340, 341,* 353,
  364, 370, *38*
Aboulafia, D. M., 469, *474*
Abrams, D. I., 57, *68*
Abrams, H. L., 572, *596*
Abrams, J. K., 94, 95, *102*
Achenbach, S., 594, *600*
Ackerman, N., 348, *363*
Adachi, S., 201, *216*
Adams, H., 283, *295,* 337, *341*
Adelman, A. G., 550, *565*
Adelstein, D. J., 70, *97*
Adenle, A. D., 115, *124*
Adenroth, C. S., 348, *363*
Adler, B. D., 20, 23, 29, 30, 31, *37, 39,*
  210, *218,* 239, *243,* 245, 246, *271*

Adler, L. P., 427, 430, *442*
Adler, O. B., 142, *156*
Adler, R. H., 359, *366*
Aeschbacher, B. C., 593, *600*
Agrawa, S. K., 554, *567*
Aguayo, S. M., 206, 207, *217*
Ahn, J. M., 21, *37,* 201, *216,* 260, *272*
Aisen, A. M., 91, *101*
Aisner, J., 94, 95, 96, *102*
Akira, M., 201, 202, 210, *216,* 260, *272*
Al-Zarka, A. M., 424, 439, *441*
Alavi, A., 391, 414, *415, 418*
Albelda, S. M., 50, *67,* 227, 236, *241*
Alberts, W. M., 359, *366*
Albin, R. J., 237, *242*
Alderman, E. L., 540, *563*
Alexander, S., 94, *102*
Alexopoulous, D., 425, *441*
Alfageme, I., 358, *365*
Alfonso, Aguiran, E. R., 346, *362*
Ali, I., 358, *365*
Allen, H. D., 560, *568*
Allen, J., 539, *563*
Allen, M. K., 137, *155*
Allen, M. S., 176, 183, *196,*
Almagor, Y., 439, *443,* 541, 550, *564, 565*

603

Almind, M., 359, *366*
Alonso, A., 358, *365*
Alpern, M. B., 81, *99*
Altin, R. S., 485, *505*
Alvarez-Castells, A., 264, *273*
Ambrose, J. A., 424, 425, 439, 440, *441, 444*
American College of Radiology, 12, *18*
American Heart Association, 423, *441*
Amidone, T., 595, *601*
Amitia, Z., 189, *197*
Ampel, N. M., 52, *67*
Anderson, C. B., 358, *365*
Anderson, D. C., 190, *197,* 298, 308, *316, 318*
Anderson, D. J., 90, *100,* 314, *318,* 360, *366*
Anderson, J. N., 145, *156*
Anderson, J. R., 237, *243*
Anderson, M. H., 552, *566*
Anderson, R. F., 284, *296*
Anderson, W., 118, *124*
Andriole, J. G., 352, 353, 354, 355, *363*
Anjos, R. T., 562, *568*
Antkowaik, J. G., 172, *195*
Antman, K. H., 335, *341*
Antonuk, L. E., 383, *388*
Appel, P. L., 525, *533*
Apple, J. S., *122*
Applefeld, M. M., 463, *474*
Appleton, C. P., 463, *474*
Aprahamian, C., 14, *18,* 525, *533*
Aquino, S. L., 262, *273,* 325, *339*
Arai, H., 304, *317*
Araj, N., 381, *388*
Aranda, C. P., 47, *66,* 247, 248, 255, 257, 258, *271, 272*
Archer, A., 24, *38,* 43, 45, *66*
Archer, D. C., 284, *295, 296*
Arenson, R. L., 371, *387*
Arger, P. H., 78, *98*
Argiro, V., 577, *597*
Ariani, M., 536, 537, 540, *562*
Armitage, J. M., 189, *197*
Armstrong, D., 23, 24, *38*
Armstrong, P., 355, *364*

Arnold, S., 173, *195*
Aronberg, D. J., 90, *100,* 333, *340,* 450, *472*
Aronchick, J. M., 30, *39,* 48, 50, 52, *66, 67,* 86, *100,* 149, *158,* 391, *415*
Aronow, A., 236, *242*
Arora, N. S., 83, *99*
Asfaw, I., 135, *155*
Askin, F. B., 262, *272*
Atallah, N., 371, *387*
Athanasoulis, C. A., 391, 414, *415, 418,* 522, *532*
Atkinson, B., 78, 79, *98*
Attar, S., 147, 148, *157*
Aufferman, W., 583, *597*
Auffermann, W., 518, *531*
Aughenbaugh, G. L., 8, *17,* 32, *39,* 200, *215*
Auh, P. R., 115, *124,* 450, *472*
Austin, J. H. M., 350, *363*

B

Baamonde, C., 93, *102*
Baasch, B. N., 107, *122*
Baber, C., *122*
Baber, C. E., 108, 113, *122, 123,* 330, *339*
Babic, U. U., 556, *568*
Babyn, P. S., 128, *153*
Baciewicz, F. A., Jr., 304, *317*
Badimon, J. J., 425, *442*
Badimon, L., 423, 425, *441, 442*
Bae, K. T., 291, *296*
Bae, W. K., 246, *271,* 358, *365*
Baert, A. L., 403, *417*
Bahnson, H. T., 189, *197*
Bahr, A. L., 132, *154*
Bai, M., 467, *474*
Bailey, P. B., 83, *99*
Bailey, W. C., 284, *296*
Baim, D. S., 547, 552, *565*
Baker, E. J., 562, *568*
Baker, H. L., Jr., 10, *17*
Baker, J. A., 384, *388*
Baker, M., 455, *473*

Author Index

Bakris, G. L., 74, 98
Bakx, A. L. M., 554, 567
Baldt, M. M., 165, 195
Baldwin, J. C., 299, 305, 316, 317
Ball, T., 148, 157
Ball, W. C., 262, 272
Banerjee, A., 587, 597
Bank, E. R., 455, 473, 484, 488, 489, 503, 505
Bankier, A. A., 165, 195
Bankoff, M. S., 463, 474
Banks, P. M., 35, 36, 40
Bansal, S., 12, 18
Baptista, J., 541, 564
Barcia, T. C., 525, 533
Barloon, T. J., 20, 37
Barnes, P. A., 81, 99
Barnes, P. F., 47, 66
Barnett, V. T., 236, 242
Barnhard, H. J., 281, 295
Baron, R. L., 36, 40, 311, 318
Barone, M., 271
Barr, J. W., 572, 596
Barrett, T. F., 144, 156
Barrio, J. L., 43, 65
Bartel, A. G., 436, 443
Barth, K. H., 404, 417
Bartiromo, G., 248, 271
Bartorelli, A. L., 439, 443
Bashi, S. A., 253, 271
Bassand, J-P., 555, 567
Bataille, D., 201, 216
Bates, F. T., 45, 66
Bates, J. M., 281, 295
Batkoff, B. W., 569
Batra, P., 41, 65, 65, 68
Batson. O. V., 107, 122
Battesti, J-P., 203, 217, 248, 271
Baumback, A., 547, 565
Baur, X., 236, 242
Baxley, W. A., 475, 477, 489, 500, 505
Baxt, W. G., 127, 152
Beache, G. M., 447, 463, 472
Beacher, J. R., 220, 223, 240, 255, 256, 272
Beal, S. L., 148, 157

Beaman, B. L., 21, 37
Beaman, L., 21, 37
Beattie, E. J., 358, 365
Beaulieu, C. F., 577, 597
Beaumont, M., 47, 66
Beaune, J., 237, 242
Becette, V., 265, 273
Becher, H., 593, 600
Bechtold, R. E., 127, 132, 152
Becker, A. E., 437, 443
Bedal, S., 200, 203, 215, 217
Beechler, C. R., 94, 102
Beekman, E., 141, 155
Beekman, R H., 558, 568
Beeley, J. M., 144, 156
Bégin, R., 203, 204, 217
Behrenot, D. M., 525, 533
Belanger, A. J., 592, 598
Belani, C. P., 61, 68
Bell, A. L. L., 43, 66
Bell, B. Y., 203, 217
Bell, D. Y., 199, 200, 215
Bell, M. R., 546, 552, 565, 566
Bellamy, E. A., 20, 37
Bellefleur, J-P., 556, 568
Bembom, M. C. B., 555, 567
Ben-Menachem, Y., 128, 153, 524, 532
Bender, T. M., 129, 153
Bendick, P. J., 520, 532
Benjamin, E. J., 592, 598
Benson, L., 558, 568
Berger, H. W., 227, 240
Berger, P. B., 546, 565
Berger, R., 353, 364
Bergeron, D., 203, 204, 217
Bergey, P., 594, 600
Bergin, C., 283, 295
Bergin, C. J., 20, 24, 37, 43, 66, 199, 200, 203, 215, 217, 248, 262, 271, 273, 306, 318, 354, 364
Bergin, K. T., 160, 195, 354, 364
Bergman, K., 128, 153
Bergmann, F., 236, 242
Berko, B., 434, 442
Berkow, A. E., 147, 156
Berlin, N. I., 70, 97

Berman, A. D., 558, *568*
Berman, D. S., 573, 587, *596, 598*
Bernadac, P., 276, *294*
Bernard, M. S., 283, *295*
Bernard, Y., 555, *567,* 558, *568*
Bernardino, M. E., 81, 94, *99, 102*
Bernatz, P. E., 90, *100*
Berquist, T. H., 83, *99,* 118, *124*
Berry, B. E., 147, *156*
Berry, C. R., 348, *363*
Berry, G. J., 20, 24, *37,* 43, 56, *66, 67,* 262, *273,* 301, 306, *316, 318*
Bertoli, C., 56, *67*
Bertozzi, P., 262, *273*
Bertrand, M. E., 550, 553, *565, 566*
Bessent, R. G., 397, *416*
Besson, A., 106, *122*
Bethel, R., 254, *272,* 307, 311, *318*
Beuscart, R., 203, 204, *217*
Beute, G. H., 81, 90, *99, 100*
Bhalla, M., 314, *318*
Bickerstaff, L. K., 517, *530*
Bidwell, J. K., 508, *530*
Biello, D. R., 394, *416*
Bigby, T. D., 28, *38*
Billingham, M., 305, *317*
Biondetti, P. R., 180, *196*
Birnbaum, B., 57, *67*
Bis, K. G., 520, *532*
Bissett, G. S., 484, 493, 503, *505*
Bittl, J. A., 547, *565*
Black, C. M., 201, *216*
Black, W. C., 142, *156*
Bladergroen, M. R., 147, *157*
Blair, D. N., 90, *101*
Blake, L., 595, *601*
Blank, N., 33, *39,* 355, *365*
Blaquiere, R. M., 20, *37*
Blennerhaset, J. B., 33, *39,* 107, *122*
Blickman, J. G., 10, *17*
Bloch, A. B., 47, *66*
Bloch, F. R., 578, *597*
Block, P. C., 556, *568*
Blume, D., 118, *124*
Blumenson, L. E., 107, *122*
Boctor, M., 203, 204, *217*

Bodey, G. P., 21, 32, *37, 39*
Bogaert, J., 403, *417*
Bogdanov, A. A., Jr., 410, *418*
Bogelzang, N. J., 113, *123*
Bogren, H. G., 595, *601*
Boison, C., 203, 204, *217*
Bolling, S. F., 162, 164, 165, *195*
Bond, J. P., 574, *596*
Bookstein, F. L., 91, *101,* 391, *415*
Boothroyd, A. E., 220, *240*
Borges-Neto, S., 587, *597*
Boring, C. C., 70, *97*
Borrione, M., 550, *565*
Bortolotti, U., 469, *474*
Bos, J. J., 14, *18*
Bostwick, J., III, 169, *195*
Botham, M. J., 358, *365*
Bouchard, G., 152, *158*
Bouchardy, L. M. 262, *272,*
Boucot, K. R., 81, *99*
Bourgouin, P. M., 91, *101,* 353, *364*
Bowker, T. J., 545, *564*
Bowley, N. B., 227, 232, *241*
Boxt, L. M., 476, 477, *505*
Boyd, A. D., 247, *271*
Boyd, D. P., 509, *530,* 577, *597*
Boyle, J. J., 108, *123*
Boyle, N. G., 427, *442*
Bradley, J. D., 227, 233, *241*
Brady, M. B., 173, *196*
Brady, T. J., 410, *418,* 517, *531*
Bragg, D. G., 36, *40*
Braidy, T. F., 353, *364*
Braman, S. S., 106, *122*
Brantigan, O. C., 287, *296*
Brasch, R. C., 260, *272*
Braun, S. D., 414, *418*
Brauner, M .W., 203, 206, 207, 209, *217, 218,* 248, *271*
Braunwald, E., 447, 455, 456, 458, 459, 462, 467, *472*
Brawley, R. K., 520, *532*
Breatnach, E., 262, *273*
Brecher, E., 5, 6, 7, *17*
Bree, R. L., 522, *532*
Bree, R., 520, *532*

Bresnahan, J. F., 552, *566*
Bressler, E. L., 348, *363*
Brett, C. M., 132, *154*
Brewer, L. A., III, 78, 79, *98*
Bridges, K. G., 132, *154*
Briethardt, G., 583, *597*
Briggs, J. E., 7, *17*
Brink, J. A., 151, *158*, 247, *271*
Brockhoff, C., 523, *532*
Broerse, J. J., 383, *388*
Brogdon, B. G., 173, *196*
Bronson, S. M., 235, *241*
Brook, M. P., 135, *154*
Brooks, R. A., 11, *18*
Bross, I. D. K., 107, *122*
Bross, I. J., 107, *122*
Brown, E., 43, *65*
Brown, J. J., 450, *472*
Brown, L. R., 8, *17*, 32, *39*, 117, 118, *124*
Brown, M. J., 28, 29, *38*
Brown, O. L., 236, *242*
Brown, R. A., 130, *154*
Brown, R. H., *273*
Brown, R. H., 269, *273, 274*, 401, *416*
Bruderman, I., 69, 70, 81, *97*
Brudin, L. H., 333, *340*
Brundage, B. H., 403, *417*
Brunt, E. M., 301, *316*
Bruwer, A. J., 235, *241*
Bryan, C. L., 304, *317*
Bryant, R. E., 30, *39*
Bryd, R. B., 79, *99*
Bryk, D. , 323, *338*
Brymer, J. F., 425, *442*
Buchbinder, M., 553, *566*
Buchbinder, S. P., 56, *67*
Bucher, T. A., 540, *563*
Buckley, J. A., 11, *18*
Buckman, R., 152, *158*
Buddemeyer, E. U., 508, *530*
Buff, S. J., 239, *243*
Bunch, P. C., 8, *17*
Buncher, C. R., 70, *97*
Bunn, P. A., Jr., 96, *103*
Burch, K. H., 22, *38*
Burch, M., 555, *567*

Burke, B., 24, *38*
Burke, C. M., 305, *317*
Burke, J. F., 145, *156*
Burke, R. M., 276, *294*
Burns, M. A., 510, *530*
Burrows, B., 275, *293*
Burton, A. C., 425, *442*
Burwell, D., 323, *338*
Busch, E., 172, *195*
Busch, H. P., 384, *388*
Buschman, D. L., 210, *218*
Bush, A., 282, *295*
Bush, R., 469, *474*
Butch, R. J., 327, *339*
Butchar, E. G., 337, *341*
Buxton, R. C., 333, *340*
Buy, J., 91, *102*
Buy, J. N., 333, *340*
Byrd, R. B., 71, 72, 73, 81, *98*

C

Cagle, J. E., Jr., 358, *365*
Cahan, W. G., 113, *123*
Cahn, A. P., 256, *272*
Calabro, F., 469, *474*
Calhoun, P., 355, *364*
Callahan, R. J., 591, *598*
Cammilleri, S., 304, *317*
Campbell, D. N., 130, 134, *154*
Cantin, A., 203, 204, *217*
Caplan, E. S., 135, *155*
Caputo, G. R., 407, *417*, 514, *530*, 580, *597*
Carette, M. F., 90, 91, *101*
Carey, J. T., 115, *123*
Carneiro, R., 546, *564*
Caroline, D. F., 202, *216*
Carpenter, H. A., 234, *241*
Carr, D. H., *218*
Carr, D. T., 71, 72, 73, 81, 79, *98, 99*
Carr, J. J., 450, 471, *472*
Carrington, C. B., 199, *215*, 335, *341*
Carroll, F. E., 389, *415*
Carrozza, J. P., 550, 553, 554, *565, 566*

Carter, B. L., 463, *474*
Carter, B. N., 148, 152, *157*
Carter, C. J., 414, *419*
Casablanca, G., 248, *271*
Casablanca, G., *271*
Casale, A. S., 189, 190, 191, *197*
Casanova, C., 235, 236, *242*
Cascade, P. N., 9, *17,* 314, *318,* 371, 376, *388*
Cascinelli, L. N., 113, *123*
Case records of the Mass. Gen. Hosp., 233, 235, *241, 242*
Caskey, C. I., 85, 86, 93, 94, *100*
Casola, G., 354, 360, 361, *364, 366, 367*
Cassagnes, J., 552, *566*
Cassidy, J. M., 528, *534*
Cassidy, S. C., 555, *567*
Castagno, A. A., 90, *101*
Castellanos, A., 572, *596*
Castellino, R. A., 20, 24, 33, *37, 39,* 43, *66,* 199, 200, *215,* 237, *242,* 355, *365*
Casteneda-Zuniga, W., 353, *364*
Castillo, M., 64, *68*
Castleman, B., 106, *122*
Castro, E. L. B., 113, *123*
Cauthen, G. M., 47, *66*
Cavallino, R. P., 525, *533*
Celo, J. S., 43, *66*
Centers for Disease Control, 41, *65*
Chadhuri, M. R., 72, *98*
Chaisson, R. E., 52, *67*
Chamberlain, D. W., 209, *218,* 262, *273, 300,* 305, 316, *317*
Chambers, C., 309, *318*
Chamides, B. K., 56, *67*
Chan, H-P., 9, *17,* 371, 376, *388*
Chan, M. C. K., 174, *196*
Chan-Yeung, M., 203, *217*
Chan-Yeung, M. M., 201, *216*
Chaney, C., 595, *601*
Chang, A. E., 117, *124*
Chang, C. H., 282, *295*
Chang, C. L., 9, *17,* 371, 376, *388*
Chang, D. B., 327, *339,* 347, *362*
Chang, J. M., 580, *597*
Chang, P., 458, *473*

Chaparro, C., 305, *317*
Chapekis, A. T., 553, *566*
Charig, M. J., 108, *123*
Charnock, G. C., 359, *366*
Chasen, M. H., 14, *18,* 525, *533*
Chazuilleres, A. F., 583, *597*
Cheah, F. K., 235, 236, *242*
Chee, P. W., 9, *17,* 371, 376, *388*
Chen, C. C., 433 *442*
Chen, J. T., 276, *294,* 436, *443*
Chen, J. T. T., 496, 497, 501, *506*
Chenevert, T. L., 91, *101*
Cherif, J., 593, *600*
Chern, M-S., 556, *567*
Cherry, K. J., 517, *530*
Chesebro, J. H., 425, *442*
Chew, F. S., 10, *17*
Chiao, P. C., 591, *598*
Child, J. S., 475, 482, 492, 493, *505*
Chiles, C., 199, 200, 203, 209, *215, 217, 218,* 299, *316*
Chin, W. S., 227, 232, *241*
Ching, W. T. W., 22, *37*
Cho, S-R., 144, *156*
Choi, B. I., 78, 79, *99*
Choi, E. W., 246, *271*
Choplin, R. H., 327, 328, *339*
Chor, P. J., 36, *40*
Chotas, H. G., 9, *17*
Chou, C. S., 129, *153*
Chow, C., 43, 45, *66*
Christiansen, W. R., 275, 281, *293*
Christoforidis, A. J., 275, 281, *294*
Chu, K., 70, *97*
Chung, J. W., 580, *597*
Cichelli, A. V., 237, *242*
Cigarroa, J. E., 523, *532*
Cink, T. M., 254, *272,* 307, 311, *318*
Clark, N., 594, *600*
Clarke, G. D., 595, *601*
Clelland, C., 299, *316*
Clemen, M. W., 553, *566*
Clements, J. L., Jr., 148, *157*
Cluzel, P., 203, *217*
Coblentz, C. L., 199, 200, 203, *215, 217,* 284, *295, 296*

Cockerham, J. T., 562, *568*
Cockerill, F. R., III, 19, 32, *37*
Codington, R., 283, *295*
Cohen, A. B., 276, *294*
Cohen, A. J., 471, *474*
Cohen, A. M., 525, *533*
Cohen, D. J., 553, *567*
Cohen, E. A., , 550, *565*
Cohen, M., 423, *441*
Cohen, M. H., 71, 81, *98*
Colan, S. D., 432, *442*
Colby, T. V., 234, *241,* 261, 262, *272, 273*
Coleman, B. G., 78, *98*
Coleman, R. E., 203, *217,* 391, 395, 402, *416*
Coles, J. C., 128, *153*
Collie, D. A., 118, *124*
Collier, D., 304, *317*
Collins, J. C., 132, *154*
Collins, J. D., 323, *338*
Collins, L. J., 592, *598*
Collins, T. J., 536, 538, 539, *562*
Colman, R. W., 237, *242*
Cologanato, A., 180, *196*
Colombo, A., 541, 550, *564, 565*
Colt, H. G., 304, *317*
Committee on Trauma and Committee on Schock, 127, *152*
Comti, C. R., 550, *569*
Conant, E. F., 331, *340*
Conces, D. J., 52, *67,* 247, 248, *271*
Conces, D. J., Jr., 359, 360, *366*
Conkle, D. M., 117, *124*
Conlan, A. A., 174, *196*
Connell, D. G., 145, *156*
Conti, P. S., 15, *18,* 84, *99*
Cook, S. L., 548, *555*
Cooke, J. P., 517, 520, 521, *531*
Cooley, D. A., 519, *531*
Cooley, T. P., 57, *68*
Cooper, D. A., 81, *99*
Cooper, E. S., 423, *441*
Cooper, J. A. D., Jr., 30, 31, *39*
Cooper, J. D., 90, *100,* 291, *296,* 297, 305, 314, *315, 317, 318*
Cooper, J. F., 135, *155*

Cooper, T. J., 413, *418*
Copin, M. C., 201, *216*
Coppage, L., 107, 108, 112, *122, 123,* 337, *341*
Coppel, D. L., 142, *156*
Corcoran, H. L., 74, *98*
Cordier, J. F., 209, *218,* 234, *241*
Corey, L., 30, *38*
Cormack, A. M., 577, *597*
Corrin, B., 201, *216*
Corson, J. M., 335, *341*
Corte, B., 201, *216*
Cortese, D. A., 83, *99*
Coselli, J. S., 519, *531*
Cosentino, A. M., 236, *242*
Cossette, R., 360, *366*
Costello, P., 33, *40,* 118, *124,* 402, *416*
Couraud, L., 305, *318*
Courtois, M., 575, *596*
Coutant-Perrone, V., 24, *38.,*
Cowen, A. R., 378, 379, *388*
Cox, E. F., 148, 152, *157*
Craber, L. F., 33, *39*
Craig, F. E., 35, 36, *40*
Cranston, P. E., 132, 134, *154*
Crass, J. R., 525, *533*
Craver, J. M., 169, *195*
Crawford, E. S., 517, 519, *530, 531*
Crawford, W. O., Jr., 139, 140, 141, *155*
Cribier, A., 536, 544, 556, *568*
Crittenden, M., 127, *152*
Cronan, J. J., 327, *339,* 358, *365*
Crook, R., 558, *568*
Crow, J., 106, 107, 112, *121,* 144, *156*
Crowe, J. K., 117, *124*
Cruz, C. J., 151, *158*
Cruz, F., 93, *102*
Cryer, H. M., 525, *533*
Crystal, G. J., 525, *533*
Cuasay, N. S., 333, *340*
Cuello, L., 147, *157*
Cullinan, P., 201, *216*
Cumberland, D. C., 555, *567*
Curry, T. S., 479, 480, 482, *505*
Curry, T. S., III, 508, *530*
Curtin, J. J., 134, *154,* 403, *417*

Curtis, A. M., 108, 112, *123*
Cyrlak, D., 471, *474*
Czarnecki, D., 353, *364*
Czuppon, A., 236, *242*

D

D'Agostino, H. B., 346, 348, 361, *362, 363, 367*
D'Agostino, R. B., 592, *598*
D'Angio, G. J., 108, *123*
Daffner, R. H., 132, *154*
Dahlberg, S. T., 590, *598*
Dahlgren, S. E., 346, *362*
Daikos, G. L., 47, *66*
Daily, P. O., 519, *531*
Dale, R. C., 255, 256, *272*
Daley, C. L., 45, 47, *66*
Dana, E. R., 471, *474*
Danchin, N., 552, *566*
Dandy, W. E., 324, *339*
Danher, J., 129, *153*
Daniel, T. M., 359, *366*
Danielson, G. K., 452, *473*
Das, P. K., 437, *443*
Dauphinee, B., 270, *274*
Davidoff, A., 14, *18*, 525, *533*
Davidson, C. J., 412, *418*, 555, *567*
Davidson, P. T., 47, *66*
Davies, S. F., 227, 233, 236, *241*
Davis, J. H., 141, *155*
Davis, J.. T., 142, *156*
Davis, R. D., 187, 189, *196*
Davis, S. D., 56, *67*, 115, 121, *124, 125*, 327, *339*
Davis, W. A., 94, *102*
Dawkins, K. O, 305, *317*
Dayaniklli, F., 591, *598*
De Bakey, M. E., 519, *531*
De Cesare, N. B., 552, *565*
De Chiro, G., 11, *18*
de Crémoux, H., 203, *217*
de Franco, A. C., 541, *564*
de Geest, H., 539, *563*

de Gracia, J., 264, *273*
de Gregorio, Ariza, M. A., 346, *362*
De Groot, M. K., 524, *532*
De Hoyos, A., 190, 191, *197*, 300, 305, 307, *316, 317. 318*
de Jeagere, P., 553, 554, *566*
de Kamp, R. A., 284, *295*
de Lassence, A., 237, *242*
De Long, D. M., 395, 402, *416*
De Lorenzo, L. J., 43, *65*
De Luca, S. A., 129, *153*
de Man, F., 539, *563*
de Mello, D. E., 304, *317*
De Muinck, E.D., 553, *566*
De Muth, W. E., Jr., 137, *155*
De Natale, R. W., 517, *530*
de Roos, A., 594, *600*
de Scheerder, I., 539, 553, *563, 566*
De Simone, S. D., 371, *387*
Dea, M. W., 487, *506*
Deanfield, J. E., 555, *567*
Dedrick, C. G., 183, *196*
Dee, P. M., 129, 145, 147, *153*
Deeb, Z. L., 525, *533*
Degreef, J. M., 203, 204, *217*
Delany, D. J., 359, *366*
Delcambre, B., 201, *216*
Delignette, A., 191, *197*, 304, 306, *317, 318*
Delorme, N., 276, *294*
Deluce, M. C., 594, *601*
Demers, C., 397, *416*
Demian, S. E., 540, *563*
Demos, T. C., 150, *158*, 510, 523, *530, 532*
den Heijer, P., 539, *562*
Denison, D. M., 282, *295*
Denne, L., 545, *564*
Denny, D. F., 525, *533*
Desanctis, R. W., 520, 523, *531, 532*
Deschamps, C., 176, 183, *196*
Desser, T. S., 90, *101*
Detrano, R., 578, *597*
Deurinckx, A. J., 594, *601*
Deutsch, A. L., 83, *99*
Deutsch, H. J., 523, *532*

Dewan, N. A., 82, 83, 84, *99,* 119, *125,* 333, *340*
Di Marco, A. F., 172, *195*
di Mario, C., 540, 541, *563, 564*
Diaconis, J. N., 508, *530*
Diamond, H. D., 33, *39*
Dichter, J. R., 20, 21, *37*
Dickie, H. A., 232, *241*
Dickson, B. A., 74, *98*
Didier, D., 528, *534*
Diethrich, E. B., 548, *565*
Dietz, R., 553, *566*
Dillon, S., 592, *599*
Diner, W. C., 147, *157*
Dinsmore, R. E., 447, 463, *472,* 517, *531*
Ditesheim, J. A., 127, 132, *152*
Dito, W. R., 234, *241*
Dixon, J., 554, *567*
Djurisic, Z., 556, *568*
Dobbins, J. T., III, 9, *17*
Dodd, G. D., 108, *123*
Dodd, G. D., III, 36, *40,* 311, *318*
Dodds, W. J., 147, *157*
Dogan, A. S., 487, *506*
Doi, K., 387, *388*
Doll, D. C., 70, 78, *97*
Dolovish, J., 309, *318*
Dombernowksy, P., 81, *99*
Donaldson, R. M., 399, *416*
Dontigny, L., 360, *366*
Dooley, B. N., 147, *157*
Doppman, J. L., 24, *38,* 117, *124*
Dorfman, G. S., 327, *339,* 358, *365*
Doroghazi, R. M., 520, *531*
Doty, D. B., 424, *441*
Douek, P., 410, *418,* 540, *563*
Dougall, A. M., 128, *153*
Douglas, J. M., 171, *195*
Douglas, J. S., 544, *564*
Douglas, P. S., 434, *442,* 592, *598*
Douglas, W. W., 200, *215*
Dowdey, J. E., 479, 480, 482, *505,* 508, *530*
Doyle, L. A., 94, 95, *102*
Drescher, P., 384, *388*
Driscoll, D., 172, *195*

Dromer, C., 305, *318*
Drosos, A. A., 235, *241*
Drouillard, J., 305, *318*
duBois, R. M., 201, *216*
DuCret, R. P., 306, *318*
Duerinckx, A. J., 427, 428, *442,* 587, *597*
Duff, J. H., 128, *153*
Duhamel, A., 201, 203, *216, 217*
Duhaylongsod, F. G., 179, 180, *196*
Dulce, M., 584, *597*
Dumler, J. S., 25, *38*
Dummer, S., 309, 310, *318*
Dumont, M., 152, *158*
Duncan-Meyer, J. 90, *100,* 333, *340*
Dunham, C. M., 14, *18,* 525, *533*
Dunne, T. T., 524, *532*
Dunnick, N. R., 96, *102*
Dunnill, M. S., 280, 281, *294*
Dupree, D. W., 135, *154*
Dupuy, D. E., 403, *417*
Duurkens, V. A., 359, *366*
Duva-Moulin, A. M., 593, *600.,*
Dwyer, A., 117, *124*
Dwyer, S. J., 9, 10, *17*
Dyrda, I., 424, *441*

E

Eagle, K. A., 523, *532*
Earls, J. P., 135, *155*
Eaton, G., 541, *564*
Eber, C. D., 262, *273*
Echols, R. M., 43, *66*
Ecker, C. P., 403, *417*
Eckles, R., 595, *601*
Edelman, J. M., 52, *67*
Edelman, R. R., 90, *101,* 427, 428, *442,* 595, *601*
Edler, I., 574, *596*
Edma, J. L., 265, *273*
Edwards, D., 220, *240*
Edwards, D. K., III, 221, 235, *241*
Edwards, J. E., 115, *124,* 235, *241*
Edwards, W. D., 437, 439, *443,* 552, *566*

Efmann, E. L., 32, *39*
Egan, T., 305, *317*
Eggen, D. A., 436, *443*
Egger, M. J., 21, *37*
Egglin, T. K., 522, *532*
Eichelberger, M. R., 128, 139, *153*
Eigler, N. L., 547, 548, *565*
Eisner, R. L., 590, *598*
El Yousef, S. B., 351, *363*
Elder, K. H., 61, *68*
Eldridge, W. J., 485, *505*
Eliraz, A., 129, *154*
Elisaf, M., 467, *474*
Elissa, L., 398, *416*
Ellegood, D., 270, *274*
Ellis, K., 144, *156*
Ellis, M. C., 135, *155*
Elmendorf, S. L., 43, *66*
Elshami, A., 47, *66*
Endo, T., 371, *388*
Endress, Z. F., 30, *39*
Engeler, C. E., 353, *364*
England, D. M., 332, *340*
Enriquez-Sarano, M., 593, *599*
Epler, G. R., 335, *341*
Epstein, D. M., 70, 78, 79, 86, *97, 98, 100*, 227, 236, *241*
Erbel, R., 540, *563*
Erdman, W. A., 408, *418*
Erdmann, E., 523, *532*
Erickson, D. R., 141, *155*
Erny, R. E., 552, *565*
Erozan, Y. S., 352, 353, 354, 355, *363*
Escaned, J., 539, 541, *562, 564*
Escobar, A., 539, *562*
Esposito, B., 132, *154*
Esposito, T., 148, 152, *157*
Esptein, D. M., 149, *158*
Essed, C. E., 439, *443*
Estella, P., 547, *565*
Esteves, C. A., 555, *567*
Estrera, A. S., 148, 152, *157,* 166, *195*
Etievent, J., 558, *568*
Ettenger, N. A., 220, *240,* 246, 248, 255, 257, 258, *271, 272,* 313, *318*
Ettinger, D. S., 96, *102*

Evangelista, A., 593, *599*
Evans, K. G., 91, *101,* 200, 201, *215,* 333, *340*
Evens, R. G., 11, *18*
Eyes, B. E., 129, *153*
Eyssen, G. E., 281, *295*
Ezdinli, E. Z., 74, *98*

F

Faber, L. P., 176, *196*
Fabian, T. C., 148, 150, *158*
Fallon, J. T., 437, *443*
Fantus, R. J., 525, *533*
Farha, P., 81, *99*
Farmer, D. W., 509, *530*
Farre, I., 203, *217*
Farris, R. H., 304, *317*
Fataar, S., 148, *158*
Fattal, P. G., 575, *596*
Federle, M. P., 132, *154,* 136, *155,* 165, *195,* 329, *339,* 517, *531*
Fedyshin, P. J., 325, *339*
Feigal, E., 57, *68*
Feigenbaum, H., 462, *473,* 574, *596*
Feigin, D. S., 467, *474*
Feinberg, S. B., 24, *38*
Feldman, F., 144, *156*
Feldman, P. S., 355, *364*
Feldmeier, J. E., 353, *364*
Felix, S. B., 541, 552, *564*
Fellows, K. E., 562, *568*
Felson, B., 72, 144, 148, 152, *98, 156, 157*
Fenoglio, J. J., 467, *474*
Fentiman, I. S., 115, *123*
Ferguson, M. K., 360, *366,* 456, *473*
Ferguson, T. B., 358, *365*
Ferrans, V. J., 446, 447, *472*
Ferraro, M. J., 20, 23, *37*
Ferrucci, J. T., 94, *102,* 327, 330, *339*
Feuerstein, I. M., 24, *38,* 43, 45, *66,* 118, *124*
Fiacaro, E. P., 591, *598*

Fiarbairn, J. F., 517, *531*
Fiel, S. B., 202, *216*
Fields, B. L., 467, *474*
Fields, J. M., 128, *153*
Fife, K. H., 30, *38*
Figley, M. M., 528, *534*
Filderman, A. E., 69, 74, 81, *97,* 107, *122,* 337, *341*
Filion, R. B., 90, *101*
Filly, R., 33, *39*
Finck, S., 463, *473*463, *474,* 579, *597*
Finger, W., 129, *153*
Fink, D., 70, *97*
Fink, I., 346, 352, *362*
Finley, J. P., 560, 562, *568*
Finley, R. J., 128, *153*
Finley, T. N., 236, *242*
Fiolkoski, J., 434, *442*
Fiore, D., 180, *196*
Firmin, D. N., 313, *318,* 427, 430, *442*
Fischl, M. A., 47, *66*
Fischman, D. L., 553, *567*
Fish, G. B., 352, *363*
Fish, G. D., 352, 353, 354, 355, *363*
Fishbein, M. C., 536, 537, 540, 553, *562, 566*
Fisher, E., 22, *38*
Fisher, E. R., 523, *532*
Fisher, M. R., 528, *534,* 580, *597*
Fisher, M. S., 202, *216*
Fisher, R. G., 128, *153,* 524, 525, *532, 533*
Fisher, W. G., 592, *599*
Fishman, D., 553, *566*
Fishman, E. K., 20, 23, 24, 25, *37, 38,* 43, 57, *66, 68,* 78, 79, *98,* 109, 112, 115, *123,* 170, *195,* 237, 240, *243*
Fishman, J. E., 61, *68*
Fishman, R. F., 550, *565*
Fitspatrick, A. P., 592, *599*
Fitzgerald, P. H., 540, *563*
Fitzgerald, P. J., 439, *443,* 540, *563*
Fitzpatrick, K., 371, *387*
Flancbaum, L., 148, 152, *157*
Fleck, E., 547, *565*
Flehinger, B. J., 70, *97*

Fleischner, F. G., 145, *156*
Fleiszer, D. M., 130, *154*
Fleming, W. H., 358, *365*
Flenley, D. C., 283, 284, 285, *295, 296*
Fletcher, E. C., 83, *99*
Fleury, J., 237, *242*
Flicker, S., 485, *505*
Fligiel, S., 239, *243*
Flisak, M. J., 150, *158*
Flores, M. R., 61, *68*
Flower, C. D. R., 220, *240,* 256, *272,* 327, *339*
Floyd, C. E., Jr., 9, *17,* 384, *388*
Flynn, T. C., 128, *153*
Fogne, L., 235, 236, *242*
Foley, D. A., 593, *600*
Foley, D. P., 539, 550, *562, 565*
Foley, M. J., 147, *157*
Foley, W. D., 14, *18,* 525, *533*
Folland, E. D., 564
Fontana, R. S., 70, *97*
Fontes, V., 560, *568*
Fontes, V. F., 555, *567*
Ford, C. M., 135, *155*
Forman, B. H., 330, *339*
Forrester, J. S, 548, *565*
Foster, G. P., 539, *563*
Foster, W. L., 283, 285, *295,* 325, 331, *339, 340*
Fowler, N. O., 462, 463, *473*
Fox, S. H., 401, *416*
Fracchia, A. A., 115, *123*
Fradet, G., 522, *532*
Frager, D., 47, *66*
Francis, I. R., 84, 90, 91, *99, 101*
Franco, I., 541, *564*
Frank, A. R., 83, *99,* 119, *125,* 333, *340*
Frank, H., 410, *418*
Frank, I., 52, *67*
Frank, M. S., 371, *388*
Fraser, R. G., 133, 135, 142, 144, *154,* 225, *240,* 275, 276, 281, *293, 295,* 332, *340*
Fraser, R. S., 25, *38,* 275, 276, 281, *293,* 332, *340*
Frederick, P. R., 132, *154*

Freifeld, A. G., 20, 24, *37*
Freireich, E. J., 32, *39*
Fretz, C. J., 94, *102*
Frick, M. P., 82, 83, 84, *99*
Fried, A. M., 227, *240*
Friedman, A. C., 202, *216*
Friedman, J., 591, *598*
Friedman, P. J. 85, *100,* 329, *339*
Friedman, S. A., 517, *531*
Frieman, D., 78, 79, *98*
Frija, J., 209, *218*
Froehlich, J., 90, 101, 437, *443*
Frola, C., 90, *100*
Fromaget, J. M., 276, *294*
Frost, A., 304, *317*
Frost, J. K., 70, *97*
Fry, D. L., 425, *442*
Fryback, D. G., 13, *18*
Fugita, N., 584, *597*
Fuhrman, C. R., 36, *40,* 262, *273,* 306, 311, *318,* 371, *387,* 391, *415*
Fujii, M., 201, *216*
Fujimura, L., 539, 540, *563*
Fujimura, O., 539, *563*
Fujisawa, H., 520, *532*
Fujita, N., 583, *597*
Fujiwara, T., 84, *99*
Fuks, J. Z., 81, *99*
Fukuda, T., 520, *532*
Fuller, J. D., 57, *68*
Fulton, D. R., 593, *599*
Funari, M., 584, *597*
Funt, S. F., 220, 240, 255, 257, 258, *272*
Fuortes, L. J., 331, *340*
Furmanski, S., 323, *338*
Furon, D., 265, *273*
Fuster, V., 423, 425, *441, 442*

G

Gaensler, E. A., 199, 213, *215, 218,* 335, *341*
Gaeta, M., 248, *271*
Gaeta, M., *271*
Galbraith, H. J. B., 280, *294*
Galgiani, J. N., 52, *67*

Galjee, M. A., 407, *418*
Galli, M., 591, *598*
Gallis, H. A., 52, *67,* 239, *243*
Galvin, J. R., 20, *37,* 331, *340,* 403, *417*
Galy, P., 78, *99*
Gamberg, P., 189, *197*
Gamsu, G., 33, *39,* 56, 57, *67,* 118, *124,* 202, 203, 210, *216, 217, 218,* 246, *271,* 283, 284, 287, *295,* 331, 332, 335, *340, 341,* 346, 348, 352, 353, *362, 363, 364,* 403, *417,* 450, *472*
Garay, S. M., 20, 23, *37,* 55, 57, *67,* 115, *124,* 247, 248, 255, 256, *271, 272*
Garcia del Castillo, H., 593, *599*
Garcia, A., 572, *596*
Garcia-Bunuel, R., 74, *98*
Garcia-Dorado, D., 593, *599*
Gard, M. F., 401, *416*
Gardner, D., 346, *362*
Garratt, K. N., 552, *566*
Garray, S. M., 246, *271*
Garvey, J. M., 236, *242*
Gatewood, R. P., Jr., 435, 436, *442*
Gatsonis, C., 90, 91, *101*
Gay, B. B., Jr., 147, *157*
Gay, S. B., 142, *156*
Gayraud, L., 305, *318*
Gazelle, G. S., 348, *363*
Ge, J., 540, *563*
Gee, J. B. L., 335, *341*
Geelhoed, G. W., 24, *38*
Gefter, W. B., 30, *39,* 52, *67,* 78, 79, 86, *98, 100,* 149, *158,* 227, 236, *241,* 331, *340,* 406, 407, *417, 418,* 450, 471, *472*
Gehlmann, H. R., 455, *473*
Geisinger, M. A., 135, *155*
Gelb, A., 276, *294*
Gelbfish, J. S., 552, *565*
Geleijns, J., 383, *388*
Geller, S. C., 522, *532*
Gelman, R., 148, *157*
Généreux, G. P., 133, 135, 142, 144, *154,* 275, 276, 281, *293,* 332, *340*
Gens, D., 148, *157*
George, B. S., 553, 554, *566, 567*
George, P. Y., 137, *155*

George, R. B. , 323, 338
Georgi, M., 384, 388
Gephardt, G. N., 190, 191, 197, 301, 316
Geraghty, J. J., 403, 417
Gerber, T., 540, 563
Germann, P. S., 165, 195
Germano, G., 591, 598
Gerson, M. C., 573, 596
Geshwind, H., 536, 544, 568
Ghahremani, G. G., 147, 156, 157
Ghossain, M. A, 91, 102.,
Gibbons, R. J., 546, 565
Giddens, D. P., 425, 442
Gierada, D. S., 291, 296
Gil-Extremera, B., 21, 37
Gilbert, H. A., 106, 122
Gilpin, J. W., 127, 132, 152
Gingrich, R. D., 20, 37
Ginsberg, R., 96, 103
Ginsberg, R. J., 90, 94, 100, 102
Girard, W. M. , 323, 338
Giraud, F., 118, 124, 201, 203, 216, 217, 403, 417
Girdany, B. R., 129, 153
Girod, D. A., 555, 567
Girone, G., 248, 271
Gitschlag, K. F., 94, 102
Giuntini, C., 322, 338
Giuseffi, J., 148, 152, 157
Glabraith, T. A., 353, 365
Glagpov, S., 425, 442
Glas, W. W., 144, 156
Glasier, C. M., 112, 123
Glaspy, F., 333, 340
Glassberg, R. M., 353, 364
Glassroth, J., 57, 61, 68
Glazer, G. M., 84, 90, 91, 99, 100, 101, 325, 339
Glazer, H. S., 8, 17, 90, 100, 115, 123, 124, 190, 197, 298, 304, 308, 314, 316, 318, 333, 340, 360, 366, 377, 379, 388, 391, 404, 415, 417, 450, 472
Gleason, R. E., 70, 97
Glickman, M. G., 525, 533
Global Program on Aids, 41, 65
Glover, J. L., 520, 532

Goar, F. G., 439, 443
Gobien, R. P.., 135, 155
Goco, R. V., 287, 296
Goddard, P. R., 283, 295
Godeau, B., 24, 38
Godwin, J. D., 218
Godwin, J. D., 52, 67, 108, 123, 206, 207, 217, 245, 246, 271, 337, 341, 403, 417, 517, 523, 531, 532
Goff, B. A., 358, 366
Goldberg, E. M., 360, 366
Goldberg, M. A., 10, 17
Goldberg, S. L., 541, 564
Golden, J., 203, 217, 262, 273
Golden, J. A., 353, 364
Goldenberg, T., 548, 565
Goldin, J. G., 270, 274
Goldman, A. L., 359, 366
Goldstein, L. D., 508, 530
Goldstein, S. A., 516, 530
Goldstraw, P., 201, 216
Golinko, R. J., 560, 568
Gomes, A. S., 394, 416
Gomez, F., 353, 364
Gong, H., 65, 68
Good, W. F., 371, 387
Goodgold, H. M., 304, 317
Goodman, L., 325, 339
Goodman, L.R., 14, 18, 135, 141, 154, 155, 173, 176, 180, 195, 196, 276, 294, 323, 339, 403, 417, 525, 533
Goodman, N. C., 593, 600
Goodman, P., 137, 155
Goodman, P. C., 56, 67, 91, 102, 136, 155, 165, 195, 333, 341, 359, 366
Goodman, P. G., 329, 339
Goodpasture, E. W., 230, 241
Gopal, A. S., 593, 599
Goralnik, C. H., 351, 363
Gordon, L., 135, 155
Gosselin, B., 201, 216, 265, 273
Gossinger, H. D., 467, 474
Gott, V. L., 520, 532
Gottschalk, A., 391, 395, 399, 415, 416
Gough, J., 280, 294
Gould, G. A., 283, 295

Gould, K. L., 423, *441*
Gould, R. G., 577, *597*
Goulding, P. L., 284, *296*
Gouse, J. C., 142, *156*
Graham, R. J., 144, *156*
Granda, M. G., 227, *240*
Granton, J., 305, *317*
Gray, H., 282, *295*
Gray, H. W., 397, *416*
Gray, J. E., 8, *17*
Gray, W. C., 359, 360, *366*
Gray, W. M., 281, *295*
Greco, F. A., 70, 78, *97*
Greco, M., 113, *123*
Green, W. M., 144, *156*
Greenberg, R. W., 91, *101*, 436, *443*
Greenberg, S. D., 47, *66*, 70, *97*
Greenblatt, D. G., 255, 256, *272*
Greene, C. E., 452, *472*
Greene, D., 94, *102*
Greene, R. E., 81, *99*
Greene, R., 5, 6, 9, *17*, 127, 128, 139, 140, 141, 142, 145, 147, *152, 155,* 352, 353, *363*
Greenough, R. L., 93, *102*
Greenspan, R. H., 391, *415*
Greenwood, L. H., 525, *533*
Grekin, T. D., 144, *156*
Grenier, P., 90, 91, *101,* 203, 206, 207, 209, *217, 218,* 220, *240,* 248, 253, *271*
Gribbin, C., 118, *124*
Griffin, D. J. , 325, *339*
Griffith, B. P., 189, *197,* 299, 307, *316, 318*
Griffith, J., 439, *443*
Grillo, H. C., 183, *196*
Grinan, N. P., 355, *365*
Grines, C L., 439, *443*
Grist, T. M., 408, *418*
Griswold, J. A., 132, 134, *154*
Grondin, C. M., 424, *441*
Groskin, S. A., 130, 132, 134, 137, 148, 149, 150, *154*
Gross, B. H., 84, 90, 91, *99, 100, 101,* 314, *318,* 325, *339*
Gross, G. W., 492, 493, 497, 502, *506*

Gross, S. C., 94, *102*
Grossman, J. E., 145, *156*
Grossman, R. F., 144, *156,* 304, 309, *317, 318*
Gruden, J. F., 56, 57, 65, *67, 68,* 260, *272*
Gruentzig, A., 535, *562*
Grujicic, S., 556, *568*
Grumbach, K., 132, *154*
Grundfest, W., 536, 537, *562*
Guagliumi, G., 539, *563*
Guest, J. L., Jr., 145, *156*
Guiberteau, M. J., 487, *506*
Guillevin, L., 234, *241*
Gulley, M. L., 35, 36, *40*
Gullo, J., 353, *364*
Gunn, J., 555, *567*
Günther-Kohfahl, S., 380, *388*
Gupta, K. B., 407, *417*
Gupta, N. C., 82, 83, 84, *99,* 119, *125,* 333, *340*
Gur, D., 371, *387*
Gurbel, P. A., 412, *418,* 555, *567*
Gurdijam, E. S., 139, *155*
Gurley, J. C., 439, *443*
Gurney, J., 45. *66*
Gurney, J. W., 6, *17,* 32, *39,* 173, *195,* 237, *242,* 323, *339,* 397, *416,* 508, *530*
Gushiken, B. J., 325, *339*
Gussenhoven, E. J., 439, *443*
Guthaner, D. F., 299, *316,* 517, 519, *530, 531,* 541, *564*
Gutierrez, F. R., 404, *417,* 455, *473,* 510, *530*

H

Ha, H. K., 361, *367*
Haacke, E. M., 427, 430, *442*
Haaga, J. R., 348, *363*
Haas, R. A., 327, *339*
Haasler, G. B., 135, *154*
Habermann, T. M., 237, *242*
Hackman, R. C., 30, *38*
Haddad, R., 94, *102*
Hadlock, F., 524, *532*

Haft, J. J., 424, 439, *441*
Haggar, A. M., 90, *101*
Hagler, D. J., 560, *568*
Hahn, P. F., 327, 330, *339*
Hall, P., 550, *565,* 592, *599*
Halls, J. M., 15, *18*
Halvorsen, R. A., 52, *67,* 325, *339*
Halvorsen, R. A., Jr., 306, *318*
Hamada, M., 450, *472*
Hamade, S., 517, *531*
Hamby, R. I., 436, *443*
Hamer, N. A. J., 78, *98*
Hamilton, G. W., 423, *441*
Hamm, C. W., 553, *566*
Hammainen, P., 304, *317*
Hammers, L. W., 90, *101*
Hammond, C. B., 108, 113, *122, 123*
Hamper, U. M., 351, *363*
Hamvas, A., 400, *416*
Han, M. C., 21, *37,* 201, *216,* 260, *272*
Handschumacher, M. D., 593, *599*
Hanfling, S. M., 469, *474*
Hanna, J. W., 327, 328, *339*
Hannah, J., 48, 55, *66, 67*
Hansell, B. M., 201, *216*
Hansell, D., 370, *387*
Hansell, D. M., 30, 31, *39,* 201, 210, *216, 218,* 235, 236, *242,* 291, *296*
Hansen, H. H., 81, *99*
Hansen, M., 81, *99*
Hansen, W. W., 578, *597*
Hansen-Flaschen, J., 33, 35, *40*
Hanson, J. S., 455, *473*
Haque, A. K., 70, 72, 78, 79, 81, *97*
Harada, J., 520, 522, *532*
Haramati, L. B., 61, *68,* 350, *363*
Haratake, J., 108, *122*
Hardesty, R. L., 189, *197,* 299, 307, *316, 318*
Hardy, K. A., 260, *272*
Harell, G., 517, *530*
Harell, G. S., 447, *472*
Harjula, A. L. J., 299, *316*
Harker, C., 361, *367*
Harkin, T. J., 220, 223, *240,* 255, 256, *272*
Harms, G. F., 8, *17*

Harris, J. A., 520, *532*
Harris, J. H., Jr., 130, *154*
Harris, K. M., 36, *40,* 310, *318*
Harris, R. D., 130, *154*
Harris, R. E., 30, *39*
Harris. L. K., 333, *341*
Harrison, N. K., 201, *216*
Hart, I. R., 107, *122*
Harter, L., 346, 352, *362*
Hartiala, J. J., 583, 595, *597, 601*
Hartigan, P. A., *564*
Hartman, A., 552, *566*
Hartman, T. E., 26, *38,* 148, 150, *157,* 201, *216,* 227, 237, 240, *241, 243,* 262, *272*
Hartnell, G. G., 558, *568*
Hartog, M., 413, *418*
Hartung, W., 280, 281, *294*
Hartunian, S. L., 127, *152*
Harvey, J. C., 358, *365*
Hasegawa, S., 410, *418*
Haskin, M. E., 325, *339*
Hatabu, H., 407, 410, *418,* 450, 471, *472*
Hatakeyama, M., 202, *217*
Hatcher, C. R., Jr., 169, *195*
Hatle, L. K., 463, *474*
Hatron, P-Y., 201, *216*
Hatttori, N., 588, *598*
Haussinger, K., 247, *271*
Havemann, K., 96, *103*
Hawkins, H. K., 593, *600*
Hawkins, R. A., 333, *340*
Hay, E., 129, *154*
Hayashi, K., 520, *532*
Hayden, C. H., 47, *66*
Hayes, S. N., 593, *599*
Haygood, T. M., 5, 7, *17*
Hayhurst, M. D., 283, 284, 285, *295, 296*
Hayward, M. W. J., 413, *418*
Heard, B. E., 275, *294*
Heater, K. 180, *196*
Hedlund, L. W., 32, *39,* 284, *296,* 330, *339*
Heelan, R., 90, 91, *101*
Heffner, J.. E., 357, 359, *365, 366*
Heiberg, E., 150, *158,* 525, *533*

Heiken, J. P., 151, *158,* 247, *271*
Heitzman, E. R., 61, *68,* 74, *98,* 107, *122,* 275, *294,* 323, 324, 325, *338*
Hellekant, C. A. G., 329, *339*
Hellenbrand, W. E., 560, *568*
Helmen, C., 455, *473*
Hemmingsson, A., 335, *341*
Hendel, R. C., 590, *598*
Hendershott, L., 304, *317*
Henkel, B., 412, *418*
Henly, W. C., 519, *531*
Henry, D. A., 128, *153*
Henschke, C. I., 56, *67,* 115, *124*
Hepper, N. G. G., 338, *341*
Herbert, F. A., 236, *242*
Herf, S. M., 83, *99*
Herfkens, R. H., 313, *318*
Herfkens, R. J., 403, 407, *417*
Herfkens, R. L., 517, *531*
Herlod, C. J., 165, *195*
Herman, S. J., 209, *218,* 262, *273,* 298, 299, 302, 304, 305, 308, *316, 317,* 348, 353, 355, *363, 364*
Hermans, W., 550, *565*
Hernandez, R. J., 455, *473*
Herndon, J., 91, *102*
Herold, C. J., 269, *273, 274,* 401, *416*
Herold, C. J., *273*
Heron, C. W., 113, 115, , *123*
Herregods, M. C., 539, *563*
Herrmann, H. C., 553, *566*
Hertz, C. H,. 574, *596*
Hertz, M. I., 30, 31, 32, *39,* 306, *318*
Hertzler, G. L., 467, *474*
Herve, P. A., 307, *318*
Hess, J., 560, *568*
Hess, K. R., 519, *531*
Hessen, I. , 323, *338*
Hessol, N. A., 56, *67*
Heyd, R L., 144, *156*
Heywang, S. H., 115, *124*
Higashihara, T., 210, *218,* 260, *272*
Higashino, S. M., 528, *534*
Higenbottam, T., 299, 300, *316*
Higgins, C. B., 447, 463, *472, 473, 474,* 518, 528, *531, 534,* 579, 580, *597*

Higgins, T. L. , 167, *195*
Hildebrand, F. L., 237, *242*
Hill, C. A., 74, 79, *98, 99*
Hillege, H. L., 553, *566*
Hillerdal, G., 335, *341*
Hillis, L. D., 545, *564*
Hillman, B. J., 13, *18*
Hindel, R., 387, *388*
Hines, J.D., 70, *97*
Hiraishi, S., 432, *442*
Hirakada, K., 108, *122*
Hirose, Y., 517, *531*
Hirota, S., 201, *216*
Hirozawa, A., 56, *67*
Hirschman, C. A, 269, *273, 274*
Hirsh, J., 414, *419*
Hirshman, C. A., *273*
Hirst, A. E., 519, *531*
Hix, W., 331, *340*
Ho, M, 354, 360, *364, 366*
Hochholzer, L., 332, *340*
Hodgson, J. McB., 439, *444*
Hoffman, J. M., 83, 91, *99,* 119, *125,* 333, *341*
Hoffmann, K. R., 377, *388*
Hofman, M., 407, *418*
Hogg, J., 276, *294*
Hoh, C. K., 333, *340*
Hoidal, J. R., 227, 233, 236, *241*
Holland, D G., 148, 149, 150, *158*
Holland, G. A., 407, 410, *417, 418*
Holland, S.A., 299, 306, *316, 318*
Holliday, R. L., 128, *153*
Hollier, L. H., 517, *530*
Holmberg, S. D., 56, *67*
Holmes, D. R., 545, 546, 552, *564, 565, 566*
Holt, S., 129, *153*
Holub, R. V., 348, 355, *363*
Holubkov, R., 545, *564*
Hom, M., 135, *155*
Honda, T., 450, *472*
Honeyman, J. C., 9, *17*
Hooper, R. G., 32, *39,* 94, *102,* 237, *243*
Hopewell, P. C., 56, 57, *67*
Hopper, K. D., 348, 352, *363*

Horowitz, S. F., 590, *598*
Horrigan, T. P., 70, *97,* 160, *195,* 354, *364*
Horvath, J. , 309, 310, *318*
Hounsfield, G. N., 10, 11, *17, 18*
Hourihane, D. O., 331, *340*
Houssfield, G. N., 577, *596*
Howard, J., 456, 458, 462, 467, *473*
Howard, T., 78, 79, *98*
Hoyt, N., 135, *155*
Hruban, R. H., 25, *38,* 262, *272,* 283, *295,* 304, *317*
Hsai, T., 578, *597*
Hsieh, J., 401, *416*
Hsu, B. Y., 221, *241*
Hsu, T. C., 129, *153*
Hu, B., 595, *601*
Huang, C. T., 43, *65*
Huang, E. K., 436, *443*
Huang, H. K., 370, *387*
Huang, L., 56, 57, *67*
Huang, R., 20, 23, *37*
Huang, T-Y, 144, *156*
Huang, W., 383, *388*
Huber, R. M., 247, *271*
Hudson, E. R., 414, *418*
Hull, R. D., 414, *419*
Humphrey, H., 236, *242*
Humphrey, L. M., 371, *387*
Hung, J-S., 556, *567*
Hunink, M. G. M., 14, *18*
Hunter, D. M., 381, *388*
Hunter, D. W., 353, *364*
Huong, D. L. T., 24, *38*
Hurd, R. N., 150, *158*
Hurley, J. D., 147, 148 , *157*
Hurst, D J., 237, *242*
Husband, J. E., 20, *37,* 113, 115, *123*
Husian, M., 353, *364*
Hussain, S., 520, *532*
Husted, J. 78, 79, *98*
Hutchins, G. M., 25, *38*
Hutton, L.C., 299, 306, *316, 318*
Hwang, S. H., 358, *365*
Hyde, P. P., 574, *596*

I

Iannaccone, G., 108, *123*
Ido, T., 84, *100*
Idolor, L., 305, *317*
Igboaka, G., 299, *316*
Ihde, D. C., 96, *102*
Iinuma, T., 377, *388*
Ikeda, M., 371, *388*
Ikeda, T., 283, *295*
Ikeda, U., 456, *473*
Ikezoe, J., 91, *101,* 227, *240,* 260, *272,* 354, 355, *364*
Ilowite, J. S., 43, *66*
Ilves, R., 90, *100*
Im, J., 78, 79, *99,* 227, *241,* 260, *272*
Im, J-G., 21, *37,* 201, *216,* 246, *271,* 284, *295,* 332, *340,* 358, *365,* 450, *472*
Imakita, S., 517, *531*
Imoto, E. M., 234, *241*
Imparto, A., 591, *598*
Indeck, M., 127, *152*
Ingrisch, H., 115, *124,* 247, *271*
Ioto, H., 203, *217*
Iozzo, R. V., 50, *67*
Irey, N. S., 31, *39*
Ishigakai, T., 371, *388*
Ishihara, T., 446, 447, *472*
Ishiwata, K., 84, *100*
Isitman, A. T., 304, *317*
Isler, R J., 352, 353, *363*
Ismail, S., 593, *600*
Isner, J. M., 424, *441,* 463, *474,* 558, *568*
Isoda, H., 410, *418*
Isom, O. W., 555, *567*
Israel, R. H., 220, 221, *240,* 255, 256, *272*
Israel, Y., 129, *153*
Isselbacher, E. M., 523, *532*
Ito, M., 84, *100*
Itoh, H., 200, *215,* 227, *241,* 260, *272*
Izumi, R., 260, *272*
Izumi, T., 200, 203, *215, 217*

J

Jachman, J. D., 544, *564*
Jackson, A., 128, *153*
Jackson, C. V., 221, *241,* 255, 256, *272*
Jackson, D. C., 414, *418*
Jackson, D. E., Jr., 93, *102*
Jackson, L.K., 81, *99*
Jacobs, D. G., 525, *533*
Jacobson, F., 133, 144, *154*
Jacobson, F. L., 64, *68*
Jaffe, R. B., 22, *38*
Jagannadharao, B., 150, *158*
Jahnke, E. J., 524, *532*
Jain, A., 536, *562*
Jain, S. P., 539, *562*
Jamieson, P. M., 139, 140, 141, *155*
Jamieson, S. W., 299, *316*
Janower, M. L., 33, *39,* 107, *122*
Janzen, D. L., 20, 28, 29, *37,* 239, *243*
Japaze, H., 74, *98*
Jasslowitz, B., 33, *39*
Jayaweera, A. R., 593, *600*
Jederlinic, P. J., 213, *218*
Jeffrey, R. B., 132, *154*
Jeffrey, R. B., Jr., 135, *154*
Jelinek, J. S., 94, 95, *102*
Jenkinson, S. G., 304, *317,* 323, *338*
Jensen, B. G., 90, *101*
Jensik, R., 358, *365*
Jiang, L., 593, *599*
Jicha, D. L., 118, *124*
Jing, B. S., 113, *123*
Joharjy, I. A., 253, *271*
Johiaddin, R. H., 528, *534*
Johkoh, T., 227, *240*
Johns, V. J., 519, *531*
Johnson, J. A., 523, *532*
Johnson, S. B., 528, *534*
Johnson, T. D., 270, *274*
Johnston, W. W., 355, *365*
Johnston-Early, A., 96, *102*
Jolles, H., 135, *155*
Jones, J. G., 144, *156*
Jones, J. M., 237, *242*
Jones, J. W., 455, *473*
Jones, M., 446, *472,* 593, *599*
Jones, R. H., 587, *597*
Jones, R. N., 335, *341*
Jost, R. G., 8, *17,* 371, 377, 379, *388,* 391, *415*
Joyce, J. W., 281, *295,* 517, *530, 531*
Joyner, C. R., 574, *596*
Julien, P. J., 313, *318,* 407, *417*
Julius, H. W., 383, *388*
Julliere, Y., 552, *566*
Julsrud, P. R., 583, 584, *597*

K

Kadowaki, K., 91, *101*
Kagan, A. R., 106, *122*
Kagan, E., 331, *340*
Kahn, D. R., 467, *474*
Kahn, F. W., 237, *242*
Kahn, O., 399, *416*
Kaiser, L. R., 90, 90, *100*
Kaji, T., 525, *533*
Kalebo, P., 403, *417*403, *417*
Kalender, W. A., 11, 14, *18*
Kalisher, L., 106, 113, *122*
Kallay, M. C., 255, 256, *272, 352, 363*
Kalman, J. M., 592, *599*
Kaltenbach, M., 552, *566*
Kaltenborn, W. T., 283, *295*
Kamp, O., 517, *531*
Kan, J. S., 555, 560, 558, 562, *567, 568*
Kanai, E., 484, *505*
Kanaoka, M., 200, *215*
Kang, E. Y., 148, 150, *157*
Kang, M. W., 361, *367*
Kao, A. K., 439, *443*
Kaplan, J. D., 400, *416*
Kaplan, L. D., 57, *68*
Kaplan, M. H.., 23, 24, *38*
Kaplan, V., 236, *242*
Karp, J., 61, *68*
Karwande, S. V., 85, *100*
Kasper, W., 412, *418*
Kassner, E G., 476, 477, 489, 500, *505*
Kastrati, A., 553, *566*
Katsura, S., 275, 281, *293*

Katz, J., 476, 477, *505*
Katz, M. H., 56, *67*
Katz, N. M, 452, *472*
Katzenstein, A. L., 234, 237, *241, 243*
Kauder, D. R., 132, *154*
Kaufmann, R. B., 437, *443*
Kaul, T. K., 467, *474*
Kavuru, M., 20, 24, *37*
Kawaguchi, K., 456, *473*
Kawashima, A., 335, *341*
Kazerooni, E. A., 194, *197,* 314, *318,* 522, *532*
Kazmier, F. J., 517, 520, 521, *531*
Keane, J. F., 562, *568*
Kearney, P. A., 528, *534*
Keegan, J., 427, 430, *442,* 595, *601*
Keer, I., 262, *273*
Keidel, W.D., 574, *596*
Keighley, C. S., 592, *599*
Keightley, A., 360, *366*
Keiper, M. D., 47, *66*
Kelley, M. J., 361, *366,* 436, *443*
Kelly, G. D., 47, *66*
Kennedy, R. L. J., 235, *241*
Kent, K.M., 424, *441,* 540, *563*
Keppler, J. S., 15, *18*
Keramati, B., 152, *158*
Kereiakes, D. J., 403, *417*
Kerley, P., 280, *294*
Kern, J. A., 50, *67*
Kerns, S. R., 142, *156*
Keshavjee, S. H., 299, *316*
Kesten, S., 305, *317*
Khaja, F., 425, *442*
Khaw, B. A., 591, *598*
Khelifa, F., 304, *317*
Khine, N. M., 333, *340*
Khlat, B., 550, *565*
Khouri, N. F., 351, 352, 353, 354, 355, *363*
Khoury, M. B., 52, *67*
Khoury, N. F., 254, *272*
Kiat, H., 591, *598*
Kier, R., 108, *123*
Kilburn, K. H., 281, *294*
Kilner, P. J., 583, *597*

Kim, I. Y., 246, *271*
Kim, W. Y., 593, *599*
Kim, Y. H., 358, *365*
Kim, Y. M., 201, *216,* 580, *597*
Kimball, B. P ., 550, *565*
Kime, S. W., 519, *531*
Kimmel, M., 70, *97*
Kincaid, O. W., 517, *531*
King, D. S., 106, *122*
King, S. B., 544, *564*
King, T. E., Jr., 206, 207, 210, *217, 218,* 265, *273*
Kirby, T. J., 190, 191, *197,* 301, *316*
Kirchner, P. T., 487, *506*
Kirk, J. M. E., 201, *216*
Kirkham, J. A., 348, *363*
Kirschner, P. A., 333, *340*
Kirsh, M. M., 525, *533*
Kirshenbaum, K. J., 525, *533*
Kishel, J., 424, *441*
Kita, N., 210, *218,* 260, *272*
Kitaishi, M., 200, 203, *215, 217,* 260, *272*
Kitatani, F., 260, *272*
Kivisaari, L, 304, *317*
Kjeldsberg, C. R., 36, *40*
Kleerup, E. B., 270, *274*
Klein, J. S., 65, *68,* 90, 91, 92, 93, 94, 96. *100,* 210, *218,* 283, 287, *295,* 357, *365*
Klotz, E., 11, 14, *18*
Klotz, T. A., 415, *419*
Klugh, G. A., 275, 281, *294*
Knapper, W. H., 115, *123*
Knight, L. C., 592, *598*
Knowles, M. C., 43, *66*
Knudson, R J., 283, *295*
Koch, C. A., 539, 540, *563*
Kofai, F., 106, *122*
Kohman, L. J., 170, *195*
Kojima, M., 456, *473*
Kondo, C., 407, *417,* 514, *530*
Koning, R., 556, *568*
Kono, M, 201, *216*
Kopecky, K. K., 247, *271*
Korchik, R., 74, *98*
Kormos, R.L., 189, *197*
Korn, R. L., 355, *364*

Korobkin, M., 325, *339*
Koschmann, E. B., 22, *38*
Koschyk, D. H., 523, *532*
Kostuk, W. J., 572, *596*
Kotzur, I. M., 4, *17*
Kouchoukos, N. T., 167, *195*
Kovach, J. A., 541, *564*
Kovacs, S. J. J., 575, *596*
Kovalski, , R., 33, 35, *40*
Kozuka, T., 210, *218,* 260, *272,* 354, 355, *364*
Kram, H. B., 525, *533*
Kramer, J., 399, *416*
Kramer, M. R., 189, *197*
Krasnow, A. Z., 304, *317*
Kreel, L., 106, 107, 112, *121, 122*
Kress, M. B., 287, *296*
Kressel, H. Y., 147, *157*
Kricsfeld, D., 593, *600*
Kriebel, D., 331, *340*
Kriegshauser, J. S., 583, 584,*597*
Kroboth, F. J., 22, *38*
Krzyaniak, R., 467, *474*
Ku, D. N., 425, *442*
Kubota, K., 84, *99, 100*
Kudsk, K., 148, 150, *158*
Kuhjda, F. P., 78, 79, *98*
Kuhlman, J. E., 20, 23, 24, 25, *37, 38,* 43, 57, *66, 68,* 78, 79, *98,* 237, 240, *243,* 304, *317*
Kulkarni, P. K., 452, *472*
Kulling, P., 203, 209, *217, 218,* 262, *272*
Kulwiec, P., 206, 207, *217*
Kumar, K., 129, *153*
Kundel, H, L., 371, *387*
Kundu, S., 298, *316*
Kuni, C. C., 306, *318*
Kuntz, R. E., 539, 541, 547, 552, 553, 554, *562, 564, 565, 566*
Kuntz, R. E. J. P., 550, *565*
Kuo, S. H., 327, *339*
Kusano, S., 432, *442*
Kussmaul, W. G., 463, *473*
Kutcher, W. L., 248, *271*
Kuwano, K., 283, *295*
Kwan, S. Y., 201, *216*

Kwong, J. S., 148, 150, *157,* 245, 248, *271*
Kypridakis, G., 78, 79, *98*

L

Lababidi, Z., 555, *567*
Lablanche, J. M., 536, 544, 550, *565, 568*
Labs, J. D., 520, *532*
Lack, E. E., 65, *68*
Ladowski, J. S., 307, *318*
Lahrs, A., 304, *316*
Lally, J. F., 525, *533*
Lambiase, R.E., 327, *339*
Lamik, N., 14, *18,* 525, *533*
Lammert, G. K., 135, *155*
Lancee, C. T., 439, *443*
Landas, S. K., 403, *417*
Landau, C., 545, *564*
Landay, M. J., 148, 152, *157,* 166, *195*
Landzberg, J. S., 547, *565*
Lane, W. W., 71, 73, *98*
Lange, P., 359, *366*
Lange, R. A., 545, *564*
Lange, W. A., 139, *155*
Langlotz, C. P., 47, *66*
Langou, R. A., 436, *443*
Laoide, R. M., 348, *363*
LaSpada Barone, M., 248, *271*
Lastoria, S., 592, *598*
Latour, M. G., 56, *67*
Latrabe, V., 305, *318*
Laurent, F., 305, *318*
Lauterbur, P.C., 578, *597*
Law, M. R., 20, *37*
Lawrason, J., 132, *154*
Laws, J. W., 275, *294*
Lawson, D. W., 330, *340*
Lawton, M A., 539, 540, *563*
Leatherman, J. W., 227, 233, 236, *241*
LeBlanc, J., 353, *364*
Lederle, F. A., 221, 223, *241*
Ledesma-Medina, J., 36, *40,* 311, *318*
Ledgerwood, A. M., 135, *155,*
Lee, A. S., 360, *366*

Lee, B. H., 246, *271*
Lee, B. H., 358, *365*
Lee, J. J., 115, *124,* 247, 260, *271, 272*
Lee, J. N., 201, *216*
Lee, K S., 26, *38,* 237, *243,* 246, 262, *271, 272,* 358, *365*
Lee, M J., 358, 359, *366*
Lee, R. J., 592, *599*
Lee, V. W., 57, *68*
Lee, Y. C., 355, *365*
Lefcoe, M S., 210, *218*
Lehmann, K. J., 384, *388*
Lehrman, S., 223, *240*
Leitman, B. S., 55, *67*
Lemmer, J. H., 358, *365*
Lenchner, G. S., 237, *242*
Lenique, F. 248, *271*
Lenoir, S., 203, 206, 207, 209, *217, 218*
Lensing, A. W. A., 397, *416*
Lentz, D., 306, *318*
Lenz, D., 262, *273*
Leon, M. B., 539, 541, 552, 553, *562, 564, 566*
Leppanen, M., 352, 353, *363*
Leppo, J. A., 590, *598*
Leroy, F., 550, *565*
Lessof, L., 331, *340*
Lester, R. G., 24, *38,* 132, 134, 141, 148, *154*
Lesur, O., 276, *294*
Letac, B., 556, *568*
Letourneau, L., 152, *158*
Leung, A. N., 338, *341*
Lev-Toaff, A. F., 202, *216*
Levin, D. C., 83, *99,* 437, *443*
Levine, B., 52, *67*
Levine, G. M., 147, *157*
Levine, G., 132, *154*
Levine, M. J., 553, 554, *566*
Levine, M. S., 147, *157*
Levine, S. J., 20, 21, *37*
Levine, S. M., 304, *317*
Levitt, R. G., 90, *100,* 115, *124,* 333, *340,* 404, *417*
Levy-Ravetch, M., 450, *472*
LeWinter, M. M., 446, 447, *472*

Lewis, A., 425, *441*
Lewis, E., 81, *99*
Lewis, J. W., Jr., 81, 90, *99, 100*
Lewis, W., 469, *474*
Leya, F., 550, 552, *565*
Li, D., 427, 430, *442*
Li, K. C., 595, *601*
Li, W., 427, 428, *442,* 595, *601*
Liberthson, R. R., 517, *531*
Libshitz, H. I., 108, 112, 113, 115, 117, *122, 123,* 239, *243,* 335, *341*
Lie, J. T., 234, *241,* 517, *530*
Lieberman, Y., 361, *366*
Liebman, H. A., 57, *68*
Light, R. N., 323, *338*
Light, R. W., 355, *365*
Lillington, G., 215, *218*
Limas, C., 74, *98*
Lin, H. C., 129, *153*
Lincoff, A. M., 553, *566*
Linder, J., 32, *39,* 237, *242,* 355, *365*
Linder, K., 591, *598*
Lindsay, J., 520, *532*
Lindsay, J. Jr., 516, *530*
Linker, D.T., *569*
Links, J. M., 269, *273*
Linton, O. W., 4, *17*
Lipchik, E. O., 14, *18,* 525, *533*
Lipscomb, K., 423, *441*
Lipton, M. J., 517, *531*
Lisa, J. R., 106, *122*
Lishko, M. M., 32, *39*
List, A. F., 70, 78, *97*
Little, A. G., 93, *102*
Little, W. C., 424, 439, *441*
Litvack, F., 536, 537, 547, 548, *562, 565*
Liu, P., 517, *531*
Livoni, J. P., 525, *533*
Llamas, J. M., 93, *102*
Lo, J. Y., 384, *388*
Lock, J. E., 562, *568*
Lodato, R. F., 33, 35, *40*
Logan, P. M., 27, *38,* 210, *218,* 227, *241*
Lohela, P., 352, 353, *363*
Loire, R., 191, *197,* 304, *317*
Loiseau, A., 248, *271*

Lombard, C., 207, *217,* 234, *241*
Long, R. W., 90, *100*
Longmore, D. B., 313, *318,* 483, 493, 505, 528, *534*
Loop, F. D., 167, *195*
Loose, R., 384, *388*
Lopez-Pujol, J., 93, *102*
Lorber, P., 323, *338*
Lorell, B. H., 447, 455, 456, 458, 459, 462, 467, *472*
Loubeyre, P., 191, *197,* 304, 306, *317,* 410, *418*
Love, L., 147, *156*
Lowe, J. E., 147, *157,* 187, *196*
Lowe, V. J., 83, 91, *99, 102,* 119, *125,* 333, *341*
Lowrey, A. H., 69, *97*
Loy, M., 469, *474*
Loyd, J., 309, 310, *318*
Loyd, J. E., 389, *415*
Lubat, E., 20, 23, *37*
Lucas, C. E., 135, *155*
Lucca, M., 467, *474*
Lucena, F. M., 355, *365*
Luck, J. C., 167, *195*
Ludington, L. G, 78, 79, *98*
Luh, K.T., 327, *339,* 355, *365*
Lund, J. T., 583, 584, *597*
Lundell, C. J., 415, *419*
Lundevall, J., 524, *532*
Lundy, J., 135, *155*
Luo, H., 553, *566*
Lutin, W., 560, *568*
Lynch, D A., 203, 206, 207, 210, *217, 218,* 254, 260, 261, 264, 270, *272, 274,* 307, 311, *318,* 335, *341*
Lynch, E. L., 206, 207, *217*

M

Maack, I., 380, *388*
Maason, D. T., 573, *596*
Mabry, M. R., 12, *18*
Macander, P. J., 554, *567*
Macaya, C., 553, 554, *566*

Macdonald, D.W., 129, *153*
MacFall, J. R., 408, *418*
Macher, A. M., 469, *474*
Machovski, A., 595, *601*
MacIntyre, N. R., 203, *217*
MacMahon, H., 371, 372, 377, 382, 384, 387, *388*
MacMillan, R. M., 485, *505*
Macnee, W., 283, *295*
Madayag, M. A., 525, *533*
Maddahi, J., 587, *598*
Madewell, J. E., 467, *474*
Madrazo, B. L., 90, 94, *100, 102*
Maglinte, D. D. T., 525, *533*
Maguire, G. P., 471, *474*
Maher, J. E., 437, *443*
Mahfood, S. S., 168, *195*
Mahon, D. J., 541, *564*
Mahon, T. G., 113, 115, *123*
Mahoney, M. C., 74, *98*
Maiello, L., 541, 550, *564, 565, 592, 599*
Maile, C. W., 108, *123,* 237, *243*
Maisch, B., 456, 462, 463, 467, *473*
Maitre, S., 403, *417*
Makino, T., 529, *534*
Makowka, L., 36, *40*
Makris, A. N., 56, *67*
Makuch, R., 117, *124*
Mallery, J. A., 439, *443*
Malmberg, P., 335, *341*
Maltby, J. D., 237, *242*
Mangiante, E. C., 148, 150, *158*
Manion, W. C., 524, *532*
Mann, H., 85, *100*
Manning, W. J., 427, 428, *442,* 592, 595, *599, 601*
Manoussakis, M. N., 235, *241*
Manson, D., 128, 145, *153, 156*
Mansour, K., 94, *102*
Manzara, C. C., 583, *597*
Marcassa, C., 591, *598*
Marchal, G., 14, *18*
Marchevsky, A., 64, *68*
Marcq, M., 78, *99*
Mardelli, T. J., 433, *442*
Marelli, A. J., 482, 493, *505*

Marglin, S. I., 237, *242*
Margolis, J., 547, *565*
Marin, M. G., 220, 221, *240,* 255, 256, *272*
Marinelli, D. L., 50, *67*
Mark, J. B. D., 28, *38*
Markarian, B., 107, *122,* 275, *294*
Markham, J., 400, *416*
Marnocha, K. E., 525, *533*
Marquette, C. H., 203, *217*
Marsan, R. E., 523, *532*
Marshall, C. H., 118, *124*
Marshall, J., 517, *531*
Marshall, S. E., 189, *197*
Martin, C. J., 275, 281, *293*
Martin, R. G., 458, *473*
Martinez, A. J., 237, *242*
Martinez, J., 528, *534*
Martini, N., 90, 91, *101*
Marx,, G.R., 593, *599*
Masuba, K., 283, *295*
Masui, T., 407, 410, *417, 418,* 463, *474,* 579, *597*
Masur, H., 19, 20, *35*
Masura, J., 555, *567*
Mathejssen, N. A., 594, *600*
Mathews, J. F., 371, 376, *388*
Mathieson, J. R., 199, 200, *215*
Mathisen, D. J., 172, 173, *195*
Matsubara, O., 529, *534*
Matsunaga, N., 520, *532*
Matsuoka, Y., 520, *532*
Matsuzawa, T., 84, *99*
Matthay, R., 28, 30, 31, *38, 39,* 69, 74, 81, 84, *97, 99,* 107, *122,* 337, *341*
Matthews, J. F., 9, *17*
Matthews, M. J., 72, 74, *98*
Matthias, P. M., 270, *274*
Mattingly, T. W., 524, *532*
Mattox, K. L., 128, 137, *153, 155*
Mauch, P., 33, *40*
Mauer, J., 305, *317*
Maurer, A. H., 592, *598*
Maurer, J. R., 190, 191, *197,* 307, 309, *318*
Mauri, F., 201, *216*

Maurice, F., 220, *240,* 253, *271*
Maus, T. P., 403, *417*
Mautner, G. C., 437, *443*
Mautner, S. L., 437, *443*
May, G. R., 118, *124*
Mayo, J., 33, *39,* 119, *125,* 212, *218*
Mayo, J. R., 148, 150, *157,* 199, 200, *215, 218,* 284, *295,* 510, 522, *530, 532*
Mayr, B., 115, *124,* 247, *271*
McAdams, H. P., 135, *155*
McAllister, H. A., 467, *474*
McCabe, R. E., 26, 29, *38*
McCaley, D. I., 247, *271*
McCarthy, M. J., 332, *340*
McCarthy, S. M., 90, *101*
McCauley, D. I., 20, 23, *37,* 55, *67,* 246, 254, *271, 272*
McClelland, R. N., 148, 152, *157*
McClennan, B. L., 151, *158*
McCloud, T. C., 183, *196,* 391, *415*
McClung, H. C., 220, 221, *240*
McCollum, C. H., 519, *531*
McConnochie, K., 283, *295*
McCort, J. J., 128, *153*
McCracken, S. , 325, *339*
McCrea, E. S., 81, *99*
McCready, V. R., 400, *416*
McCrindle, B. W., 555, *567*
McCrory, R., 148, *157*
McDermott, V. G., 414, *418*
McDonald, J. B., 33, *39*
McElvein, R. B., 128, *153*
McGavran, M. H., 70, *97*
McGhie, J. 593, *599*
McGill, H. C., 436, *443*
McGonigal, M. D., 132, *154*
McGorisk, G., 592, *598*
McGuinnes, G., 47, 55, *66, 67,* 201, *216,* 220, 223, *240,* 240, *243,* 255, 256, *272*
McIvor, J., 355, *364*
McKennan, M., 148, *157*
McKenzie, F. N., 299, 306, *316, 318*
McKillop, J. H., 397, *416*
McKnight, R. C., 455, *473*
McLean, A., 283, 284, *295, 296*
McLelland, R., 239, *243*

McLoud, T. C., 20, *37,* 90, 91, *101,* 106, 113, *122,* 199, 202, 209, *215, 217,* 314, *318,* 327, 335, *339, 341,* 353, *364,* 517, *531*
McManus, B. M., 455, *473,* 493, *506*
McNamara, A. E., 269, *273*
McNamara, D. G., 475, *505*
McNamara, J. J., 517, *530*
McNamara, M. T., 580, *597*
McNeil, B. J., 394, *416*
McNitt-Gray, M F., 270, *274*
McVeigh, E. R. 594, *600*
Meary, E., 333, *340*
Medina, J. L., 129, *153*
Medina, L. S., 304, 313, *316, 318*
Meduri, G. U., 45, 46, *66*
Meema, H. E., 129, *153*
Meheswaran, B., 541, *564*
Mehta, A., 301, *316*
Mehta, R. C., 96, *103*
Meinertz, T., 412, *418*
Melamed, M.R., 70, *97*
Mellins, H. , 323, *338*
Melton, L. J., 517, *530*
Melville W. G., 520, *532*
Mencini, R. A., 358, *365*
Mendelson, D. S., 333, *340*
Mensch, J., 307, *318*
Menu, Y., 253, *271*
Mera, S. L., 283, *295*
Mercer, C. D., 174, *196*
Mercier, C., 360, *366*
Meredith, J. W., 127, 132, *152*
Mergner, W., 237, *242*
Merigan, T. C., 28, *38*
Merriam, M. A., 327, *339,* 358, *365*
Merrick, S. H., 436, *443*
Mesa, J. E., 536, 538, 539, *562*
Metcalf, J. P., 32, *39*
Metha, A., 190, 191 *197*
Mettler, F. A., 487, *506*
Metz, C. E., *388*
Metz, C. E., 94, *102*
Metzger, R. A., 78, *98*
Mewissen, M. W., 403, *417*
Meyer, C. R., 93, *102*

Meyer, H., 523, *532*
Meyer, P. R., Jr., 130, 132, *154*
Meyer, R., 541, 522, *564*
Meyer, R. D., 22, *37*
Meyers, J. D., 30, *38*
Meziane, M. A., 25, *38,* 283, *295*
Millar, A. B., 220, *240,* 262, *273*
Millard, F. J. C., 275, 281, *293*
Miller, D. L., 452, *472,* 529, *534*
Miller, F. A., 593, *599*
Miller, F. B., 525, *533*
Miller, F. F., 283, 287, *295*
Miller, J. I., 94, *102*
Miller, K. S., 352, *363*
Miller, M H., 128, 129, 132, 134, 136, 142, 145, *153, 154*
Miller, R. R., 27, 28, 29, 33, *38, 39,* 91, *101,* 119, *125,* 200, 201, 203, 210, 212, *215, 216, 217, 218,* 248, *271,* 283, 284, *295, 296,* 333, 338, *340, 341,* 354, *364*
Miller, S. W., 10, *17,* 447, 455, 456, 462, 467, *472,* 517, *531*
Miller, W., 47, *66*
Miller, W. E., 71, 72, 73, 81, 83, *98, 99*
Miller, W. L., 469, *474*
Miller, W. T., 48, 50, 52, *66, 67,* 78, 79, 86, *98, 100,* 132, 149, *154, 158*
Miller, W. T., Jr., 52, *67*
Millis, R., 115, *123*
Mills, L. J., 148, 152, *157*
Mills, R. J., 281, *295*
Mills, S. R., 414, *418*
Milne, E. N. C., 19, *37,* 108, *122,* 572, *596*
Milner, L. B., 353, *364*
Milroy, F., 358, *365*
Minagi, H., 151, *158*
Minami, H., 360, *366*
Miniati, M. , 322, *338*
Minna, J. D., 237, *242*
Minty, B. D., 144, *156*
Mintz, B. J., 94, *102*
Mintz, G. S., 516, *530,* 540, 541, *563, 564*
Minutoli, A., 248, *271*
Miravitlles, M., 264, *273*

Mirvis, S. E., 14, *18*, 96, *102*, 148, 152, *157, 158*, 508, 525, *530, 533*
Mitchell, S. E., 404, *417*, 555, 562, *567*, 568
Mitzner, W., 269, *273*, 274
Mitzner, W., *273*
Miyamoto, A., 537, *562*
Miyazawa, N., 90, *100*
Mizuno, K., 537, *562*
Mladinich, C. R., 348, *363*
Mintz, G. S., 592, *599*
Modiaddin, R. H., 583, *597*
Mogavaro, L., 247, *271*
Mohiaddin, R. H., 313, *318*, 483, 493, *505*
Molina, P. L., 314, *318*, 360, *366*, 371, *388*, 510, *530*
Mompoint, D., 203, 206, 207, *217*
Moncada, R., 455, *473*
Mones, J. M., 64, *68*
Mongtomery, R. D., 78, *98*
Montefusco, C. M., 298, *316*
Montesi, S. A., 353, *364*
Montgomery, D. H., 592, *598*
Moody, M., 96, *102*
Moody, P., 127, *152*
Moore, A. D. A., 206, 207, *217*
Moore, A. V., 237, *243*
Moore, A. V., Jr., 361, *366*
Moore, E. H., 209, *217*, 353, *364*, 436, *443*
Moore, K. L, 446, *472*
Moore, P. T., 352, 358, *364, 365*
Mootz, A. R., 166, *195*
Moran, F., 281, *295*
Moran, J. F., 90, *100*, 182, *196*, 333, *340*, 404, *417*, 519, *531*
Morgan, A. S., 148, 152, *157*
Morgan, D. B., 132, 134, *154*
Morgan, P. W., 14, *18*, 525, *533*
Morganroth, J. , 433 *442*
Morganstern, M J., 129, *153*
Mori, K., 90, *100*
Mori, M., 20, *37*
Morimoto, S., 91, *101*, 260, *272*, 354, 355, *364*
Morisoli, S., 484, *505*

Mornex, J. F., 304, *317*
Mornex, J., 191, *197*
Morris, E. J., 528, *534*
Morris, J. C., 64, *68*
Morrish, W. F., 262, *273*, 305, *317*
Morrison, M. C., 358, 359, *366*
Morse, S. S., 525, *533*
Moscucci, M., 553, *567*
Moser, E. S., Jr., 144, *156*
Moser, R. J., III, 404, *417*
Moses, D. C., 391, *415*
Moshage, W. E., 594, *600*
Moskovic, E., 210, *218*
Moskowitz, H. , 323, *338*
Mossman, B. T., 335, *341*
Mostbeck, G., 584, *597*
Motta, A. O., 525, *533*
Mouelhi, M. M., 206, 207, *217*
Moulton, A. L., 358, *365*
Moulton, J. S., 352, *364*
Moulton, M. S., 358, *365*
Mountain, C., 333, *340*
Mountain, C. F., 85, 86, *100*
Mourand, J-L., 558, *568*
Mouroux, J., 90, *101*
Muakkassa, F. F., 132, 134, *154*
Mueller, P. R., 10, *17*, 327, 330 *339*, 356, 358, 359, *365, 366*
Muhm, J. R., 117, *124*
Muka, E., 8, *17*, 377, *388*, 391, *415*
Mulder, D. S., 130, *154*
Mulhern, C.B., 78, *98*
Mullen, W. L., 540, *563*
Muller, J. E., 456, *473*
Muller, D. W. M., 546, *565*
Müller, N. L., 20, 26, 27, 28, 29, 30, 31, 33, *37, 38, 39*, 91, *101*, 118, 119, *124, 125*, 145, 148, 150, *156, 157*, 199, 200, 201, 203, 206, 207, 209, 210, 212, 215, *215, 216, 217, 218*, 240, *243*, 245, 246, 248, 262, 269, *271, 272, 273*, 276, 283, 284, 287, *294, 295, 296*, 322, 333, 338, *338, 340, 341*, 354, *364*
Muller, N. L., *218*
Mulopulos, G. P., 74, *98*

Mulvagh, S. L., 593, *600*
Munk, P. A., 212, *218*
Munk, P. L., 33, *39,* 119, *125, 174, 196,*
Munoz, F., 358, *365*
Munster, A. M., 135, *155*
Muntz, H. G., 358, *366*
Murch, C. R., *218*
Murdoch, J., 203, *217*
Murgo, J. P., 538, 539, *562*
Murray, K. A., 36, *40*
Murray, R. J., 237, *242*
Murry, R. C., 479, 480, 482, *505,* 508, *530*
Musselman, M. M., 144, *156*
Musset, D., 90, 91, *101,* 220, *240,* 253, *271,* 403, *417*
Muto, P., 592, *598*
Myers, J. L., 200, *215,* 234, *241,* 261, 262, *272, 273,* 304, *317,*

N

Naclerio, E. A., 147, *157*
Nadich, D. P., 246, 248, 24*1, 271*
Nadimpalli, S. R., 525, *533*
Nagai, S., 200, 203, *215, 217*
Nahmias, C., 284, *296*
Nahum, H., 253, *271*
Naidech, H. J., 485, *505*
Naidich, D. P., 20, 23, *37,* 47, 55, *66,* 67, 115, 118, 119, *124, 125,* 206, 207, *217,* 220, *240, 243,* 247, 254, 255, 256, 257, 258, *271, 272*
Naito, H., 517, *531*
Nakajima, Y., 525, *533*
Nakamura, F., 539, *563*
Nakamura, S., 541, *564*
Nakayama, D. K., 128, *153*
Naketa, H., 108, *122*
Nalesnik, M., 36, *40*
Nanda, N.C., 435, 436, *442*
Narkiewicz,-Jodko, J. B., 593, *600*
Narodick, B.G., 147, 148, *157*
Nash, G., 239, *243*
Nassar, W. K., 455, *473*

Nath, H., 5, *17*
Nath, P.H., 284, *296*
National Cancer Institute Cooperative Early Lung Cancer Group, 70, *97*
National Heart, Lung and Blood Institute, 276, 277, *294*
National Reserch Council, 70, *97*
Neff, C. C., 330, *340*
Neitzel, U., 380, *388*
Nelems, B., 91, *101,* 333, *340*
Nelson, M. E., 182, *196*
Nesbitt, J. C., 173, *196*
Nesto, R. W., 542, *564*
Netto, D., 540, *563*
Newell, J. D., 254, *272,* 307, 311, *318*
Newell, J. D., Jr., 270, *274*
Newman, B. M., 142, *156*
Newman, G. E., 395, 402, 414, *416, 418, 419*
Newman, K. B., 270, *274*
Newman, L. S., 254, 270, *272, 274,* 307, 311, *318*
Newmark, G., 247, *271*
Nichol, K. L., 221, 223, *241*
Nichols, D. M., 248, *271,* 283, *295*
Nicklaus, T. M., 275, 281, *293*
Nicolas, V., 523, *532*
Nienaber, C. A., 523, *532,* 577, 579, *596, 597*
Nierman, D. M., 43, *66*
Niklason, L. T., 9, *17,* 371, 376, *388*
Nishimura, K., 200, 203, *215, 217,* 260, *272*
Nishimura, R. A., 439, *443*
Nishimura, T., 517, *531*
Nissen, S. E., 439, *443,* 541, *564*
Nolop, K. B., 333, *340*
Noma, S., 260, *272*
Nomura, F., 90, *100*
Nordenstrom, B., 346, 354, *362, 364*
Norman, G., 284, *296*
Normand J-P., 152, *158*
Novelline, R. A., 132, *154*
Nowels, K. W., 355, *364*
Numano, F., 529, *534*
Nunn, A., 591, *598*

Author Index

O

O'Brian, M. J., 57, *68*
O'Connell, D. M., 351, *363*
O'Connor, B. K., 558, *568*
O'Donovan, P. B., 190, *197*
O'Malley, P. 56, *67*
O'Malley, T. O., 129, *153*
O'Moore, P. V., 327, *339,* 356, 358, *365,*
O'Sullivan, M., 584, *597*
Oca, O., 172, *195*
Ochsner, J. L., 147, *156*
Oddson, T. A., 330, *339*
Oestmann, J. W., 9, *17*
Offord, K. P., 90, *100*
Ogawa, S., 433 *442*
Ogden, J. A., 129, *153*
Ognibene, A. J., 234, *241*
Ognibene, F. P., 19, *37,* 239, *243*
Oh, K. S., 129, 145, *153, 156*
Ohman, E. M., 555, *567*
Ohshima, K, ., 456, *473*
Ohtani, H., 591, *598*
Okada, R. D., 517, *531*
Okazawa, M., 269, *273*
Okuyama, A., . 90, *100*
Older, R.A., 414, *418*
Oldham, H. N., 519, *531*
Oldham, H. N., Jr., 187, 189, *196*
Oldham, S. A. A., 64, *68*
Olivari, M. T., 306, *318*
Oliver, J. H., 371, *387,* 391, *415*
Oliver, T. W., Jr., 94, *102*
Olofsson, P. A., 518, *531*
Olsen, G. A., 355, *365*
Olson, M. C., 510, *530*
Omehara, I., 529, *534*
Orford, R., 236, *242*
Orrego, H., 129, *153*
Orringer, M. B., 90, *100,* 91, 93, *101, 102,*
    185, 186, *196,* 358, *365,* 525, *533*
Orsinelli, D. A., 592, *598*
Orszulak, T. A., 517, 520, 521, *531*
Ortiz, C. R., 255, 256, *272*

Osborn, H., 129, *153*
Osborn, M. J., 469, *474*
Osborne, D., 245, 246, *271*
Oser, A., 132, *154*
Oskoui, R., 520, *532*
Osteen, R. T., 69, *97*
Osterlind, K., 96, *102*
Ostrow, D., 200, *215*
Ostrow, D. N., 33, *39,* 200, 201, 212, *215,*
    218, 248, *271*
Ostrow, L. B., 93, *102*
Otsuji, H., 202, *217*
Otto, C. M., 523, *532*
Otulana, B. A., 299, *316*
Ovenfors, C. O., 65, *68,* 403, *417*
Owaki, T., 432, *442*

P

Pacheco, A., 235, 236, *242*
Packard, M. E., 578, *597*
Padley, S. P. G., 20, 28, 29, 30, 31, *37, 39,*
    210, *218,* 239, *243,* 245, 246, *271*
Padovani, B., 90, *101*
Pae, W. E., 167, *195*
Pagani, J J., 239, *243*
Page, A., 360, *366*
Paine, S., 395, 402, *416*
Paine, S. S., 333, *341*
Painter, J. A., 540, *563*
Pairolero, P. C., 90, *100,* 176, 183, *196,*
    517, *530*
Pais, S. O., 508, *530*
Pal, J. M., 130, *154*
Palacios, I. F., 556, *568*
Palder, S., 128, *153*
Palder, S. B., 145, *156*
Palla, A., 399, *416*
Pan, J. F., 347, *362*
Pandian, N. G., 540, *563,* 593, *599*
Pandolfo, I., 248, *271*
Pang, D., 132, *154*
Panicek, D. M., 119, *124*
Papiris, S. A., 235, *241*
Pappas, P. G., 54, *67*

Paré, J. A. P., 133, 135, 142, 144, *154,* 225, *240,* 275, 276, 281, *293,* 332, *340*
Paré, P. D., 133, 135, 142, 144, *154,* 225, *240,* 275, 276, 281, *293,* 332, *340*
Parenti, C. M., 221, 223, *241*
Parisi, A. F., *564*
Park, J. H., 78, 79, *99,* 580, *597*
Park, J. M., 361, *367*
Parker, D. R., 57, *68*
Parker, L. A., 359, *366*
Parker, S. H., 352, *363*
Parmley, L. F., 524, *532*
Parness, I. A., 432, *442*
Parrish, D. M., 594, *600*
Paschal, C. B., 427, 430, *442*
Pasquini, L., 432, *442*
Pass, H. I., 19, *37,* 117, 118, *124*
Pasternac, A., 424, *441*
Pastores, S. M., 47, *66*
Patel, A. M., 237, *242*
Patrick, L. M., 139, *155*
Patterson, G. A., 90 *100,* 194, *197,* 298, 308, *316, 318*
Patterson, R. E., 590, *598*
Patton, A. S., 330, *340*
Patton, D. D., 3, *16, 17*
Patz, D. F., 333, *341*
Patz, E. F., 83, 91, *99,* 119, *125*
Patz, E. F., Jr., 91, *102,* 359, *366*
Paujabi, M., 130, 132, *154*
Paul, M. E., 128, *153*
Paulson, D. F., *122*
Pavlidis, N. A., 467, *474*
Payne, W. S., 71, 72, 73, 79, 81, 90, *98, 99, 100*
Paz, R., 313, *318*
Pearcy, E. A., 359, 360, *366*
Pearlberg, J. L., 81, 90, 94, *99, 100, 101, 102*
Pearson, A. C., 592, *598*
Pearson, F. G., 90, *100*
Peck, W. W., 584, *597*
Pejcic, P., 556, *568*
Pelc, L. R., 595, *601*
Pelc, N. J., 313, *318,* 407, *417*
Peller, P. J., 135, *155*

Pelletier, L. C., 360, *366*
Pellett, J. R., 145, *156*
Peltier, L. F., 144, *156*
Pemberton, A. H., 147, 148, *157*
Pena, N., 358, *365*
Penketh, R., 300, *316*
Penn, I., 35, *40,* 310, *318*
Pennell, D. J., 427, 430, *442,* 595, *601*
Pennes, D. R., 90, *100*
Pennington, D. G., 304, *317*
Perchet, H., 593, *600*
Pereiras, R., 572, *596*
Perlman, S. B., 96, *103*
Perlmutt, L. M., 414, *418*
Perloff, J. K., 475, 482, 491, 493, 495, 497, 501, *505, 506*
Perry, J. J., 94, 95, *102*
Perusse, K. R., 135, *155*
Peshock, R. M., 408, *418*
Petasnick, J. P., 523, *532*
Peter, R. H., 436, *443*
Peters, J., 220, 221, *240*
Petersen, B., 577, *596*
Peterson, R. R., 450, *472*
Peuchot, M., 113, 117, *123*
Peyser, P. A., 437, *443*
Pflugfelder, P. W., 514, *530*
Phalen, J. J., 82, 83, 84, *99*
Phillips, D. A., 14, *18,* 525, *533*
Philpott, G W., 358, *365*
Piacenza, G., 90, *100*
Piana, R. N., 553, *567*
Piccione, W., Jr., 176, *196*
Pichard, A. D., 540, 541, *563, 564,* 592, *599*
Pickren, J. Q., 107, *122*
Pickren, J. W., 71, 73, *98*
Picozzi, V. J., 469, *474*
Piehler, J. M., 90, *100*
Piepho, A., 523, *532*
Pierce, J. A., 281, *295*
Pierce, W. S., 166, *195*
Pierson, R. N., 43, *66*
Piessens, J., 539, *563*
Pietra, G. G., 33, 35, *40,* 71, 78, 79, *98*
Pigeau, I., 333, *340*

Pilon, V. A., 43, *66*
Pinkerton, C. A., 550, 552, *565*
Pinto, F. J., 540, *563*
PIOPED Investigators, 394, 397, *416*
Pistolesi, M., 322, *338*
Pitchenik, A. E., 43, *65*
Platt, M. R., 148, 152, *157*
Platt, R. T., 323, *338*
Pluda, J. M., 24, *38*, 43, 45, *66*
Podransky, A. E., 136, *155*, 329, *339*
Poe, R. H., 220, 221, *240*, 255, 256, *272*, 352, *363*
Poirson, F., 91, *102*
Polacin, A., 14, *18*
Polansky, S. M., 391, *415*
Pollack, I. F., 132, *154*
Pollak, J. S., 404, *417*
Polu, J M., 276, *294*
Poncelot, B. P., 595, *601*
Poole, G. V., 132, 134, *154*
Popma, J. J., 539, 541, 552, *562, 564, 565*, 592, *599*
Popovic, Z., 556, *568*
Popp, R. L., 463, *474*, 540, *563*
Port, R. B., 147, *155*
Porter, D. K., 93, *102*
Porter, T. R., 540, *563*, 593, *600*
Poschl, G. P., 165, *195*
Posniak, H. V., 150, *158*, 510, 523, *530, 532*
Postlethwait, R. W., 147, *157*
Potkin, B. N., 439, *443*
Pottage, J. C., 54, *67*
Potts, J. M., 587, *597*
Poulsen, J. K., 593, *599*
Powderly, W. G., 54, *67*
Powell, R. D. Jr., 32, *39*
Pratt, P. C., 275, 276, 277, 280, 281, 283, 285, *294, 295*
Predd, P. C., 281, *294*
Pressler, V., 517, *530*
Price, J. S., 378, 379, *388*
Primack, S. L., 26, 27, *38*, 201, *216*, 227, 237, 240, *241, 243*, 522, *532*
Prince, C. R., 592, *599*
Priviteri, C. A., 147, *157*

Proto, A. V., 144, *156*
Pugatch, R. D., 275, *293*
Puig, A. S., 147, *157*
Purut, C. M., 164, *195*
Putman, C. E., 28, 32, *38, 39,* 52, *67,* 118, 122, *124,* 141, *155,* 203, *217,* 276, *294,* 330, *339*

Q

Quebbeman, E. J., 135, *154*
Quinn, D. L., 93, *102,* 221, *241,* 255, 256, *272*
Quinn, J. R., 577, *597*
Quinn, M. F., 415, *419*
Quint, L. E., 84, 90, 91, 93, *99, 101, 102,* 194, *197*
Qureshi, S. A., 562, *568*

R

Raasch, B. N., 323, 324, 325, *338*
Rabahie, G. N., 518, *531*
Radclifee, R., 592, *598*
Radecki, P. D., 202, *216*
Rajagopalan, R., 305, *317*
Ramee, S. R., 536, 538, 539, *562*
Ramenofsky, M. L., 128, *153*
Ramirez, J., 194, *197,* 308, *318*
Ramsey, R. G., 30, *38*
Rand, R. P., 169, *195*
Randall, P. A., 170, *195*
Randolph, J. G., 128, 139, *153*
Rankin, J. S., 519, *531*
Rao, K. C. V. G., 139, 140, 141, *155*
Raphael, M. J., 399, *416*
Raply, D. D., 397, *416*
Rapoport, S., 90, *101*
Rappaport, D. C., 209, *218,* 298, *316,* 302, 304, 308, *316*
Raptopoulos, V., 14, *18,* 525, *533*
Rath, G. S., 221, *241*
Ratto, G. B., 90, *100*
Raval, V. A., 144, *156*

Ravasini, R., 180, *196*
Ravin, C. E., 9, *17,* 52, *67,* 276, *294,* 371, 384, *387, 388,* 391, *415*
Ray, C. S., 202, *216,* 331, *340*
Raymond, R. E., 541, *564*
Reagan, K., 476, 477, *505*
Reddy, K.G., 439, *444*
Reddy, S. C., 22, *38*
Redepenning, L. S., 82, 83, 84, *99*
Redman, H. C., 408, *418*
Redmond, J., 94, 95, *102*
Reed, E. C., 32, *39*
Reed, J. C., 327, 328, *339*
Rees, S., 528, *534*
Reich, H., 358, *365*
Reicheck, N., 594, *600*
Reichek, N., 434, *442*
Reicher, M. A., 221, 235, *241*
Reichert, C. M., 469, *474*
Reid, J. M., 574, *596*
Reid, L., 275, 277, 281, *293, 294*
Reider, H. L., 47, *66*
Reidy, J. F., 562, *568*
Reigh, S. B., 281, *294*
Reinig, J. W., 529, *534*
Reisser, J. R., 148, 150, *158*
Reitz, B. A., 189, 190, 191, *197*
Remington, J. S., 21, *37*
Remy, J., 118, *124,* 201, 203, 204, 210, *216, 217, 218,* 265, *273,* 403, 404, *417*
Remy-Jardin, M., 118, *124,* 201, 203, 209, 210, *216, 217, 218,* 265, *273,* 403, 404, *417*
Ren, H., 304, *317*
Rennard, S. I., 32, *39*
Rensetti, A. D., 275, 281, *293*
Renston, J. P., 172, *195*
Repace, J. L., 69, *97*
Revel, D., 191, *197,* 304, 306, *317, 318,* 410, *418*
Revel, V., 209, *218*
Revzani, L., 180, *196*
Reynolds, J., 142, *156*
Rezai, K., 487, *506*
Rhea, J. T., 129, 132, *153, 154*
Rhoades, E. R., 30, *39*

Rhodes, G., 333, *340*
Ribeiro, E. E., 546, *564*
Rice, L. W., 358, *366*
Rice, T. W., 135, *155,* 190, 191, *197,* 301, *316*
Richardson, J. D., 128, *153,* 525, *533*
Richardson, P., 14, *18,* 525, *533*
Richardson, P. C., 331, *340*
Richenbacher, W. E., 166, *195*
Rickdeschel, J. C., 458, *473*
Rioux, M., 152, *158*
Risher, R. G., 14, *18*
Risius, B., 135, *155*
RITA Trial Pariticpants, 545, *564*
Ritchie, C. J., 401, *416*
Rizzi, M. C., 353, *364*
Ro, J. A. E., 74, *98*
Road, J., 215, *218*
Robbins, R. A., 32, *39,* 237, *242*
Robboy, S. J., 237, *242*
Roberge, R. J., 129, *153*
Roberts, L., 276, *294*
Roberts, W. C., 447, 458, 469, *472, 473,* 519, *531*
Robin, E. D., 414, *419*
Robinson, L. A., 358, *365*
Robotham, J. L., 273
Rocchini, A. P., 558, *568*
Rockoff, S. D., 56, *67,* 331, 335, *340, 341*
Rodan, B. A., 108, *123*
Rodgers, B. M., 359, *366*
Rodgers, R. F., 338, *341*
Rodrigues, E., 587, *598*
Rodriguez, A., 127, 148, 152, *152, 157, 158*
Rodriguez, J. L., 43, *65*
Rodriguez, V., 21, *37*
Rodriguez-Morales, G., 148, *157*
Roe, D., 394, *416*
Roelandt, J. R. T. C., 540, *563*
Rogers, L. F., 147, *157*
Rogers, W. J., 594, *600*
Roggli, V., 209, *218,* 283, 285, *295*
Roggli, V. L., 70, *97,* 331, *340*
Rohatgi, P., 331, *340*
Rollins, R. J., 145, *156*

Rom, W. N., 47, *66*, 255, 256, *272*
Romani, S., 180, *196*
Romero, J. V., 355, *365*
Root, J. D., 314, *318*
Rosato, E. F., 147, *157*
Rose, C. S., 210, *218*
Rosen, A., 332, *340*, 450, *472*
Rosen, M. J., 64, *68*
Rosen, P., 23, 24, *38*
Rosen, S. T., 96, *103*
Rosenberg, S. A., 33, *39*
Rosenberger, A., 142, *156*
Rosenblatt, M. B., 106, *122*
Rosenblum, J., 550, *565*
Rosengart, T. K., 555, *567*
Rosenow, E. C., 237, *242*
Rosenow, E. C., III, 19, 32, *37*
Rosenthal, A., 558, *568*
Rosenthal, D. I., 10, *17*
Rossman, C., 309, *318*
Roth, J. A., 19, *37*
Rothenberg, R., 56, *67*
Rothpearl, A., 47, *65*
Roubin, G. S., 544, 553, *564*, *566*, *567*
Rouviere, H., 107, *122*
Rowe, M. I., 128, *153*
Rowell, N. P., 400, *416*
Rowlands, J. A., 381, *388*
Royal, H. D., 313, *318*
Royston, D., 144, *156*
Rubens, M B., 201, *216*
Rubin, G. D., 221, 235, *241*, 577, *597*
Rubin, J. M., 180, *196*
Rubin, R. H., 20, 23, *37*
Rubin, S. A., 69, *96*, 147, *157*
Rubinstein, W., 450, *472*
Ruggiero, R., 304, *317*
Rusch, V. W., 337, *341*
Ruskin, J. A., 323, *339*
Russi, E. G., 248, *271*
Russi, E. V., *271*
Rutherford, R. B., 130, 134, *154*
Ryan, C. J., 338, *341*
Ryan, K., 353, *364*
Ryan, T. J., 547, *565*
Rybak, B. J., 57, *67*

Ryu, J. H., 237, *242*

S

Sabbath, H. N., 425, *442*
Sabeti, V., *388*
Sachs, D. P. L., 234, *241*
Sachs, P. B., 135, *155*
Sacknoff, R., 132, *154*
Saeed, M., 594, *600*
Saegesser, F., 106, *122*
Safi, H. J., 519, *531*
Safian, R. D., 552, 558, *565*, *568*
Sagel, S. S., 8, *17*, 90, *100*, 115, *123*, 151, *158*, 314, *318*, 333, *340*, 360, *366*, 377, 379, *388*, 391, *415*, 450, *472*, 510, *530*
Sahn, S. A., 115, *123*, 321, 322, 327, 337, *338*, *339*, *341*, 359, *366*
Saini, A., 107, *122*
Saini, S., 327, 330, *339*, 358, *365*, 517, *531*
Sais, G. J., 52, 61, *67*, *68*
Saito, Y., 90, *100*
Saka, H., 90, *100*, 360, *366*
Sakai, F., 284, *295*
Sakai, S., 90, *100*
Sakamoto, I., 520, *532*
Sakatani, M., 201, 210, *216*, *218*
Sako, M., 201, *216*
Sakuma, H., 595, *601*
Saldana, M. J., 43, 64, *65*, *68*
Saleh, S. S., 355, *365*
Salinas, M., 455, *473*
Salustri, A., 593, *599*
Salvatierra, A., 93, *102*
Samdarshi, T. E., 435, 436, *442*
Samet, J. M., 69, 70, 81, *97*
Samson, L., 203, 204, *217*
Samuelson, S. L., 360, *366*
Sanada, S., 387, *388*
Sanborn, T. A., 547, *565*
Sanchez, R. B., 348, *363*
Sanders, C., 281, 284, *294*, *296*
Sanders, S. P., 432, *442*

Sandler, C. M., 132, 134, 141, 148, *154*
Sandler, M. A., 81, 90, 94, *99, 100, 102*
Santiago, S. M., 223, *240*
Santiago, S., 221, 223, *241*
Sapin, P. M., 528, *534,* 593, *599*
Saracci, R., 70, *97*
Saravolatz, L. D., 22, *38,*
Sartori, F., 180, *196*
Sasagawa, M., 90, *100*
Satoh, T., 456, *473*
Satomura, K., 537, *562*
Savage, M., 553, *566*
Savage, M. P., 553, *567*
Savage, P. J., 221, *241,* 255, 256, *272*
Sayek, I., 359, *366*
Sayre, J. W., 9, 10, *17*
Scatarige, J. C., 109, 112, 115, *123*
Schachar, R., 323, *338*
Schaefer, C. M., 9, *17*
Schaff, H. V., 452, *473*
Schaff, J. T., 221, *241*
Schaner, E. G., 117, *124*
Schatz, R. A., 553, *567*
Schauble, J. F., 520, *532*
Schicha, H., 523, *532*
Schiebler, M. L., 410, *418*
Schiele, F., 555, *567*
Schild, H. H., 141, *156*
Schimpf, P. P., 139, 140, 141, *155*
Schinco, M. A., 132, *154*
Schinella, R., 57, *67*
Schlant, R. C., 467, *474*
Schlegel, W., 467, *474*
Schmidt, D. A., 552, *565*
Schmidt, W., 129, *153*
Schnapp, L. M., 56, *67*
Schnell, F. R., 30, *39*
Schnitt, S. J., 552, *565*
Scholes, J. V., 55, *67*
Scholl, D. G., 147, *157*
Scholten, E. T., 107, *122*
Schomig, A., 553, *566*
Schuchmann, G. G., 145, *156*
Schulman, A., 148, *158*
Schulman, L. L., 28, *38*
Schultz, S., 357, *365*

Schuster, D. P., 400, *416*
Schvartzman, R., 300, *316*
Schwab, C. W., 132, *154*
Schwartz, A. M., 56, *67*
Schwartz, A., 331, *340*
Schwartz, D., 558, *568*
Schwartz, D. A., 331, *340*
Schwartz, D. S., 61, *68*
Schwartz, M. L., 36, *40,* 206, 207, *217,* 310, *318*
Schwartz, R. S., 437, *443*
Scorpio, R., 14, *18,* 525, *533*
Scott, I. R., 333, *340*
Scott, J., 299, *316*
Scott, J. M., 174, *196*
Scott, W. W., Jr., 11, *18*
Sears, T., 540, *563*
Seatman, M. C., 262, *273*
Seaton, K. G., 359, *366*
Sechtem, U., 447, 463, *472,* 514, 523, *530, 532*
Sedney, M. I., 554, *567*
Seed, W. A., 355, *364*
Seese, B., 594, *600*
Sefczek, D. M., 525, *533*
Sefczek, R. J., 525, *533*
Segal, S. L., 237, *242*
Seino, Y., 456, *473*
Seissler, W., 11, 14, *18*
Seksik, L., 90, *101*
Semenkovich, J. W., 151, *158,* 190, *197,* 298, 308, *316, 318*
Senda, K., 360, *366*
Serota, M. L., 28, *38*
Serruys, P. W., 553, 554, *566*
Set, P. A. K., 220, *240,* 256, *272*
Sexton, S., 115, *123*
Shachar, G. B., 558, *568*
Shackelford, G. D., 455, *473*
Shackford, S. R., 140, *155*
Shah, J. P., 113, *123*
Shandling, B., 145, *156*
Shanzer, S., 94, *102*
Shapiro, S. R., 555, *567*
Shatney, C. H., 148, *157*

Shaw, C., 69, 74, 81, 97, 107, 108, 112, 122, 123, 337, 341
Shaw, R. E., 550, 565
Sheedy, P. F., 403, 417, 437, 443
Shefer, A., 548, 565
Sheiman, R. G., 525, 533
Shelhamer, J. H., 19, 20, 21, 36, 37, 239,
Shellock, F. G., 484, 505
Shelton, D. K., Jr., 93, 102
Shelton, R. W., 81, 99
Shen, Z., 593, 599
Shepard, J. O., 90, 101, 183, 196, 209, 217, 314, 318, 353, 364
Shepherd, F. A., 94, 102
Sheppard, M. N., 235, 236, 242
Sher, S., 56, 67
Sherman, C. T., 536, 537, 562
Sherman, R. G., 14, 18
Sherrier, R. H., 209, 218
Shibuya, H., 529, 534
Shields, J. B., 525, 533
Shim, Y., 227, 241, 260, 272
Shimizu, T., 201, 216
Shimokata, K., 90, 100
Shin, M. S., 81, 99
Shinella, R., 20, 23, 37
Shinozaki, T., 141, 155
Shiota, T., 593, 599
Shipley, R. T., 74, 98
Shirakawa, S., 588, 598
Shoemaker, W. C., 525, 533
Shor, M. J., 333, 340
Shorr, R. M., 127, 152
Shuford, W. H., 519, 528, 531, 534
Shuman, W. P., 90, 101, 337, 341
Shumway, N. E., 519, 531
Sicililan, L., 213, 218
Sider, L., 52, 57, 61, 67, 68, 70, 71, 72, 73, 74, 78, 79, 81, 97
Sides, D. M., 56, 57, 67
Siegel, M. J., 112, 123, 304, 316
Siegel, R. J., 536, 537, 540, 562
Siegleman, S. S., 11, 18, 20, 24, 25, 37, 38, 43, 66, 237, 243, 254, 262, 272
Siglow, V., 523, 532
Silbert, D., 307, 318

Silva, L. A., 546, 564
Silva, W. E., 14, 18, 525, 533
Silveman, D. I., 592592,
Silver, M. A., 469, 474
Silver, M., 132, 154
Silver, S. F., 210, 218
Silver, T. M., 391, 415
Silverman, D. I., 592, 598
Silverman, J. M., 313, 318, 407, 417
Silverman, N. E., 299, 316
Silverman, P. M., 245, 246, 271, 401, 416, 447, 472
Silverman, S. G., 330, 339, 358, 365
Simari, R. D., 546, 565
Simeone, J. F., 327, 330, 339, 356, 358, 365
Simmons, J. T., 65, 68
Simon, A. L., 572, 596
Simon, G., 275, 280, 281, 293, 294
Simons, D. B., 437, 443
Simpson, G. L., 21, 37
Sinak, L. J., 469, 474
Singer, S. J., 399, 416
Singh, S. P., 5, 17
Siotrzonek, P., 467, 474
Sisler, J., 215, 218
Sisson, J. H., 237, 243
Sivak, E. D., 169, 195
Sivit, C. J., 56, 67
Skeens, J. L., 262, 273, 306, 318
Sköldebrand, C. G., 517, 531
Skrbensky, G. T., 165, 195
Skupin, A., 353, 364
Slasky, B. S., 36, 40, 310, 318
Slater, E., 520, 531
Slatsky, B. S., 371, 387
Slavia, G., 106, 107, 112, 121
Slone, R. M., 291, 296
Smart, C., 70, 97
Smith, D., 353, 364
Smith, I. E., 220, 240, 256, 272
Smith, J. E., 555, 567
Smith, J. O., 148, 157
Smith, L. J., 237, 243
Smith, M. D., 57, 61, 68, 528, 534
Smith, P. K., 164, 195

Smith, T. P., 414, *418*
Smyth, B. T., 129, *153*
Snider, D. E., 47, *66*
Snider, G. L., 221, *241,* 355, *365*
Snow, N., 160, *195*
Snow, N. J., 70, *97*
Snyder, L. S., 30, 31, *39*
Sobonya, R. E., 275, *293*
Soergel, K. H., 235, *242*
Sollitto, R., 90, *101*
Solomon, C., 150, *158*
Solomon, D. A., 359, *366*
Solomon, J., 275, *294*
Solomon, S. L., 360, *366,* 450, *472*
Solomon, S. L., *388*
Somerville, J., 528, *534*
Sommers, S. C., 235, *242*
Sonoi, H., 539, *563*
Sostman, H. D., 90, *10,* 395, 402, 408, *416, 418*
Soto, B., 476, 477, 489, 500, *505*
Soule, A. B., 436, *443*
Soulen, R. L., 463, *473*
Sousa, E. M. R., 555, *567*
Souther, S., 528, *534*
Southworth, H., 455, *473*
Speckman, J. M., 246, *271*
Spencer, H., 106, 107, *121*
Spielman, R. P., 579, *597*
Spielmann, R. P., 523, *532*
Spigos, D. G., 333, *340*
Spitaels, S., 593, *599*
Spizarny, D. L., 183, *196*
Spjut, H. J., 70, *97*
Spodick, D. H., 446, 447, *472*
Spouge, D., 284, *295*
Spratling, L., 94, *102*
Sprawls, P., Jr., 509, *530*
Spray, T. L., 447, 458, 469, *472, 473*
Squires, T. S., 70, *97*
Sridhar, K. S., 61, *68*
St. Goar, F. G., 540, *563*
Stack, R. S., 555, *567*
Stadius, M. L., 540, *563*
Stahel, R. A., 96, *103*
Stahl, M. G., 32, *39,* 237, *242*

Standen, J. R., 283, *295*
Standerfer, R. J., 359, *366*
Stanely, J. H., 352, *363*
Stanford, W., 20, *37,* 403, *417*
Stanger, P., 555, *567*
Stanley, J. H., 352, 353, 354, 355, *363*
Stanton, M. C., 230, *241*
Staples, C. A., 91, *101,* 199, 200, *215,* 283, 283, *295, 296*
Stark, D. D., 94, *102,* 136, *155,* 165, *195,* 327, 329, *339,* 463, *473*
Stark, P., 106, 113, *122,* 127, 128, 130, 133, 134, 135, 142, 144, 145, 147, *152, 154,* 262, *273*
Starnes, V. A., 189, *197*
Stavens, B. R., 525, *533*
Stavropoulos, C., 47, *66*
Stears, J., 8, *17*
Stears, J. G., 8, *17*
Steckel, R. J., 323, *338*
Steffen, W., 553, *566*
Stein, D. S., 45, 46, *66*
Stein, H. L., 519, *531*
Stein, M. G., 33, *39,* 119, *125,* 212, *218*
Stein, P. D., 391, 414, *415, 416, 418*
Steinberg, F. L., 522, *532*
Steinberg, I., 519, *531*
Steiner, E., 327, 330, *339*
Steiner, R. E., 227, 232, *241*
Steiner, R. M., 485, 492, 493, 497, 502, *505, 506*
Stelling, C. B., 73, 74, *98*
Stembridge, V. A., 140, *155*
Stenlund, R., 113, *123*
Stephenson, L.W., 86, *100*
Stern, A., 440, *444*
Stern, C. A., 236, *242*
Stern, E. J., 269, 273, *274,* 276, *294,* 348, *363,* 523, *532*
Sternfeld, M., 129, *154*
Stertzer, S. H., 550, *565*
Stevenson, C. S., 455, *473*
Stewart, B. K., 9, 10, *17*
Stewart, E. T., 147, *157*
Stewart, J. T., 545, *564*
Stewart, S., 300, *316*

Stinson, E. B., 21, *37*, 519, *531*
Stirling, G. A., 78, *58*
Stitik, F. P., 85, 86, 93, 94, *100, 102,* 254, *272,* 351, 352, 353, 354, 355, *363*
Stockberger, S. M., 52, *67*
Stoddard, M. F., 592, *599*
Stoehr, C., 262, *273* 306, *318*
Stone, D. J., 43, *65*
Stone, P. H., 456, *473*
Stoneburner, R., 56, *67*
Stoney, R. J., 518, *531*
Stowell, D. W., 275, 281, *293*
Strange, C., 327, *339*
Stratemeier, E. J., 517, *531*
Strauss, E. B., 525, *533*
Strauss, G. M., 70, *97*
Strauss, H. W., 591, *598*
Strauss, L. G., 84, *99*
Strickland, B., 262, *273*
Strong, J. P., 436, *443*
Strunk, H., 141, *156*
Stulbarg, M., 203, *217*
Sturtz, K. W., 348, *363*
Suarez, M., 43, *65*
Suffredini, A. F., 65, *68*
Sugarbaker, D. J., 70, *97*
Sugimoto, T., 539, *563*
Sullivan, I. D., 555, *567*
Sundaram, M., 150, *158,* 525, *533*
Sunder-Plassmann, L., 247, *271*
Suneja, R., 439, *444*
Sunshine, J. H., 11, 12, *18*
Suratt, P. M., 83, *99*
Sussman, R., 248, *271*
Sussman, S. K., 353, *364*
Suster, B., 47, *66*
Sutherland, G., 593, *600*
Sutinen, S., 275, 281, *294*
Sutton, F. J., 463, *473*
Suzuki, J., 514, *530,* 580, *597*
Suzuki, S., 529, *534*
Svensson, L. G., 519, *531*
Svindland, A., 425, *442*
Swensen, S., 32, *39*
Swensen, S. J., 8, *17,* 200, 201, *215, 216*
Sybers, J. L., 232, *241*

Sybers, R. G., 232, *241,* 519, 528, *531, 534*
Szyfelbein, W. M., 352, 353, *363*

T

Tabakin, B. S., 455, *473*
Tabrah, F., 436, *443*
Tada, S., 520, 522, *532*
Tait, D., 400, *416*
Takamiya, M., 517, *531*
Takano, M., 377, *388*
Takasugi, J. E., *218*
Takehara, Y., 594, *600*
Takeuchi, N., 227, *240*
Takita, H., 172, *195*
Talavera, W., 43, *65*
Taliercio, C. P., 456, 458, 462, 467, *473*
Tamaki, N., 588, *598*
Tampas, J. P., 436, *443,* 455, *473*
Tan, C. S., 333, *340*
Tan, K. P., 348, *363*
Tange, J. D., 230, *241*
Tannenbaum, M A., 425, *441*
Tapper, D. P., 237, *242*
Tapson, V. F., 412, *418*
Tardif, J-C., 436, *442*
Tardivon, A. A., 403, *417*
Tarver, R. D., 52, 57, *67,* 248, *271,* 359, 360, *366,* 523, *532*
Tashkin, D. P., 270, *274*
Tateno, Y., 377, *388*
Tavares, N J., 518, *531*
Tavel, M. E., 455, *473*
Taylor, J. R., 237, *242*
Taylor, K., 436, *442*
Teague, R. B., 220, 221, *240*
Tedder, M., 187, *196*
Teefy, S. A., 151, *158*
Teien, D. E., 593, *599*
Teigen, C., 23, *38*
Teigen, C. L., 403, *417*
Teirstein, A. S., 64, *68*
Teklu, B., 281, *295*

Templeton, P. A., 43, 45, 66, 85, 86, 93, 94, 100, 147, 148, 157, 170, 195, 209, 217
Tenaglia, A. N., 544, 564
Tenholder, M. F., 32, 39, 94, 102, 237, 243, 404, 417
Tennant, S. N., 554, 567
Teplick, J. G., 325, 339
Terp, K., 593, 599
Terriff, B. A., 201, 216
Tespili, M., 539, 563
Thaete, F, L., 371, 387, 391, 415
Theissen, P., 523, 532
Theodore, J., 189, 197, 305, 306, 317, 318
Theodoropoulos, S., 313, 318
Theordore, J., 262, 273
Theros, E. G., 71, 72, 73, 74, 78, 79, 81, 98
Thieme, T., 541, 552, 564
Thomas, F., 132, 154
Thomas, G. A., 304, 317
Thomas, H. A., 525, 533
Thomas, J. L., 81, 99
Thomas, L. M., 139, 155
Thomason, R., 467, 474
Thompson, A. B., 237, 243
Thompson, B. M., 129, 153
Thompson, K. R., 281, 295
Thompson, R., 517, 531
Thompson, W. M., 325, 339
Thornbury, J. R., 13, 18
Thorsen, M. K., 323, 339
Thrall, J. H., 12, 18
Thurlbeck, W. M., 200, 215, 275, 276, 280, 281, 293, 294
Tierney, L. M., Jr., 28, 38
Tikkakoski, T., 352, 353, 363
Tobe, S., 305, 317
Tobias, J., 221, 223, 241
Tobias, M. J., 107, 122
Tobis, J. M., 439, 443, 541, 564
Tobler, J., 115, 124
Tocino, I., 128, 129, 132, 134, 136, 142, 145, 153, 156
Tocino, I. M., 132, 154
Toews, G. B., 19, 20, 36

Tofler, G. H., 456, 473
Tolly, T. L., 353, 364
Tomaru, T., 539, 563
Tomashefski, J. F., 70, 97, 525, 533
Tong, K. T., 201, 216
Tong, T., 70, 97
Tonsfeldt, D., 129, 153
Tood, T. R. J., 90, 100
Toombs, B. D., 132, 134, 141, 148, 154
Topol, E. J., 546, 550, 552, 553, 565, 566
Torenbeek, R., 517, 531
Toronto Lung Transplant Group, 313, 318
Torrents, C., 264, 273
Torstveit, J., 359, 366
Trambert, M. A., 221, 241
Trapnell, D. H., 119, 125
Trasolini, N. C., 170, 195
Trastek, V. F., 176, 183, 196
Travis, W. D., 234, 241
Trento, A., 299, 316
Tribble, C. G., 359, 366
Triebwasser, J. H., 30, 39
Trinidad, S., 106, 122
Trinkle, J. K., 128, 153
Trueblood, H. W., 519, 531
Trulock, E. P., 298, 299, 300, 313, 316, 318
Tsai, S. H., 147, 157
Tscholakoff, D., 447, 463, 472
Tschomper, B. A., 254, 272, 307, 311, 318
Tsikaderis, D., 555, 567
Tuhrim, S., 94, 102
Tullis, E., 309, 318
Tumeh, S. S., 399, 416
Turner, M. A., 147, 156
Turner-Warwick, M., 262, 273
Tuzcu, M., 541, 564
Tylen, U., 306, 318
Tynan, M., 560, 568
Tynan, M. J., 562, 568

U

Uchida, Y., 539, 563

Ueda, E., 201, *216*
Uetani, M., 520, *532*
Ulreich, S., 237, *243*
Umans, V. A., 550, *565*
Umbria, S., 358, *365*
Underwood, G. H., 94, *102*
Underwood, R., 528, *534*
Unger, J. M., 145, *156*
Unni, K. K., 338, *341*
Unruh, H., 358, *365*
Unruh, L., 359, *366*
Urman, M. K., 427, 428, *442*
Uttamchandani, R. B., 47, *66*

V

Vaitkus, P. T., 463, *473*
Valbracht, C., 552, *566*
Valdivieso, M., 21, *37*, 81, *99*
Valere, D., 248, *271*
Valeyre, D., 203, *217*, 234, *241*
Valsecchi, O., 539, *563*
van Beek, E. J. R., 397, *416*
van de Brekel, J. A., 359, *366*
Van der Linden, L. P., 554, *567*
van der Loos, C. M., 437, *443*
van der Vorde, F., 86, *100*
van der Wal, A. C., 438, *443*
Van der Wall, E. E., 594, *600*
van Dijk, P., 594, *600*
van Dijk, R. B., 553, *566*
van Ingel, G. J., 455, *473*
Van Peenen, H. J., 517, *530*
van Rossum, A. C., 407, *418*, 517, *531*
van Son, J. A. M., 452, *473*
van Sonnenberg, E., 330, *340*, 346, 354, 360, 361, *362*, *364*, *366*, *367*
Vandiviere, H. M., 227, *240*
Vannan, M. A., 436, *442*
Vannier, M. W., 247, *271*
Vanwijck, E., 403, *417*
Varela, P., 592, *598*
Varney, R. R., 361, *367*
Vaughn, L. M., 359, *366*
Vazquez, de Prada, J. A., 593, *599*

Vedal, S., 201, *216*, 283, 287, *295*
Veith, F. J., 298, *316*
Vellet, A. D., 174, *196*
Venable T. C., 554, *567*
Vendrell, M., 264, *273*
Verazin, G., 172, *195*
Verdant, A., 360, *366*
Veronesi, V., 113, *123*
Verschakelen, J. A., 403, *417*
Verska, J. J., 78, 79, *98*
Veveris, J. J., 592, *598*
Viadara, E., 107, *122*
Vidal, R., 264, *273*
Villalba, M., 135, *155*
Villavieja, Atance, J. L., 346, *362*
Vincent, R. G., 71, 73, *98*
Virginia, M., 555, *567*
Viskum, K., 359, *366*
Vita, V. T. D., 24, *38*
Vix, V. A., 248, *271*
Vlahakes, G. J., 528, *534*
Vliestra, R. E., 545, *564*
Vlymen, W. J., 147, *157*
Vock, P., 11, 14, *18*, 32, *39*, 245, 246, *271*
Voeller, G. R., 148, 150, *158*
Volkman, D. J., 529, *534*
Vollmer, R. T., 70, *97*
Volta, S., 248, *271*
von Bibra, H., 593, *600*
von Kodolitsch, Y., 523, *532*, 577, 579, *596*, *597*
von Oppell, U. O., 524, *532*
von Schulthess, G. K., 528, *534*
VonRoenn, J. H., 57, 61, *68*
Voorhees, W. D., 553, 554, *566*, *567*
Vucinic, M., 556, *568*
Vujic, I., 135, *155*
Vyborny, C., 371, 372, 377, 382, 384, *388*
Vyborny, C. J., *388*

W

Wachsberg, R. H., 352, *363*
Wagner, R. B., 139, 140, 141, *155*, 173, *196*

Wahl, G. W., 255, 256, *272*
Wahl, R. L., 84, 90, 91, 93, *99, 102*
Wain, J. C., 314, *318*
Wain, J. C., Jr., 172, 173, *195*
Wain, S. L., 331, *340*
Wakely, P. E., 562, *568*
Waldhausen, J. A., 574, *596*
Waldron, J. A., Jr., 210, *218*
Walker, S., 47, *66*
Walker-Renard, P. B., 359, *366*
Wall, S. D., 132, *154*
Wallace, J. M., 48, 55, 65, *66, 67, 68,* 83, *99*
Wallace, S., 113, *123*
Wallaert, B., 201, 203, *216, 217*
Waller, B. F., 456, 458, 462, 467, *473*
Wallin, J., 403, *417*
Wallwork, J., 299, 300, *316*
Walsh, F. W., 359, *366*
Walsh, T. J., 28, *38*
Waltman, A. C., 522, *532*
Wang, S., 578, *597*
Warburton, R. K., 436, *443*
Ward, C., 528, *534*
Ward, D. E., 552, *566*
Ward, R. E., 128, *153*
Wareing, T. H., 167, *195*
Warnes, C. A., 439, *443*
Warnock, M., 260, *272*
Warren, R. L., 528, *534*
Warren, S. E., 558, *568*
Wasser, L. S., 43, *65*
Watanabe, A., 90, *100*
Watanabe, A. T., 135, *154*
Watkins, M. W., 446, 447, *472*
Wattinne, L, 203, *217,* 403, 404, *417*
Waxman, K., 132, *154*
Way, D., 210, *218*
Webb, W. R., 33, *39,* 56, 57, 65, *67, 68,* 90, 91, 92, 93, 94, 96, *100, 101,* 118, 119, *124, 125,* 136, *155,* 200, 201, 203, 212, *215, 217, 218,* 246, 255, 260, 262, 269, *271, 272, 273, 274,* 276, 283, 287, *294, 295,* 325, 329, 332, *339, 340,* 348, *363,* 403, *417,* 450, *472*

Webber, M. M., 394, *416*
Weber, W., 141, *156*
Wechsler, R. J., 176, 180, *196*
Wedeen, V. J., 447, 463, *472,* 595, *601*
Weens, H. S., 519, *531*
Weiland, L. H., 90, *100*
Weinaker, A., 276, *294*
Weinshelbaum, A., 281, *294*
Weinstein, H., 590, *598*
Weir, I. H., 145, *156*
Weisbrod, G. L., 262, *273,* 298, 302, 304, 305, 308, *316, 317,* 348, 353, 355, *363, 364*
Weisbrod, L., 302, 308, *316*
Weiss, A. J., 57, 61, *68*
Weiss, W., 81, *99*
Weissberg, D., 361, *366*
Weisskoff, R. M., 595, *601*
Weissleder, R., 410, *418*
Weissman, N. J., 539, *563*
Welch, G., 132, *154*
Wellington, C., 284, *295*
Wellner, L. J., 118, *124*
Wells, A. U., 201, *216*
Welsh, E. V., 201, *216*
Wendland, M. F., 594, *600*
Wentworth, J. E., 280, *294*
Wesiborg, G. L., 209, *218*
Westbrook, B. M., 469, *474*
Westcott, J., 90, 91, *101*
Westcott, J. L., 56, *67,* 330, *339,* 352, 353, 354, 355, *363*
Westcott, M. A., 52, *67*
Weston, M., 558, *568*
Wetzel, R. C., *273*
Wexler, L., 517, 519, *530, 531,* 587, *597*
Wheat, L. J., 52, *67*
Wheeler, P. S., 25, *38*
Whitacre, M., 96, *102*
Whitcomb, M. E., 106, *122*
White, A., 130, 132, *154*
White, C. J., 536, 538, 539, *562*
White, C. S., 43, 45, 61, *66, 68,* 147, 148, *157*
White, C. W., 424, *441*
White, D. A., 30, 31, *39*

White, R. D., 514. *530*
White, R. I., 93, *102*, 555, 562, *567, 568*
White, R. I., Jr., 404, *417*
Whitley, J. E., 96, *102,* 508, *530*
Whitley, N. O., 81, 96, *99, 102,* 463, *473*
WHO-MONICA Project, 423, *441*
Whyte, R. I., 194, *197*
Wichter, T., 583, *597*
Wicks, C. M., 352, *363*
Wiesen, E. J., 525, *533*
Wilde, R. P. H., 558, *568*
Willard, J. E., 540, *563*
Williams, A. J., 221, 223, *240, 241*
Williams, D. M., 522, *532*
Williams, F. H., 5, 6, 12, *17,* 572, *596*
Williams, J. R., 118, *124,* 140, *155*
Williams, M. P., 108, 113, 115, *123*
Williams, T. M., 50, *67*
Williamson, B. R. J., 142, *156*
Willing, S. J., 525, *533*
Willis, R., 106, *121*
Wills, J. S., 525, *533*
Wilson, M. A., 96, *103*
Wilson, W. R., 19, 32, *37*
Wimbush, K. J., 90, *100*
Windebank, W. J., 413, *418*
Winning, A. J., 355, *364*
Winsett, M. Z., 147, *157*
Winters, S. L., 440, *444*
Winton, T., 304, *316*
Winton, T. L., 298, *316*
Wirth, R. L., 20, 24, *37,* 43, *66*
Wismer, G. L., 517, *531*
Wisoff, H. C., 436, *443*
Withers, C., 360, *366*
Witte, R. J., 32, *39,* 237, *242*
Wittich, G. R., 355, 361, *364, 367*
Woefel, M., 56, *67*
Wohlmuth, D. A., 525, *533*
Wolfe, W. G., 159, 179, 180, *194, 196,* 519, *531*
Wolff, S. D., 57, *68,* 240, *243*
Wolfman, N. T., 127, 132, *152*
Wolverson, M. K., 150, *158,* 525, *533*
Wong-You-Chong, J. J., 128, *153*
Woodring, J. H., 72, 73, 74, *98,* 115, 116, *124,* 227, *240,* 323, *339,* 525, *533*
Woods, B. O., 335, *341*
Woolner, L. B., 71, 72, 73, 79, 81, *98, 99*
Workman, A., 378, 379, *388*
World Health Organization, 70, *97*
Worman, L.W., 147, 148, *157*
Worsley, D . F., 391, *415*
Worthy, S. A., 148, 150, *157*
Wright, A. R., 118, *124*
Wright, C. B., 424, *441*
Wright, G. A., 595, *601*
Wu, H. D., 327, *339*
Wu, J-J., 556, *567*
Wueflein, R. D., 519, *531*
Wyman, S. M., 145, *156*

X

Xie, F., 540, *563,* 593, *600*
Xu, X. W., 377, *388*
Xu, X. W., *388*

Y

Yacoub, M. H., 313, *318*
Yakamura, S., 592, *599*
Yakes, W. F., 352, *363*
Yamada, I., 529, *534,* 593, *599*
Yamada, S., 84, *100*
Yamada, T., 520, 522, *532*
Yamaguchi, T., 519, *531*
Yamamoto, H., 305, *317*
Yamamoto, S., 202, *216,* 260, *272*
Yamashita, C., 305, *317*
Yamazaki, F., 299, *316*
Yanagihara, K., 432, *442*
Yang, P.C. 327, *339,* 347, 355, *362, 365*
Yang, W. C., 94, *102*
Yano, K., 450, *472*
Yap, J., 348, *363*
Yashiro, K., 432, *442*
Yee, J., 281, *294*
Yellin, A., 361, *366*

Yellin, E. O., 361, *366*
Yesner, R., 70, *97*
Yeterian, A., 32, *39*
Yilling, F. P., 467, *474*
Yock, P. G., 540, *563*
Yoko-Yama, K., 202, *216*
Yokoi, K., 90, *100*
Yoon, B., 74, *98*
Yoon, H. K., 21, *37*
Yorkston, J., 383, *388*
Yoselevitz, M., 525, *533*
Yoshikawa, J., 432, *442*
Yoshimura, H., 202, *217*
Yoshimura, H., *388*
Young, I. R., 15, *18*
Youngberg, A. D., 119, *125*
Yousem, D. M., 109, 112, *123*
Yousem, S. A., 262, *273,* 301, 306, *316, 318*
Yu, A. C., 22, *38*
Yu, C. J., 327, *339,* 347, *362*
Yu, V. L. 22, *38*
Yucel, E. K., 522, *532*

Yuda, T., 304, *317*

Z

Zairns, C., 425, *442*
Zamel, N., 276, *294,* 304, *317*
Zangeneh, M., 467, *474*
Zegel, H. G., 147, *157*
Zelch, M. G, 135, *155*
Zeman, R. K., 401, *416*
Zerhouni, E. A., 25, *38,* 85, 86, 91, 93, 94, *100, 101,* 108, *122,* 269, *273, 274,* 283, *295,* 401, *416,* 594, *600*
Zidar, J. P., 544, *564*
Zidulka, A., 353, *364*
Zilla, P., 524, *532*
Zinn, W. L., 246, *271*
Zinreich, E. S., 115, *123*
Zornoza, J., 21, *37*
Zuger, J. H., 361, *366*

SUBJECT INDEX

A

Acquired immunodeficiency syndrome (AIDS), 24, 41–65
Adult respiratory distress syndrome (ARDS), 162
Advanced multiple-beam equalization radiography (AMBER), 373, 383–384
Alpha$_1$-antitrypsin deficiency, 276, 292
and lung transplantation, 313
Alveolitis, extrinsic allergic, 209–211, 214
American College of Radiology, 12
Appropriateness Criteria for Imaging and Treatment Decisions, 12
American Roentgen Ray Society, 6
Anastomosis, tracheal, dehiscence of, 307–309
Angiography,
aortic, 508–509, 524–529
cardiac, 572
pulmonary, 413–415
Angiosarcoma, 584
diffuse pulmonary hemorrhage, 237
Anomalous pulmonary venous return, 482
Antiglomerular basement membrane disease, 230–234
Aorta,
aneurysm, 508, 516
coarctation of, 482, 488–489, 503, 528, 560

[Aorta]
dissection, 511, 519–524, 579–580
penetrating atherosclerotic ulcer, 524–528
Takayasu's arteritis, 528–529
traumatic ruputure, 512–513, 517–518
Arch, aortic,
double, 488, 490
right-sided, 488
Arteries, bronchial, 322
Artery, coronary,
angioscopy, 535–541
bypass grafting, complications of, 167–169
calcification in, 436
disease, 423–441
electron beam CT, 436–439
intravascular ultrasound, 539–544
intravenous thrombolysis, 554–555
magnetic resonance imaging, 595
mechanical recanalization, 548–553
percutaneous transluminal coronary angioplasty (PTCA), 535–539, 541–555
selective coronary thrombolysis, 554–555
stents, 553–554
Arthritis, rheumatoid,
and interstitial lung disease, 200
and diffuse pulmonary hemorrhage, 234
Asbestos, and pleural plaques, 331

Asbestosis, 202–204, 214
Aspergillus, 25
  air-crescent sign, 25
  airway invasive, 26–27
  angioinvasive, 25–26, 237–238
  CT halo sign, 25
  in AIDS, 52
  in transplant patient, 194, 310
Aspiration, 160, 183
Asthma, 267, 269–270
Atelectasis,
  postoperative, 176
  in trauma patient, 142
Atherosclerosis, 425, 438–440

B

Balloon, intra-aortic counterpulsation, 165–166
Barotrauma, 161
Blastomycosis,
  in AIDS, 52
  in transplant patient, 194
Blebs, 279
Bleomycin, 30, 112
Boerhaave syndrome, 147, 187
Bronchi,
  rupture, 145–146
  stricture formation after anastomosis, 194
Bronchiectasis, 220–221, 225–226, 228–230, 254–255, 259
  after lung transplantation, 305
Bronchiolitis obliterans, 260–262
  after heart-lung transplantation, 305–307
  with organizing pneumonia (BOOP), 261–262
  in posttransplantation population, 307
Bronchiolitis,
  constrictive, 262–264
  proliferative, 261–262
  respiratory, 264–265
Bronchography, 6
Bronchoscopy,
  in endobronchial neoplasm, 115

[Bronchoscopy]
  in focal bronchial disease, 247
  in hemoptysis, 221, 255
  of tracheal anastomosis, 308
Bullae,
  bullectomy, 287
  classification of, 277

C

Candidiasis, 28, 194, 237–239
  in lung transplantation, 310
Carcinoma, bronchogenic, 115
  adenocarcinoma, 73–83, 88–89, 95
    acinar, 73
    bronchioloalveolar cell, 73–74, 78, 82–83
    papillary, 73
    solid, 73
  asbestos exposure in, 69
  bronchorrhea in, 78
  bronchoscopy in, 82
  calcification in, 74
  chest wall invasion in, 90, 333
  cigarette smoking in, 69
  diagnosis of, 81–84
  in hemoptysis, 223
  in HIV-infected patients, 61–62
  large cell, 84–85, 91
  mediastinal invasion in, 90–91
  metastasis from, 71, 81, 93–95
  nodal involvement in, 91
  Pancoast tumor, 73
  pleural effusion in, 333–334, 358
  positron emission tomography in, 83, 88–89
  radon exposure in, 69
  risk factors for, 69–70
  screening radiography, 70
  small cell, 81, 86–87, 94
  squamous cell, 71–78, 92–93
  staging of, 12, 85–86, 90–91, 93–94
  superior vena cava syndrome in, 72
  thoracotomy in, 82
  transthoracic needle aspiration in, 82, 354

[Carcinoma, bronchogenic]
World Health Organization pathological classification of, 70–71
Carcinomatosis, lymphangitic (see Lung metastasis, lymphangitic)
Cardiomyopathy, 579–580, 582
Catheter, Swan-Ganz, 164–165
Catheters, central venous, 162–164
CD4 cell count, 43, 47–48, 56–57
Chronic obstructive pulmonary disease (COPD), 293
and lung transplantation, 313
Chylothorax, 135
postoperative, 188
Coagulation, disseminated intravascular, and diffuse pulmonary hemorrhage, 237
Coccidioidomycosis,
in AIDS, 52
in transplant patient, 194
Compression, of data, 387
Computed tomography (CT),
bronchus sign, 248, 254
electron beam, 436–439, 485–486, 577–578, 594
helical, 11, 118, 121, 246, 577, 593–594
history of, 10–11
split pleura sign, 329
Cryptococcosis,
in AIDS, 52
in transplant patients, 194
Cyclophosphamide, 31
Cyst, pericardial, 463, 466–467
Cytomegalovirus, 28–29
in AIDS, 54–55
in diffuse pulmonary hemorrhage, 239
in lung transplantation, 304, 310
Cytosine arabinoside, 31

D

Defect, septal,
atrial, 478, 482–483, 489–492, 497, 562

[Defect, septal]
ventricular, 480, 483, 486, 492, 562
Diaphragm,
rupture, 148–152, 518
paralysis, 169
hernia, 467–468
Digitizer, laser film, 377, 384
Ductus arteriosus,
patent, 493–494
persistent, 558–560
Dysplasia, arrhythmogenic right ventricular, 580, 583

E

Ebstein's anomaly, 497, 501
Echocardiography,
contrast, 593
Doppler, 480, 482, 516, 583
stress, 576
transesophageal, 482, 516, 574–575, 592
of aortic dissection, 523–524, 577
of coronary arteries, 435–436
transthoracic, 575
of aorta, 516
of congenital heart disease, 577
of coronary arteries, 432–435
of ventricular function, 576
Edema, pulmonary,
cardiogenic, 32
noncardiogenic, 32
Efficacy, clinical, 13
Effusion, pleural,
catheter drainage of, 355–359
chest radiography of, 323–325
computed tomography of, 323–325
differentiation from ascites on CT, 325–326
exudative, 322–323
magnetic resonance imaging of, 327
malignant, 115–116, 358–359
parapneumonic, 327, 355–356
transudative, 322–323
ultrasonography of, 327
Eisenmenger's complex, 492

Embolism,
  fat, 144
  pulmonary (see Embolus, pulmonary)
  septic, 22, 46
  systemic air, 353
Embolus, pulmonary,
  chest radiography in, 391
  computed tomography in, 400–409
  magnetic resonance imaging in, 404–412
  probability crteria, 394–398, 402
  pulmonary angiography in, 413–415
  ventilation-perfusion imaging in, 391–403
Emphysema,
  centrilobular, 276–279, 285–286
  chest radiograph in, 280–281
  CT findings in, 283–287
  historical observations, 6
  panlobular, 276–277, 285, 288
  paraseptal, 276–277, 287, 289
  paracicatricial, 276–277, 290
  pulmonary function testing in, 281
  severity of, 280
Empyema, 327–330
  catheter drainage of, 355–358
  complication of abscess drainge, 361–362
  differentiation from lung abscess, 328
  postoperative, 176–179, 182
  posttraumatic, 135–136
Enterobacter, 21
  in lung transplantation, 310
Epstein-Barr virus,
  association with lymphoproliferative disorder, 311
  in lung transplantation, 310
Escherichia coli, 21
Esophagus,
  rupture, 147, 187
  surgery, 185–187

F

18f-Fluorodeoxyglucose (FDG), 15, 83
Fibroma, pleural, 332

Fibrosis, idiopathic pulmonary, 200–202
  and lung transplantation, 313
Fibrothorax, 335
Fick principle, 477
Film, radiographic, 8, 373–374
Fissures, interlobar, 325
Fistula,
  bronchocutaneous, 180
  bronchopleural, 176
  complication of abscess drainage, 361–362
  esophageal pericardial, 469
Flail chest, 128
Forestier, Jacques, 6

G

Goodpasture's syndrome (see Antiglomerular basement membrane disease)
Granuloma,
  eosinophilic, 204, 206–209
  transthoracic needle biopsy in, 351
Great vessels, congenitally corrected L-transposition of, 484, 498–501
Gunshot wound, 137–139

H

Haemophilus influenzae, 45
Hamartoma, 248
  transthoracic needle biopsy in, 351
Heart,
  herniation, 173
  transplantation, 189–190, 237
Heart disease, congenital, 475–506, 584, 587
Hemoptysis, 220–225, 227, 234–235, 255–258
Hemorrhage, diffuse alveolar, 32–33
Hemosiderosis, idiopathic pulmonary, 231, 235–236
Hemothorax, 134
  postoperative, 182
Herpes simplex, 29–30
  in lung transplantation, 310

Histiocytosis, pulmonary Langerhans cell, 204, 206–209, 214
Histoplasmosis,
  in AIDS, 52–53
  in transplant patient, 194
Human immunodeficiency virus (HIV), 41–47
  in diffuse pulmonary hemorrhage, 239
Hypertrophy, lipomatous, of the atrial septum, 584

I

Imaging,
  radionuclide, cardiac, 572–573, 587, 590–592
  storage phosphor, 8–9, 377–380, 384
  ventilation-perfusion, 391–403
Immunosuppression, 19–20
Indirect immunofluorescent (IFA) test, 22
Inhalation injury, trimellitic anhydride, 236

K

Kaposi's sarcoma, 42–43, 56
  in diffuse pulmonary hemorrhage, 239–240
  metastatic, 108
  pericardial involvement, 469
  staging system of, 57–59
Kawasaki's disease, 432
Klebsiella, 21

L

Larynx, laceration, 160
Legionella pneumophila, 20–21
Leukemia, 33, 115
  in diffuse pulmonary hemorrhage, 237
Lipoma,
  cardiac, 584, 590
  pleural, 333
Listeria monocytogenes, 21

Lung,
  abscess, catheter drainage of, 361–362
  arteriovenous malformation, 390, 403–404, 407–408
  cancer (*see* Carcinoma, bronchogenic)
  contusion, 139–141
  hemorrhage,
    after abscess drainage, 361
    after transbronchial biopsy, 314–315
  laceration, 139–140, 166
  metastasis, 106
    calcification in, 108, 111
    from bladder carcinoma, 107–108
    from breast cancer, 106, 108, 111, 114–116, 120
    from chondrosarcoma, 108
    from choriocarcinoma, 106, 108
    from colorectal carcinoma, 106–108, 115
    from gastric carcinoma, 106, 115
    from leiomyosarcoma, 110
    from melanoma, 106, 108, 115, 117
    from osteosarcoma, 106–108, 117
    from ovarian carcinoma, 106–108, 115
    from prostate carcinoma, 106–107, 115
    from renal cell carcinoma, 109
    from synovial cell sarcoma, 106–108, 115
    from testicular carcinoma, 108–109, 113
    from thyroid carcinoma, 106
      medullary cancer, 108
      papillary cancer, 108
    hematogenous, 107
    lymphangitic, 32–34, 107, 119–120, 212–214
    sterilized, 113
  torsion, 144, 173–174
  transplantation, 190–194
Lung disease,
  drug-induced, 30–31

[Lung disease]
  penicillamine toxicity, 236
Lupus erythematosus, systemic, 231, 234
Lymphangioleiomyomatosis, 209–210, 214
Lymphocele, 135
Lymphography, and diffuse pulmonary hemorrhage, 237
Lymphoma, 33, 35, 115
  AIDS-related, 57, 60
  pleural involvement in, 337, 358
  transthoracic needle biopsy in, 351, 355
Lymphoproliferative disorder, following lung transplantation, 311

M

Magnetic resonance arteriography, of coronary arteries, 426–432
Magnetic resonance imaging,
  cardiac, 578–587
  contraindications, 483
  of thoracic aorta, 578–580
Malignancy, radiation-induced, 118
Mediastinitis, postoperative, 169–172
Mesothelioma, 335–338
  transthoracic needle biopsy in, 351
Metastases,
  cardiac, 584
  endobronchial, 106, 115–117
  mediastinal nodal, 106, 113
  hilar nodal, 106, 113
  pericardial, 584
Methotrexate, 30–31, 112
Mitral valve, valvuloplasty, 555–557
Mucormycosis, 28
Mycobacterium, nontuberculous, 42
  Mycobacterium avium-intracellulare (*MAI*), 47–48, 50
  Mycobacterium kansasii, 47, 50, 53
Myocardium,
  infarction, 423–425, 456, 537, 545, 580–581, 594–595
  motion, 594

[Myocardium]
  perfusion, radionuclide imaging, 573
Myxoma, atrial, 584

N

Needle aspiration, transthoracic,
  coaxial technique, 350
  contraindications to, 344
  complications of, 352–354
  cutting needles for, 347–348
  fine-aspirating needles for, 347–348
  in AIDS, 65
  in bronchogenic carcinoma, 82
  indications for, 344
Nocardia asteroides, 20–21, 23

O

Omentum, intrathoracic, after lung transplantation, 313–314
Output, cardiac, 477

P

Pacemaker, 166–167, 483
Panbronchiolitis, 260
Pendelluft, 128
Pericarditis, 455–462, 579
  constrictive, 463, 579
  radiation-induced, 458
Pericardium, 446–472
  congenital absence of, 452–455
  cyst, 463, 466–467
  metastatic involvement of, 115, 458–459, 469–470
  normal anatomy, 446–451
  primary tumor of, 467
Pleura,
  chemical pleurodesis of, 359
  diffuse thickening of, 335
  lymphatic drainage of, 322
  metastases to, 337–338
  plaques, 331–332
  pseudotumor, 324
Pneumatocele, posttraumatic, 142

Pneumoconiosis, of coal workers, 203–204, 214
Pneumocystis carinii, 24–25, 42–46, 194
  in lung transplantation, 310
Pneumomediastinum, 145, 162
Pneumonectomy, complications, 172–185
Pneumonia,
  chronic eosinophilic, 213–215
  cryptogenic organizing (*see* Bronchiolitis oblilterans with organizing pneumonia)
  desquamative interstitial, 200, 214
  lymphocytic interstitial, 42, 64
  pneumococcal, 232
  postoperative, 182–183
  usual interstitital, 200–202, 214
Pneumonitis,
  hypersensitivity, 209–211
  nonspecific interstitital, 42, 63–65
Pneumopericardium, 469
Pneumothorax,
  catheter drainage of, 359–360
  complication of catheter placement, 164–165, 361
  complication of transthoracic needle biopsy, 352, 359–360
  in ARDS, 162
  posttraumatic, 132–134, 145
  tension, 133, 145, 177
Positron emission tomography (PET), 15–16
  in bronchogenic carcinoma, 83
  of solitary pulmonary nodule, 119
Postpneumonectomy syndrome, 183–184
Posttransplantation lymphoproliferative disorder (PTLD), 35–36
Procarbazine, 30
Prospective investigation of pulmonary embolism diagnosis (PIOPED), 391, 394, 397, 402, 414
Proteinosis, alveolar, 210, 212, 214
Pseudomonas, 21–22, 48–49
  in lung transplantation, 310
Pulsus paradoxus, 462

Q

Quantum mottle, 379, 382

R

Radiation exposure, 5, 379
Radiography,
  computed (*see* Imaging, storage phosphor)
  selenium-detector, 380–382
Rashkind procedure, 477
Rastelli conduit, 502
Rejection,
  acute pulmonary, 299–305
  classification of, 301
Research, outcomes, 13
Resolution, spatial, 371–372, 391
Response, reimplantation, 298–301
Ribs, fractures, 128–129
Ring, vascular, 488

S

Sarcoidosis, 203, 205–206, 214
  emphysema in, 290
Scapula, fractions, 129–130
Scleroderma, and interstitital lung disease, 200
Sestamibi, 590–591
Shunt,
  left-to-right, 487, 489–493
  right-to-left, 487, 493, 495
Sign,
  split pleura, 329
  swinging heart, 462
Silicosis, 203–204, 207–208, 214
Single-proton emission computed tomography (SPECT), 398–400, 573–574, 588
Spine, fractures, 130–132
Staphylococcus aureus, 22, 45
  in lung transplantation, 310
Sternum,
  fractures, 130
  osteomyelitis, 171
Streptococcus pneumoniae, 21–22, 45–46

Strongyloides stercoralis, 56
Surgery, lung volume reduction, 287–293
Swyer-James syndrome, 262, 264

T

Takayasu's arteritis, 528–529
Tamponade, cardiac, 456–458, 462–465
Technology, assessment of, 13
Teleradiology, 9
Tetralogy of Fallot, 493, 495–496, 502
Thallium-201, 573, 590–591
Thoracic duct, disruption, 135
Thoracostomy, tube, 165–166, 168
Thrombolysis, intravenous, 545
Thymoma, distinction from lymphoma on transthoracic needle biopsy, 355
Tomography, 7
Toxoplasma gondii, 56
Trachea,
  rupture, 145, 160
  stenosis, 162
Transplantation,
  bone marrow, 20–21, 237
  heart, 35, 237
  heart-lung, 35, 305–307
  lung, 297–315
tuberculosis, 231
  hemoptysis in, 227
  history of, 5
  in AIDS, 47, 50–51
  infection in the immunocompromised host, 23–24

[Trachea]
  military screening for, 7
  mycobacterium tuberculosis, 23
Tumor,
  carcinoid, 224
  cardiac, 584, 588
  localized fibrous, of the pleura, 332–333

U

Ultrasound, intravascular, 439–440, 535, 539–541, 592

V

Valve, aortic,
  bicuspid, 495–499
  stenosis of, 495–499, 558
  valvuloplasty, 556
Valve, pulmonic,
  stenosis, 481, 497, 500
  valvuloplasty, 555
Valvuloplasty, balloon, 555–559
Varicella-zoster virus, 30
  in lung transplantation, 310
Ventilation, one-lung, 184
Ventricular function, 487

W

Wegener's granulomatosis, 231, 234

X

X-ray, discovery of, 3–4